Network Pharmacology of Natural Products, 2nd Edition

Network Pharmacology of Natural Products, 2nd Edition

Guest Editors

Alexander George Panossian
Karl Wah-Keung Tsim

MDPI

Basel • Beijing • Wuhan • Barcelona • Belgrade • Novi Sad • Cluj • Manchester

Guest Editors
Alexander George Panossian
Phytomed AB
Västervik
Sweden

Karl Wah-Keung Tsim
Center for Chinese Medicine
The Hong Kong University of
Science and Technology
Hong Kong
China

Editorial Office
MDPI AG
Grosspeteranlage 5
4052 Basel, Switzerland

This is a reprint of the Special Issue, published open access by the journal *Pharmaceuticals* (ISSN 1424-8247), freely accessible at: https://www.mdpi.com/journal/pharmaceuticals/special_issues/4TE37Y2AD8.

For citation purposes, cite each article independently as indicated on the article page online and as indicated below:

Lastname, A.A.; Lastname, B.B. Article Title. *Journal Name* **Year**, *Volume Number*, Page Range.

ISBN 978-3-7258-8301-1 (Hbk)
ISBN 978-3-7258-8302-8 (PDF)
https://doi.org/10.3390/books978-3-7258-8302-8

Contents

About the Editors

Alexander George Panossian

Alexander George Panossian, Ph.D., Dr.Sc, has been the Head of Research and Development of Phytomed AB in Sweden since 2016. He has multiple advanced degrees in bioorganic chemistry and the chemistry of natural and physiologically active compounds.

He completed his doctorate in organic chemistry at the Yerevan State University in Armenia in 1971 and obtained his scientific degrees from the Moscow Institute of Bioorganic Chemistry in 1975 and the Moscow Institute of Fine Chemical Technology in 1986.

Dr. Panossian was appointed as full professor of bioorganic chemistry and the chemistry of natural and physiologically active compounds in the Russian Federation, and later served as Director of the Laboratory of Quality Control of Drugs at the Medical Drug Agency of the Republic of Armenia (1993–2003).

In 2003, he moved to Sweden to act as head of research and development at the Swedish Herbal Institute.

Additionally, he had the honor of participating as a guest scientist in the Laboratory of Nobel Laureate Bengt Samuelsson at the Karolinska Institute in Stockholm (1982–1983), at Munich University (1993–1995), and at King's College in London (1996).

He was the editor-in-chief of *Phytomedicine, International Journal of Phytopharmacology* and *Phytotherapy* (Elsevier, Germany) from 2014 to 2017.

He has authored or co-authored approximately 200 articles in peer-reviewed journals. His main research interest is focused on plant adaptogens, anti-stress compounds that are involved in the regulation of the neuroendocrine and immune systems.

Karl Wah-Keung Tsim

Karl Wah-Keung Tsim is the Chair Professor of Division of Life Science, Director of Center for Chinese Medicine and Director of Shenzhen Key Laboratory of Edible & Medicinal Bioresources at The Hong Kong University of Science and Technology (HKUST).

Prof. Karl Tsim received his BSc and MPhil from The Chinese University of Hong Kong, and his PhD in Molecular Neurobiology from the University of Cambridge, UK. After his post-doctoral training at Medical School of Stanford University, USA, he joined HKUST in 1992.

Prof. Tsim developed a molecular technique to determine the genetic and chemical properties of Chinese herbs. He has published approximately 500 scientific papers and serves as the editor for many scientific journals internationally. His works on Chinese herbal medicine have twice been recognized with the Research Excellence in Natural Sciences award from the Ministry of Education of China.

Prof. Tsim is the Founding Chairman of Hong Kong Association of Biotechnology in Chinese Medicine. He also serves as an adviser/consultant/member to various organizations, both nationally and internationally, in the standardization of Chinese herbs, including the WHO and HKSAR Government in Testing and Certification of Chinese herbs. He is an active entrepreneur and the founding director of several biotech companies.

Preface

Natural products remain a cornerstone of drug discovery, yet their true therapeutic potential is often underestimated when evaluated through single-target, reductionist frameworks. Increasing evidence demonstrates that botanicals, traditional herbal medicines, and their constituent compounds exert synergistic and pleiotropic effects by modulating interconnected molecular pathways. Network pharmacology, together with systems biology, multi-omics technologies, and advanced computational tools, provides a robust conceptual and methodological foundation to capture this complexity.

This Research Topic focuses on elucidating the multi-target, multi-component mechanisms underlying natural product bioactivity. By integrating in silico network analysis, artificial intelligence, omics-based profiling, and experimental validation, the contributions in this collection aim to advance a systems-level understanding of how natural products influence the biological networks relevant to complex and multifactorial diseases. The scope encompasses inflammatory, metabolic, infectious, neurodegenerative, and stress-related disorders, as well as mechanisms of drug resistance and resilience-supporting pharmacology.

Collectively, this Preface frames a shift toward holistic, translational, and mechanism-driven natural product research, supporting the development of rational, effective, and integrative therapeutic strategies consistent with modern drug discovery paradigms.

Alexander George Panossian and Karl Wah-Keung Tsim
Guest Editors

pharmaceuticals

Editorial

Network Pharmacology and Natural Products in Modern Drug Discovery: Emerging Trends, Challenges, and Future Directions

Alexander Panossian

Phytomed AB, Sjöstadsvägen 6A, 59344 Västervik, Sweden; ap@phytomed.se

The past decade has witnessed a paradigm shift in pharmacological research, moving from reductionist, single-target drug discovery toward systems-based, multitarget therapeutic strategies. This transition has largely been driven by advances in network pharmacology (NP), multi-omics technologies, and artificial-intelligence-based drug discovery [1–4]. The collection of recent publications in *Pharmaceuticals* (2025–2026) shown in Supplementary Table S1 reflects this transformation, highlighting the expanding role of natural products, traditional herbal medicines, and integrative pharmacology in addressing complex diseases (Figure 1) [3–15].

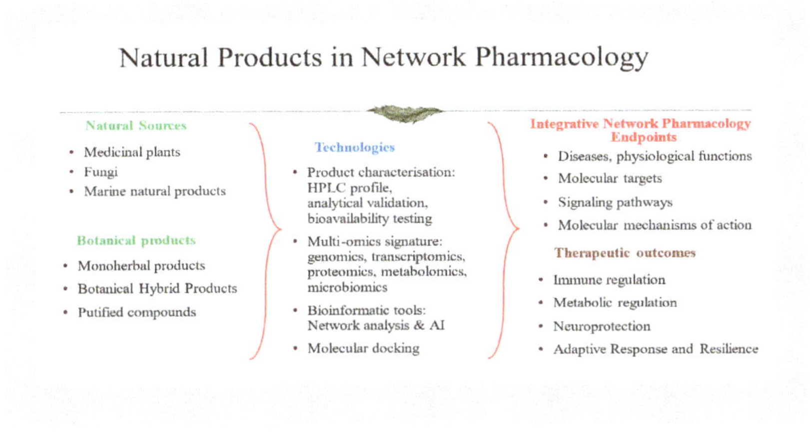

Figure 1. The natural sources of botanical products, technologies, integrative network pharmacology endpoints, and therapeutic outcomes covered in publications in this Special Issue.

An expert community in China [2] has officially recognized NP under the guidelines of the Communist Party focused on modernizing the archaic theories of TCM through a holistic/integrative approach, since the reductionistic/differential approach based on another archaic theory pertaining to Galenic preparations is not always suitable for new-drug discovery due to multitarget effects, complex botanical combinations, and purified compounds [4]. Notably, both approaches are complementary and essential for achieving the desired goal [4].

This Special Issue includes 12 original articles and 2 reviews (Supplementary Table S1) on NP of botanicals from seven Asian countries predominantly implementing traditional medical systems (including China, Japan, South Korea, and Saudi Arabia) and Western countries following mainly conventional medicine paradigms (such as the USA, the UK, and Sweden), representing a variety of ethnic groups and political views. In this context, as declared by Sune K. Bergström, one of the Nobel Laureates in Medicine in 1982, "science does not know any national borders. The scientists of the world are forming an invisible network with a very free flow of scientific information—a freedom accepted by the countries of the world irrespective of political systems or religions. . .." [16].

These studies collectively emphasize multitarget mechanisms, computational drug discovery, experimental validation, and translational potential [17]. Moreover, they underscore the importance of systems-level understanding in treating multifactorial diseases such as neurodegeneration, inflammation, metabolic disorders, and infectious diseases. This editorial synthesizes the key findings and contributions of these publications, outlines recent developments in the field, identifies knowledge gaps, and proposes future research directions.

A major development across these studies is the transition from single-target drug discovery to multitarget network pharmacology. This approach reflects the complex nature of chronic diseases and supports the therapeutic use of multi-component natural products.

The review on Cordyceps and cordycepin highlights the fact that multiple signaling pathways—including PI3K–Akt, AMPK–mTOR, MAPK, and NF-κB—serve as mechanistic hubs underlying pleiotropic bioactivity. These pathways regulate immune responses, metabolism, and cellular resilience, supporting the notion that these compounds are adaptogenic [4].

The studies on traditional complex Botanical Herbal Product (BHPs) demonstrate multitarget mechanisms [18]:

- BHP Banhasasim-Tang, composed of eight botanicals and used to treat irritable bowel syndrome, was found to operate via TNF signaling and apoptosis pathways as central mechanisms, as validated through in vivo models [8];
- BHP Qingfei Tongluo Jiedu, composed of nine botanicals and used for the treatment of pneumonia, regulates macrophage polarization via the butyrate–GPR109A–MAPK pathway, demonstrating immunomodulatory activity [15];
- BHP XuanYunNing, composed of 10 botanicals and used for the treatment of Meniere's disease, a rare inner-ear disorder characterized by symptoms such as vertigo and hearing loss, disrupts a pathological cycle driven by JAK-STAT signaling, inflammation, and metabolic dysfunction [9];
- BHP Dahuang Xiaoshi -M (DXT-M), composed of three botanicals and used as a hepatoprotective agent in the treatment of liver injuries, demonstrated significant effectiveness in ameliorating liver pathologies, correcting abnormal liver function biomarkers, and regulating the CYP/GST-ROS axis [12].

Monoherbal botanical products, such as *Gynostemma pentaphyllum* [13], *Artemisia scoparia* [7], *Aronia melanocarpa* [14], and *Vitis vinifera* berry oligomeric polytcianodins [10], contain many active phytochemicals and exhibit multitarget effects; for instance, *Gynostemma pentaphyllum* exhibits dual-pathway modulation capacity, involving inflammatory signaling and renin–angiotensin system regulation, useful for COVID-19 treatment.

In several studies in this collection, multi-omics analyses were employed to identify molecular mechanisms and biomarkers. Even purified compounds such as Schisandrin B [11] and cordycepin [4] demonstrate multitarget action. The review on Cordycepin highlights how systems-level network analysis complements reductionist molecular pharmacology, fostering a holistic understanding of adaptogenic mechanisms [4].

These findings illustrate the shift toward holistic pharmacological frameworks.

Another significant trend is the integration of computational predictions with experimental validation. Most studies combine network pharmacology tools, molecular docking, molecular dynamics simulations, and in vitro/in vivo validation. This complementary

https://doi.org/10.3390/ph19050653

approach represents a methodological advancement, improving prediction reliability and translational potential.

The integration of multi-omics technologies—including transcriptomics, proteomics, metabolomics, and microbiomics—has further transformed natural-product research. These approaches allow comprehensive analysis of biological systems and identification of novel therapeutic targets [17]. Multi-omics integration in herbal medicine research enables the identification of pathway-level interactions, thereby facilitating the development of precision therapeutics [3].

The therapeutic areas covered in several of these studies center on inflammatory and infectious diseases. The study on Qingfei Tongluo Jiedu demonstrated immune regulation through macrophage polarization, providing a novel therapeutic approach for drug-resistant pneumonia [15].

Similarly, the study on *Gynostemma pentaphyllum* revealed dual-mechanistic pathways involving immunological and renin–angiotensin system regulation useful for COVID-19 therapy [13].

These findings highlight the growing importance of immunomodulatory natural products.

Natural products are attracting an increasing amount of attention for their potential role in treating neurodegenerative disorders. The bibliometric analysis of natural products used for treating cognitive disabilities demonstrated rapid growth in this research field, with an annual growth rate of 12.36% from 1971 to 2024 [6]. This bibliometric study on cognitive disabilities identifies research trends, highlights knowledge gaps, and suggests future directions. The authors identified Alzheimer's disease as the dominant research focus, followed by oxidative stress, neuroprotection, and molecular-docking approaches. Emerging trends include ferroptosis, UPLC-Q-TOF-MS, and network pharmacology methodologies [6]. However, the study also highlighted several gaps, including the underrepresentation of autism spectrum disorders and traumatic brain injuries as well as limited clinical validation of computational findings. These findings underscore the need for increased research on various cognitive disorders.

Natural products also show promise in regard to metabolic and chronic diseases. The review on Cordyceps discusses the adaptogenic effects in stress-related and aging-related disorders through metabolic and mitochondrial regulation [4], identifying multitarget adaptogenic mechanisms, highlighting regulatory challenges, and proposing a resilience-based therapeutic category. This research supports the use of natural compounds for preventive medicine and resilience-based therapeutics.

One of these publications' major conceptual contributions is their recognition of adaptogens as resilience-supporting agents [3,4]. The authors of the review on Cordyceps propose a new regulatory category for resilience-supporting physiological modulators, emphasizing homeostasis rather than disease-specific treatment [4].

This concept aligns with preventive medicine and personalized healthcare.

Another important concept is multi-component drug synergy [18]. Herbal formulations often contain multiple compounds acting synergistically.

The study on *Gynostemma pentaphyllum* demonstrates the complementary actions of flavonoids and saponins, reinforcing the concept of polypharmacology [13].

This approach may improve therapeutic efficacy and reduce adverse effects. Two studies in this Special Issue demonstrate that

- *Aronia melanocarpa* berries can effectively overcome 5-FU resistance in colorectal cancer cells by targeting the TLR3/NF-κB pathway [14];
- Oligomeric proanthocyanidins from French grape (*Vitis vinifera* L.) seed extract can overcome chemotherapy resistance by targeting the integrin pathway in individuals with hepatocellular carcinoma [10].

https://doi.org/10.3390/ph19050653

Recent innovations include artificial intelligence and machine learning, molecular docking and dynamics simulations, multi-omics integration, and systems biology approaches. These technologies and approaches are transforming natural-product drug discovery.

Despite significant advances, there are still several knowledge gaps [1,2,19]:

- *Limited Clinical Evidence*: Most studies remain preclinical, highlighting the need for randomized clinical trials.
- *Standardization Challenges*: Variability in herbal preparations complicates reproducibility.
- *Bioavailability Issues*: The review on Cordyceps highlights the importance of low systemic concentrations of cordycepin, suggesting indirect mechanisms and emphasizing the need for pharmacokinetic studies.
- *Mechanistic complexity*.

Future research should emphasize clinical translation, multi-omics integration, AI-driven drug discovery, precision medicine, and regulatory-framework development.

The publications in this Special Issue demonstrate rapid advancement in natural-product pharmacology driven by network pharmacology, computational approaches, and systems biology. These studies collectively support a shift toward multitarget therapeutic strategies for complex diseases.

Future research should emphasize clinical translation, mechanistic understanding, and regulatory harmonization to fully realize the potential of natural products in modern pharmacotherapy.

Supplementary Materials: The following supporting information can be downloaded at https://www.mdpi.com/article/10.3390/ph19050653/s1. Supplement S1 on the website. Table S1: Overview of the network-pharmacology studies in the Special Issue "Network Pharmacology of Natural Products, 2nd Edition".

Funding: This research received no external funding.

Data Availability Statement: No new data were created or analyzed in this study.

Acknowledgments: The authors acknowledge their use of artificial intelligence (AI) technology (ChatGPT for iOS, version 1.202, model 2025, OpenAI, L.L.C.) as an assistive tool for language refinement and drafting support. All scientific interpretation, synthesis, and final editorial decisions remain the responsibility of the authors. AI-proposed methodological options were critically assessed and either adopted or rejected by the author. All concepts and interpretations are solely the author's, originating from practical observations.

Conflicts of Interest: The author is self-employed through Phytomed AB, serving as the founder and owner of this Research and Development company, and declares that the research was conducted in the absence of any commercial or financial relationships that could be construed as potential conflicts of interest.

References

1. Panossian, A. Trends and Pitfalls in the Progress of Network Pharmacology Research on Natural Products. *Pharmaceuticals* **2025**, *18*, 538. [CrossRef] [PubMed]
2. Li, S.; Xiao, W. General expert consensus on the application of network pharmacology in the research and development of new traditional Chinese medicine drugs. *Chin. J. Nat. Med.* **2025**, *23*, 129–142. [CrossRef]
3. Panossian, A.; Lemerond, T. Two Sides of the Same Coin for Health: Adaptogenic Botanicals as Nutraceuticals for Nutrition and Pharmaceuticals in Medicine. *Pharmaceuticals* **2025**, *18*, 1346. [CrossRef] [PubMed]
4. Panossian, A. Pleiotropic Bioactivity of Caterpillar Fungus, Orange Cordyceps, and Cordycepin: Insight from Integrated Network Pharmacology and Food and Drug Regulatory Framework. *Pharmaceuticals* **2026**, *19*, 519. [CrossRef] [PubMed]
5. Santiago-de-la-Cruz, J.A.; Rivero-Segura, N.A.; Alvarez-Sánchez, M.E.; Gomez-Verjan, J.C. Network Pharmacology and Machine Learning Identify Flavonoids as Potential Senotherapeutics. *Pharmaceuticals* **2025**, *18*, 1176. [CrossRef] [PubMed]

6. Albratty, M.; Halawi, M.; Albarrati, A.M. Natural Products for Drug Discovery in Cognitive Disabilities: Bibliometric Hotspots, Research Trends, Conceptual Framework, and Future Directions. *Pharmaceuticals* **2025**, *18*, 983. [CrossRef] [PubMed]
7. Guo, M.; Ma, Y.; Wang, L.; Ge, R.; Wang, Y.; Ma, G.; Du, G.; Li, L. Network Pharmacology Analysis and Experimental Study of Yinchen Against Neuroinflammation in Ischemic Stroke. *Pharmaceuticals* **2025**, *18*, 1852. [CrossRef] [PubMed]
8. Choi, W.-G.; Ko, S.-J.; Shim, J.-H.; Bae, C.-H.; Kim, S.; Park, J.-W.; Kim, B.-J. Integrative In Silico and In Vivo Analysis of Banhasasim-Tang for Irritable Bowel Syndrome: Mechanistic Insights into Inflammation-Related Pathways. *Pharmaceuticals* **2025**, *18*, 1123. [CrossRef] [PubMed]
9. Jin, Z.; Wang, C.; Gao, Y.; Tao, X.; Wu, C.; Guo, S.; Huang, J.; Zhou, J.; Qiao, C.; Chai, K.; et al. Systems Network Integration of Transcriptomic, Proteomic, and Bioinformatic Analyses Reveals the Mechanism of XuanYunNing Tablets in Meniere's Disease via JAK-STAT Pathway Modulation. *Pharmaceuticals* **2025**, *18*, 1266. [CrossRef] [PubMed]
10. Noma, T.; Li, Y.; Wada, Y.; Morine, Y.; Ikemoto, T.; Saito, Y.; Yamada, S.; Teraoku, H.; Shimada, M.; Goel, A. Oligomeric Proanthocyanidins Reverse Lenvatinib Resistance in Hepatocellular Carcinoma Through ITGA3-Mediated Pathway. *Pharmaceuticals* **2025**, *18*, 1361. [CrossRef] [PubMed]
11. Gao, M.; Liu, F.; Feng, X.; Wang, M.; Zhang, Z.; Li, H.; Wang, C.; Sun, J. Schisandrin B Alleviates Lipid Metabolism Disorders and Apoptosis of MAFLD via Modulation of PPARγ-PCK1 and Caspase-3 Signaling Pathways. *Pharmaceuticals* **2025**, *18*, 1441. [CrossRef] [PubMed]
12. Kong, X.; Wang, X.; Ren, H.; Yao, Y.; Zhang, H.; Li, H.; Li, H.; Cheng, Y.; Song, Z.; Pei, M.; et al. The Hepatoprotective Properties of the Revised Formulation of Dahuang Xiaoshi Tang, an Ancient Chinese Herbal Decoction, Are Probed by Integrated Metabolomics and Network Pharmacology. *Pharmaceuticals* **2025**, *18*, 1534. [CrossRef] [PubMed]
13. Kim, M.H.; Won, J.A.; Yu, J.S.; Kim, S.M.; Lee, D.K.; Piao, X.-L.; Yoo, H.H. Therapeutic Potential of *Gynostemma pentaphyllum* (Thunb.) Makino Against COVID-19 Identified Through Network Pharmacology. *Pharmaceuticals* **2025**, *18*, 1851. [CrossRef] [PubMed]
14. Duan, H.; Noma, T.; Goel, A. Aronia Berry Extract Inhibits Cancer Stemness and Overcomes 5-Fluorouracil Resistance by Targeting TLR3/NF-κB Signaling in Colorectal Cancer. *Pharmaceuticals* **2026**, *19*, 261. [CrossRef] [PubMed]
15. Liu, Z.; Fan, Q.; Sun, R.; Jiang, Y. Qingfei Tongluo Jiedu Formula Regulates M2 Macrophage Polarization via the Butyric Acid-GPR109A-MAPK Pathway for the Treatment of *Mycoplasma pneumoniae* Pneumonia. *Pharmaceuticals* **2026**, *19*, 212. [CrossRef] [PubMed]
16. The Nobel Prize. Sune K. Bergström. Banquet Speech. Available online: https://www.nobelprize.org/prizes/medicine/1982/bergstrom/speech/ (accessed on 30 March 2026).
17. Panossian, A.; Efferth, T. Network Pharmacology of Adaptogens in the Assessment of Their Pleiotropic Therapeutic Activity. *Pharmaceuticals* **2022**, *15*, 1051. [CrossRef] [PubMed]
18. Panossian, A.; Lemerond, T.; Efferth, T. State-of-the-Art Review on Botanical Hybrid Preparations in Phytomedicine and Phytotherapy Research: Background and Perspectives. *Pharmaceuticals* **2024**, *17*, 483. [CrossRef] [PubMed]
19. Panossian, A. Challenges in phytotherapy research. *Front. Pharmacol.* **2023**, *14*, 1199516. [CrossRef] [PubMed]

https://doi.org/10.3390/ph19050653

pharmaceuticals

MDPI

Article

Aronia Berry Extract Inhibits Cancer Stemness and Overcomes 5-Fluorouracil Resistance by Targeting TLR3/NF-κB Signaling in Colorectal Cancer

Hongxia Duan [1], Takayuki Noma [1,2] and Ajay Goel [1,3,*]

[1] Department of Molecular Diagnostics and Experimental Therapeutics, Beckman Research Institute of City of Hope, Biomedical Research Center, Monrovia, CA 91016, USA; hongxiaduan666@gmail.com (H.D.); takayukinoma1994@gmail.com (T.N.)
[2] Department of Surgery, Tokushima University, Tokushima 770-8503, Japan
[3] City of Hope Comprehensive Cancer Center, Duarte, CA 91010, USA
* Correspondence: ajgoel@coh.org; Tel.: +1-626-218-3452

Abstract

Background: Colorectal cancer (CRC) remains a major clinical challenge, in part due to the limited efficacy of 5-fluorouracil (5-FU)-based chemotherapy, which is often compromised by the emergence of acquired resistance. Aronia berry extract (ABE), a phenolic-rich natural compound, has gained increasing attention for its anticancer and chemosensitizing properties. This study aimed to investigate whether ABE can overcome 5-FU resistance (5-FU-R) in CRC and to elucidate the molecular mechanisms underlying its therapeutic effects. **Methods**: We conducted a series of in vitro experiments using 5-FU-R CRC cell lines to evaluate the synergistic effects of combined ABE and 5-FU treatment. Genome-wide transcriptomic profiling was performed to identify key regulatory pathways associated with chemoresistance and to determine potential ABE-responsive targets. Findings were further validated using patient-derived 3D organoids (PDOs). **Results**: Co-treatment with ABE and 5-FU significantly reduced the effective concentration of 5-FU required to inhibit 5-FU-R CRC cells, yielding a Bliss synergy score greater than 10. The combination markedly suppressed cell viability, clonogenic potential, migration, and invasion. ABE also reduced cancer stemness, as evidenced by reduced CD44, Nanog, and Oct4 expression. Functional inhibition of Toll-like receptor 3 (TLR3) impaired spheroid growth, and PDO experiments corroborated these findings, demonstrating reduced organoid growth, diminished survival, and decreased NF-κB expression following ABE treatment. **Conclusions**: Our findings reveal that ABE effectively overcomes 5-FU resistance in CRC by targeting the TLR3/NF-κB signaling axis. This study highlights ABE as a safe, accessible, and promising adjunctive strategy to enhance therapeutic responses in 5-FU-resistant CRC.

Keywords: aronia berry extract; colorectal cancer; 5-fluorouracil; synergistic anticancer effect

1. Introduction

Colorectal cancer (CRC) remains one of the most commonly diagnosed malignancies and a leading cause of cancer-related mortality worldwide, with an estimated more than a million new cases and approximately 903,859 deaths annually [1]. Despite improvements in early detection and therapeutic interventions, CRC continues to pose a significant clinical burden, particularly in advanced stages. Current standard-of-care treatment strategies involve surgery followed by adjuvant chemotherapy for high-risk stage II and stage III patients, as well as systemic therapy for those with stage IV disease, aimed at eradicating minimal residual disease and improving overall survival [2–4].

Among available chemotherapeutic agents, 5-fluorouracil (5-FU) remains the standard of care for CRC treatment and serves as the backbone of most combination regimens. However, its long-term efficacy is severely limited by the development of intrinsic or acquired chemoresistance. Alarmingly, more than 90% of patients with metastatic CRC ultimately fail to respond to 5-FU-based therapies, resulting in disease progression and poor clinical outcomes [5]. Resistance to 5-FU is a multifactorial process involving alterations in drug metabolism, dysregulation of apoptotic signaling, enhanced DNA repair capacity, and enrichment of therapy-resistant tumor cell subpopulations. These challenges underscore the urgent need to identify novel, mechanism-based approaches to overcome chemoresistance and restore therapeutic sensitivity in CRC.

Natural products and dietary phytochemicals have emerged as promising candidates for cancer prevention and therapy due to their pleiotropic biological activities and favorable safety profiles [6–8]. Aronia berry (*Aronia melanocarpa*), a polyphenol-rich fruit native to North America, has gained increasing attention for its potent antioxidant, anti-inflammatory, and anticancer properties. Aronia berries contain exceptionally high concentrations of phenolic compounds, including anthocyanins, flavonoids, and phenolic acids, which collectively contribute to their bioactivity. Among these, cyanidin-3-O-galactoside, quercetin, and chlorogenic acid have been identified as key bioactive constituents with demonstrated antitumor effects [9–11].

Cyanidin-3-O-galactoside, the predominant anthocyanin in aronia berry, exhibits strong antiproliferative, antioxidant, and anti-inflammatory activities and has been shown to suppress CRC cell growth in multiple preclinical models [12–16]. Quercetin, another abundant flavonoid, exerts broad anticancer effects by modulating apoptosis, oxidative stress, cell cycle progression, and oncogenic signaling pathways, including the PI3K/AKT and MAPK cascades [17,18]. Chlorogenic acid further contributes to aronia berries' anticancer potential by inhibiting tumor cell proliferation, migration, and invasion through the regulation of key signaling mediators, including p53, p38 MAPK, JNK, c-Myc, and reactive oxygen species (ROS) [16]. Collectively, these findings suggest that aronia-derived polyphenols act on multiple molecular targets relevant to tumor growth and survival.

Importantly, accumulating evidence indicates that aronia berry constituents may also impact cancer stem cells (CSCs), a subpopulation of tumor cells characterized by self-renewal capacity, tumor-initiating potential, and intrinsic resistance to chemotherapy. CSCs are increasingly recognized as key drivers of CRC recurrence, metastasis, and treatment failure. Previous studies have demonstrated that aronia juice selectively inhibits P19 mouse embryonal carcinoma stem cells by upregulating the tumor suppressors p53 and p73, highlighting a potential role for aronia-derived compounds in CSC-targeted therapy [19]. Moreover, aronia polyphenols have been shown to enhance the cytotoxic efficacy of gemcitabine in AsPC-1 pancreatic cancer cells, further supporting their ability to function as chemosensitizing agents that potentiate conventional anticancer therapies [20].

Despite substantial evidence supporting the antitumor and chemosensitizing properties of aronia berry components, their role in modulating 5-FU resistance (5-FU-R) in CRC has not yet been investigated. Addressing this gap is particularly important given the central role of 5-FU in CRC management and the pressing need for strategies capable of reversing resistance. In the present study, we conducted a comprehensive evaluation of the effects of aronia berry extract (ABE) on 5-FU-R CRC. Specifically, we sought to determine whether ABE can restore sensitivity to 5-FU and to elucidate the underlying molecular mechanisms. By integrating in vitro functional assays, genome-wide transcriptomic profiling, and validation using patient-derived three-dimensional organoid models, this study

https://doi.org/10.3390/ph19020261

aims to define the therapeutic potential of ABE and to provide mechanistic insights that may inform the development of novel adjuvant strategies to overcome chemoresistance in CRC.

2. Results

2.1. The Treatment of ABE and 5-FU Shows Synergistic Inhibition in 5-FU-R CRC Cells

We initially utilized the two 5-FU-R cell lines as described in our prior study [21]. Notably, the half maximal inhibitory concentration (IC50) of 5-FU was substantially higher in 5-FU-R HCT116 and 5-FU-R SW480 cells compared to their respective parental cell lines (Figure S1). Specifically, IC_{50} values in parental HCT116 and SW480 cells were 15.38 μM and 11.96 μM, respectively, whereas both 5-FU-R cell lines exhibited IC_{50} values exceeding 160 μM. We next evaluated whether ABE could restore 5-FU sensitivity in 5-FU-R CRC cells. Cells were treated with increasing concentrations of ABE (0–120 μg/mL) and 5-FU (0–60 μM), either alone or in combination. At identical 5-FU concentrations, the addition of ABE consistently enhanced growth inhibition compared with 5-FU monotherapy, indicating increased chemosensitivity. Combination treatment resulted in a synergistic reduction in cell viability. Bliss synergy analysis identified an optimal ABE:5-FU ratio of 60:40, yielding synergy scores > 10 in both cell lines. Notably, the presence of ABE markedly reduced the effective 5-FU concentration required to achieve comparable inhibitory effects. At this ratio, inhibitory rates reached 45.37% in 5-FU-R HCT116 cells (Figure 1A–C) and 49.28% in 5-FU-R SW480 cells (Figure 1D–F). Therefore, subsequent experiments were performed using 60 μg/mL ABE and 40 μM 5-FU.

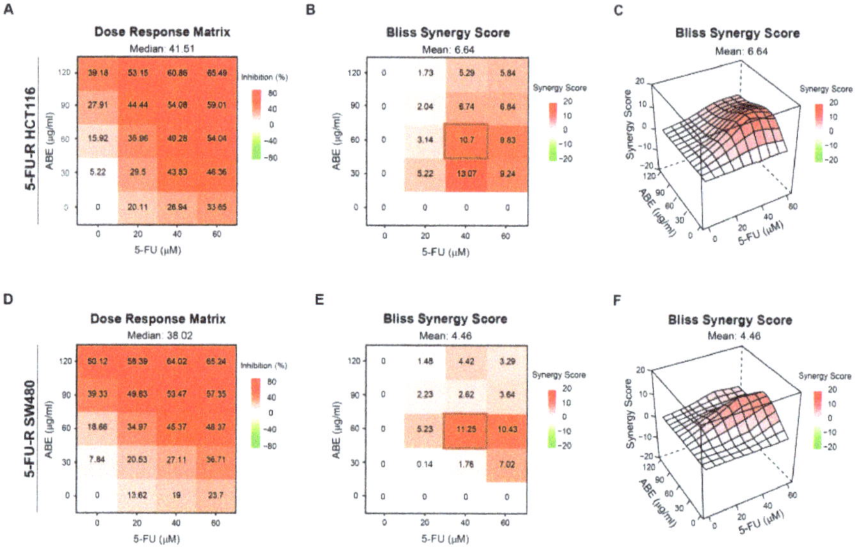

Figure 1. Identification of the ABE treatment synergistically inhibiting the growth of 5-FU-R CRC cells. Percentage of growth inhibition of 5-FU-R HCT116 cell lines (**A**) and 5-FU-R SW480 cell lines (**D**) treated in multiple combinations of ABE (0, 30, 60, 90, 120 μg/mL) and 5-FU (0, 20, 20, 60 μM). The dose–response matrix was measured using the MTT assay. Bliss synergy values were calculated from data in (**B**,**E**), accessed as a 3D-contour (**C**,**F**) drug dose–response model comparing cell viability following treatment with ABE in 5-FU-R CRC cells. The synergy score is shown in red (>0) and green (<0). The red box highlights the optimal ABE:5-FU combination (60 μg/mL ABE and 40 μM 5-FU) showing the highest Bliss synergy score (>10), which was therefore selected for subsequent experiments.

https://doi.org/10.3390/ph19020261

2.2. The Combination of ABE and 5-FU Inhibits Cell Proliferation, Migration, and Invasion in 5-FU-R CRC Cell Lines

To assess the potential of ABE to enhance chemosensitivity to 5-FU in 5-FU-R CRC cells, we conducted a series of functional assays, including colony formation, wound-healing, and invasion assays. To evaluate the impact of the combination of ABE and 5-FU on CRC cell proliferation, we treated 5-FU-R HCT116 and 5-FU-R SW480 cells with 5-FU (40 μM) and ABE (60 μg/mL), either separately or in combination, for 48 h. We performed a colony formation assay, which demonstrated a significant reduction in clonogenicity with the combination of 5-FU and ABE compared to individual treatments in 5-FU-R HCT116 cells (Combination vs. 5-FU: Fold change = 2.26, $p < 0.01$; Combination vs. ABE: Fold change = 1.64, $p < 0.01$) and 5-FU-R SW480 cells (Combination vs. 5-FU: Fold change = 2.24, $p < 0.01$; Combination vs. ABE: Fold change = 1.63, $p < 0.01$, Figure 2A). To determine whether the combination of 5-FU and ABE had a greater impact on the motility and invasive potential of CRC cells, we conducted wound-healing and transwell assays. The wound-healing assay revealed that the combination of 5-FU and ABE significantly inhibited cell migration to a greater extent than individual treatments in both 5-FU-R HCT116 (Combination vs. 5-FU: Fold change = 2.74, $p < 0.01$; Combination vs. ABE: Fold change = 2.13, $p < 0.01$) and 5-FU-R SW480 cells (Combination vs. 5-FU: Fold change = 2.00, $p < 0.01$; Combination vs. ABE: Fold change = 1.83, $p < 0.01$, Figure 2B). The trans well assay showed that a combination of 5-FU and ABE shows a significantly more significant reduction in invasion than individual treatment in both 5-FU-R HCT116 (Combination vs. 5-FU: Fold change = 8.63, $p < 0.01$; Combination vs. ABE: Fold change = 3.00, $p < 0.01$) and 5-FU-R SW480 cells (Combination vs. 5-FU: Fold change = 1.80, $p < 0.01$; Combination vs. ABE: Fold change = 1.49, $p < 0.01$, Figure 2C). Consistent with the previous results, our findings demonstrated that the combination of 5-FU and ABE significantly reduced the proliferation, migration, and invasion abilities of CRC cells.

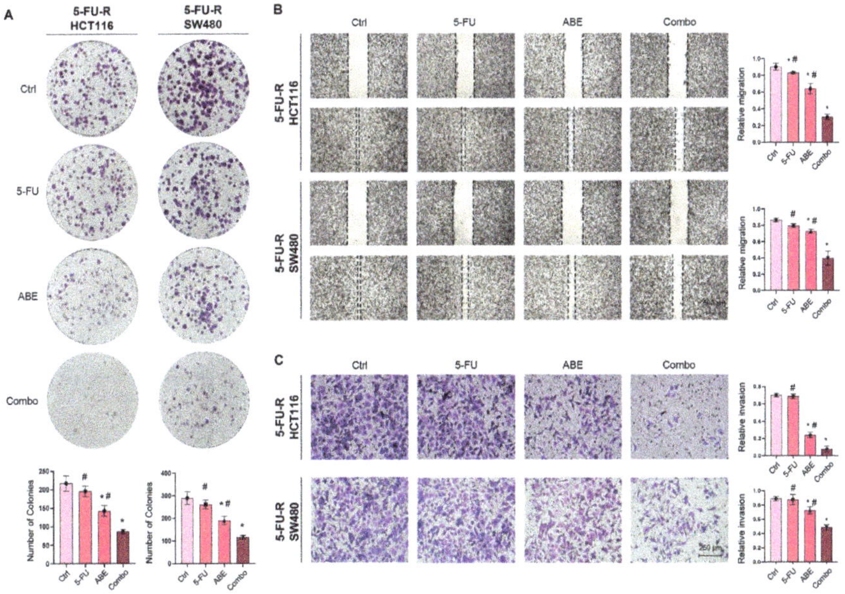

Figure 2. Aronia berry exhibits anti-proliferative, anti-migratory, and anti-invasive effects in 5-FU-R CRC cells. (**A**) A colony-formation assay was performed to evaluate the clonogenicity of each group

https://doi.org/10.3390/ph19020261

after 48 h of treatment. Representative images of colonies in 6-well plates were taken, and the number of colonies was counted. (**B**) A wound-healing assay was performed on 5-FU-R CRC cells treated with 5-FU, ABE, or their combination for 48 h. Representative images of the wound and the healing areas (marked in black) were obtained, and the percentage of wound closure was measured. (**C**) A transwell assay was performed on 5-FU-R CRC cells treated with 5-FU, ABE, or their combination for 48 h, and the number of invading cells was counted in 3 randomly selected fields on the membrane. * p indicates $p < 0.05$ vs. control group; # p indicates $p < 0.05$ vs. combination group.

2.3. ABE, in Combination with 5-FU, Prevents Cell Stemness

CSCs within the tumor bulk possess the unique capacity to self-renew, differentiate, and initiate tumor formation. Therefore, CSCs drive tumor recurrence, metastasis, and drug resistance by generating new tumor cells [22,23]. Spheroids have emerged as a helpful tool that more closely simulates the in vivo organization of solid tumors than the standard in vitro monolayer culture approach, and provides a better in vitro platform to study the enhanced properties of tumor cells [24]. Using a sphere formation assay, we evaluated the effects of combined 5-FU and ABE treatment on spheroid morphology and viability in CRC cells. Compared with untreated cells or cells treated with either agent alone, co-treatment with 5-FU and ABE markedly disrupted spheroid formation and significantly reduced overall spheroid size in both 5-FU-R HCT116 and 5-FU-R SW480 cells (Figure 3A,B, $p < 0.05$). To determine whether alterations in CSC-associated gene expression accompanied these phenotypic changes, we next examined key stemness markers. CD44 is a well-established surface marker of CRC CSCs, whereas Oct4 and Nanog are core transcription factors essential for maintaining pluripotency and self-renewal [25,26]. Quantitative gene expression analysis revealed that combined treatment significantly reduced transcript levels of *CD44*, *OCT4*, and *NANOG* compared with untreated controls or single-agent treatments (Figure 3C). Consistent with these findings, Western blot analysis of spheroid lysates showed marked downregulation of CD44, Oct4, and Nanog in the combination group compared with the untreated and 5-FU-treated groups (Figure 3D).

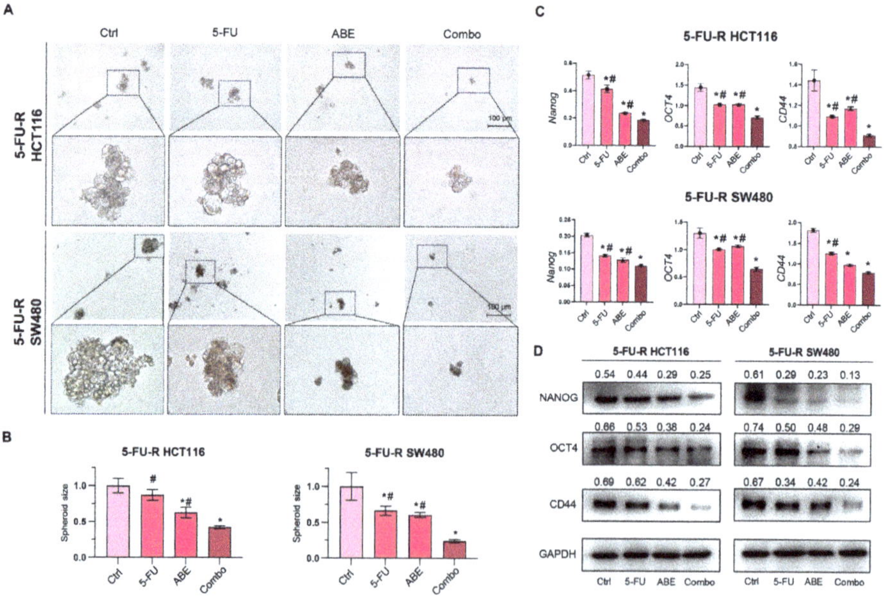

Figure 3. The combination treatment of 5-FU and ABE reduces cell stemness in 5-FU-R CRC cells. (**A**) 5-FU-R HCT116 and 5-FU-R SW480 cell lines were used for spheroid formation experiments after

https://doi.org/10.3390/ph19020261

treatment with 5-FU, ABE, or their combination for 48 h. Representative images of spheroids were taken. (**B**) Quantification of spheroid size following the indicated treatments. Combined treatment with 5-FU and ABE significantly reduced spheroid size compared with untreated controls or monotherapy in both cell lines. (**C**) Quantitative gene expression analysis of CSC-associated markers (*CD44*, *OCT4*, and *NANOG*) in spheroids following treatment with 5-FU, ABE, or their combination for 48 h. Transcript levels were normalized to the internal control and expressed relative to the untreated group. (**D**) Western blot analysis of CSC-associated proteins (CD44, OCT4, and NANOG) in spheroid lysates following the indicated treatments. Representative immunoblots and corresponding densitometric quantification normalized to GAPDH are shown. Data are presented as mean ± SD. * p indicates $p < 0.05$ vs. control group; # p indicates $p < 0.05$ vs. combination group.

Collectively, these results indicate that ABE enhances the anti-tumor efficacy of 5-FU by suppressing CSC-associated stemness properties at both the transcriptional and protein levels in 5-FU-resistant CRC cells. Collectively, these results indicate that ABE potentiates the anti-tumor effects of 5-FU by suppressing CSC-associated stemness programs at both transcriptional and protein levels, providing mechanistic support for the observed chemosensitization in 5-FU-resistant CRC cells.

2.4. The Toll-like Receptor 3 (TLR3) Expression Is Positively Correlated with 5-FU Resistance in CRC Cells

To investigate the mechanism associated with 5-FU-R in CRC cells, we performed a genome-wide transcriptomic analysis using RNA-seq in parental and 5-FU-R HCT116 and SW480 cell lines (GSE196900). In this analysis, we identified 657 upregulated genes in the 5-FU-R HCT116 cell line vs. the HCT116 cell line and 3060 upregulated genes in the 5-FU-R SW480 cell line vs. the SW480 cell line. 117 genes were upregulated in both 5-FU-R HCT116 and 5-FU-R SW480 cells compared with their parental cells. Furthermore, we performed a Kyoto Encyclopedia of Genes and Genomes (KEGG) pathway analysis of the differentially up-regulated genes in 5-FU-R versus parental CRC cells (Figure 4A). We selected the top 7 significant signaling pathways based on their p-value. It was observed that several important cancer-associated signaling pathways, including the TLR3 signaling pathway and cytokine pathway, were significantly suppressed in 5-FU-R CRC cells compared with parental cells (Figure 4B). In our study, we observed that the TLR3 signaling pathway is enriched and activated in 5-FU-R cells; the relative mRNA expression of *TLR3* in 5-FU-R HCT116 (fold change = 1.46, $p < 0.01$, Figure 4C) and 5-FU-R SW480 cells (fold change = 3.24, $p < 0.01$, Figure 4D) was significantly higher compared with parental CRC cells.

Activation of TLR3 signaling in 5-FU–R CRC cells by poly (I:C) stimulation resulted in increased spheroid formation, as evidenced by enlarged adherent spherical clusters (Figure 4E). Furthermore, pharmacological inhibition of TLR3 significantly enhanced sensitivity to 5-FU in both 5-FU–R HCT116 and SW480 cells, as demonstrated by reduced cell viability compared with control-treated cells ($p < 0.01$; Figure 4F,G). Collectively, these results indicate that TLR3 activation is associated with enhanced cancer stem-like phenotypes and contributes to chemoresistance in 5-FU-resistant CRC cells.

https://doi.org/10.3390/ph19020261

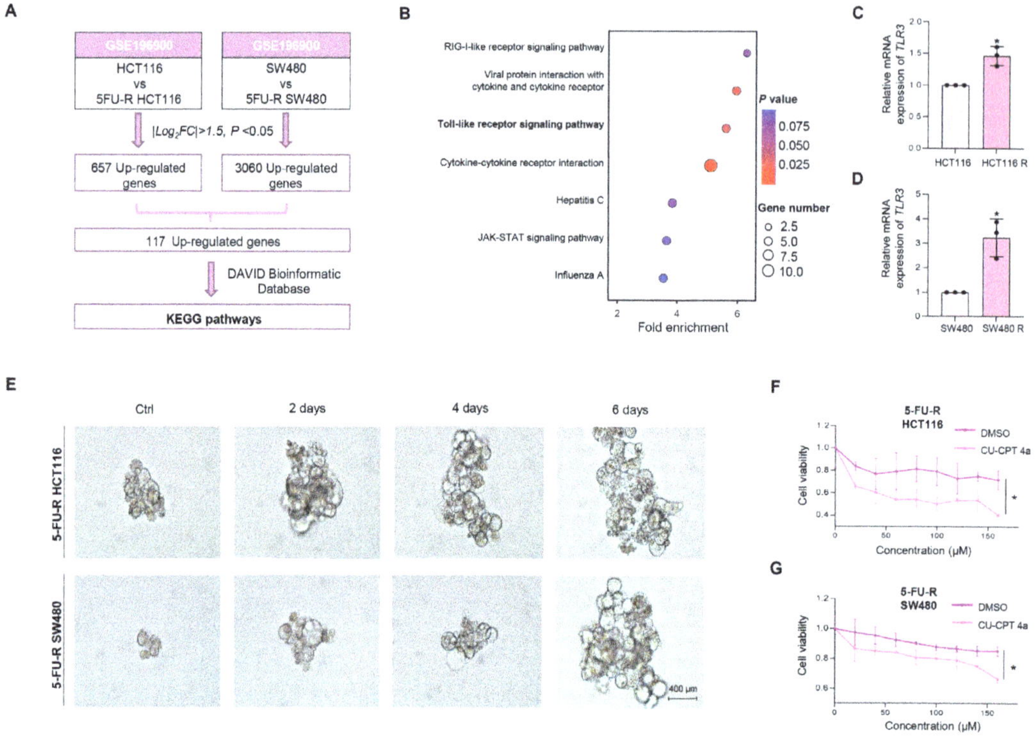

Figure 4. The expression of TLR3 is positively correlated with 5-FU-Resistance in CRC cells. (**A**) Schematic overview of the transcriptomic analysis workflow comparing parental and 5-FU-R HCT116 and SW480 CRC cell lines using RNA-sequencing data (GSE196900). Differentially upregulated genes were identified using the criteria of $\log_2$ fold change ($\log_2$FC) > 1.5 and $p < 0.05$, and overlapping upregulated genes between the two 5-FU-R cell lines were determined. (**B**) Scatter plot of KEGG pathway enrichment analysis based on genes upregulated in 5-FU-R CRC cells compared with their parental counterparts. The size of each circle represents the number of differentially expressed genes in the corresponding pathway, while the color scale indicates the enrichment *p*-value. (**C**) qRT-PCR analysis showing increased relative *TLR3* mRNA expression in 5-FU-R HCT116 cells compared with parental HCT116 cells. (**D**) qRT-PCR analysis of *TLR3* mRNA expression in 5-FU-R SW480 cells relative to parental SW480 cells. Gene expression levels were normalized to *GAPDH* and expressed relative to parental control. (**E**) Representative phase-contrast images showing morphological changes and enhanced formation of adherent spheroid-like clusters in 5-FU-R CRC cells following stimulation with the TLR3 agonist poly (I:C) (1 μg/mL) for the indicated time points. (**F**) Cell viability analysis of 5-FU-R HCT116 cells treated with 5-FU in the presence of DMSO or the TLR3 inhibitor CU-CPT 4a, as determined by the MTT assay. (**G**) Cell viability analysis of 5-FU-R SW480 cells treated with 5-FU following inhibition of TLR3 signaling using CU-CPT 4a. Data are presented as mean ± SD. * $p < 0.05$ vs. parental cells or DMSO-treated control, as indicated.

2.5. Combined Treatment with 5-FU and ABE Down-Regulates Cell Stemness Through the TLR3/NF-κB Axis

As mentioned above, the TLR3 activation may promote the capacity of 5-FU-R CRC cells to form spheroids. The cellular responses to TLR3 activation are widely acknowledged to be primarily regulated by the NF-κB signaling pathway [27]. Given that NF-κB activation drives pro-survival and stemness-associated pathways, we hypothesized that NF-κB signaling plays a pivotal role in TLR3-mediated CSC phenotypes. Consistent with this concept, Western blot analyses demonstrated that combination treatment with 5-FU

https://doi.org/10.3390/ph19020261

and ABE resulted in the most pronounced reduction in both TLR3 and NF-κB expression compared with untreated cells or cells treated with either agent alone (Figure 5A). Although 5-FU monotherapy partially reduced TLR3 levels, combination treatment achieved markedly greater suppression. Because nuclear translocation of NF-κB is a critical step for transcriptional activation, we further examined NF-κB localization in cytoplasmic and nuclear fractions. Notably, combined treatment significantly decreased NF-κB levels in both compartments in both CRC cell lines (Figure 5B), indicating effective inhibition of NF-κB nuclear translocation and signaling activity.

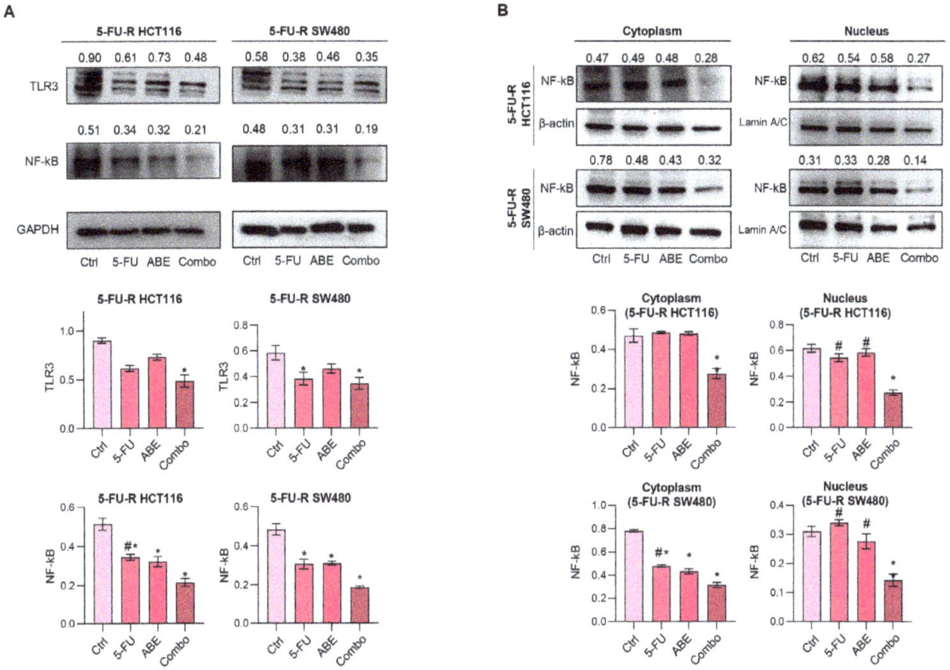

Figure 5. The combination treatment of 5-FU and ABE has been shown to regulate the TLR3/NF-κB axis in 5-FU-R CRC cell lines. (**A**) Western blot analysis of TLR3 and NF-κB protein expression in 5-FU-R HCT116 and SW480 cells treated with 5-FU, ABE, or their combination for 48 h. Combined treatment resulted in a marked reduction in TLR3 and NF-κB protein levels compared with untreated cells or either monotherapy. Representative immunoblots and corresponding densitometric quantification normalized to GAPDH are shown. (**B**) Western blot analysis of NF-κB expression in cytoplasmic and nuclear fractions of 5-FU-R CRC cells following treatment with 5-FU, ABE, or their combination for 48 h. Combined treatment significantly reduced NF-κB levels in both the cytoplasm and the nucleus, indicating inhibition of NF-κB activation and nuclear translocation. β-actin was used as a loading control for cytoplasmic fractions, and Lamin A/C was used as a nuclear loading control. Quantitative densitometric analyses are shown below each blot. Data are presented as mean ± SD. * *p* indicates $p < 0.05$ vs. control group; # *p* indicates $p < 0.05$ vs. combination group.

Together, these findings suggest that ABE enhances 5-FU efficacy by suppressing CSC-associated stemness via inhibition of the TLR3/NF-κB signaling axis.

2.6. The Combination of 5-FU and ABE Suppressed the Growth of PDOs

Three-dimensional organoid culture systems have become indispensable tools for modeling different facets of cancer biology, especially for investigating drug responses and evaluating treatment effectiveness [28–30]. In this study, patient-derived organoid

(PDO) models from two CRC patients were used to validate the anti-tumor effects of combined ABE and 5-FU treatment. The combination significantly reduced organoid size and viability compared with single-agent treatments (Figure 6A). In addition, *TLR3* mRNA expression was significantly suppressed in PDOs following combination treatment ($p < 0.01$, Figure 6B). Immunofluorescence analysis further demonstrated reduced NF-κB staining in the combination-treated organoids (Figure 6C), corroborating the mechanistic findings observed in CRC cell lines.

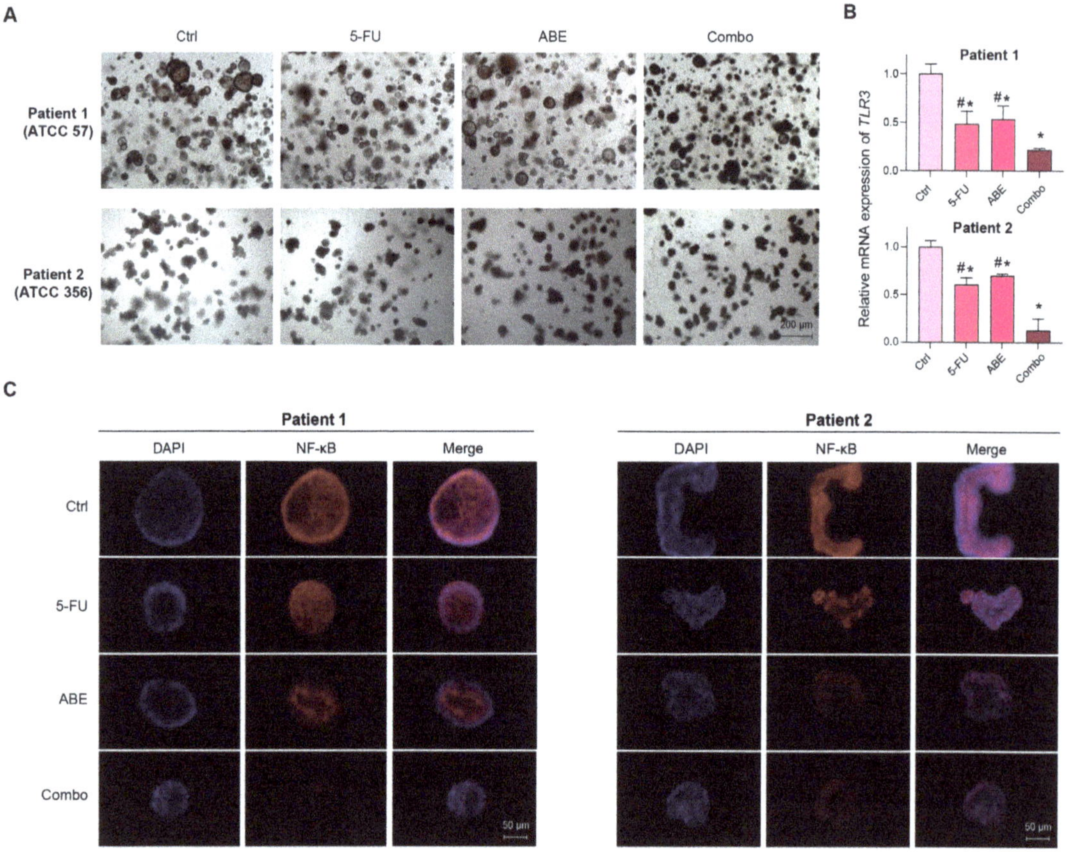

Figure 6. The combination of 5-FU and ABE effectively exhibits anti-cancer activity in CRC patient-derived organoid models. (**A**) Representative bright-field images of colorectal cancer PDOs treated with 5-FU, ABE, or their combination for 48 h. Combined treatment markedly reduced organoid size and overall growth compared with untreated controls or either monotherapy. (**B**) qRT-PCR analysis of *TLR3* mRNA expression in CRC PDOs following the indicated treatments. Transcript levels were normalized to *GAPDH* and expressed relative to the untreated control. (**C**) Representative confocal immunofluorescence images showing NF-κB expression in CRC organoids treated with DMSO, 5-FU, ABE, or the combination for 48 h. Reduced NF-κB staining was observed in organoids treated with the combination therapy compared with single-agent treatments. * *p* indicates $p < 0.05$ vs. control group; # *p* indicates $p < 0.05$ vs. combination group.

3. Discussion

CRC is the third most common cancer and a significant cause of morbidity and mortality worldwide [31]. Despite advances in early detection and therapeutic strategies, CRC remains a major cause of cancer-related mortality, largely due to disease recurrence and

https://doi.org/10.3390/ph19020261

the emergence of chemoresistance. Among currently available chemotherapeutic agents, 5-FU continues to serve as the backbone of CRC treatment; however, intrinsic and acquired resistance severely limit its long-term efficacy [32–34]. Multiple signaling pathways, including PI3K/AKT, FOXO1, FZD6, and NF-κB, have been implicated in the molecular mechanisms underlying chemoresistance [35–41]. Accumulating evidence indicates that tumor spheroids and cancer stem-like cells play central roles in therapeutic resistance, tumor heterogeneity, and disease relapse [42,43]. These high-risk cell populations exhibit enhanced self-renewal capacity and pronounced resistance to cytotoxic agents, highlighting the importance of targeting stemness-associated pathways. Accordingly, targeting these resistant stem-like tumor cells may represent a promising strategy to improve treatment efficacy in high-risk CRC patients, including those with metastatic disease.

Natural products have shown promise in cancer therapy by minimizing toxicity to healthy tissues and overcoming drug resistance [44–46]. In this study, we investigated whether ABE could enhance 5-FU sensitivity in 5-FU–resistant CRC cells. Combined treatment with ABE significantly reduced the effective concentration of 5-FU, yielding a Bliss synergy score exceeding 10. Moreover, the combination of ABE and 5-FU effectively suppressed cell viability, clonogenic capacity, migration, and invasion in CRC cells. This dual treatment also reduced stemness-associated markers, including CD44, Nanog, and Oct4, indicating attenuation of cancer stem-like properties. The results from the PDO model support the dual-drug efficacy. 5-FU and ABE combination treatment of PDOs resulted in a significant reduction in organoid growth and the number of alive organoids. The decreased survival rate is associated with reduced NF-kB levels.

To elucidate the molecular mechanisms underlying ABE-mediated chemosensitization, we analyzed RNA-seq profiles from parental and 5-FU–R CRC cells. Pathway enrichment analysis revealed significant activation of Toll-like receptor signaling, with marked upregulation of *TLR3* in resistant cells. TLR3 has been reported to activate NF-κB through both MYD88-dependent and MYD88-independent pathways [47,48]. Consistent with this concept, our Western blot analyses demonstrated that ABE, particularly in combination with 5-FU, markedly reduced TLR3 and NF-κB expression. Importantly, subcellular fractionation revealed decreased NF-κB levels in both the cytoplasm and the nucleus, indicating effective suppression of NF-κB nuclear translocation and transcriptional activity. These findings support a functional link between TLR3 inhibition and attenuation of downstream NF-κB signaling. KEGG pathway enrichment analysis additionally suggested involvement of the JAK/STAT signaling cascade. STAT3 is known to stabilize nuclear NF-κB activity [48,49] and regulate cancer malignancy [50,51]. Although phosphorylated STAT3 was not directly evaluated in the present study, TLR signaling showed more substantial fold enrichment in our pathway analysis, guiding our mechanistic focus toward TLR3. Nevertheless, these findings suggest potential crosstalk between the TLR3/NF-κB and STAT3 pathways, warranting further investigation in future studies. NF-κB signaling has been widely implicated as a central regulator of chemoresistance through its ability to promote cancer cell survival, inflammatory signaling, epithelial–mesenchymal transition, and maintenance of cancer stem-like properties [52,53]. Persistent NF-κB activation has been reported to confer resistance to 5-FU by upregulating anti-apoptotic genes and stemness-associated transcriptional programs [54]. Therefore, NF-κB suppression represents an attractive therapeutic strategy to overcome drug resistance.

Notably, natural products such as ABE are unlikely to target a single signaling pathway exclusively; instead, they may exert broader regulatory effects across interconnected oncogenic networks. Consistent with this concept, recent reviews have demonstrated that plant-derived natural products and their analogs can modulate NF-κB signaling at multiple regulatory levels, including membrane receptors, upstream kinases, and NF-

https://doi.org/10.3390/ph19020261

κB subunits [55,56], and can also regulate Toll-like receptor signaling via suppression of MyD88/NF-κB cascades [57]. Together, these reports support the notion that natural products can target NF-κB and TLR pathways, reinforcing our observation that ABE suppresses TLR3/NF-κB signaling in 5-FU-resistant CRC cells. In this context, the pronounced reduction in NF-κB observed following combined ABE and 5-FU treatment provides a mechanistic basis for the enhanced chemosensitivity and CSC suppression identified in our study. Several limitations of this study should be acknowledged. First, a well-recognized challenge of natural product–based therapies is the difficulty in standardizing complex extracts for clinical application. Aronia berry extract contains diverse bioactive compounds, including anthocyanins, flavonols, and phenolic acids, which have been reported to inhibit topoisomerase I/II activity [58–61]. While our findings demonstrate the therapeutic potential of ABE, future studies should focus on isolating active components and developing standardized formulations. Another limitation is that, although patient-derived organoids were used to enhance clinical relevance, they were not derived from 5-FU–resistant tumors. While our PDO data support synergistic efficacy of ABE and 5-FU, further validation using resistant organoid models and in vivo studies will be essential to confirm translational applicability.

In summary, our study documented that the combination of 5-FU and ABE inhibits CRC stem cell proliferation. The mechanism involves inhibition of stemness and NF-κB signaling and is supported by in vitro data. This article provides valuable insights into ABE's potential to overcome 5-FU resistance in CRC. These findings add to the growing evidence for ABE's potential as a novel therapy for CRC, especially for patients with 5-FU resistance.

4. Materials and Methods

4.1. Cell Culture

The human CRC cell lines, HCT116 and SW480, were purchased from the American Type Culture Collection (ATCC, Manassas, VA, USA). The cell lines were cultured in Dulbecco's Modified Eagle Medium (DMEM; Gibco, Waltham, MA, USA) supplemented with 10% fetal bovine serum (FBS; Gibco), 100 U/mL penicillin (Gibco), and 1% streptomycin (Sigma-Aldrich, St. Louis, MO, USA). The cells were grown at 37 °C in a humidified atmosphere containing 5% CO_2 and harvested using 0.05% trypsin-0.03% EDTA (Invitrogen, Thermo Fisher Scientific, Waltham, MA, USA). 5-FU-R cell lines, 5-FU-R HCT116 and 5-FU-R SW480, were established by continuously culturing the cells with increasing doses of 5-FU, as described previously [21,62].

4.2. Herbal Preparations

Aronia Berry extract (ABE; Aronia Berry Complex, EuroPharma USA, Green Bay, WI, USA) was employed in this study. This extract is derived from the fruit of *Aronia melanocarpa* and prepared in 70% ethanol, standardized to contain 40% polyphenols. This powdered extract, derived from the fruit of black chokeberry (native to North America), offers a characteristic sensory profile ranging from purple to dark red. The extract is dissolved in dimethyl sulfoxide to obtain stock solutions, which are then diluted to appropriate levels in the culture media.

4.3. Reagents

Poly (I:C) was obtained from InvivoGen (San Diego, CA, USA), and CU-CPT 4a was purchased from MedChemExpress (MCE; Monmouth Junction, NJ, USA). 5-fluorouracil (Sigma-Aldrich, St. Louis, MO, USA) was dissolved in dimethyl sulfoxide (DMSO, Sigma-Aldrich) for use in this study. The stock solution of 5-fluorouracil and ABE was stored at

https://doi.org/10.3390/ph19020261

−20 °C in opaque containers and diluted with complete culture medium to achieve the desired experimental concentrations before each application.

4.4. Cell Counting MTT (3-(4,5-Dimethylthiazol-2-yl)-2,5-diphenyltetrazolium Bromide) Assays

To confirm the 5-FU resistance, we compared the proliferation rates of 5-FU-R and parental cell lines by treating them with increasing doses of 5-FU. Cells were seeded at a density of 5×10^3 cells per well in 96-well flat-bottom plates and incubated for 24 h. Subsequently, they were exposed to escalating concentrations of 5-FU (0–160 μM). After 48 h of treatment, the supernatant was removed, and each well was supplemented with 90 μL of DMEM and 10 μL of MTT solutionas previously described [63,64]. The plates were then incubated for an additional 4 h, and the absorbance of the final product was measured at 490 nm (OD490) using a microplate reader (Tecan Trading AG, Männedorf, Switzerland). To evaluate the combined impact of ABE and 5-FU on CRC cell proliferation, cells were seeded at 3×10^3 cells/well in 100 μL of complete medium in 96-well plates and grown for 24 h. Following this, the cells were exposed to appropriate concentrations of 5-FU (40 μM), ABE (60 μg/mL), and their combination. Proliferation was assessed at different time points using the MTT assay.

4.5. TLR3 Activation and Inhibition Assays

TLR3 activation was achieved by treating 5-FU–resistant CRC cell lines with poly (I:C) (InvivoGen) as a specific TLR3 ligand. Cells were exposed to poly (I:C) for 2–6 days, and spheroid formation was monitored under adherent culture conditions. To inhibit TLR3 signaling, cells were treated with the TLR3 inhibitor CU-CPT 4a (MCE). Following inhibitor treatment, cells were subsequently exposed to 5-FU, and cell viability was assessed using the MTT assay.

4.6. Drug Response Testing

The CRC cell lines were cultured in 96-well plates at a density of 5×10^3 cells per well and incubated for 24 h prior to drug introduction. Subsequent treatment involved exposing the cells to varying concentrations of 5-FU (0, 20, 40, and 60 μM) and ABE (0, 30, 60, 90, 120, and 150 μg/mL), individually and in various combinations, for 48 h. Cell viability was evaluated using the MTT assay as mentioned above. To analyze the combined effects of the drugs, synergy scores were computed utilizing SynergyFinder 3.0 (https://synergyfinder.fimm.fi, accessed on 28 January 2026), a user-friendly tool tailored for interactive assessment and visualization of combination treatment outcomes.

4.7. Colony Formation Assay

Colony formation assays were performed as previously described [9,11,65]. 5×10^2 cells per well were seeded in 6-well flat-bottom plates, followed by treatment with 5-FU (40 μM), ABE (60 μg/mL), or their combination for 48 h. Colony formation was allowed to proceed for 10 to 14 days, with the culture medium refreshed every 3 days. Upon completion of the incubation period, the cell colonies were fixed with methanol for 30 min and subsequently stained with 1% crystal violet (Thermo Fisher Scientific, Waltham, MA, USA). Quantification of colony numbers was performed using ImageJ software (version 1.53; National Institutes of Health, Bethesda, MD, USA).

4.8. The Wound Healing Assay

The wound healing assay was performed as previously described [9,11,65]. 5×10^5 cells per well were seeded in 6-well flat-bottom plates after 48 h of treatment with 5-FU, ABE, or their combination. Upon reaching 90% to 100% confluence, a controlled scratch was created in the monolayer using a sterile 200 μL micropipette tip, followed by a wash with serum-

https://doi.org/10.3390/ph19020261

free medium to remove detached cells. Subsequently, the cells were cultured in medium devoid of FBS. Photographs of cellular migration were captured 24 h post-wounding, and the percentage of wound closure was quantified using ImageJ.

4.9. Invasion Assays

Invasion assays were conducted as previously described [9,11,65]. BioCoat Matrigel Invasion Chambers with 8.0 μm Pore Polyester Membrane (BD Biosciences, Franklin Lakes, NJ, USA) were used. Following treatment with 5-FU, ABE, or their combination for 48 h, 5×10^4 cells per well were seeded in 24-well flat-bottom plates for the invasion assay. Subsequently, the cells were placed onto inserts in serum-free medium and transferred to wells containing culture medium supplemented with 10% FBS. After 72 h of incubation, the cells that had invaded the bottom surface of the membrane were fixed and stained using a Diff-Quick staining kit (Thermo Fisher Scientific). Quantification of the stained cells was performed under a microscope.

4.10. Spheroid Formation Assay

Spheroid formation assays were performed as previously described [64]. After 48 h of treatment with 5-FU, ABE, and their combination, 5-FU-R HCT116 and 5-FU-R SW480 cells were seeded in ultra-low attachment plates at a density of 500–1000 cells per well in serum-free DMEM-F12 medium (STEMCELL Technologies, Vancouver, BC, Canada) containing epidermal growth factor (EGF; STEMCELL Technologies), basic fibroblast growth factor (bFGF; Gibco), and B27 supplement (Gibco). After 7–10 days, the spheroids were observed under a bright-field microscope at 40× magnification and counted using ImageJ.

4.11. Genome-Wide Transcriptomic Profiling and Pathway Enrichment Analysis

Genome-wide mRNA expression profiling was conducted to compare parental CRC cells with their 5-FU-R counterparts [66]. Total RNA was isolated and used for next-generation sequencing library preparation with the SureSelect XT HS2 mRNA Library Preparation Kit (Agilent Technologies, Santa Clara, CA, USA), using up to 1 μg of input RNA per sample in accordance with the manufacturer's instructions. The raw Fastq files and the processed, filtered count matrix for mRNA sequencing were deposited in the NCBI GEO database under accession GSE196900. RNA sequencing was performed on an Illumina NovaSeq 6000 platform (Illumina, San Diego, CA, USA). Initial base calling was carried out using Illumina Real-Time Analysis software (RTA3, version 3.4.4), followed by conversion to FASTQ format using bcl2fastq (version 2.20.0.422). Low-quality bases at the 5′ and 3′ ends of reads were removed based on Phred quality scores prior to downstream processing. The filtered reads were aligned to the human reference genome (GRCh38) using the STAR aligner (version 2.7.8a) with default alignment settings [67]. After alignment, the final BAM files were quantified using the Partek E/M algorithm [68], and gene-level annotations were assigned based on Ensembl transcript release 102. Normalization and differential expression analysis were subsequently performed using the DESeq2 package to identify transcriptional differences between 5-FU-R and parental CRC cells [69]. Genes exhibiting an absolute $\log_2$ fold change greater than 1 with a nominal p-value < 0.05 were considered differentially expressed. To explore the biological significance of the identified differentially expressed genes (DEGs), pathway enrichment analysis was performed using KEGG pathways through DAVID Bioinformatics Resources (https://davidbioinformatics.nih.gov/summary.jsp, accessed on 22 Janually 2025).

4.12. Protein Isolation and Western Blot

Total protein was extracted from CRC cell lines treated with 5-FU, ABE, or their combination for 48 h. The cells were collected using a plastic scraper and rinsed three times with cold phosphate buffered solution (PBS; Gibco). Subsequently, the cells were lysed using ice-cold RIPA protein extraction solution supplemented with a protease inhibitor cocktail (Thermo Fisher Scientific). Protein concentration was determined using the BCA method (Thermo Fisher Scientific). Equal amounts of protein samples (50 μg) were resolved via SDS-PAGE using 10% Mini-PROTEAN TGXTM Precast Gels (BIO-RAD, Hercules, CA, USA) and then transferred onto a 0.45 μm PVDF membrane (Cytiva, Marlborough, MA, USA). The membrane was blocked with 5% bovine serum albumin (BSA; Sigma-Aldrich) in Tris-buffered saline (BIO-RAD) containing 0.1% Tween-20 (Sigma-Aldrich) for 1 h at room temperature. Primary antibodies, including anti-CD44 (1:1000, 5023S; Cell Signaling Technology [CST], Danvers, MA, USA), anti-Nanog (1:1000, 9505; CST), anti-Oct4 (1:1000, 9532S; CST), anti-TLR3 (1:1000, PA5-20183; Thermo Fisher Scientific), anti-P65 (1:1000, 3034; CST), anti-GAPDH (1:2000, 5174T; CST), anti-β-actin (1:5000, 58169S; CST), and anti-Lamin A/C (1:1000, 10298-1-AP; Proteintech, Rosemont, IL, USA) were incubated with the membranes at 4 °C overnight. After three washes with TBST, the membrane was incubated with the appropriate anti-rabbit (1:2000, 7074; CST) or anti-mouse (1:2000, 7076; CST) secondary antibodies for 1 h at room temperature. Blots were visualized using an HRP-based chemiluminescence kit (Thermo Fisher Scientific) and Gel Imaging Systems (BIO-RAD). GAPDH, β-actin, and Lamin A/C protein were used as internal controls, and protein band intensities were quantified using ImageJ. The original Western blot images are provided in Figure S2.

4.13. *Quantitative Reverse Transcription PCR (qRT-PCR)*

Total RNA extraction was performed using the Qiagen miRNeasy Kit (Qiagen, Hilden, Germany). cDNA synthesis was performed by reverse transcription of total RNA using the High-Capacity cDNA Reverse Transcription Kit (Thermo Fisher Scientific). RT-PCR assays were performed using the QuantStudio 6 Flex RT-PCR System (Applied Biosystems, Foster City, CA, USA) according to the manufacturer's protocols and the SensiFAST SYBR Lo-ROX Kit (Bioline, London, UK). Relative mRNA expression levels were calculated using the $2^{-\Delta\Delta Ct}$ method and normalized to β-actin, the internal control. The primers used in the study are detailed in Table S1.

4.14. *Nuclear Protein Extraction*

CRC cells were harvested after treatment and washed twice with cold PBS. Nuclear protein extraction was performed using a standard hypotonic lysis protocol. Briefly, cell pellets were resuspended in 500 μL hypotonic buffer [20 mM Tris-HCl, pH 7.4, 10 mM NaCl, 3 mM $MgCl_2$, 0.5 mM DTT] supplemented with protease and phosphatase inhibitor cocktails (Sigma-Aldrich, cat. #P8340; Thermo Fisher Scientific, cat. #78420) and incubated on ice for 15 min. Subsequently, 25 μL of 10% Nonidet P-40 (Sigma-Aldrich) was added, followed by centrifugation at 1000× *g* for 10 min at 4 °C. The resulting nuclear pellet was washed once, then lysed in 180 μL of complete lysis buffer provided in the transcription factor extraction kit, according to the manufacturer's instructions, as previously described [10]. Nuclear protein concentrations were determined prior to downstream analyses.

4.15. *Patient-Derived CRC Tumor Organoids*

Patient-derived CRC organoids were purchased from the American Type Culture Collection (ATCC; Manassas, VA, USA) and cultured according to previously published procedures [65]. For the culture of human organoids, the Human Complete Feeding Medium (hCPLT) comprised IntestiCult Organoid Growth Medium (STEMCELL Technologies, Vancouver, BC, Canada) supplemented with Y-27632 (1:1000; STEMCELL Technologies). The Human Wash Medium with BSA consisted of Advanced DMEM/F-12 (STEMCELL Technologies), 10 mM HEPES, 1× GlutaMAX Supplement (Gibco), 100 μg/mL Primocin

https://doi.org/10.3390/ph19020261

(InvivoGen), and 0.1% BSA (Sigma-Aldrich). CRC organoids were seeded in 24-well plates, forming domes within 40 μL of Matrigel (Corning, Tehama County, CA, USA), and cultured in 700 μL of the hCPLT. Subsequently, the organoids were divided into four treatment groups, and appropriate concentrations of ABE, 5-FU, and their combination were administered. After a 3-day treatment period, the number and size of the organoids were assessed by microscopy (magnification ×40), with measurements obtained using ImageJ software. Harvested organoids were also aliquoted for total RNA extraction.

4.16. Immunofluorescence Assays

For the immunofluorescence assay, the organoids were treated with 5-FU, ABE, or a combination of both for 48 h. The organoids were subsequently fixed with 4% paraformaldehyde for 10 min at room temperature, then permeabilized with 0.5% Triton X-100 (Thermo Fisher Scientific) for 10 min at room temperature. To remove endogenous peroxides, the slides were treated and subsequently blocked in TBST (Tris-buffered saline (Thermo Fisher Scientific) containing Tween-20 (Sigma-Aldrich)) containing 3% BSA (Sigma-Aldrich) for 1 h at room temperature. The slides were then incubated overnight at 4 °C with an anti-NF-kB Polyclonal antibody, followed by incubation with a FITC-labeled secondary antibody (1:1000, A-21202; Thermo Fisher Scientific) for 1 h at 37 °C. After the incubation periods, the organoids were subjected to three additional washes with PBS (Gibco), each lasting 5 min. Finally, the organoid nucleus was stained with DAPI (Thermo Fisher Scientific), and all images were captured using a Carl Zeiss fluorescent microscope (Zeiss, Oberkochen, Germany).

4.17. Statistical Analysis

Statistical analyses were conducted using GraphPad Prism v. 6.0 software (GraphPad Software, San Diego, CA, USA). Student's *t*-test was employed to assess the significance of differences between any two groups, while one-way analysis of variance (ANOVA) was utilized to evaluate differences across multiple comparisons. Each experiment was independently performed in triplicate using biological replicates, and data were expressed as mean ± standard deviation. A significance level of $p < 0.05$ was adopted to determine statistical significance.

5. Conclusions

We have introduced a novel perspective on ABE's potential to address 5-FU resistance in CRC cells, through a comprehensive series of experiments using 5-FU-resistant cell cultures and patient-derived tumor organoids. Furthermore, our observations indicate a pivotal role for the TLR3/NF-κB axis in mediating stemness and 5-FU resistance in CRC, and ABE mitigates this resistance by downregulating TLR3 and its associated signaling pathways in CRC cells. These findings underscore a promising, economically feasible strategy to enhance therapeutic efficacy in CRC.

Supplementary Materials: The following supporting information can be downloaded at: https://www.mdpi.com/article/10.3390/ph19020261/s1. Table S1: List of primers for RT-qPCR used in this study. Figure S1: Dose–response curves illustrating the sensitivity of parental and 5-FU-R CRC cell lines to 5-FU treatment. Figure S2: The original WB images.

Author Contributions: H.D., T.N. and A.G. conceived and designed the experiments. H.D. performed the experiments and analyzed the data. H.D., T.N. and A.G. wrote and edited the manuscript. All authors have read and agreed to the published version of the manuscript.

Funding: This work was supported by the following grants from the National Cancer Institute, National Institutes of Health: CA181572, CA184792, CA187956, CA214254, CA271443, and CA296639.

https://doi.org/10.3390/ph19020261

Institutional Review Board Statement: The study was conducted in accordance with the Declaration of Helsinki and was approved by the Ethics Committee of the Beckman Research Institute of the City of Hope (protocol code 23228, date 1 November 2025).

Informed Consent Statement: Not applicable.

Data Availability Statement: The original contributions presented in this study are included in the article/Supplementary Material. Further inquiries can be directed to the corresponding author.

Acknowledgments: The authors thank Junyong Weng, Yudai Higuchi, Toshiaki Takahashi, and Yuan Li for their thoughtful discussions and advice during this project.

Conflicts of Interest: The authors disclose no potential conflicts of interest.

Abbreviations

ABE	Aronia berry extracts
CRC	colorectal cancer
CSCs	Cancer stem cells
DMSO	Dimethyl sulfoxide
FC	Fold Change
GEO	Gene Expression Omnibus
IC50	50% inhibitory concentration
KEGG	Kyoto Encyclopedia of Genes and Genomes
MTT	3-(4,5-Dimethylthiazol-2-yl)-2,5-diphenyltetrazolium bromide
qRT-PCR	Quantitative reverse transcription PCR
RT	room temperature
TLR3	Toll-like receptor 3
WB	Western blotting
5-FU	5-fluorouracil
5-FU-R	5-fluorouracil-resistance

References

1. Bray, F.; Laversanne, M.; Sung, H.; Ferlay, J.; Siegel, R.L.; Soerjomataram, I.; Jemal, A. Global cancer statistics 2022: Globocan estimates of incidence and mortality worldwide for 36 cancers in 185 countries. *CA Cancer J. Clin.* **2024**, *74*, 229–263. [CrossRef]
2. Benson, A.B., 3rd; Schrag, D.; Somerfield, M.R.; Cohen, A.M.; Figueredo, A.T.; Flynn, P.J.; Krzyzanowska, M.K.; Maroun, J.; McAllister, P.; Van Cutsem, E.; et al. American Society of Clinical Oncology recommendations on adjuvant chemotherapy for stage II colon cancer. *J. Clin. Oncol.* **2004**, *22*, 3408–3419. [CrossRef] [PubMed]
3. Luo, X.J.; Zhao, Q.; Liu, J.; Zheng, J.B.; Qiu, M.Z.; Ju, H.Q.; Xu, R.H. Novel Genetic and Epigenetic Biomarkers of Prognostic and Predictive Significance in Stage II/III Colorectal Cancer. *Mol. Ther.* **2021**, *29*, 587–596. [CrossRef]
4. Akgul, O.; Cetinkaya, E.; Ersoz, S.; Tez, M. Role of surgery in colorectal cancer liver metastases. *World J. Gastroenterol.* **2014**, *20*, 6113–6122. [CrossRef]
5. Tirendi, S.; Marengo, B.; Domenicotti, C.; Bassi, A.M.; Almonti, V.; Vernazza, S. Colorectal cancer and therapy response: A focus on the main mechanisms involved. *Front. Oncol.* **2023**, *13*, 1208140. [CrossRef] [PubMed]
6. Link, A.; Balaguer, F.; Goel, A. Cancer chemoprevention by dietary polyphenols: Promising role for epigenetics. *Biochem. Pharmacol.* **2010**, *80*, 1771–1792. [CrossRef]
7. Reuter, S.; Gupta, S.C.; Park, B.; Goel, A.; Aggarwal, B.B. Epigenetic changes induced by curcumin and other natural compounds. *Genes Nutr.* **2011**, *6*, 93–108. [CrossRef] [PubMed]
8. Weng, W.; Goel, A. Curcumin and colorectal cancer: An update and current perspective on this natural medicine. *Semin. Cancer Biol.* **2022**, *80*, 73–86. [CrossRef]
9. Asahi, Y.; Xu, C.; Okuno, K.; Taketomi, A.; Goel, A. The anticancer effects of Aronia berry extract are mediated by Chk1 and p53 in colorectal cancer. *Phytomedicine* **2024**, *135*, 156086. [CrossRef]
10. Li, Y.; Xu, C.; Han, H.; Pascual-Sabater, S.; Fillat, C.; Goel, A. Aronia Berry Extract Modulates MYD88/NF-kB/P-Glycoprotein Axis to Overcome Gemcitabine Resistance in Pancreatic Cancer. *Pharmaceuticals* **2024**, *17*, 911. [CrossRef]

https://doi.org/10.3390/ph19020261

11. Li, Y.; Xu, C.; Weng, W.; Goel, A. Combined treatment with Aronia berry extract and oligomeric proanthocyanidins exhibit a synergistic anticancer efficacy through LMNB1-AKT signaling pathways in colorectal cancer. *Mol. Carcinog.* **2024**, *63*, 2145–2157. [CrossRef]
12. Bermudez-Soto, M.J.; Larrosa, M.; Garcia-Cantalejo, J.M.; Espin, J.C.; Tomas-Barberan, F.A.; Garcia-Conesa, M.T. Up-regulation of tumor suppressor carcinoembryonic antigen-related cell adhesion molecule 1 in human colon cancer Caco-2 cells following repetitive exposure to dietary levels of a polyphenol-rich chokeberry juice. *J. Nutr. Biochem.* **2007**, *18*, 259–271. [CrossRef]
13. Dai, J.; Patel, J.D.; Mumper, R.J. Characterization of blackberry extract and its antiproliferative and anti-inflammatory properties. *J. Med. Food* **2007**, *10*, 258–265. [CrossRef]
14. Gill, N.K.; Rios, D.; Osorio-Camacena, E.; Mojica, B.E.; Kaur, B.; Soderstrom, M.A.; Gonzalez, M.; Plaat, B.; Poblete, C.; Kaur, N.; et al. Anticancer Effects of Extracts from Three Different Chokeberry Species. *Nutr. Cancer* **2021**, *73*, 1168–1174. [CrossRef]
15. Liang, Z.; Liang, H.; Guo, Y.; Yang, D. Cyanidin 3-O-galactoside: A Natural Compound with Multiple Health Benefits. *Int. J. Mol. Sci.* **2021**, *22*, 2261. [CrossRef]
16. Wang, L.; Pan, X.; Jiang, L.; Chu, Y.; Gao, S.; Jiang, X.; Zhang, Y.; Chen, Y.; Luo, S.; Peng, C. The Biological Activity Mechanism of Chlorogenic Acid and Its Applications in Food Industry: A Review. *Front. Nutr.* **2022**, *9*, 943911. [CrossRef] [PubMed]
17. Shriwas, P.; Chen, X.; Kinghorn, A.D.; Ren, Y. Plant-derived glucose transport inhibitors with potential antitumor activity. *Phytother. Res.* **2020**, *34*, 1027–1040. [CrossRef] [PubMed]
18. Reyes-Farias, M.; Carrasco-Pozo, C. The Anti-Cancer Effect of Quercetin: Molecular Implications in Cancer Metabolism. *Int. J. Mol. Sci.* **2019**, *20*, 3177. [CrossRef] [PubMed]
19. Ren, Y.; Frank, T.; Meyer, G.; Lei, J.; Grebenc, J.R.; Slaughter, R.; Gao, Y.G.; Kinghorn, A.D. Potential Benefits of Black Chokeberry (*Aronia melanocarpa*) Fruits and Their Constituents in Improving Human Health. *Molecules* **2022**, *27*, 7823. [CrossRef]
20. Thani, N.A.; Keshavarz, S.; Lwaleed, B.A.; Cooper, A.J.; Rooprai, H.K. Cytotoxicity of gemcitabine enhanced by polyphenolics from *Aronia melanocarpa* in pancreatic cancer cell line AsPC-1. *J. Clin. Pathol.* **2014**, *67*, 949–954. [CrossRef]
21. Roy, S.; Zhao, Y.; Yuan, Y.C.; Goel, A. Metformin and ICG-001 Act Synergistically to Abrogate Cancer Stem Cells-Mediated Chemoresistance in Colorectal Cancer by Promoting Apoptosis and Autophagy. *Cancers* **2022**, *14*, 1281. [CrossRef]
22. Caglar, H.O.; Biray Avci, C. Alterations of cell cycle genes in cancer: Unmasking the role of cancer stem cells. *Mol. Biol. Rep.* **2020**, *47*, 3065–3076. [CrossRef]
23. Li, H.; Feng, Z.; He, M.L. Lipid metabolism alteration contributes to and maintains the properties of cancer stem cells. *Theranostics* **2020**, *10*, 7053–7069. [CrossRef]
24. Lamichhane, A.; Thakuri, P.S.; Rafsanjani Nejad, P.; Tavana, H. Modeling adaptive drug resistance of colorectal cancer and therapeutic interventions with tumor spheroids. *Exp. Biol. Med.* **2021**, *246*, 2372–2380. [CrossRef]
25. Ozawa, M.; Ichikawa, Y.; Zheng, Y.W.; Oshima, T.; Miyata, H.; Nakazawa, K.; Guan, H.B.; Shiozawa, M.; Akaike, M.; Watanabe, K.; et al. Prognostic significance of CD44 variant 2 upregulation in colorectal cancer. *Br. J. Cancer* **2014**, *111*, 365–374. [CrossRef]
26. Yang, L.; Shi, P.; Zhao, G.; Xu, J.; Peng, W.; Zhang, J.; Zhang, G.; Wang, X.; Dong, Z.; Chen, F.; et al. Targeting cancer stem cell pathways for cancer therapy. *Signal Transduct. Target. Ther.* **2020**, *5*, 8. [CrossRef]
27. Pradere, J.P.; Dapito, D.H.; Schwabe, R.F. The Yin and Yang of Toll-like receptors in cancer. *Oncogene* **2014**, *33*, 3485–3495. [CrossRef] [PubMed]
28. Avci, C.B.; Bagca, B.G.; Shademan, B.; Takanlou, L.S.; Takanlou, M.S.; Nourazarian, A. The future of cancer therapy: Exploring the potential of patient-derived organoids in drug development. *Front. Cell Dev. Biol.* **2024**, *12*, 1401504. [CrossRef] [PubMed]
29. Clevers, H. Modeling Development and Disease with Organoids. *Cell* **2016**, *165*, 1586–1597. [CrossRef] [PubMed]
30. Janapati, Y.K.; Junapudi, S. Progress in experimental models to investigate the in vivo and in vitro antidiabetic activity of drugs. *Anim. Models Exp. Med.* **2024**, *7*, 297–309. [CrossRef]
31. Siegel, R.L.; Miller, K.D.; Wagle, N.S.; Jemal, A. Cancer statistics, 2023. *CA Cancer J. Clin.* **2023**, *73*, 17–48. [CrossRef] [PubMed]
32. Del Rio, M.; Molina, F.; Bascoul-Mollevi, C.; Copois, V.; Bibeau, F.; Chalbos, P.; Bareil, C.; Kramar, A.; Salvetat, N.; Fraslon, C.; et al. Gene expression signature in advanced colorectal cancer patients select drugs and response for the use of leucovorin, fluorouracil, and irinotecan. *J. Clin. Oncol.* **2007**, *25*, 773–780. [CrossRef] [PubMed]
33. Singh, U.; Kokkanti, R.R.; Patnaik, S. Beyond chemotherapy: Exploring 5-FU resistance and stemness in colorectal cancer. *Eur. J. Pharmacol.* **2025**, *991*, 177294. [CrossRef] [PubMed]
34. Vodenkova, S.; Buchler, T.; Cervena, K.; Veskrnova, V.; Vodicka, P.; Vymetalkova, V. 5-fluorouracil and other fluoropyrimidines in colorectal cancer: Past, present and future. *Pharmacol. Ther.* **2020**, *206*, 107447. [CrossRef]
35. Chen, H.; Deng, J.; Hou, T.W.; Shan, Y.Q. Villosol reverses 5-FU resistance in colorectal cancer by inhibiting the CDKN2A gene regulated TP53-PI3K/Akt signaling axis. *J. Ethnopharmacol.* **2024**, *325*, 117907. [CrossRef]
36. Gan, D.; Yang, C.; Shen, X.; Shi, J.; Wang, R.; Zhu, L.; Li, H.; Luo, J.; Zhao, T.; Li, J.; et al. GIPC1 Restrains the Progression and Chemoresistance of Colorectal Cancer by Regulating TTC7B/mTOR/NF-kappaB Axis. *Int. J. Biol. Sci.* **2026**, *22*, 786–801. [CrossRef]

https://doi.org/10.3390/ph19020261

37. He, Z.; Yang, J.; Zhang, Y.; Zhang, T.; Guo, T.; Jin, L.; Mao, Y.; Wang, T. FZD6 promotes 5-fluorouracil resistance through inhibiting pyroptosis in colorectal cancer. *Carcinogenesis* **2025**, *46*, bgaf041. [CrossRef]
38. Liu, Q.; Zhang, Y.; Li, H.; Gao, H.; Zhou, Y.; Luo, D.; Shan, Z.; Yang, Y.; Weng, J.; Li, Q.; et al. Squalene epoxidase promotes the chemoresistance of colorectal cancer via (S)-2,3-epoxysqualene-activated NF-kappaB. *Cell Commun. Signal.* **2024**, *22*, 278. [CrossRef]
39. Wang, Y.; Chang, Z.; Sun, Z.; Wang, L.; Li, J.; Li, G.; Wang, Y.; Zhang, J.; Ai, L.; Zhang, Z.; et al. Targeting the ARL4C/RAP1/PI3K-Akt-mTOR signaling loop promotes ARL4C ubiquitination and reverses oxaliplatin resistance in colorectal cancer. *Theranostics* **2026**, *16*, 99–122. [CrossRef]
40. Yan, S.; Hu, X.; Wu, Y.; Ye, W.; Zhu, Y.; He, Y.; Zhan, F.; Wu, W.; Ma, Z. ITGA4 Contributes to 5-Fluorouracil Resistance by Up-Regulating PI3K/AKT Signaling: Evidence from Network Pharmacology, Molecular Docking and Experimental Verification. *Drug Des. Dev. Ther.* **2025**, *19*, 4105–4122. [CrossRef]
41. Wang, D.; Yang, L.; Yu, W.; Wu, Q.; Lian, J.; Li, F.; Liu, S.; Li, A.; He, Z.; Liu, J.; et al. Colorectal cancer cell-derived CCL20 recruits regulatory T cells to promote chemoresistance via FOXO1/CEBPB/NF-kappaB signaling. *J. Immunother. Cancer* **2019**, *7*, 215. [CrossRef]
42. Banerjee, V.; Sharda, N.; Huse, J.; Singh, D.; Sokolov, D.; Czinn, S.J.; Blanchard, T.G.; Banerjee, A. Synergistic potential of dual andrographolide and melatonin targeting of metastatic colon cancer cells: Using the Chou-Talalay combination index method. *Eur. J. Pharmacol.* **2021**, *897*, 173919. [CrossRef] [PubMed]
43. Liu, Y.; Zhao, C.; Wang, G.; Chen, J.; Ju, S.; Huang, J.; Wang, X. SNORD1C maintains stemness and 5-FU resistance by activation of Wnt signaling pathway in colorectal cancer. *Cell Death Discov.* **2022**, *8*, 200. [CrossRef]
44. Newman, D.J.; Cragg, G.M. Natural Products as Sources of New Drugs over the Nearly Four Decades from 01/1981 to 09/2019. *J. Nat. Prod.* **2020**, *83*, 770–803. [CrossRef] [PubMed]
45. Hashem, S.; Ali, T.A.; Akhtar, S.; Nisar, S.; Sageena, G.; Ali, S.; Al-Mannai, S.; Therachiyil, L.; Mir, R.; Elfaki, I.; et al. Targeting cancer signaling pathways by natural products: Exploring promising anti-cancer agents. *Biomed. Pharmacother.* **2022**, *150*, 113054. [CrossRef]
46. Chen, T.; Xiao, Z.; Liu, X.; Wang, T.; Wang, Y.; Ye, F.; Su, J.; Yao, X.; Xiong, L.; Yang, D.H. Natural products for combating multidrug resistance in cancer. *Pharmacol. Res.* **2024**, *202*, 107099. [CrossRef] [PubMed]
47. Fitzpatrick, J.M.; Minogue, E.; Curham, L.; Tyrrell, H.; Gavigan, P.; Hind, W.; Downer, E.J. MyD88-dependent and -independent signalling via TLR3 and TLR4 are differentially modulated by Delta(9)-tetrahydrocannabinol and cannabidiol in human macrophages. *J. Neuroimmunol.* **2020**, *343*, 577217. [CrossRef]
48. Krajka-Kuzniak, V.; Belka, M.; Papierska, K. Targeting STAT3 and NF-kappaB Signaling Pathways in Cancer Prevention and Treatment: The Role of Chalcones. *Cancers* **2024**, *16*, 1092. [CrossRef]
49. Ishteyaque, S.; Singh, G.; Yadav, K.S.; Verma, S.; Sharma, R.K.; Sen, S.; Srivastava, A.K.; Mitra, K.; Lahiri, A.; Bawankule, D.U.; et al. Cooperative STAT3-NFkB signaling modulates mitochondrial dysfunction and metabolic profiling in hepatocellular carcinoma. *Metabolism* **2024**, *152*, 155771. [CrossRef]
50. Hashemi, M.; Abbaszadeh, S.; Rashidi, M.; Amini, N.; Talebi Anaraki, K.; Motahhary, M.; Khalilipouya, E.; Harif Nashtifani, A.; Shafiei, S.; Ramezani Farani, M.; et al. STAT3 as a newly emerging target in colorectal cancer therapy: Tumorigenesis, therapy response, and pharmacological/nanoplatform strategies. *Environ. Res.* **2023**, *233*, 116458. [CrossRef]
51. Yue, Y.; Zhang, Q.; Wang, X.; Sun, Z. STAT3 regulates 5-Fu resistance in human colorectal cancer cells by promoting Mcl-1-dependent cytoprotective autophagy. *Cancer Sci.* **2023**, *114*, 2293–2305. [CrossRef]
52. Ma, Q.; Hao, S.; Hong, W.; Tergaonkar, V.; Sethi, G.; Tian, Y.; Duan, C. Versatile function of NF-kB in inflammation and cancer. *Exp. Hematol. Oncol.* **2024**, *13*, 68. [CrossRef]
53. Rinkenbaugh, A.L.; Baldwin, A.S. The NF-kappaB Pathway and Cancer Stem Cells. *Cells* **2016**, *5*, 16. [CrossRef]
54. Li, Y.; Zhao, B.; Peng, J.; Tang, H.; Wang, S.; Peng, S.; Ye, F.; Wang, J.; Ouyang, K.; Li, J.; et al. Inhibition of NF-kappaB signaling unveils novel strategies to overcome drug resistance in cancers. *Drug Resist. Updat.* **2024**, *73*, 101042. [CrossRef] [PubMed]
55. Chang, S.N.; Dey, D.K.; Oh, S.T.; Kong, W.H.; Cho, K.H.; Al-Olayan, E.M.; Hwang, B.S.; Kang, S.C.; Park, J.G. Phorbol 12-Myristate 13-Acetate Induced Toxicity Study and the Role of Tangeretin in Abrogating HIF-1alpha-NF-kappaB Crosstalk In Vitro and In Vivo. *Int. J. Mol. Sci.* **2020**, *21*, 9261. [CrossRef]
56. Chang, S.N.; Khan, I.; Dey, D.K.; Cho, K.H.; Hwang, B.S.; Bae, K.B.; Kang, S.C.; Park, J.G. Decursinol angelate ameliorates 12-O-tetradecanoyl phorbol-13-acetate (TPA) -induced NF-kappaB activation on mice ears by inhibiting exaggerated inflammatory cell infiltration, oxidative stress and pro-inflammatory cytokine production. *Food Chem. Toxicol.* **2019**, *132*, 110699. [CrossRef]
57. Fakhri, S.; Moradi, S.Z.; Yarmohammadi, A.; Narimani, F.; Wallace, C.E.; Bishayee, A. Modulation of TLR/NF-kappaB/NLRP Signaling by Bioactive Phytocompounds: A Promising Strategy to Augment Cancer Chemotherapy and Immunotherapy. *Front. Oncol.* **2022**, *12*, 834072. [CrossRef]
58. Bandele, O.J.; Clawson, S.J.; Osheroff, N. Dietary polyphenols as topoisomerase II poisons: B ring and C ring substituents determine the mechanism of enzyme-mediated DNA cleavage enhancement. *Chem. Res. Toxicol.* **2008**, *21*, 1253–1260. [CrossRef]

https://doi.org/10.3390/ph19020261

59. D'yakonov, L.U.D.; Dzhemilev, U.M. Advances in the Chemistry of Natural and Semisynthetic Topoisomerase I/II Inhibitors. *Stud. Nat. Prod. Chem.* **2017**, *54*, 21–86. [CrossRef]
60. Bandele, O.J.; Osheroff, N. (-)-Epigallocatechin gallate, a major constituent of green tea, poisons human type II topoisomerases. *Chem. Res. Toxicol.* **2008**, *21*, 936–943. [CrossRef]
61. Neukam, K.; Pastor, N.; Cortes, F. Tea flavanols inhibit cell growth and DNA topoisomerase II activity and induce endoreduplication in cultured Chinese hamster cells. *Mutat. Res.* **2008**, *654*, 8–12. [CrossRef]
62. Toden, S.; Okugawa, Y.; Jascur, T.; Wodarz, D.; Komarova, N.L.; Buhrmann, C.; Shakibaei, M.; Boland, C.R.; Goel, A. Curcumin mediates chemosensitization to 5-fluorouracil through miRNA-induced suppression of epithelial-to-mesenchymal transition in chemoresistant colorectal cancer. *Carcinogenesis* **2015**, *36*, 355–367. [CrossRef]
63. Mosmann, T. Rapid colorimetric assay for cellular growth and survival: Application to proliferation and cytotoxicity assays. *J. Immunol. Methods* **1983**, *65*, 55–63. [CrossRef]
64. Noma, T.; Li, Y.; Wada, Y.; Morine, Y.; Ikemoto, T.; Saito, Y.; Yamada, S.; Teraoku, H.; Shimada, M.; Goel, A. Oligomeric Proanthocyanidins Reverse Lenvatinib Resistance in Hepatocellular Carcinoma Through ITGA3-Mediated Pathway. *Pharmaceuticals* **2025**, *18*, 1361. [CrossRef]
65. Okuno, K.; Garg, R.; Yuan, Y.C.; Tokunaga, M.; Kinugasa, Y.; Goel, A. Berberine and Oligomeric Proanthocyanidins Exhibit Synergistic Efficacy Through Regulation of PI3K-Akt Signaling Pathway in Colorectal Cancer. *Front. Oncol.* **2022**, *12*, 855860. [CrossRef]
66. Toden, S.; Ravindranathan, P.; Gu, J.; Cardenas, J.; Yuchang, M.; Goel, A. Oligomeric proanthocyanidins (OPCs) target cancer stem-like cells and suppress tumor organoid formation in colorectal cancer. *Sci. Rep.* **2018**, *8*, 3335. [CrossRef] [PubMed]
67. Dobin, A.; Davis, C.A.; Schlesinger, F.; Drenkow, J.; Zaleski, C.; Jha, S.; Batut, P.; Chaisson, M.; Gingeras, T.R. STAR: Ultrafast universal RNA-seq aligner. *Bioinformatics* **2013**, *29*, 15–21. [CrossRef] [PubMed]
68. Xing, Y.; Yu, T.; Wu, Y.N.; Roy, M.; Kim, J.; Lee, C. An expectation-maximization algorithm for probabilistic reconstructions of full-length isoforms from splice graphs. *Nucleic Acids Res.* **2006**, *34*, 3150–3160. [CrossRef]
69. Love, M.I.; Huber, W.; Anders, S. Moderated estimation of fold change and dispersion for RNA-seq data with DESeq2. *Genome Biol.* **2014**, *15*, 550. [CrossRef] [PubMed]

https://doi.org/10.3390/ph19020261

pharmaceuticals

Article

Qingfei Tongluo Jiedu Formula Regulates M2 Macrophage Polarization via the Butyric Acid-GPR109A-MAPK Pathway for the Treatment of *Mycoplasma pneumoniae* Pneumonia

Zhilin Liu , Qiuyue Fan, Ruohan Sun and Yonghong Jiang *

Longhua Clinical Medical College, Shanghai University of Traditional Chinese Medicine, 725 Wanping South Road, Xuhui District, Shanghai 200032, China; l15125018790@163.com (Z.L.); 17803850740@163.com (Q.F.); 19966517461@163.com (R.S.)
* Correspondence: jyh203225@126.com

Abstract

Background: *Mycoplasma pneumoniae* pneumonia (MPP) is a common community-acquired pneumonia in children. Increasing drug resistance highlights the need for more effective treatments with fewer side effects. The Qingfei Tongluo Jiedu formula (QTJD) has demonstrated clinical efficacy against MPP; however, its underlying mechanisms remain unclear. This study aimed to explore the mechanism of QTJD on MPP using network pharmacology and in vitro experiments. **Methods**: Network pharmacology was used to identify the active compounds and signaling pathways of QTJD in MPP. QTJD-containing serum was prepared, and primary mouse lung and bone marrow cells were isolated to examine the effects of QTJD on macrophage polarization through butyric acid. Cell viability assays, flow cytometry, and quantitative reverse transcription-polymerase chain reaction were performed. $GPR109^{-/-}$ cells were used to confirm the receptor mediating butyric acid's action, and Western blotting was employed to assess the MAPK signaling pathway. **Results**: QTJD promoted macrophage polarization and alleviated the inflammatory response caused by *Mycoplasma pneumoniae*. High-performance liquid chromatography-electrospray ionization mass spectrometry combined with network pharmacology identified 20 active compounds. Protein-protein interaction analysis revealed 10 core target, including JUN and Tumor Necrosis Factor (TNF), while enrichment analysis highlighted pathways such as Mitogen-Activated Protein Kinase (MAPK) and Phosphoinositide 3-Kinase-Protein Kinase B. Experimental validation demonstrated that QTJD reduced M1 markers (CD86, CXCL10) by increasing butyrate levels ($p < 0.01$) and enhanced M2 markers (CD206, Arg-1, MRC-1), promoting M2 polarization. QTJD inhibited ERK1/2, p38, and JNK1/2 ($p < 0.01$). In $GPR109A^{-/-}$ mice macrophages, QTJD suppressed p38 and JNK1/2 ($p < 0.01$) but showed no effect on ERK1/2 ($p > 0.05$), confirming involvement of the butyrate-GPR109A-MAPK pathway. **Conclusions**: QTJD effectively alleviates MPP by regulating macrophage polarization through the butyrate-GPR109A-MAPK pathway. Future studies should explore how QTJD modulates pulmonary immunity through gut microbiota and butyrate production and elucidate its immunoregulatory mechanisms along the gut-lung axis using multi-omics approaches.

Keywords: *Mycoplasma pneumoniae*; network pharmacology; macrophage polarization; butyric acid; GPR109A

1. Introduction

MPP is the most common community-acquired pneumonia in children, the pathogenesis of which remains unclear, and is usually self-limiting with a good prognosis [1]. However, in severe cases, it can cause inflammatory reactions in the lungs and throughout the body, inducing asthma and affecting multiple systems, including the gastrointestinal tract, circulatory system, and nervous system. In critical cases, it can be life-threatening [2]. The *Mycoplasma pneumoniae* (MP) outbreak cycle occurs every 3–7 years [3]; however, isolation and protective measures during the coronavirus disease 2019 epidemic reduced exposure to MP and infection detection [4,5], resulting in a delayed re-emergence of MPP [6]. The current treatment of choice for MPP is anti-inflammatory with macrolide antibacterial drugs, including azithromycin and clarithromycin [7], which can relieve symptoms of MPP. However, their gastrointestinal irritation, which causes intestinal flora disorders, can lead to adverse effects such as cardiovascular and liver damage [8]. In recent years, the prevalence of macrolide-resistant MP has increased worldwide, particularly in parts of Asia, especially China, where it exceeds 90% [3,9]. Second-line antibiotics, such as quinolones and tetracyclines, have potential adverse effects in children younger than 8 years [10,11]. Furthermore, the clinical efficacy of current treatment regimens has decreased, making the search for highly effective treatment with minimal side effects crucial for the diagnosis and prognosis of MPP.

Macrophages are the most numerous immune effectors in the lungs and critical cells in innate immunity [12]. Macrophages can be classically and alternatively activated to polarize into M1 and M2 phenotypes, respectively. The phosphorylation of ERK1/2, JNK1/2, and p38 pathways in MAPK is a key response in macrophage polarization [13,14]. Signal transducer and activator of transcription 1 is a critical factor in M1 macrophage polarization and is associated with the upregulation of interleukin 6 (IL-6), tumor necrosis factor-alpha (TNF-α), and Cluster of Differentiation 86 (CD86), which are involved in the clearance of pathogens, mediation of reactive oxygen species-induced tissue injury, and impaired tissue rejuvenation. In contrast, signal transducer and activator of transcription 6 and 3 proteins play essential roles in M2 polarization. It upregulates the expression of IL-10, arginase 1, mannose receptor (MRC-1), and Cluster of Differentiation 206 (CD206) [15], which promotes tissue repair and healing, removes fragmented and apoptotic cells, and possesses strong phagocytic and pro-regulatory properties, thus effectively inhibiting inflammation and serving as a critical factor in alleviating pneumonia. It also has phagocytic, solid, and pro-peritoneal properties and can effectively suppress inflammatory response in a meaningful way to alleviate pneumonia [16].

The intestinal tract is the largest immune organ of the body, containing hundreds of millions of bacteria, archaea, fungi, viruses, and protozoa. The interaction between the altered intestinal flora and respiratory flora disorders through the mucosal immune system is referred to as the "intestinal-pulmonary axis." Diversity and abundance of the flora are both reduced in pneumonia [17]. A preclinical trial analyzed by 16S rRNA gene sequencing found similar results. The abundance of intestinal *Rumenococci*, *Clostridium butyricum*, *Lactobacillus*, and *Bifidobacterium* in the affected children was lower than that in healthy children, and the abundance of intestinal *Rumenococci* and *C. butyricum* in children with wheezing MPP was considerably lower [18]. *Ruminococcus luteus* and *C. butyricum* are important butyric acid-producing bacteria [19]. Butyric acid is a short-chain fatty acid produced by intestinal anaerobic bacteria in the proximal colon (including the ascending and transverse colons) through the fermentation of indigestible dietary fibers and carbohydrates [20]. It plays an important role in maintaining energy and immune homeostasis in the body. It can activate G-protein-coupled receptors (GPCRs) and inhibit histone deacetylase (HDAC) by affecting the migration of immune cells [21]. GPCRs form the largest and

https://doi.org/10.3390/ph19020212

most functionally diverse superfamily of membrane proteins in eukaryotic organisms [22]. Butyric acid primarily regulates immunity and metabolism by activating GPR41, GPR43, and GPR109A [23], with GPR109A showing high specificity and sensitivity to butyric acid. Among short-chain fatty acids (SCFAs), only butyric acid can activate GPR109A at a low threshold. GPR109A is expressed in the immune system in monocytes, macrophages, and neutrophils [24], where it functions by regulating pathways such as mitogen-activated protein kinase (MAPK), phosphoinositide 3-kinase (PI3K), and mechanistic target of rapamycin (mTOR). MAPK is a crucial pathway mediating inflammatory responses and is involved in macrophage polarization induction [25].

Clinically, the Qingfei Tongluo formula has been used to treat MPP for decades, with its efficacy validated in both clinical practice [26] and in vivo/in vitro studies [27–29]. Building upon this foundation, the modified Qingfei Tongluo Jiedu formula (QTJD) has been developed, comprising the following nine herbal components: *Cortex mori* (Sang Bai Pi), *Cortex lycii* (Di Gu Pi), *Polygonum cuspidatum* (Hu Zhang), *Scutellaria barbata* (Ban Zhi Lian), *Persicae semen* (Tao Ren), *Pheretima* (Di Long), *Perillae fructus* (Su Zi), *Lepidii semen* (Ting Li Zi), and *Glycyrrhiza uralensis* (Gan Cao). Some studies have demonstrated the efficacy of QTJD in suppressing systemic inflammatory responses induced by MP infection. In vivo and in vitro investigations have revealed that QTJD exerted therapeutic effects against MPP by increasing butyrate-producing bacteria in the intestinal tract of mice, elevating butyrate levels, and activating the GPR109A receptor to inhibit the NLRP3-caspase-1-IL-1β pathway [30]. Notably, individual herbs with channel-collateral regulating properties, such as *P. cuspidatum* and *S. barbata*, exhibit direct inhibitory effects against MP in vitro. In a previous study, this formula significantly reduced TNF-α and IL-6 levels, inhibited NF-κB activation, and decreased LOX-1 and PLA2 expression, while upregulating RvD1 and PD1 levels in MPP model mice [31]. QTJD, as a traditional Chinese medicine compound, has demonstrated promising clinical efficacy in treating MPP. It offers a potentially effective alternative or complementary therapy that is less likely to induce drug resistance, addressing the global public health crisis of rising antibiotic resistance rates during MPP treatment. Moreover, this represents a shift from traditional "direct bactericidal" approaches toward "host modulation", controlling infection by reshaping the gut microbiota and regulating immune balance. The efficacy of QTJD offers novel biological insights, particularly through mechanisms such as the "gut-lung axis." As a multi-targeted, holistic treatment, this traditional Chinese herbal formula may simultaneously achieve comprehensive effects: reducing inflammatory damage, repairing the intestinal barrier, and modulating systemic immunity.

This study aimed to explore the mechanism of action of QTJD on MPP using network pharmacology and in vitro experiments. We hypothesized that QTJD affects macrophage polarization through butyrate-GPR109A regulation of inflammatory pathways.

2. Results

2.1. HPLC/ESI-MS Determined the Active Ingredients in QTJD

A total of 20 active ingredients were identified, including Syringaldehyde, Gancaonin U, Glyinflanin A, Quercetin-3-*O*-β-D-glucose-7-*O*-β-D-gentiobiosiden, Arachic acid, Luteolin, Resveratrol, Apigenin, Luteolin 7-*O*-glucuronide, Gancaonin A, Glycyrrhizin, Sinapinic acid, Citric acid, Amygdalinic acid, Tryptophan, Mulberroside C, Licuraside, Polydatin, Rosmarinic acid, and Glycyrrhizic Acid (Appendix A).

https://doi.org/10.3390/ph19020212

2.2. *Network Pharmacology Results Analysis*

2.2.1. Potential Targets of QTJD for the Treatment of MPP

To explore the potential targets of QTJD for treating MPP, 20 chemicals were imported into the SwissTargetPrediction (STP) database after obtaining the CAS numbers or structures-data file of potentially active compounds from PubChem. Compounds with prediction scores greater than 0 were selected for further analysis, ultimately mapping a list of potential drug targets for QTJD-active compounds (Figure 1a). To identify disease targets, we searched the Online Mendelian Inheritance in Man, GeneCard, DrugBank, and Genetic Association Databases using the keyword "*Mycoplasma pneumoniae*" and obtained the disease targets after deduplication. Candidate component targets and MPP-related targets were imported into the Venny online software to construct the intersecting targets of the QTJD and MPP, and 92 intersecting targets were found out of 257 QTJD targets and 1767 MPP targets (Figure 1b,c).

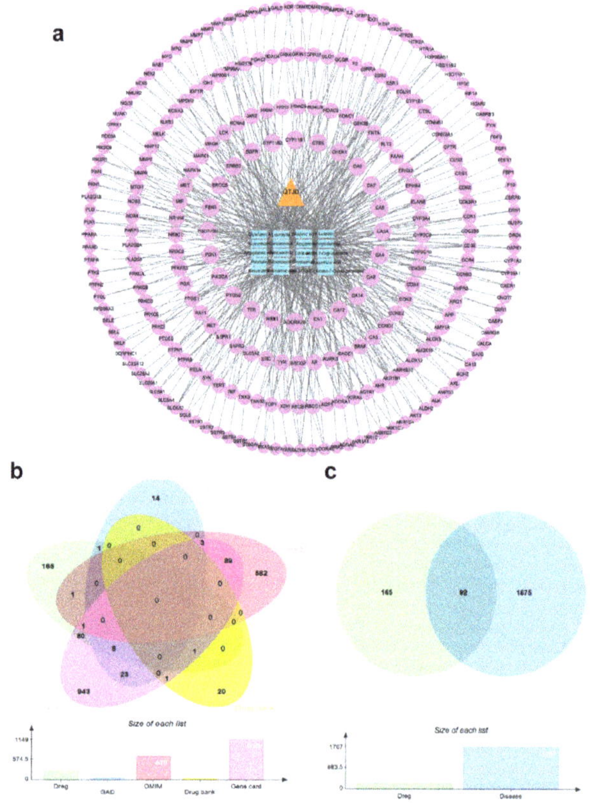

Figure 1. (**a**) Network of the relationship between the active ingredient and target of the Qingfei Tongluo Jiedu formula. (Note: purple circular nodes represent the drug targets, blue diamond nodes represent the active ingredient of the Qingfei Tongluo Jiedu formula, and orange triangles represent the Qingfei Tongluo Jiedu formula.) (**b**) Venn diagram of *Mycoplasma pneumoniae* pneumonia-related targets in four disease databases and datasets. (**c**) Venn diagram of targets appearing in the intersection of the four disease databases, in which the target is the active ingredient of Qingfei Tongluo Jiedu formula.

https://doi.org/10.3390/ph19020212

2.2.2. Protein–Protein Interaction (PPI) Network Construction

To study and visualize the linkage of drug-disease common targets, we imported drug–disease common targets into the STRING database, specifying "human" as a protein species. We set the minimum interaction threshold to 0.4 and generated protein-protein interaction (PPI) networks (Figure 2).

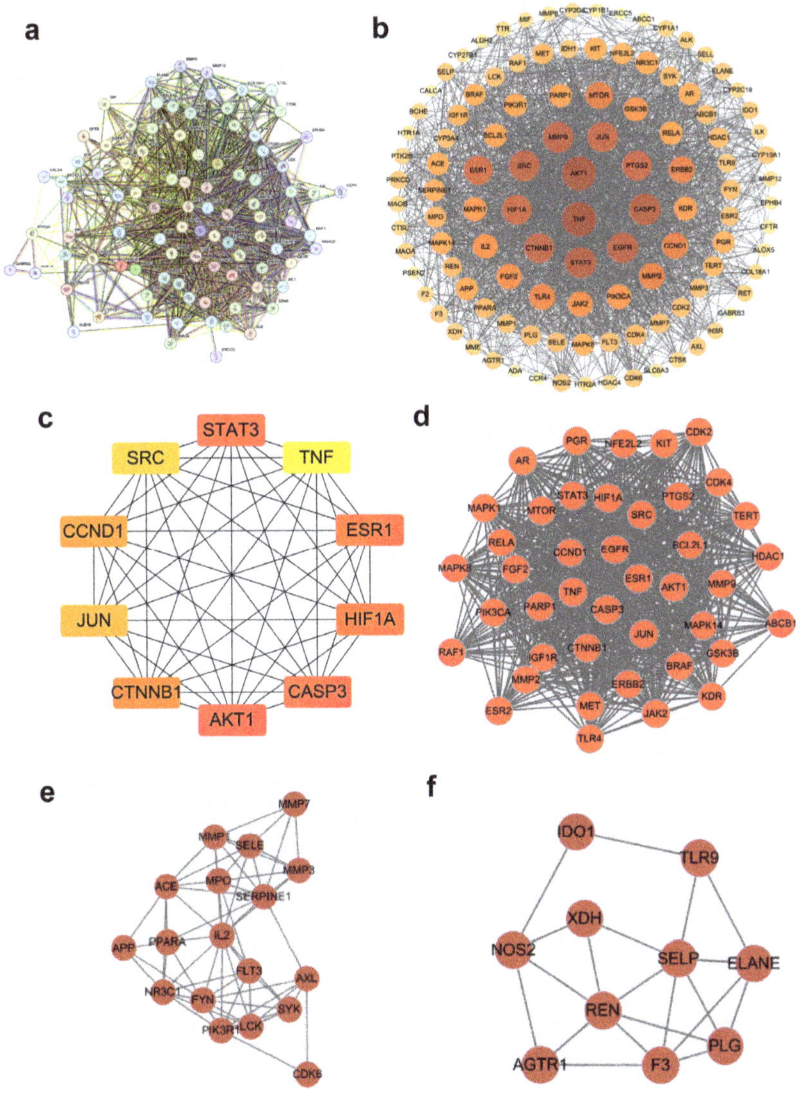

Figure 2. Protein–protein interaction (PPI) network analysis of cross-targets involved in *Mycoplasma pneumoniae* pneumonia (MPP) treatment with Qingfei Tongluo Jiedu formula. (**a**,**b**) PPI networks of cross-targets. (**c**) Top 10-ranked hub target. (**d**) Three protein clusters were obtained in the MCODE plugin analysis ((**e**,**f**) are all part of subgraph (**d**)).

2.2.3. GO and KEGG Pathway Enrichment Analysis

To further explore the potential pathways for QTJD treatment of MPP, GO and KEGG were used to perform enrichment analysis using the DAVID database, and the results

https://doi.org/10.3390/ph19020212

were visualized using a bioinformatics platform. The statistical significance threshold for enrichment analysis was set at $p \leq 0.05$ (Figure 3), and KEGG analyzed the top 40 pathways. The darker red color indicates higher significance. KEGG analysis results revealed 163 pathways, including pathways in cancer, PI3K-Akt, MAPK, HIF-1, T cell receptor, TNF, and AGE-RAGE, involving cancer, immunity, infection, metabolism, and cellular signaling. Among these, inflammatory pathways such as MAPK, PI3K-Akt, and TNF signaling may be relevant pathways in the mechanism of QTJD treating MPP (Figure 3e). Activation of the MAPK pathway led to macrophage M1 polarization and exacerbated the inflammatory response, suggesting that QTJD has the potential to regulate MPP-induced macrophage polarization (Figure 3f).

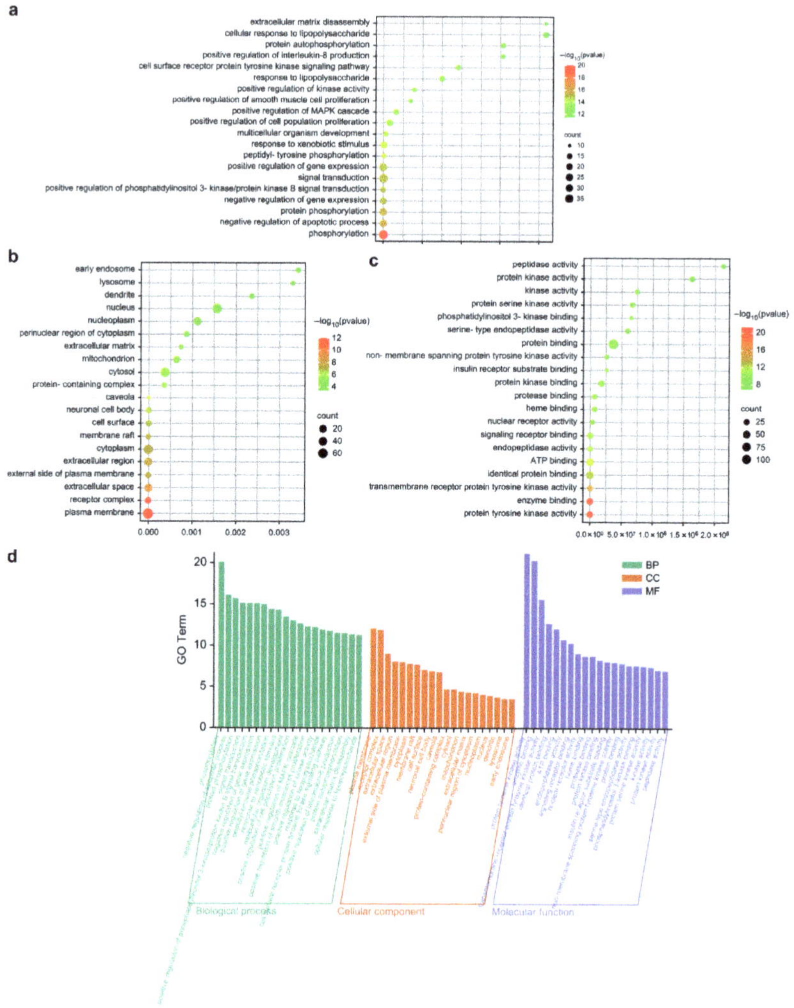

Figure 3. *Cont.*

https://doi.org/10.3390/ph19020212

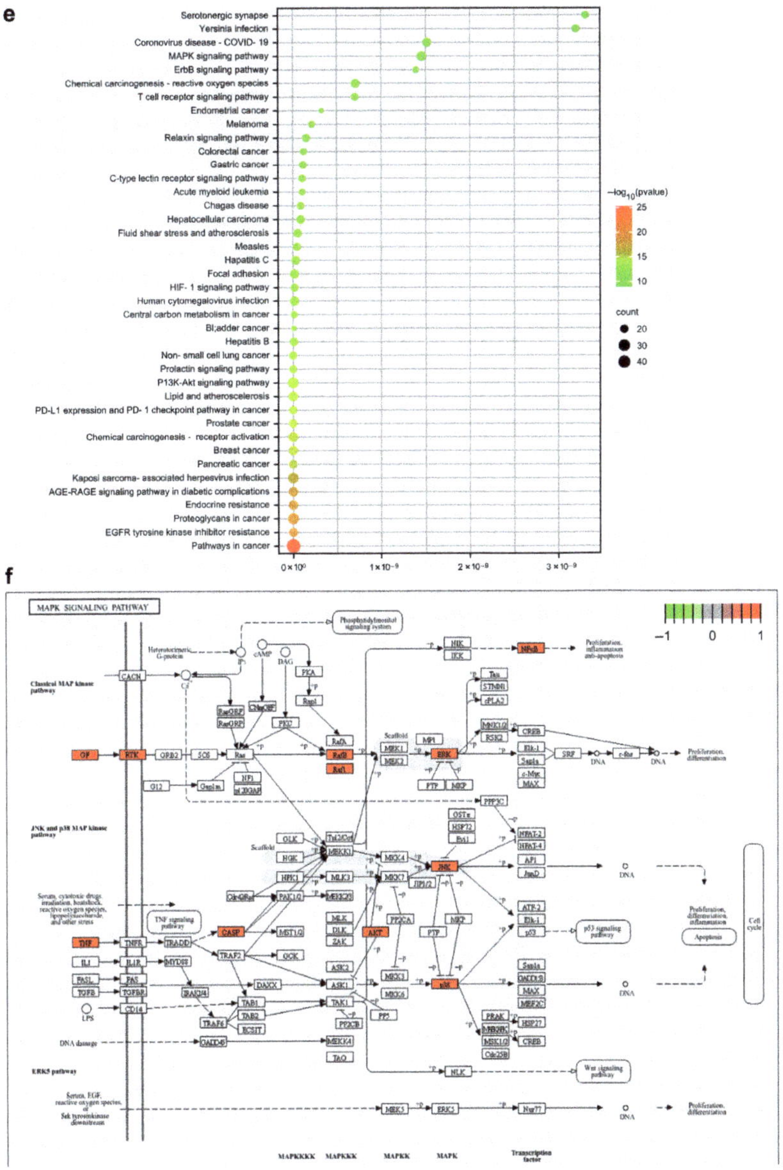

Figure 3. Cross-targets involved in *Mycoplasma pneumoniae* pneumonia (MPP) treatment with the Qingfei Tongluo Jiedu formula. (**a**) Gene Ontology (GO) enrichment analysis of the biological process (BP) bubble map. (**b**) GO enrichment analysis of the cellular component (CC) bubble map. (**c**) GO enrichment analysis of the molecular function (MF) bubble map. (**d**) GO enrichment analysis (the first 20 results of the enrichment analysis of BP, CC, and MF are shown in green, purple, and orange, respectively). (**e**) Kyoto Encyclopedia of Genes and Genomes (KEGG) enrichment analysis bar graphs (the first 40 results) in cross-target areas. (**f**) Mitogen-Activated Protein Kinase (MAPK) pathway diagram.

https://doi.org/10.3390/ph19020212

2.2.4. Molecular Docking Results

Ten key ccore target (STAT3, AKT1, CASP3, ESR1, HIF1A, CTNNB1, CCND1, JUN, SRC, TNF) and nine representative active compounds from QTJD (Luteolin, Apigenin, Gancaonin U, Gancaonin A, Rosmarinic acid, Glycyrrhizin A, Resveratrol, Amygdalinic acid, Mulberroside C) were subjected to molecular docking. All binding energies were negative. Notably, GPCRs exert their effects by regulating the MAPK pathway [32–34], and JUN serves as a key protein in the PPI network and a core target in MAPK. To validate the downstream pathways of QTJD in treating MPP, we employed JUN alongside all key compounds of QTJD (Luteolin, Apigenin, Gancaonin U, Gancaonin A, Rosmarinic acid, Glycyrrhizin A, Resveratrol, Mulberroside C). All compounds yielded affinity values below −1.2 kcal/mol, as demonstrated through 3D and 2D visualizations (Figure 4). These results indicate that QTJD may exert its effects through the MAPK pathway.

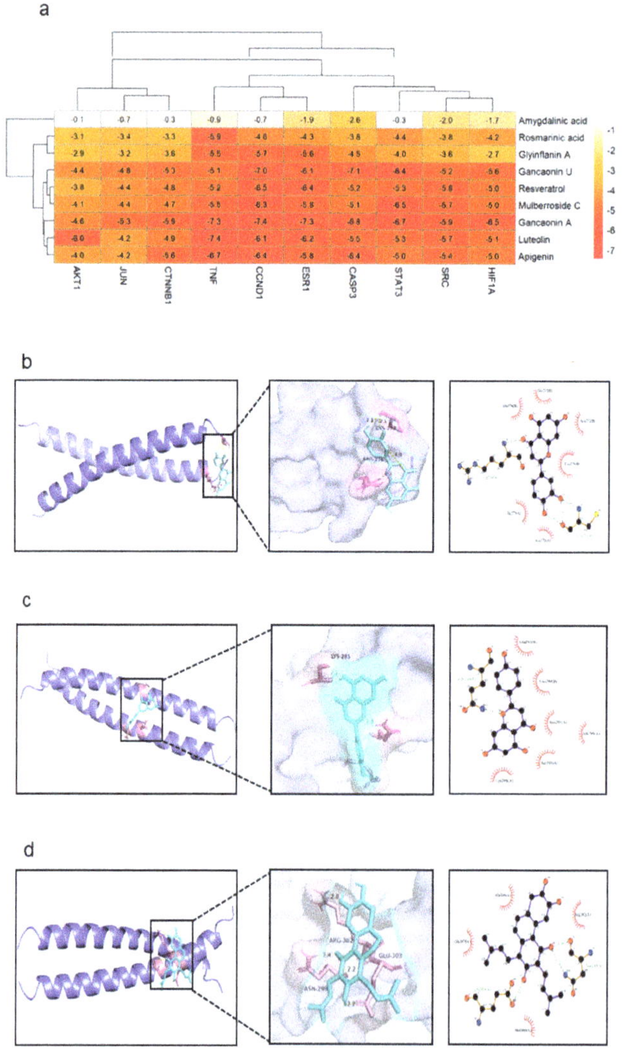

Figure 4. *Cont.*

https://doi.org/10.3390/ph19020212

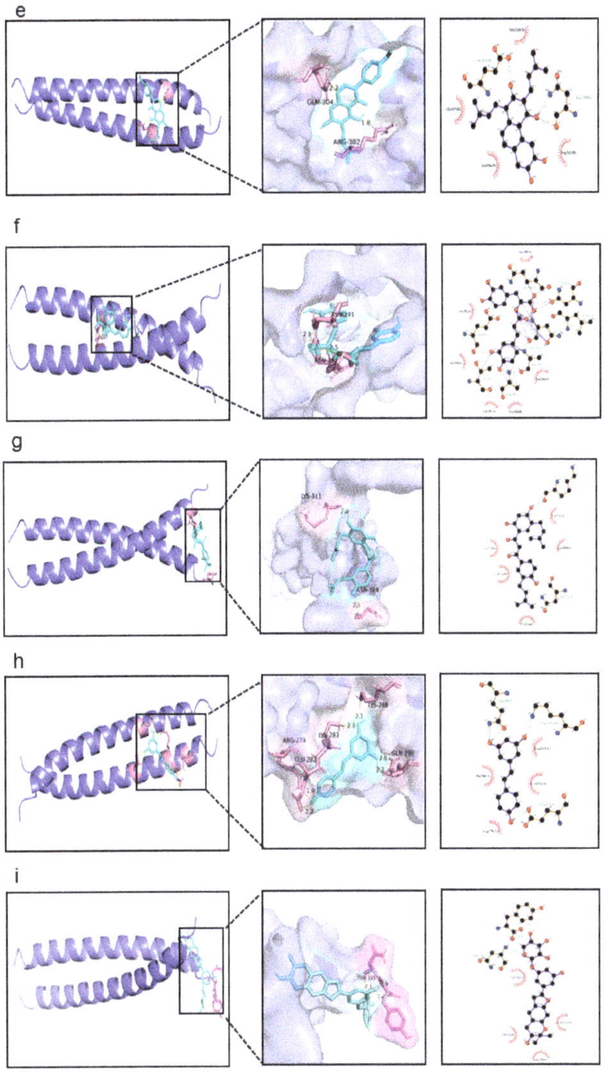

Figure 4. (**a**) Heatmap of molecular docking between 10 key target genes and 9 key active compounds of QTJD. (**b**) JUN–Luteolin; (**c**) JUN–Apigenin; (**d**) JUN–Gancaonin U; (**e**) JUN–Gancaonin A; (**f**) JUN–Rosmarinic acid; (**g**) JUN–Glycyrrhizin A; (**h**) JUN–Resveratrol; (**i**) JUN–Mulberroside C.

2.3. Cell Experiment Results

2.3.1. QTJD Parties Inhibit MPP Inflammatory Responses

To screen the optimal drug-containing serum concentration for the subsequent study, we first determined the macrophage inhibition rate of the blank control group, MP model group, and QTJD high-, medium-, and low-dose groups using CCK-8. The macrophage inhibition rate = $[(Ac - As)/(Ac - Ab)] \times 100\%$, where As represents experimental group absorbance, Ac represents MP group absorbance, and Ab represents control group absorbance. Compared with the blank group, the AM inhibition rate of the MP group was higher ($p < 0.01$). However, the macrophage inhibition rate in the high-dose group was significantly lower than that of the model group ($p < 0.05$). The difference in macrophage inhibition rates between the medium- and low-dose groups and the model group was not significant (Figure 5).

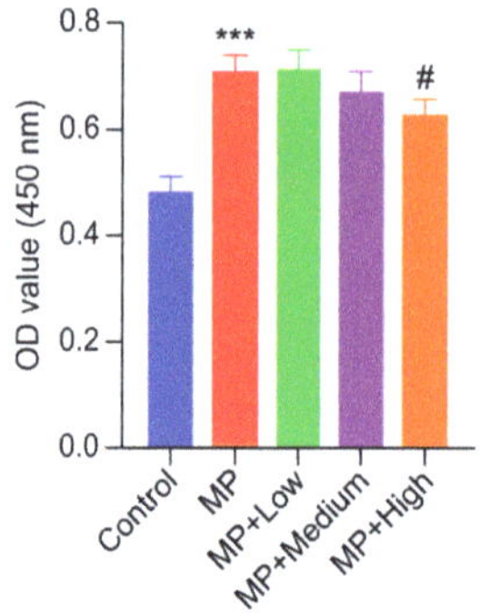

Figure 5. Cell inhibition rate of serum-containing drug at various concentrations ($n = 3$). Note: Compared with the control group, *** $p < 0.001$; compared with the model group, # $p < 0.05$. MP, *Mycoplasma pneumoniae*.

2.3.2. QTJD Modulates Macrophage Polarization via Butyric Acid

Our preliminary clinical and animal studies have found that QTJD increases the abundance of butyric acid-producing bacteria, including *Rumenococci* and *C. butyricum*, in the intestinal microbiota, thereby raising butyric acid levels in vivo. To investigate whether QTJD regulates macrophage polarization by increasing butyric acid concentration for MPP treatment, we extracted lung macrophages from mice using alveolar lavage fluid. We used butyric acid as a positive control. The results showed that in MP-infected macrophages, QTJD significantly increased macrophage cell viability ($p < 0.05$) (Figure 6a). It significantly decreased the expression of CD86 and CXCL10 (M1 markers) while significantly increasing the expression of CD206 and Arg-1 and MRC-1 (M2 markers) ($p < 0.01$) (Figure 6b,c). QTJD also induced an increase in the anti-inflammatory cytokine IL-10 in macrophages, inhibited the production of pro-inflammatory cytokines IL-6 and TNF-a (Figure 6d), and promoted macrophage polarization to the M2, which had the same effect as that of the butyric acid group, with no substantial difference between the two groups. Collectively, QTJD increased butyric acid levels, favored macrophage polarization to the M2 phenotype, and inhibited macrophage polarization to the M1 phenotype.

2.3.3. QTJD Regulates Macrophage Polarization via Butyric Acid-GPR109A

GPR109A is a receptor through which butyric acid acts, and the results of the in vivo experiments showed that QTJD operated through the butyric acid-GPR109A pathway with niacin serving as a specific GPR109A activator. To verify that QTJD regulates macrophage polarization through butyric acid-GPR109A, we extracted bone marrow macrophages from wild-type mice and GPR109A$^{-/-}$ mice, respectively. The results showed that the wild-type bone marrow macrophages in MP-infected macrophage conditions in the QTJD, butyric acid, and nicotinic acid groups significantly increased cell viability and decreased expression of CD86 and CXCL10 (M1 markers). They also show significantly increased CD206, Arg-1, and MRC-1 (M2 marker) ($p < 0.01$) expression, induced an increase in macrophage IL-10, inhibited IL-6 and TNF-α production, and promoted macrophage polarization to M2, similar to the results in lung macrophages. GPR109A$^{-/-}$ bone marrow macrophages showed opposite results, with no remarkable differences in cell viability, CD86 and CXCL10 (M1 markers), CD206, Arg-1, and MRC-1 (M2 markers), or the cytokine IL-10, IL-6, and TNF-α levels among macrophages in the MP model, QTJD, butyric acid, and nicotinic acid groups. Thus, QTJD promoted macrophage polarization to the M2

https://doi.org/10.3390/ph19020212

phenotype through the butyric acid-GPR109A pathway to alleviate the inflammatory response (Figure 7).

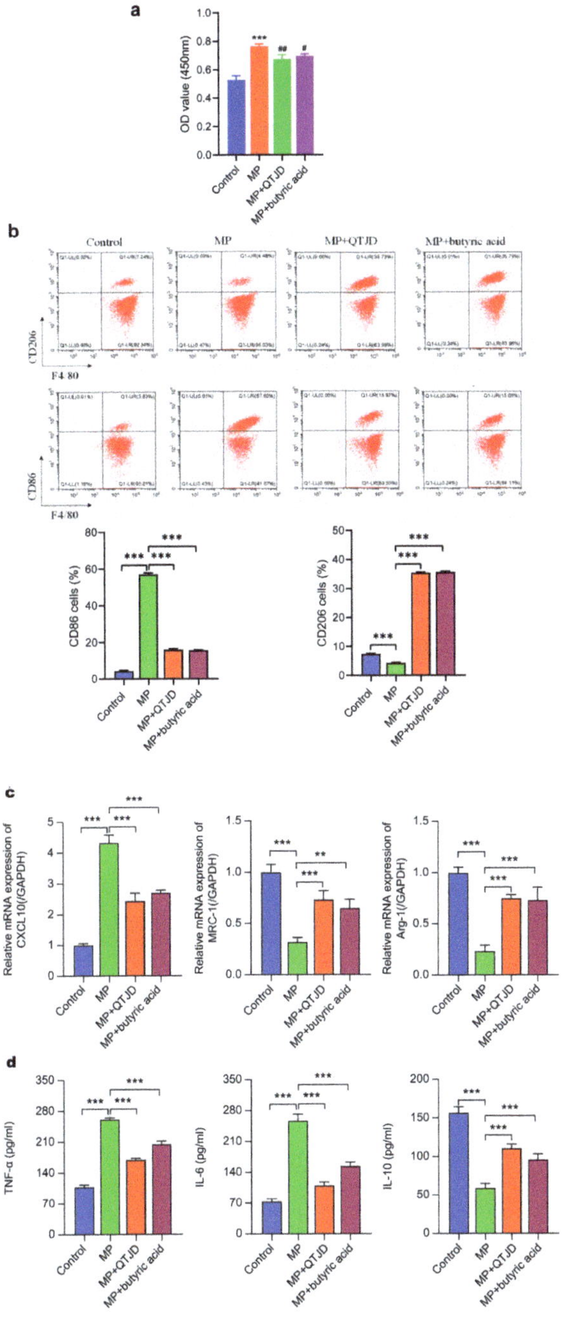

Figure 6. Qingfei Tongluo Jiedu formula (QTJD) enhances M2 macrophage polarization by butyric acid in vitro. (**a**) Macrophage activity was significantly reduced in the QTJD and butyric acid groups

https://doi.org/10.3390/ph19020212

of lung macrophages compared with the model group ($p < 0.05$). (**b**) Flow cytometry analysis of lung macrophages decreased CD86 (M1 marker) expression and significantly increased CD206 (M2 marker) ($p < 0.01$) expression in QTJD and butyric acid compared with the model group. (**c**) Quantitative reverse transcription–polymerase chain reaction (RT-PCR) analysis of lung macrophages with QTJD and butyric acid significantly decreased the expression of CXCL10 (M1 markers) and significantly increased the expression of Arg-1, MRC-1 (M2 marker) compared with the model group ($p < 0.01$). (**d**) QTJD and butyric acid induced an increase in IL-10 expression in macrophages compared with the model group ($p < 0.01$) and inhibited interleukin (IL)-6 and tumor necrosis factor (TNF)-α production ($n = 3$). Note: compared with the control group, *** $p < 0.001$, ** $p < 0.01$; compared with the model group, ## $p < 0.01$, # $p < 0.05$. MP, *Mycoplasma pneumoniae.*

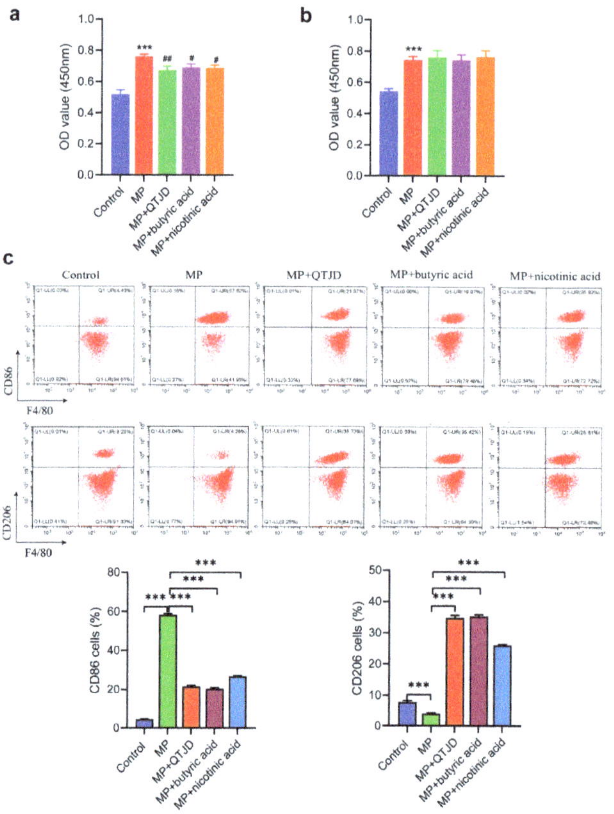

Figure 7. *Cont.*

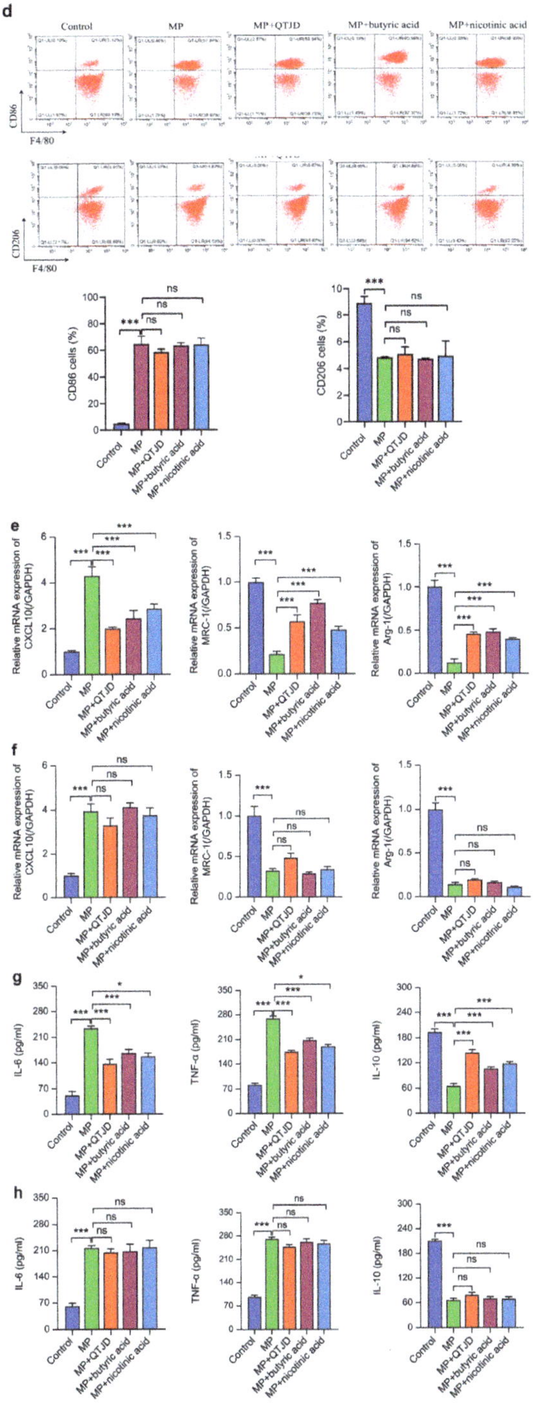

Figure 7. Qingfei Tongluo Jiedu formula (QTJD) enhances M2 macrophage polarization via butyric acid-GPR109A in vitro. (**a**) Macrophage activity in wild-type bone marrow macrophages was significantly reduced in the QTJD, butyric acid, and nicotinic acid groups compared with the model group

($p < 0.05$). (**b**) No considerable difference was found in the activity of macrophages in the QTJD, butyric acid, and nicotinic acid groups compared to the model group in GPR109A$^{-/-}$ bone marrow macrophages. (**c**) Flow cytometry analysis of wild-type bone marrow macrophages remarkably decreased the expression of CD86 and significantly increased the expression of CD206 in the QTJD. (**d**) The expression of CD86 and CD206 in the QTJD, butyric acid, and nicotinic acid groups in the GPR109A$^{-/-}$ bone marrow macrophage cells, compared with the model group expression, was not significantly different. (**e**) Quantitative reverse transcription–polymerase chain reaction (RT-PCR) detection of wild-type bone marrow macrophages substantially decreased the expression of CXCL10, remarkably increasing the expression of Arg-1 and MRC-1 in the QTJD, butyric acid, and nicotinic acid groups compared to the model group ($p < 0.01$). (**f**) GPR109A$^{-/-}$ bone marrow macrophages were significantly more sensitive to the expression of CD86 and CD206 in the QTJD, butyric acid, and nicotinic acid groups compared to the model group ($p < 0.01$). No significant difference was found in CXCL10, MRC-1, and Arg-1 expression in QTJD, butyric acid, and nicotinic acid groups. (**g**) In wild-type bone marrow macrophages, QTJD, butyric acid, and nicotinic acid groups induced an increase in the macrophage interleukin (IL)-10. (**h**) They inhibited the production of IL-6 and tumor necrosis factor (TNF)-a, compared with the model group. No considerable difference was found in cytokine IL-10, IL-6, and TNF-α content in GPR109A$^{-/-}$ bone macrophages compared to the model group in QTJD, butyric acid, and nicotinic acid groups ($n = 3$). ns = not significant; MP, *Mycoplasma pneumoniae*. Note: Compared with the control group, *** $p < 0.001$, * $p < 0.05$; compared with the model group, $^{\#\#}$ $p < 0.01$, $^{\#}$ $p < 0.05$.

2.3.4. Effect of QTJD on MAPK Pathway

The previous network pharmacology analysis pathways through which QTJD acted for MPP treatment highlight the MAPK pathway as an important pathway involved in cellular immunity and macrophage polarization. To further explore how QTJD regulates macrophage polarization through the butyric acid-GPR109A pathway, we extracted bone marrow macrophages from the wild-type mice and the GPR109A$^{-/-}$ mice, respectively. The results indicated that in wild-type bone marrow macrophages, the QTJD, butyric acid, and nicotinic acid groups significantly inhibited the ERK1/2, p38, and JNK1/2 pathways compared with the model group ($p < 0.01$) (Figure 8a). No significant difference was observed in the effect of GPR109A$^{-/-}$ bone marrow macrophages on the ERK1/2, p38, and JNK1/2 pathways in the butyric acid and nicotinic acid groups compared with the model group. In comparison with the model group, no significant difference was observed in the effect of QTJD on the ERK1/2 pathway. However, QTJD significantly inhibited the p38 and JNK1/2 pathways compared with the model, butyric acid and nicotinic acid groups ($p < 0.01$) (Figure 8b). In brief, GPR109A affects macrophage polarization primarily through MAPK, particularly ERK1/2.

https://doi.org/10.3390/ph19020212

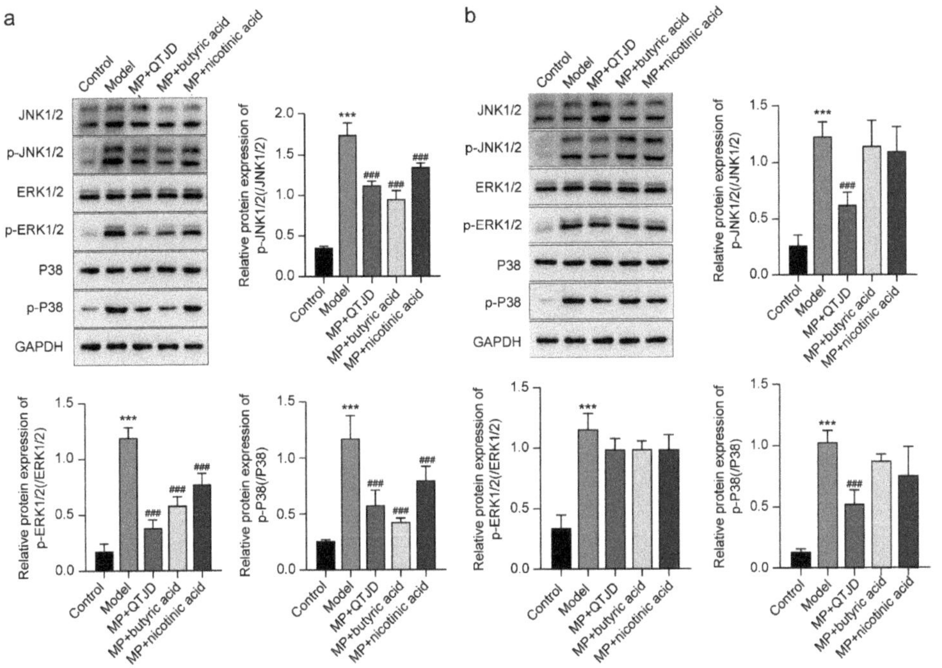

Figure 8. Protein levels of each pathway in MAPK. (**a**) Effect of the model, Qingfei Tongluo Jiedu formula (QTJD), butyric acid, and nicotinic acid groups on MAPK protein expression in wild-type bone marrow macrophages. (**b**) Effect of the model, QTJD, butyric acid, and nicotinic acid groups on MAPK protein expression in GPR109A$^{-/-}$ bone marrow macrophages (n = 3). Note: compared with the control group, *** $p < 0.001$; compared with the model group, ### $p < 0.001$. MP, *Mycoplasma pneumoniae*.

3. Discussion

This study identified the mechanism by which QTJD treats MPP through network pharmacology and in vitro validation. The results indicate that QTJD inhibits macrophages by regulating the butyrate-GPR109A-MAPK axis, preventing M1 polarization of macrophages and suppressing IL-6 and TNF-α expression (Figure 9). This study reveals that QTJD alleviates MPP through the gut microbiota metabolite butyrate-GPR109A-MAPK pathway, providing a novel therapeutic approach for MPP.

3.1. Network Pharmacology Analysis of Compound Mass Spectrometry Components and Key Pathway Screening

Macrolide antibiotics, including azithromycin, are the first-line drugs for the treatment of MPP [35]. However, refractory mycoplasma infections and severe MPP are gradually increasing due to the interference of antibiotics with intestinal dysbiosis as well as the increase in resistance of MPP [36,37]. Therefore, it is crucial to seek a highly effective treatment modality. Based on the foundation of TCM combined with clinical practice, the group proposed treating MPP using the theory of "complex disease," represented by QTJD, composed of *Cortex mori*, *Cortex lycii*, *P. cuspidatum*, *S. barbata*, *Persicae semen*, *Pheretima*, *Perillae fructus*, *Lepidii semen*, and *G. uralensis*. This formula has proven effective in treating MPP in the clinic, but the mechanism of action remains unclear.

https://doi.org/10.3390/ph19020212

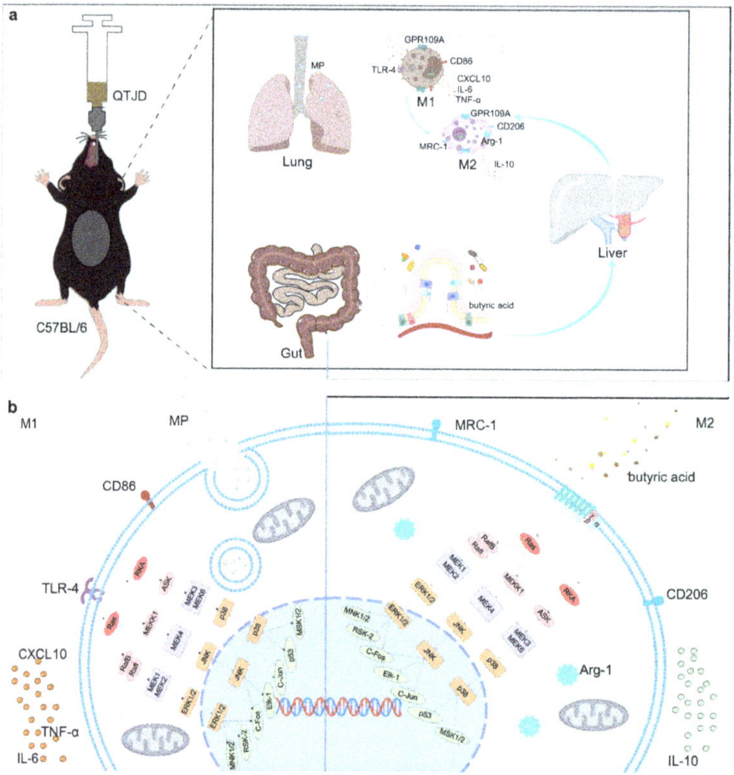

Figure 9. Mechanism of Qingfei Tongluo Jiedu formula (QTJD) in the treatment of *Mycoplasma pneumoniae* pneumonia (MPP). (**a**) MP infection reduces the abundance of butyrate-producing bacteria, leading to decreased butyrate concentrations. This failure to effectively activate GPR109A results in M1 macrophage polarisation, release of inflammatory cytokines, and exacerbated pulmonary inflammatory responses. QTJD increases the abundance of beneficial gut bacteria, particularly butyrate-producing strains, elevates butyrate levels, and activates the GPR109A receptor. (**b**) By elevating butyrate concentrations, QTJD activates GPR109A to inhibit the MAPK pathway, specifically suppressing ERK1/2 expression. This converts macrophages towards an anti-inflammatory M2 phenotype, diminishing pro-inflammatory cytokine release and thereby mitigating inflammatory responses.

The multi-component and multi-target characteristics of TCM compounding have both favorable and unfavorable effects. Alternatively, individualized treatment, multi-drug compounding and reconciliation, and multi-method action [38,39] are clinically effective with minimal side effects. However, the active ingredients and mechanism of action of TCM compounds are difficult to clarify. In this study, 20 active ingredients, including eugenol, glycyrrhizin, quercetin, arachidonic acid, lignoceric acid, and albuterol, were determined in QTJD using an HPLC/ESI-MS assay and network pharmacology. These compounds were found to regulate the MAPK signaling pathway when treating MPP.

3.2. QTJD Treats MPP by Regulating Macrophage Polarization via the Butyrate-GPR109A Axis

The innate immune system is the first weapon of invading microorganisms [40]. Macrophages are considered the vanguard of the immune response in the lungs and are critical regulators of host innate immunity during bacterial infections and pneumonia. Following MPP infection, tracheal macrophages promote lymphangiogenesis of VEGF-C and VEGF-D, suggesting that macrophages play a crucial role in lymphangiogenesis

https://doi.org/10.3390/ph19020212

during acute inflammation [41]. Additionally, macrophages can be classically or alternatively activated to polarize into pro-inflammatory M1-type and anti-inflammatory M2-type cells, respectively, which is an essential pathway for macrophages in immune regulation [42]. Liang et al. [43]. demonstrated that Yes-associated protein 1 (YAP1) inhibitors alleviate lipopolysaccharide (LPS)-induced pulmonary inflammatory injury by promoting M2 macrophage polarization. Similarly, our results showed that QTJD inhibited MP-induced macrophage activation and significantly reduced the expression of M1 markers, such as CD86, CXCL10, MRC-1, and other M1 markers, while significantly increasing the expression of CD206, Arg-1, and other M2 markers, alleviating the inflammatory response caused by MPP.

The immune crosstalk between intestinal flora and lung microbiota primarily operates in three ways, including direct migration of immune cells (ILC2s, ILC3s, TH17) [44,45], metabolites transported to the lungs via blood circulation (SCFAs), and soluble microbial fraction transfer [46,47]. Our preliminary clinical and animal experiments have demonstrated that QTJD can regulate the dysbiosis of the intestinal flora caused by MPP, increase the abundance and production of butyric acid in the intestine, and enhance butyric acid production. Butyric acid plays a vital role in immunomodulation. A small portion of it can be transported to the lungs through the hepatic portal vein, where it plays a role in the circulatory system [48]. Most of the butyric acid can be used in the intestines to regulate immune cells and cytokine production, including ILC2s and Treg/TH17 cells. Therefore, in this experiment, we prepared QTJD-containing sera that included immune cell migration and the transfer of soluble microbial components. The results showed no significant difference between the QTJD-containing serum group and the butyric acid group in regulating the polarization of lung macrophages. The in vitro experiments demonstrated that QTJD could exert its effects by increasing butyric acid.

The mechanism of action of butyric acid includes the inhibition of histone deacetylase (HDAC) [49] to regulate gene expression and the activation of G protein-coupled receptors (GPR41, GPR43, and GPR109A). Previous animal experiments conducted by our research group showed that butyric acid inhibited the NLRP3-caspase-1-IL-1β pathway by activating the GPR109A receptor and the treatment of MPP. Our research obtained similar results, specific GPR109A activator niacin promoted macrophage M2-type polarization and inhibited inflammatory response, which was not remarkably different from the butyric acid or QTJD groups. Conversely, the GPR109A$^{-/-}$ macrophages, QTJD group, butyric acid group, and niacin group did not show significant differences compared with the MP model group, which proved that QTJD regulated macrophage polarization primarily through the butyric acid-GPR109A.

3.3. Mechanism of MAPK Signaling Pathway Mediating Macrophage Polarization Regulation by GPR109A

The butyric acid-GPR109A receptor can regulate MAPK, PI3K, mTOR, and other pathways. Among them, MAPK is a group of evolutionarily conserved serine-threonine kinases that can be classified into four subfamilies, each representing one of the four classical MAPK pathways [50]. MAPK also plays a vital role in regulating systemic macrophage polarization [51,52]. In the locomotor system, osteoarthritis is aggravated by LPS and IFN-γ, which activate the MAPK signaling pathway, including p-JNK, p-ERK, and p-P38, to increase the M1 phenotype [53]. Simultaneously, ginsenoside (Kin) dose-dependently inhibits MAPK signaling, reducing its activation and highly expressing CD206 and Arg-1, phenotypic markers of M2; repolarized M1 macrophages to M2 phenotype, which could be helpful in treating osteoarthritis [54]. In the context of metabolic diseases, puerarin can reduce the release of inflammatory mediators by inhibiting the activation of p38 MAPK and ERK1/2, exert anti-inflammatory effects, enhance the expression of IL-10

https://doi.org/10.3390/ph19020212

and Arg-1, and increase the polarization of macrophages to the M2 phenotype, which synergistically improves diabetic wounds [55]. Ou-mei pills are also validated to inhibit the MAPK signaling pathway through a combination of network pharmacology and experimental validation, increasing the M2 phenotype for treating IBD [56]. The exact mechanism is also observed in macrophages in the lungs, where they can regulate the polarization of lung macrophages by inhibiting the MAPK signaling pathway to treat chronic lung diseases. To further clarify the mechanism of action of QTJD, based on KEGG pathway analysis and the results of several studies, we used Western blotting to explore the MAPK pathway downstream of GPR109A. The results showed that GPR109A could inhibit the MAPK pathway, particularly ERK1/2. Similarly, multiple in vitro studies have consistently demonstrated that macrophage M2 polarization can be regulated through the ERK1/2 pathway of the MAPK signaling cascade [57,58], suggesting that QTJD can regulate macrophage polarization through the butyric acid-GPR109A-MAPK (ERK1/2) pathway to alleviate MPP. Additionally, GPR109A macrophages did not activate JUN1/2 and p38 of MAPK, possibly due to the multi-targeting of the herbal complex, and the multi-method action inhibited the JUN1/2 and p38 pathways of MAPK, among other macrophage responses.

3.4. Advantages and Limitations

This study combines network pharmacology with in vitro experiments to provide insights into the immunomodulatory mechanisms of traditional Chinese medicine in treating MP infection. It offers an alternative or complementary therapeutic approach targeting the "gut-lung axis" for MPP treatment, which is holistic, regulates the entire system, and is less likely to induce drug resistance. However, several limitations exist in the research process. First, although our prior animal studies demonstrated that QTJD and butyrate increased fecal butyrate concentrations in MPP-infected mice, this study did not address butyrate levels in drug-containing serum. Additionally, interspecies differences in gut microbiota composition and butyrate concentrations may exist between rats and mice. Second, to explore QTJD's potential as an alternative or adjunct therapy against antibiotic resistance beyond its immunomodulatory effects, our team should conduct further studies on resistance and antimicrobial activity. Due to the multi-targeted and multi-pathway nature of traditional Chinese medicine, the precise mechanisms of action for QTJD and its individual herbal components remain difficult to determine. Therefore, the specific pathways and mechanisms of QTJD and its intestinal metabolites (including butyrate) within the lung-gut axis remain to be elucidated. This can be explored through methods such as histological tracing, fluorescent labeling, and isotope analysis. Concurrently, multi-omics analysis and single-cell sequencing technologies can further clarify the mechanisms of action of individual compounds within QTJD.

4. Materials and Methods

4.1. Instruments and Reagents

The instruments and reagents used in this study are as follows: Sodium butyrate (Beijing Solarbio Technology Co., Beijing, China; IS0190), MP international standard strain MPFH (ATCC, Manassas, VA, USA, catalogue number ATCC15531), MP strain culture medium PPLO (catalogue number: LA7090), procured from Beijing Solarbio Technology Co., Ltd. Niacin (Beijing, China, batch number: 20220803) procured from Sinopharm Chemical Reagent Co., Ltd. (Shanghai, China). Fetal bovine serum (GIBCO, Waltham, MA, USA), RPMI-1640 (Biosharp, Beijing, China), CCK-8 (Biosharp), penicillin-streptomycin mixture (100×) (Solarbio, Beijing, China), DM (Biosharp), FBS (Gibco, USA), M-CSF (Solarbio), erythrocyte lysate (Solarbio), fluorescence quantitative polymerase chain reaction

https://doi.org/10.3390/ph19020212

instrument (Shanghai Hongshi Medical Science & Technology Co., Ltd., Shanghai, China), Palm Centrifuge (Biyuntian, Shanghai, China), trypsin-EDTA (0.25%) (Solarbio), vortex mixer, ultra-clean bench (Su Jing Antai, Suzhou, China), and ultra-micro spectrophotometer (Wuyi Technology, Hangzhou, China).

4.2. Preparation of QTJD

QTJD consisted of *Morus alba* bark (Sang Bai Pi), *Lycium barbarum* bark (Di Gu Pi), *P. cuspidatum* root (Hu Zhang), *S. barbata* root (Ban Zhi Lian), *Prunus persica* seed (Tao Ren), *Pheretima* (Di Long), *Perilla frutescens* fruit (Su Zi), *Lepidium semen* (Ting Li Zi), and *G. uralensis* (Gan Cao), purchased from Longhua Hospital affiliated with Shanghai University of Traditional Chinese Medicine (Shanghai, China). The drugs conformed to the standards described in the 2020 edition of the Pharmacopoeia of the People's Republic of China. Clinically, MP frequently affects children. Referencing the pharmacopoeia, the total dosage ranged between 1/2 and 2/3. Based on clinical practice, the dry weight ratio of the QTJD formulation was 2:2:2:2:2:2:2:2:1, with a total dry weight of 51 g for the nine herbs. The components of QTJD are listed in Table 1. The herbal materials for the clear decoction were soaked for half an hour. After soaking, the materials underwent two rounds of decoction. The resulting decoction liquids were filtered and concentrated to 27.3 mL of crude drug decoction. Drying yielded 15.5 g of dry extract, with a calculated dry extract yield of 30.4%. with a drug-to-extract ratio (DER) of 3.29:1 [59] (i.e., 3.29 g crude drug yields 1 g dry extract). The dry extract was thoroughly ground with a 0.5% sodium carboxymethylcellulose solution and diluted to a final concentration of 0.56 g/mL (dry extract basis) to prepare an oral suspension.

Table 1. QTJD composition.

Chinese Name	Latin Name	English Name	Plant Part Used	Weights (g)	Pharmacopeial Dosage (g)
Sangbaipi	*Morus alba* L.	MORI CORTEX	root and rhizome	6	6–12
Digupi	*Lycium chinense* Mill.	LYCIICORTEX	root and rhizome	6	9–15
Huzhang	*Polygonum cuspidatum* Siebold & Zucc.	POLYGONI CUSPIDATI RHIZOMA ET RADIX	root and rhizome	6	9–15
Taoren	*Prunus persica* (L.) Batsch	PERSICAE SEMEN	seed	6	5–10
Banzhilian	*Scutellaria barbata* D. Don	SCUTELLARIAE BARBA TAE HERBA	whole plant	6	15–30
Dilong	*Pheretima aspergillum* (E. Perrier)	PHERETIMA	earthworm	6	5–10
Zisuzi	*Perilla frutescens* (L.) Britt.	PERILLAE FRUCTUS	seed	6	3–10
Tinglizi	*Descurainia sophia* (L.) Webb ex Prantl.	DESCURAINIAE SEMEN LEPIDII SEMEN	seed	6	3–10
GanCao	*Glycyrrhiza uralensis* Fisch	LICORICE	root and rhizome	3	2–10

Abbreviation: QTJD—Qingfei Tongluo Jiedu formula.

4.3. The Active Components of QTJD Were Analyzed Using High-Performance Liquid Chromatography–Electrospray Ionization Mass Spectrometry (HPLC/ESI-MS)

Positive and negative ion modes were determined by HPLC/ESI-MS for the mixed aqueous extract of nine herbal medicines, as reported in our previous report (Appendix A).

4.4. Network Pharmacology

4.4.1. Screening of QTJD-Active Ingredients

The Chemical Abstracts Service (CAS) numbers of the active ingredients determined by HPLC/ESI-MS were obtained by searching the PubChem database (https://pubchem.ncbi.nlm.nih.gov/) [60]. Subsequently, the CAS numbers were input into the SwissTargetPrediction platform (http://www.swisstargetprediction.ch/, accessed on 19 January 2026) [61–63] to predict and complement their associated protein targets. Finally, compounds obtained from various databases were combined, and any duplicate entries were eliminated using the UniProt database (https://www.uniprot.org/) [64] to convert the names of targets associated with these. The validated compounds and drug targets were imported into Cytoscape 3.7.1 software (Informer Technologies, Inc., Los Angeles, CA, USA) [65], and a "compound-target" network diagram was created.

4.4.2. Identification of Disease-Related Targets

Using "MPP" as the keyword, we used the OMIM database (https://omim.org/), the DrugBank database (https://go.drugbank.com/) [66,67], the GeneCards database (https://www.genecards.org/) [68], the GAD database (https://geneticassociationdb.nih.gov/) (accessed on 21 July 2024) [69], etc., to identify the targets of "*Mycoplasma pneumoniae*", and obtained the disease targets after deduplication. Candidate targets and MP-associated targets were imported into Venny2.1.0 online software (https://bioinfogp.cnb.csic.es/tools/venny/, accessed on 19 January 2026) to construct a clear-lung and clear-vessel solution and create a Venn diagram of the intersecting targets of QTJD and MPP.

4.4.3. Building a Protein–Protein Interaction (PPI) Network

The PPI network was constructed by importing the common intersecting target proteins of QTJD and MPP into the STRING database (https://www.string-db.org/) [70]. The species was set to "*Homo sapiens*", and the confidence level was set to >0.4. The PPI network was visualized using Cytoscape 3.7.1. Hub target and potential functional modules were further analyzed using the plugins cytoHubba and MCODE.

4.4.4. Gene Ontology (GO) and Kyoto Encyclopedia of Genes and Genomes (KEGG) Pathway Enrichment Analysis

To elucidate the effects of the candidate components of QTJD on MPP, GO and KEGG enrichment analyses were performed using the DAVID database (https://davidbioinformatics.nih.gov/) [71,72], and the results were visualized using a bioinformatics platform (bioinformatics.com.cn). The significance threshold for the enrichment analysis was set at $p \leq 0.05$. The DAVID data were analyzed in R 4.3.3 (R Foundation for Statistical Computing, Vienna, Austria) [73–76] to map the pathways and enrich the intersecting targets onto the pathway maps.

4.4.5. Molecular Docking

Retrieve the three-dimensional structures of active compounds and their corresponding target proteins from the PubChem database and the Protein Data Bank (https://www.rcsb.org/), respectively. AutoDock 4 software (The Scripps Research Institute, La Jolla, CA, USA) [77] was used to perform flexible docking of key targets in the intersecting targets with the core components in QTJD. A negative binding energy indicates that the compound exhibits binding activity towards the receptor. A binding energy below −1.2 kcal/mol signifies strong binding activity [78]. And PyMol 3.0 software (Schrödinger, LLC, New York, NY, USA) [79] was used to visualize the docking sites in three dimensions and use Ligplot^{+} 2.2.5 [80] for 2D visualization.

4.5. *QTJD-Containing Serum Preparation*

Forty SPF-grade Sprague-Dawley rats (male, 6 weeks old, weighing 200 ± 10 g) were purchased from Shanghai Slaughter Laboratory Animal Co. (Shanghai, China) and acclimatized for 1 week. The rats were randomly categorized into four groups: high-dose (High group), medium-dose (Medium group), low-dose (Low group), and blank (CON group) (n = 10). Sample size calculations were based on prior animal studies evaluating butyrate concentrations in mouse feces following MP infection and after QTJD treatment. Calculations were performed using software (version 3.1.9.7, G*Power) [81]. QTJD was administered by gavage, and the dose conversion for rats was performed using a pharmacological experimental method. The total crude drug amount of QTJD is 51 g. Based on a standard human body weight of 70 kg, the human dose is calculated as 0.73 g crude drug/kg/day. According to the body surface area-based dose equivalent conversion principle (using a human-to-rat coefficient of 6.3), the rat clinical equivalent dose is calculated to be approximately 4.6 g crude drug/kg/day. Based on this, three experimental dose groups—low, medium, and high—were established at approximately 1, 2, and 4 times the clinical equivalent dose, respectively. The low-dose group received QTJD 1.4 g dry extract/kg/day (4.6 crude drug/kg/day), the medium-dose group received QTJD 2.8 g dry extract/kg/day (9.2 crude drug/kg/day), and the high-dose group received QTJD 5.6 g dry extract/kg/day (18.4 crude drug/kg/day) at a concentration of 0.56 g/mL (dry extract basis), with the volume of the drug by gavage set at 2 mL/day. The blank group was administered 2 mL/200 g of saline once daily for 7 days. Samples with improper drug administration, issues during blood collection (e.g., incorrect timing, severe hemolysis, clotting, or contamination), or inadequate serum processing were excluded to ensure consistent and reliable serum quality. No samples were excluded in this study. At the final dose, rats were given 3% pentobarbital intraperitoneally to anesthetize them. Blood was collected from the abdominal aorta and labeled. The serum was centrifuged and inactivated in a water bath. The serum was then filtered and stored in a refrigerator at −80 °C for subsequent in vitro experiments.

4.6. Cell Experiments

4.6.1. MP Culture

After thawing, the MP strain was introduced into the liquid culture medium, and 1 mL of the bacterial solution was aspirated and maintained at 37 °C under 5% CO_2. The culture is complete when the medium changes from red to translucent yellow without precipitation.

4.6.2. Cell Culture

Acquisition of Lung Macrophages

Alveolar-derived macrophages (AM) were obtained by collecting alveolar lavage fluid from wild-type C57BL/6 mice (n = 5). One milliliter of pre-cooled lavage fluid [90% Dulbecco's modified Eagle medium (DMEM)—high glucose, 10% FBS, 1% double antibody, and 100 ng/mL macrophage colony-stimulating factor (M-CSF)] was injected into the lungs, and the infusion was repeated four to five times. The collected lung lavage fluid was centrifuged, and the supernatant was discarded, resulting in a precipitation of cells. The cells were resuspended and inoculated with 90% DMEM high glucose medium, 10% FBS, 1% double antibody, and 100 ng/mL M-CSF culture medium at 37 °C. The culture system was subsequently incubated at 37 °C for 24 h, after which the unattached cells were washed away. The remaining adherent cells were AM cells. The blank control group was cultured with normal serum. The MP group was cultured with normal serum and infected with 1 mL of MP at 1×10^7 CCU/mL for 3 h. The butyrate and nicotinic acid groups had 1 mM butyrate and nicotinic acid, respectively, added to the cell culture medium and incubated for 12 h, then infected with 1 mL of MP at 1×10^7 CCU/mL for 3 h. QTJD group: Cell culture medium supplemented with low, medium, and high concentrations (10%) of Chinese herbal medicine-containing serum. After incubation for 12 h, cells were infected with 1 mL of MP at a concentration of 1×10^7 CCU/mL for 3 h. The cell activity was determined by CCK-8 after 24 h of incubation.

https://doi.org/10.3390/ph19020212

Acquisition of Bone Marrow-Derived Macrophages (BMDM)

Bilateral femurs and tibiae from C57BL/6 and GPR109a knockout (GPR109A$^{-/-}$) mice (*n* = 5) were isolated to obtain BMDM. The femur was obtained by stripping the leg muscles from the hind limbs of mice and transferring it to pre-cooled phosphate-buffered saline (PBS) containing 2% bis-antibodies. The femoral epiphysis was washed three times, and the femur was rinsed repeatedly using 5 mL of pre-cooled wash solution. The rinsing solution was collected, filtered through a 70 μm cell sieve to remove residual bone and tissue, and then centrifuged at 4 °C, 280× *g*. The supernatants were discarded, and the BMDM were cultured in a 37 °C implantation solution (DMEM + 10% FBS). The supernatant was discarded, and the precipitate was resuspended in a 37 °C planting solution (DMEM + 10% FBS +1% dual antibody + 100 μg/mL M-CSF) and incubated at 37 °C in an incubator. The cells were categorized into the normal control serum group, MP model group, QTJD serum group, butyric acid group, and nicotinic acid group. Bone marrow-derived macrophages were collected (days 5–7) for CCK-8, flow cytometry, polymerase chain reaction, enzyme-linked immunosorbent assay (ELISA), and protein blotting.

4.6.3. CCK-8 Method to Screen for Optimal Concentration of QTJD-Containing Serum

Cells in the logarithmic growth phase were digested with trypsin. A total of 100 μL was transferred into a 96-well culture plate at a density of 5×10^3 cells/well. The cells were divided into the MP model group and the QTJD high-, medium-, and low-dose groups. Each cell type was inoculated into three identical wells as duplicate wells per plate. A total of 100 μL of culture medium was used as a blank control. The cells were then cultured in 5% CO2 at 37 °C for 0 and 48 h. Subsequently, CCK-8 and serum-free essential medium were mixed in a volume ratio of 1:10 and incubated in an incubator for 1 h. Absorbance at 450 nm was measured using an enzyme meter, and the value for each plate was recorded.

4.6.4. Macrophage Activity Assay

Cells were treated with the blank control, MP, QTJD (optimal concentration), and butyrate group for 0 and 48 h. Cell Counting Kit-8 (CCK-8) solution was mixed with serum-free essential basal medium at a 1:10 volume ratio. A 100 μL aliquot of this mixture was added to each well containing the test samples and incubated at 37 °C in a 5% CO_2 incubator for 1 h. Absorbance at 450 nm was measured using a microplate reader and recorded.

4.6.5. Flow Cytometry: Detection of CD86\CD206 Level

The cells were collected into centrifuge tubes, washed 2–3 times with PBS, and resuspended by adding PBS. Except for the blank group, the dyes M0: F4/80, M1: CD80, and M2: CD206 were added and incubated at 4 °C for 30 min. The cells were subsequently washed, PBS was added, and the samples were centrifuged. The supernatant was discarded, and a machine assay was performed. The data were analyzed using FlowJo10.8.1 (FlowJo™ v10.8 Software, BD Life Sciences, Lakes, NJ, USA) [82].

4.6.6. RT-PCR: Detection of CXCL10, MRC-1, Arg-1 Levels

Tissue was lysed with Trizol reagent, and total ribonucleic acid was extracted and examined for concentration and purity. Complementary deoxyribonucleic acid (cDNA) was synthesized by reverse transcription using a reverse transcription kit. A volume of 2 μL of cDNA was used as the template, and SYBR Green was used to detect CXCL10, MRC-1, and Arg-1 levels in the sample. The amplification was carried out by SYBR Green under the following reaction conditions: 95 °C for 10 min, 95 °C for 15 s, 60 °C for 1 min, 40 cycles. This was followed by 95 °C for 15 s, 95 °C for 1 min, and 95 °C for 15 s. Amplification was

https://doi.org/10.3390/ph19020212

carried out according to the $2^{-\Delta\Delta Ct}$ method. The primers required for the experiment are shown in Table 2.

Table 2. Primer sequences for QRT-PCR.

Gene	Forward Strand	Reverse Strand
CXCL10	CCAAGTGCTGCCGTCATTTT	CTCAACACGTGGGCAGGATA
MRC1	TGTCCATTGCACTTTGAGGGA	CGTGGATCTCCGTGACACTC
ARG1	CGCACACCATGCTCAACCTC	GGCCTCTTAGAGACACCAGC
GAPDH	CTCAGGAGAGTGTTTCCTCGT	TTTGCCGTGAGTGGAGTCAT

Abbreviation: CXCL10, C-X-C motif chemokine ligand 10; MRC1, Mannose receptor C type 1; ARG1, Arginase-1; GAPDH, Glyceraldehyde-3-phosphate dehydrogenase.

4.6.7. ELISA: Determination of TNF-α, IL-6 and IL-10 in the Supernatants

The optical density of the samples was measured at the corresponding wavelengths using the Elabscience kit instructions (Wuhan, China).

4.6.8. Western Blot Analysis of MAPK

Macrophage-containing samples were lysed in radioimmunoprecipitation assay buffer with phosphatase/protease inhibitors, followed by protein quantification using the bicinchoninic acid assay. After denaturation (100 °C, 5 min), equal protein amounts mixed with loading buffer were separated by sodium dodecyl sulfate–polyacrylamide gel electrophoresis and transferred to polyvinylidene fluoride membranes. Membranes were blocked with 5% bovine serum albumin (1 h), subsequently incubated overnight at 4 °C with primary antibodies targeting p38MAPK, p-p38MAPK, p44/42MAPK, p-p44/42MAPK, SAPK/JNK/, p-SAPK/JNK, Tubulin, and β-Actin. After washing, membranes were probed with horseradish peroxidase-conjugated secondary antibodies (anti-rabbit or anti-mouse immunoglobulin G [IgG], 1 h, RT). Protein bands were visualized via the Odyssey Infrared Imaging System and quantified using ImageJ software (National Institutes of Health, Bethesda, MD, USA) [83] for grayscale analysis.

4.6.9. Statistical Analysis

Data were processed and plotted using GraphPad Prism 10.1.2 software (GraphPad Software, San Diego, CA, USA) [84]. Normally distributed quantitative data were expressed as mean ± standard deviation. Intergroup differences were analyzed using one-way analysis of variance (ANOVA) for normally distributed data, followed by Tukey's multiple comparison test. Non-normally distributed data were analyzed using the Kruskal–Wallis test. Differences were considered statistically significant when the P value was less than 0.05.

5. Conclusions

This study confirms that QTJD can improve MPP-induced lung injury by regulating macrophage polarization through the core mediator of the gut–lung axis mediator butyric acid-GPR109A-MAPK. These findings offer an innovative immunotherapy for treating MPP. Building upon future research into drug resistance, it holds promise for pioneering a highly promising non-antibiotic treatment pathway to address the increasingly urgent challenge of drug-resistant severe MPP. Future follow-up studies should integrate multi-omics and single-cell sequencing technologies to investigate the mechanism of QTJD in regulating "flora-metabolism-immunity" and further evaluate the therapeutic potential of QTJD in other inflammatory lung diseases. These findings indicate the importance of optimizing

https://doi.org/10.3390/ph19020212

the active ingredients of QTJD to provide a new direction for clinical and anti-inflammatory drug development.

Author Contributions: Conceptualization, Z.L.; methodology, Z.L.; software, Z.L.; validation, Y.J.; formal analysis, R.S. and Q.F.; resources, Y.J.; data curation, Z.L. and Q.F.; writing—original draft preparation, Z.L.; writing—review and editing, Y.J.; visualization, Z.L.; supervision, Y.J.; project administration, Y.J.; funding acquisition, Y.J. All authors have read and agreed to the published version of the manuscript.

Funding: This research was funded by the National Natural Science Foundation of China, Nos. 82174127 and 82374515.

Institutional Review Board Statement: The animal study protocol was approved by the Institutional Animal Care and Use Committee of SHRM (Approval number SYXK(hu)2021-0007 and retrospective approval date 7 October 2023).

Informed Consent Statement: Not applicable.

Data Availability Statement: The original contributions presented in this study are included in the article. Further inquiries can be directed to the corresponding author.

Conflicts of Interest: The authors declare no conflicts of interest.

Abbreviations

The following abbreviations are used in this manuscript:

MPP	*Mycoplasma pneumoniae* pneumonia
QTJD	Qingfei Tongluo Jiedu formula
PPI	Protein–protein interaction
GPR109A	G-protein-coupled receptor 109A
MAPK	Mitogen-activated protein kinase
mTOR	Mechanistic target of rapamycin
TNF	Tumor necrosis factor
IL	Interleukin
STAT	Signal transducer and activator of transcription
CD	Cluster of Differentiation
HPLC/ESI-MS	High-performance liquid chromatography–electrospray ionization mass spectrometry
CAS	Chemical Abstracts Service
GAD	Genetic Association Database
GO	Gene Ontology
KEGG	Kyoto Encyclopedia of Genes and Genomes
PI3K/Akt	Phosphoinositide 3-Kinase/Protein Kinase B
GPCRs	G-protein-coupled receptor
SCFAs	Short-chain fatty acids
16SrDNA	16S rRNA genes
NF-κB	Nuclear factor kappa-light-chain-enhancer of activated B cells
LOX-1	Lectin-like oxidized low-density lipoprotein receptor 1
PLA2	Phospholipase A2
RvD1	Resolvin D1
PD1	Programmed cell death protein 1
$GPR109^{-/-}$	G-protein-coupled receptor 109 knockout mice
FBS	Fetal bovine serum
RPMI	Roswell Park Memorial Institute (medium)
CCK-8	Cell Counting Kit-8
DMEM	Dulbecco's modified Eagle medium
M-CSF	Macrophage colony-stimulating factor

https://doi.org/10.3390/ph19020212

Appendix A

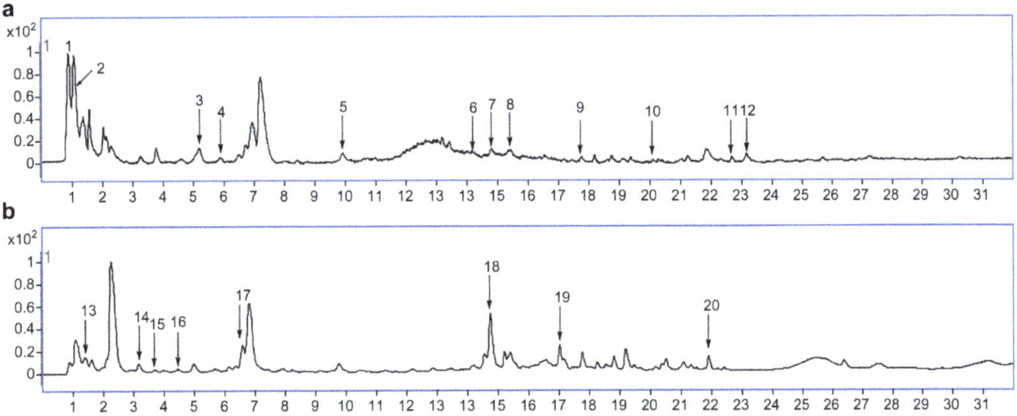

Figure A1. The aqueous extract of QTJD was characterised by HPLC/ESI-MS. (**a**) Active constituents 1–12 (**b**) Active constituents 13–20.

Title of data: Determination of active ingredients in QTJD by HPLC/ESI-MS method.

Description of data: The water extract of nine mixed Chinese medicinal materials was measured by high-performance liquid chromatography coupled with electrospray mass spectrometry (HPLC/ESI-MS) in positive-ion and negative mode. Twenty compounds (1–20), with retention times of 0.9 min, 1.1 min, 5.2 min, 5.9 min, 10.0 min, 14.2 min, 14.8 min, 15.4 min, 17.8 min, 21.0 min, 22.7 min, 23.1 min, 1.4 min, 3.2 min, 3.7 min, 4.4 min, 14.5 min, 14.7 min, 17.0 min, and 21.8 min, were identified: Syringaldehyde (1), Gancaonin U (2), Glyinflanin A (3), Quercetin-3-*O*-β-D-glucose-7-*O*-β-D-gentiobiosiden (4), Arachic acid (5), Luteolin (6), Resveratrol (7), Apigenin (8), Luteolin 7-*O*-glucuronide (9), Gancaonin A (10), Glycyrrhizin (11), Sinapinic acid (12), Citric acid (13), Amygdalinic acid (14), Tryptophan (15), Mulberroside C (16), Licuraside (17), Polydatin (18), Rosmarinic acid (19) and Glycyrrhizic Acid (20). These 20 compounds were unambiguously identified by comparing the retention times and the MS data with the reference standards.

References

1. Wang, Y.S.; Zhou, Y.L.; Bai, G.N.; Li, S.X.; Xu, D.; Chen, L.N.; Chen, X.; Dong, X.Y.; Fu, H.M.; Fu, Z.; et al. Expert consensus on the diagnosis and treatment of macrolide-resistant *Mycoplasma pneumoniae* pneumonia in children. *World J. Pediatr. WJP* **2024**, *20*, 901–914. [CrossRef]
2. Yang, S.; Lu, S.; Guo, Y.; Luan, W.; Liu, J.; Wang, L. A comparative study of general and severe *Mycoplasma pneumoniae* pneumonia in children. *BMC Infect. Dis.* **2024**, *24*, 449. [CrossRef]
3. Meyer Sauteur, P.M.; Beeton, M.L.; Uldum, S.A.; Bossuyt, N.; Vermeulen, M.; Loens, K.; Pereyre, S.; Bébéar, C.; Keše, D.; Day, J.; et al. *Mycoplasma pneumoniae* detections before and during the COVID-19 pandemic: Results of a global survey, 2017 to 2021. *Eurosurveillance* **2022**, *27*, 2100746. [CrossRef] [PubMed]
4. Chen, Y.; Jia, X.; Gao, Y.; Ren, X.; Du, B.; Zhao, H.; Feng, Y.; Xue, G.; Cui, J.; Gan, L.; et al. Increased macrolide resistance rate of *Mycoplasma pneumoniae* correlated with epidemic in Beijing, China in 2023. *Front. Microbiol.* **2024**, *15*, 1449511. [CrossRef] [PubMed]
5. Kutty, P.K.; Jain, S.; Taylor, T.H.; Bramley, A.M.; Diaz, M.H.; Ampofo, K.; Arnold, S.R.; Williams, D.J.; Edwards, K.M.; McCullers, J.A.; et al. *Mycoplasma pneumoniae* Among Children Hospitalized with Community-acquired Pneumonia. *Clin. Infect. Dis.* **2019**, *68*, 5–12. [CrossRef]
6. Meyer Sauteur, P.M.; Beeton, M.L. *Mycoplasma pneumoniae*: Delayed re-emergence after COVID-19 pandemic restrictions. *Lancet Microbe* **2024**, *5*, e100–e101. [CrossRef]

https://doi.org/10.3390/ph19020212

7. Bradley, J.S.; Byington, C.L.; Shah, S.S.; Alverson, B.; Carter, E.R.; Harrison, C.; Kaplan, S.L.; Mace, S.E.; McCracken, G.H., Jr.; Moore, M.R.; et al. The management of community-acquired pneumonia in infants and children older than 3 months of age: Clinical practice guidelines by the Pediatric Infectious Diseases Society and the Infectious Diseases Society of America. *Clin. Infect. Dis.* **2011**, *53*, e25–e76. [CrossRef]
8. Gao, L.; Sun, Y. Laboratory diagnosis and treatment of *Mycoplasma pneumoniae* infection in children: A review. *Ann. Med.* **2024**, *56*, 2386636. [CrossRef] [PubMed]
9. Kim, K.; Jung, S.; Kim, M.; Park, S.; Yang, H.J.; Lee, E. Global Trends in the Proportion of Macrolide-Resistant *Mycoplasma pneumoniae* Infections: A Systematic Review and Meta-analysis. *JAMA Netw. Open* **2022**, *5*, e2220949. [CrossRef]
10. Cai, F.; Li, J.; Liang, W.; Wang, L.; Ruan, J. Effectiveness and safety of tetracyclines and quinolones in people with Mycoplasma pneumonia: A systematic review and network meta-analysis. *eClinicalMedicine* **2024**, *71*, 102589. [CrossRef]
11. Meyer Sauteur, P.M.; Beeton, M.L. Pneumonia outbreaks due to re-emergence of *Mycoplasma pneumoniae*. *Lancet Microbe* **2024**, *5*, e514. [CrossRef]
12. Xue, Y.; Wang, M.; Han, H. Interaction between alveolar macrophages and epithelial cells during *Mycoplasma pneumoniae* infection. *Front. Cell. Infect. Microbiol.* **2023**, *13*, 1052020. [CrossRef]
13. Shao, J.; Li, J.; Weng, L.; Cheng, K.; Weng, W.; Sun, Q.; Wu, M.; Lin, J. Remote Activation of M2 Macrophage Polarization via Magneto-Mechanical Stimulation to Promote Osteointegration. *ACS Biomater. Sci. Eng.* **2023**, *9*, 2483–2494. [CrossRef]
14. Zhao, K.; Huang, Z. TIMP1 promotes microglia M2 polarization through MAPK pathway to ameliorate early brain injury after ischemia. *Hereditas* **2025**, *162*, 119. [CrossRef]
15. Chen, S.; Lu, Z.; Wang, F.; Wang, Y. Cathelicidin-WA polarizes E. coli K88-induced M1 macrophage to M2-like macrophage in RAW264.7 cells. *Int. Immunopharmacol.* **2018**, *54*, 52–59. [CrossRef] [PubMed]
16. Wen, J.H.; Li, D.Y.; Liang, S.; Yang, C.; Tang, J.X.; Liu, H.F. Macrophage autophagy in macrophage polarization, chronic inflammation and organ fibrosis. *Front. Immunol.* **2022**, *13*, 946832. [CrossRef] [PubMed]
17. Koenen, M.H.; de Groot, R.C.A.; de Steenhuijsen Piters, W.A.A.; Chu, M.; Arp, K.; Hasrat, R.; de Bruijn, A.; Estevão, S.C.; van der Vries, E.; Langereis, J.D.; et al. *Mycoplasma pneumoniae* carriage in children with recurrent respiratory tract infections is associated with a less diverse and altered microbiota. *eBioMedicine* **2023**, *98*, 104868. [CrossRef] [PubMed]
18. Jiang, Y.; Bao, C.; Zhao, X.; Chen, Y.; Song, Y.; Xiao, Z. Intestinal bacteria flora changes in patients with *Mycoplasma pneumoniae* pneumonia with or without wheezing. *Sci. Rep.* **2022**, *12*, 5683. [CrossRef]
19. Vital, M.; Karch, A.; Pieper, D.H. Colonic Butyrate-Producing Communities in Humans: An Overview Using Omics Data. *mSystems* **2017**, *2*, 10-1128. [CrossRef]
20. Kircher, B.; Woltemate, S.; Gutzki, F.; Schlüter, D.; Geffers, R.; Bähre, H.; Vital, M. Predicting butyrate- and propionate-forming bacteria of gut microbiota from sequencing data. *Gut Microbes* **2022**, *14*, 2149019. [CrossRef]
21. Chun, J.; Toldi, G. The Impact of Short-Chain Fatty Acids on Neonatal Regulatory T Cells. *Nutrients* **2022**, *14*, 3670. [CrossRef]
22. van der Hee, B.; Wells, J.M. Microbial Regulation of Host Physiology by Short-chain Fatty Acids. *Trends Microbiol.* **2021**, *29*, 700–712. [CrossRef]
23. Sivaprakasam, S.; Prasad, P.D.; Singh, N. Benefits of short-chain fatty acids and their receptors in inflammation and carcinogenesis. *Pharmacol. Ther.* **2016**, *164*, 144–151. [CrossRef] [PubMed]
24. Tan, J.K.; McKenzie, C.; Mariño, E.; Macia, L.; Mackay, C.R. Metabolite-Sensing G Protein-Coupled Receptors-Facilitators of Diet-Related Immune Regulation. *Annu. Rev. Immunol.* **2017**, *35*, 371–402. [CrossRef] [PubMed]
25. Zheng, X.; Jiang, Q.; Han, M.; Ye, F.; Wang, M.; Qiu, Y.; Wang, J.; Gao, M.; Hou, F.; Wang, H. FBXO38 regulates macrophage polarization to control the development of cancer and colitis. *Cell. Mol. Immunol.* **2023**, *20*, 1367–1378. [CrossRef]
26. Xiao, Z.; Jiang, Y.; Gao, X.; Lin, S.; Lin, Y.; Liu, X.; Tan, D.; Jiang, Z. Comparison of the ameliorative effects of Qingfei Tongluo formula and azithromycin on *Mycoplasma pneumoniae* pneumonia. *J. Nat. Med.* **2017**, *71*, 685–692. [CrossRef]
27. Liu, X.; Wang, M.; Kan, Q.; Lin, Y.; Jiang, Z. Qingfei Tongluo Formula Mitigates *Mycoplasma pneumoniae* Infection via the PERK Signaling Pathway. *Dis. Markers* **2022**, *2022*, 9340353. [CrossRef]
28. Jiang, Y.H.; Yu, J.E.; Guo, A.H.; Li, X.; Lin, Y.; Jiang, Z.Y.; Xiao, Z. Ameliorative effects of Qingfei Tongluo formula on experimental mycoplasmal pneumonia in mice. *J. Nat. Med.* **2016**, *70*, 145–151. [CrossRef] [PubMed]
29. Chen, Y.; Jiang, Y.; Liu, X.; Chen, X.; Fan, Q.; Xiao, Z. Polydatin alleviates mycoplasma pneumoniae-induced injury via inhibition of Caspase-1/GSDMD-dependent pyroptosis. *Int. J. Med. Microbiol.* **2023**, *313*, 151586. [CrossRef]
30. Jiang, Y.-H.; Chen, Y.-L.; Fan, Q.-Y.; Liu, X.-H. Intervention effect of Qingfei Tongluo Formula on pyroptosis of *Mycoplasma pneumoniae*-induced human normal lung epithelial cells BEAS-2B via regulating Caspase-1. *J. Guangzhou Univ. Chin. Med.* **2023**, *40*, 450–460.
31. Lü, J.-J.; Zhao, X.-Y.; Jiang, Y.-H. Effects of Polygonum cuspidatum, Scutellaria barbata, and Cryptotympana pustulata extracts on inflammatory factors and lipid metabolism signaling molecules in MPP mice. *J. Emerg. Tradit. Chin. Med.* **2020**, *29*, 1344–1347.

32. Goldsmith, Z.G.; Dhanasekaran, D.N. G protein regulation of MAPK networks. *Oncogene* **2007**, *26*, 3122–3142. [CrossRef] [PubMed]
33. Naor, Z.; Benard, O.; Seger, R. Activation of MAPK cascades by G-protein-coupled receptors: The case of gonadotropin-releasing hormone receptor. *Trends Endocrinol. Metab. TEM* **2000**, *11*, 91–99. [CrossRef]
34. Yan, Q.; Wang, W.; Fan, Z.; Wei, Y.; Yu, R.; Pan, T.; Wang, N.; Lu, W.; Li, B.; Fang, Z. Chickpea-resistant starch exhibits bioactive function for alleviating atopic dermatitis via regulating butyrate production. *Int. J. Biol. Macromol.* **2025**, *303*, 140661. [CrossRef]
35. National institute for Health and Care Excellence (NICE). *Pneumonia (Community-Acquired): Antimicrobial Prescribing (NICE Guideline NG138)*; NICE: Manchester, UK, 2019. Available online: https://www.nice.org.uk/guidance/ng138/resources/pneumonia-communityacquired-antimicrobial-prescribing-pdf-66141726069445 (accessed on 16 October 2023).
36. Abeles, S.R.; Jones, M.B.; Santiago-Rodriguez, T.M.; Ly, M.; Klitgord, N.; Yooseph, S.; Nelson, K.E.; Pride, D.T. Microbial diversity in individuals and their household contacts following typical antibiotic courses. *Microbiome* **2016**, *4*, 39. [CrossRef]
37. Dethlefsen, L.; Relman, D.A. Incomplete recovery and individualized responses of the human distal gut microbiota to repeated antibiotic perturbation. *Proc. Natl. Acad. Sci. USA* **2011**, *108*, 4554–4561. [CrossRef]
38. Li, L.; Yao, H.; Wang, J.; Li, Y.; Wang, Q. The Role of Chinese Medicine in Health Maintenance and Disease Prevention: Application of Constitution Theory. *Am. J. Chin. Med.* **2019**, *47*, 495–506. [CrossRef]
39. Jafari, S.; Abdollahi, M.; Saeidnia, S. Personalized medicine: A confluence of traditional and contemporary medicine. *Altern. Ther. Health Med.* **2014**, *20*, 31–40. [PubMed]
40. Wang, Z.; Hou, Y.; Liu, P.; Wu, R.; Yang, J.; Fan, S.; Peng, Z.; Han, X.; Su, B.; Zhang, C. Membrane integrity changes upon viral infection activate sphingomyelinase SMPDL3B to restrict cGAS-STING signaling via cGAMP degradation. *Immunity* **2025**, *58*, 2670–2684.e10. [CrossRef]
41. Chen, X.; Ma, L.; Liu, X.; Wang, J.; Li, Y.; Xie, Q.; Liang, J. *Clostridium butyricum* alleviates dextran sulfate sodium-induced experimental colitis and promotes intestinal lymphatic vessel regeneration in mice. *Ann. Transl. Med.* **2022**, *10*, 341. [CrossRef]
42. Bai, X.; Guo, Y.R.; Zhao, Z.M.; Li, X.Y.; Dai, D.Q.; Zhang, J.K.; Li, Y.S.; Zhang, C.D. Macrophage polarization in cancer and beyond: From inflammatory signaling pathways to potential therapeutic strategies. *Cancer Lett.* **2025**, *625*, 217772. [CrossRef]
43. Liang, L.; Xu, W.; Shen, A.; Fu, X.; Cen, H.; Wang, S.; Lin, Z.; Zhang, L.; Lin, F.; Zhang, X.; et al. Inhibition of YAP1 activity ameliorates acute lung injury through promotion of M2 macrophage polarization. *MedComm* **2023**, *4*, e293. [CrossRef]
44. Burrows, K.; Ngai, L.; Chiaranunt, P.; Watt, J.; Popple, S.; Forde, B.; Denha, S.; Olyntho, V.M.; Tai, S.L.; Cao, E.Y.; et al. A gut commensal protozoan determines respiratory disease outcomes by shaping pulmonary immunity. *Cell* **2025**, *188*, 316–330.e312. [CrossRef] [PubMed]
45. Pu, Z.; Peng, Y.; Chen, X.; Ma, Y.; Liu, Y.; Li, X. "Heat-dissipating, lung-moistening, and constipation-relieving" effects of Siraitiae Fructus total saponins regulated through Gut-lung Axis. *Phytomedicine Int. J. Phytother. Phytopharm.* **2025**, *150*, 157755. [CrossRef] [PubMed]
46. Mjösberg, J.; Rao, A. Lung inflammation originating in the gut. *Science* **2018**, *359*, 36–37. [CrossRef] [PubMed]
47. Zhao, S.; Zhang, H.; Zhu, H.; Zhao, T.; Tu, J.; Yin, X.; Yang, S.; Zhang, W.; Zhang, F.; Zhang, M.; et al. Gut microbiota promotes macrophage M1 polarization in hepatic sinusoidal obstruction syndrome via regulating intestinal barrier function mediated by butyrate. *Gut Microbes* **2024**, *16*, 2377567. [CrossRef]
48. Cummings, J.H.; Pomare, E.W.; Branch, W.J.; Naylor, C.P.; Macfarlane, G.T. Short chain fatty acids in human large intestine, portal, hepatic and venous blood. *Gut* **1987**, *28*, 1221–1227. [CrossRef]
49. Schioppa, T.; Nguyen, H.O.; Tiberio, L.; Sozio, F.; Gaudenzi, C.; Passari, M.; Del Prete, A.; Bosisio, D.; Salvi, V. Inhibition of Class I Histone Deacetylase Activity Blocks the Induction of TNFAIP3 Both Directly and Indirectly via the Suppression of Endogenous TNF-α. *Int. J. Mol. Sci.* **2022**, *23*, 9752. [CrossRef]
50. Van Gerrewey, T.; Chung, H.S. MAPK Cascades in Plant Microbiota Structure and Functioning. *J. Microbiol.* **2024**, *62*, 231–248. [CrossRef]
51. Luo, B.; Ding, X.; Hu, Y.; Tian, M.; Wu, J.; Shi, H.; Lu, X.; Xia, X.; Guan, W.; Jiang, W. Shikonin hastens diabetic wound healing by inhibiting M1 macrophage polarisation through the MAPK signaling pathway. *Mol. Immunol.* **2025**, *177*, 73–84. [CrossRef]
52. Zhao, M.; Qin, S.; Wang, J.; Zheng, S.; Ma, X.; Xu, W. Cirsii Herba glycoprotein promotes macrophage M1 polarization through MAPK and NF-κB signaling pathways via interaction with TLR4. *Int. J. Biol. Macromol.* **2025**, *296*, 139687. [CrossRef] [PubMed]
53. Yuan, Z.; Jiang, D.; Yang, M.; Tao, J.; Hu, X.; Yang, X.; Zeng, Y. Emerging Roles of Macrophage Polarization in Osteoarthritis: Mechanisms and Therapeutic Strategies. *Orthop. Surg.* **2024**, *16*, 532–550. [CrossRef] [PubMed]
54. Zhou, F.; Mei, J.; Han, X.; Li, H.; Yang, S.; Wang, M.; Chu, L.; Qiao, H.; Tang, T. Kinsenoside attenuates osteoarthritis by repolarizing macrophages through inactivating NF-κB/MAPK signaling and protecting chondrocytes. *Acta Pharm. Sin. B* **2019**, *9*, 973–985. [CrossRef]
55. Li, S.; Yang, P.; Ding, X.; Zhang, H.; Ding, Y.; Tan, Q. Puerarin improves diabetic wound healing via regulation of macrophage M2 polarization phenotype. *Burn. Trauma* **2022**, *10*, tkac046. [CrossRef]

https://doi.org/10.3390/ph19020212

56. Yan, S.; Wei, H.; Jia, R.; Zhen, M.; Bao, S.; Wang, W.; Liu, F.; Li, J. Wu-Mei-Wan Ameliorates Murine Ulcerative Colitis by Regulating Macrophage Polarization. *Front. Pharmacol.* **2022**, *13*, 859167. [CrossRef]
57. Pang, X.; Wang, S.S.; Zhang, M.; Jiang, J.; Fan, H.Y.; Wu, J.S.; Wang, H.F.; Liang, X.H.; Tang, Y.L. OSCC cell-secreted exosomal CMTM6 induced M2-like macrophages polarization via ERK1/2 signaling pathway. *Cancer Immunol. Immunother. CII* **2021**, *70*, 1015–1029. [CrossRef]
58. Wei, Y.; Liang, M.; Xiong, L.; Su, N.; Gao, X.; Jiang, Z. PD-L1 induces macrophage polarization toward the M2 phenotype via Erk/Akt/mTOR. *Exp. Cell Res.* **2021**, *402*, 112575. [CrossRef]
59. Monagas, M.; Brendler, T.; Brinckmann, J.; Dentali, S.; Gafner, S.; Giancaspro, G.; Johnson, H.; Kababick, J.; Ma, C.; Oketch-Rabah, H.; et al. Understanding plant to extract ratios in botanical extracts. *Front. Pharmacol.* **2022**, *13*, 981978. [CrossRef]
60. Kim, S.; Chen, J.; Cheng, T.; Gindulyte, A.; He, J.; He, S.; Li, Q.; Shoemaker, B.A.; Thiessen, P.A.; Yu, B.; et al. PubChem 2025 update. *Nucleic Acids Res.* **2025**, *53*, D1516–D1525. [CrossRef]
61. Daina, A.; Michielin, O.; Zoete, V. SwissTargetPrediction: Updated data and new features for efficient prediction of protein targets of small molecules. *Nucleic Acids Res.* **2019**, *47*, W357–W364. [CrossRef] [PubMed]
62. Daina, A.; Zoete, V. Testing the predictive power of reverse screening to infer drug targets, with the help of machine learning. *Commun. Chem.* **2024**, *7*, 105. [CrossRef]
63. Gfeller, D.; Michielin, O.; Zoete, V. Shaping the interaction landscape of bioactive molecules. *Bioinformatics* **2013**, *29*, 3073–3079. [CrossRef] [PubMed]
64. Coudert, E.; Gehant, S.; de Castro, E.; Pozzato, M.; Baratin, D.; Neto, T.; Sigrist, C.J.A.; Redaschi, N.; Bridge, A. Annotation of biologically relevant ligands in UniProtKB using ChEBI. *Bioinformatics* **2023**, *39*, btac793. [CrossRef]
65. Shannon, P.; Markiel, A.; Ozier, O.; Baliga, N.S.; Wang, J.T.; Ramage, D.; Amin, N.; Schwikowski, B.; Ideker, T. Cytoscape: A software environment for integrated models of biomolecular interaction networks. *Genome Res.* **2003**, *13*, 2498–2504. [CrossRef] [PubMed]
66. Knox, C.; Wilson, M.; Klinger, C.M.; Franklin, M.; Oler, E.; Wilson, A.; Pon, A.; Cox, J.; Chin, N.E.L.; Strawbridge, S.A.; et al. DrugBank 6.0: The DrugBank Knowledgebase for 2024. *Nucleic Acids Res.* **2024**, *52*, D1265–D1275. [CrossRef]
67. Wishart, D.S.; Knox, C.; Guo, A.C.; Cheng, D.; Shrivastava, S.; Tzur, D.; Gautam, B.; Hassanali, M. DrugBank: A knowledgebase for drugs, drug actions and drug targets. *Nucleic Acids Res.* **2008**, *36*, D901–D906. [CrossRef] [PubMed]
68. Stelzer, G.; Rosen, N.; Plaschkes, I.; Zimmerman, S.; Twik, M.; Fishilevich, S.; Stein, T.I.; Nudel, R.; Lieder, I.; Mazor, Y.; et al. The GeneCards Suite: From Gene Data Mining to Disease Genome Sequence Analyses. *Curr. Protoc. Bioinform.* **2016**, *54*, 1.30.1–1.30.33. [CrossRef]
69. Becker, K.G.; Barnes, K.C.; Bright, T.J.; Wang, S.A. The genetic association database. *Nat. Genet.* **2004**, *36*, 431–432. [CrossRef]
70. Szklarczyk, D.; Kirsch, R.; Koutrouli, M.; Nastou, K.; Mehryary, F.; Hachilif, R.; Gable, A.L.; Fang, T.; Doncheva, N.T.; Pyysalo, S.; et al. The STRING database in 2023: Protein-protein association networks and functional enrichment analyses for any sequenced genome of interest. *Nucleic Acids Res.* **2023**, *51*, D638–D646. [CrossRef]
71. Sherman, B.T.; Hao, M.; Qiu, J.; Jiao, X.; Baseler, M.W.; Lane, H.C.; Imamichi, T.; Chang, W. DAVID: A web server for functional enrichment analysis and functional annotation of gene lists (2021 update). *Nucleic Acids Res.* **2022**, *50*, W216–W221. [CrossRef]
72. Huang, D.W.; Sherman, B.T.; Lempicki, R.A. Systematic and integrative analysis of large gene lists using DAVID bioinformatics resources. *Nat. Protoc.* **2009**, *4*, 44–57. [CrossRef]
73. R Core Team. *R: A Language and Environment for Statistical Computing*; R Foundation for Statistical Computing: Vienna, Austria, 2018.
74. Carlson, M. *org.Hs.eg.db: Genome Wide Annotation for Human*; Bioconductor: Boston, MA, USA, 2023.
75. Wickham, H. *ggplot2: Elegant Graphics for Data Analysis*; Springer: New York, NY, USA, 2016.
76. Yu, G.; Wang, L.-G.; H, Y.; He, Q.-Y. clusterProfiler: An R package for comparing biological themes among gene clusters. *OMICS J. Integr. Biol.* **2012**, *16*, 284–287. [CrossRef] [PubMed]
77. Morris, G.M.; Huey, R.; Lindstrom, W.; Sanner, M.F.; Belew, R.K.; Goodsell, D.S.; Olson, A.J. AutoDock4 and AutoDockTools4: Automated docking with selective receptor flexibility. *J. Comput. Chem.* **2009**, *30*, 2785–2791. [CrossRef] [PubMed]
78. Fu, X.; Xu, Y.; Han, X.; Lin, X.; Wang, J.; Li, G.; Fu, X.; Zhang, M. Exploring the Mechanism of Canmei Formula in Preventing and Treating Recurrence of Colorectal Adenoma Based on Data Mining and Algorithm Prediction. *Biol. Proced. Online* **2025**, *27*, 4. [CrossRef]
79. Bramucci, E.; Paiardini, A.; Bossa, F.; Pascarella, S. PyMod: Sequence similarity searches, multiple sequence-structure alignments, and homology modeling within PyMOL. *BMC Bioinform.* **2012**, *13*, S2. [CrossRef]
80. Laskowski, R.A.; Swindells, M.B. LigPlot+: Multiple ligand-protein interaction diagrams for drug discovery. *J. Chem. Inf. Model.* **2011**, *51*, 2778–2786. [CrossRef]
81. Faul, F.; Erdfelder, E.; Buchner, A.; Lang, A.G. Statistical power analyses using G*Power 3.1: Tests for correlation and regression analyses. *Behav. Res. Methods* **2009**, *41*, 1149–1160. [CrossRef]
82. FlowJo, LLC. *FlowJo*, Version 10.8.1; FlowJo: Ashland, OR, USA, 2023.

83. Schneider, C.A.; Rasband, W.S.; Eliceiri, K.W. NIH Image to ImageJ: 25 years of image analysis. *Nat. Methods* **2012**, *9*, 671–675. [CrossRef] [PubMed]
84. GraphPad Software Inc. *GraphPad Prism*, Version 10.1.2; GraphPad: San Diego, CA, USA, 2023.

https://doi.org/10.3390/ph19020212

pharmaceuticals

MDPI

Article

Network Pharmacology Analysis and Experimental Study of Yinchen Against Neuroinflammation in Ischemic Stroke

Minmin Guo [1,†], Yijie Ma [1,†], Linlin Wang [2], Ruipeng Ge [1], You Wang [1], Gefei Ma [1], Guanhua Du [1] and Li Li [1,*]

1 Beijing Key Laboratory of Innovative Drug Discovery and Polymorphic Druggability Research for Cerebrovascular Diseases, Institute of Materia Medica, Chinese Academy of Medical Sciences and Peking Union Medical College, Beijing 100050, China; guominmin@imm.ac.cn (M.G.); mayijie@mail.com.edu.cn (Y.M.); geruipeng@imm.ac.cn (R.G.); wangyou@imm.ac.cn (Y.W.); magefei@imm.ac.cn (G.M.); dugh@imm.ac.cn (G.D.)

2 Xinjiang Key Laboratory of Uygur Medicine, Xinjiang Institute of Materia Medica, Urumqi 830011, China; wanglinlin20@mails.ucas.ac.cn

* Correspondence: lili@imm.ac.cn

† These authors contributed equally to this work.

Abstract: Objective: Ischemic stroke (IS) is an acute neurologic injury in which inflammatory responses play a key role. Yinchen, a common medicinal plant used in Traditional Chinese Medicine (TCM), has been proven to possess strong anti-inflammatory effects. However, its efficacy in treating IS remains unclear. In this study, we aimed to investigate the therapeutic potential of Yinchen for IS and the material basis of this potential. **Methods:** The main active components in *Artemisia scoparia* extract (ASE, the extract of Yinchen), were identified by HPLC and MS. The targets of Yinchen and IS were obtained from public databases. Network pharmacology, molecular docking, and experimental investigation were further applied to acquire the core constituents in Yinchen that work against the neuroinflammation that occuring during IS. The neurological outcomes were evaluated in a transient Middle Cerebral Artery Occlusion (tMCAO) rat model. Additionally, the changes in the inflammatory responses in both the ischemic brain and in lipopolysaccharide (LPS)-treated microglial cells were examined using real-time qPCR. **Results:** Four active compounds of ASE, including isochlorogenic acid C (ICGA-C), isochlorogenic acid B (ICGA-B), isochlorogenic acid A (ICGA-A), and chlorogenic acid (CGA), were identified by HPLC and MS. Network pharmacology predicted that 103 compounds of Yinchen had 198 intersection targets with IS. The top five of these targets were TNF, STAT3, IL1B, AKT1, and SRC. Molecular docking results demonstrated that the abovementioned four compounds detected in ASE showed good interaction with all of the above five core targets. Moreover, both the four compounds and ASE were observed to attenuate NO release and suppress the release of various inflammatory factors (TNF-α, IL-1β, IL-6, and MCP-1) in a dose-dependent manner in LPS-induced BV2 microglial cells. ASE was further found to exert neuroprotective effects against ischemia–reperfusion (I/R) injury and inhibit the production of inflammatory factors in tMCAO rats. **Conclusions:** Yinchen exerts an anti-neuroinflammatory effect on IS, and its constituents with high scores binding to five core targets contribute to this effect. This supports its potential as an anti-inflammatory agent for the treatment of IS.

Keywords: Yinchen; *Artemisia scoparia* extract; neuroinflammation; ischemic stroke; network pharmacology; molecular docking

1. Introduction

Stroke is a temporary or permanent cerebrovascular occlusion caused by a reduction in local blood supply or local thrombosis, leading to a neurological deficit attributed to an acute focal injury of the central nervous system, which is characterized by high morbidity, a high recurrence rate, and high mortality. It is divided into ischemic stroke (IS) and hemorrhagic stroke. The incidence of IS accounts for 60–70% of all strokes and is one of the leading causes of disability worldwide [1]. Cerebral ischemia can cause neuronal hypoxia, energy depletion, and other problems in a short time, and can ultimately lead to excitotoxicity, calcium overload, apoptosis, inflammation, oxidative stress, and other pathological reactions [2]. Timely recovery of blood flow at the ischemic site has become one of the primary principles in the treatment of stroke, but it also increases the risk of ischemia–reperfusion (I/R) injury due to the generation of harmful free radicals such as the superoxide, hydroxyl, and peroxynitrite radicals [3]. In the United States, recombinant tissue plasminogen activator (r-tPA) remains the sole Food and Drug Administration (FDA)-approved therapy for IS. However, its narrow therapeutic window (less than 4.5 h) and risks such as hemorrhagic transformation significantly limit its use, with only a small percentage of patients benefiting from it [4]. Therefore, from the perspective of pathogenesis, such as inflammation, there exists a great incentive to explore new methods and new drugs for the treatment of IS [5]. In cell-based therapy, the acute phase of IS is marked by inflammation and excitotoxicity, creating a hostile microenvironment that compromises graft survival and integration. As the injury progresses to the subacute phase, inflammation subsides, while blood–brain barrier (BBB) repair and angiogenesis begin, opening a more permissive window for successful graft integration [6]. Thus, suppressing the inflammatory response may help extend this "window of receptivity" following a stroke.

Studies have shown that the degree of inflammatory response in IS is the main factor affecting the prognosis of patients. In the early stage of cerebral ischemia, hypoxia leads to neuronal necrosis and the release of damage-associated molecular patterns (DAMPs), activating microglia and astrocytes and triggering the release of pro-inflammatory cytokines such as tumor necrosis factor-α (TNF-α), interleukin-1β (IL-1β), and other chemokines [7]. These molecules disrupt the blood–brain barrier and promote peripheral immune cell infiltration [8]. TNF-α, along with IL-1β and interleukin-6 (IL-6), is recognized as one of the principal pro-inflammatory cytokines [9]. Following ischemic injury, microglia rapidly initiate localized TNF-α synthesis within the brain parenchyma. This initial response is amplified by subsequent infiltration of peripheral inflammatory cells into the ischemic zone, driving excessive TNF-α production through combined cellular interactions [10]. In addition, one study showed that IL-1β blocking was effective in improving experimental I/R brain injury in mice, and the cerebral anti-inflammatory effect was mediated by a reduction in neutrophilic infiltration and matrix metalloproteinase-2 (MMP-2) tissue levels in the infarcted parenchyma [11]. A clinical study found that baseline inflammatory cytokines, including TNF-α, IL-6, and IL-1β, were independent predictors of late recurrence of IS, suggesting that targeted therapy may benefit high-risk patients with elevated baseline inflammation [12]. For patients who are found to be genetically or biochemically affected by cryptogenic stroke, starting TNF blockade to prevent the development of strokes is essential [13]. Therefore, the search for a novel anti-inflammatory strategy to treat IS is not only beneficial but critical, especially one that has a longer treatment window than current therapies, based mainly on the principle of reperfusion. Recently, Traditional Chinese Medicine (TCM) has attracted more and more attention in the world because of its unique advantages, such as its wide range of sources, potential for systematic treatment, and fewer side effects than other therapies. Thus, in view of the pathogenesis and pathological process of IS, finding effective drugs from TCM has become a focus of current research, which is of great significance for the clinical prevention and treatment of this disease.

The herb Yinchen, which comprises the dried aerial parts of *Artemisia scoparia* Waldst. et Kit. or *Artemisia capillaris* Thunb., is included in the 'Chinese Pharmacopoeia'. The main chemical compositions of Yinchen include flavonoids, coumarins, chromones, steroids, volatile oil, and phenolic acid, and *Artemisia scoparia* has a wide range of pharmacological activities, such as anticancer, anti-inflammatory, antibacterial, liver-protective, antiatherogenic, antiviral, and neuroprotective functions [14]. In the past, Yinchen was mostly used in clinical practice to protect the liver and gallbladder, with the effects of clearing heat and removing jaundice [15]. But a growing number of studies have shown that *Artemisia scoparia* extract (ASE, the extract of Yinchen) has a certain effect on anti-inflammation and anti-oxidation, which can play a role in inhibiting the production of nitric oxide (NO), prostaglandin E2 (PGE2), TNF-α, IL-6, monocyte chemotactic protein-1 (MCP-1), and reactive oxygen species (ROS) [16]. Zhengan Xifeng Decoction, a TCM prescription written by Zhang Xichun, is composed of *Achyranthes bidentata*, Longgu, *Paeonia lactiflora*, *Scrophularia ningpoensis*, *Asparagus cochinchinensis*, Yinchen, and other TCMs. It is one of the most commonly used prescriptions for the treatment of yin deficiency and yang hyperactivity syndrome in patients with IS. It can reduce the toxic effect of excitatory amino acids and inhibit the expression of endothelin-1 (ET-1) and TNF-α, which play a role in neuroprotection [17]. However, the potential therapeutic effects of Yinchen and its effective active ingredients in the prevention and treatment of IS are still unknown and worth further investigation.

Network pharmacology is a drug discovery approach integrating systems biology, network biology, multi-pharmacology, and other disciplines. It emphasizes that the process of drug action in the body is a complex network, which is a 'multi-component, multi-target, and multi-channel' process, and is consistent with the characteristics of TCM. Through the bridge of the intersecting 'targets', we can systematically reflect on the complex relationship between TCM components and diseases, explore their mechanisms of action, and analyze the potentially effective components of TCM [18]. Molecular docking technology can quickly and effectively elucidate the pharmacological basis of drugs and improve the accuracy of predictions through computer simulation of the binding modes and affinities between the active components and targets of TCM [19].

Therefore, this study employed a network pharmacology approach to identify key targets and pathways underlying the therapeutic effects of Yinchen against IS and utilized the molecular docking technique to investigate the interactions between the active components identified in Yinchen and Yinchen–IS-associated core targets. Using the lipopolysaccharide (LPS)-induced BV2 microglial cell inflammatory model for in vitro research, the anti-inflammatory activities of these monomeric active compounds and ASE were detected. Furthermore, using a transient Middle Cerebral Artery Occlusion (tMCAO) rat model for in vivo research, the neuroprotective effect of ASE against I/R injury and its anti-inflammatory activity were investigated. Overall, this study is anticipated to provide a theoretical basis for the application of Yinchen in the treatment of IS and contribute to its therapeutic potential as an innovative treatment modality for IS.

2. Results

2.1. Identification of Bioactive Components from Yinchen

Using High Performance Liquid Chromatography–High Resolution Electrospray Ionization Mass Spectrometry (HPLC-HRESIMS) and High Performance Liquid Chromatography–Ultraviolet (HPLC-UV) analyses, four compounds, including chlorogenic acid (CGA) (1), isochlorogenic acid B (ICGA-B) (2), isochlorogenic acid A (ICGA-A) (3), and isochlorogenic acid C (ICGA-C) (4) were identified in ASE (Figure 1, Table 1 and Table S1). In addition, according to an HPLC analysis and HRMS data, the four characteristic constituents in ASE were identified with their reference standards (Figures S1–S5). Consistent with the results of previous studies, the contents of isochlorogenic acids A, B, and C in ASE were relatively high, while the flavonoid components were extremely low [16]. Therefore, the four compounds identified by the HPLC-HRESIMS and HPLC-UV analyses were the major representative compounds of ASE.

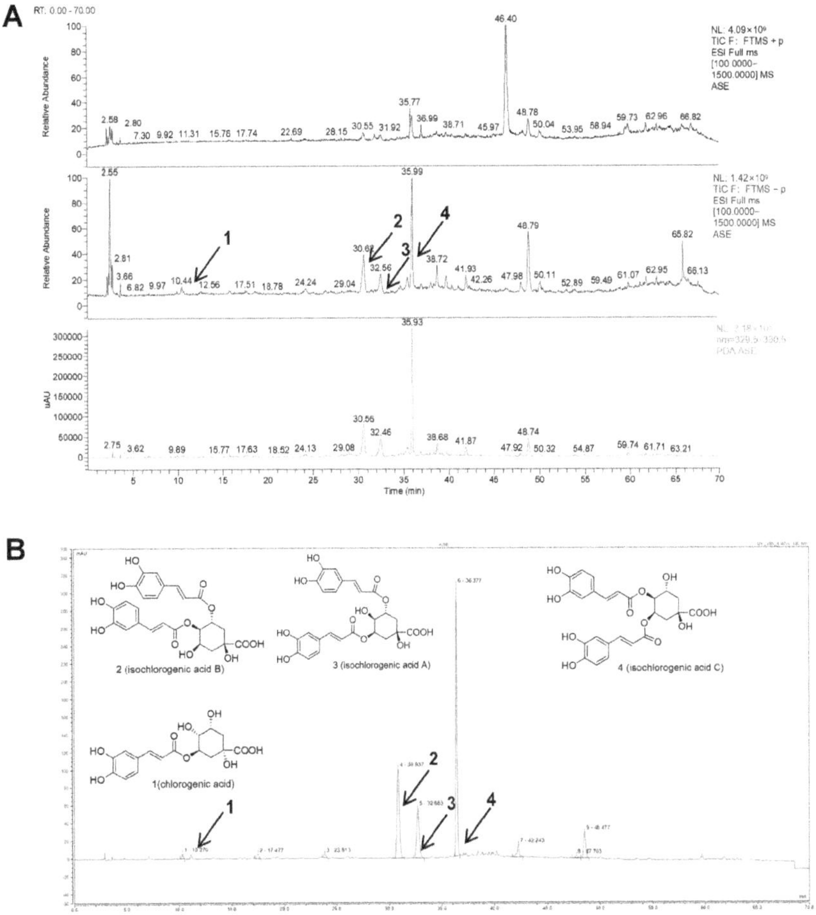

Figure 1. HPLC-HRESIMS and HPLC-UV (diode array detector (DAD)) analyses of ASE. (**A**) (+)/(−) HRESIMS ion current profiles of the ASE and HPLC-UV analysis monitored at 330 nm. (**B**) HPLC-UV (DAD) analysis of the ASE monitored at 330 nm. (1) chlorogenic acid, (2) isochlorogenic acid B, (3) isochlorogenic acid A, and (4) isochlorogenic acid C.

Table 1. HPLC-HRESIMS data analyses of major constituents of ASE.

No.	Name	Formula	t_R (min)	(+)-HRESIMS *m/z*		(−)-HRESIMS *m/z*	
				Found	Calculated	Found	Calculated
1	Chlorogenic acid	$C_{16}H_{18}O_9$	10.62	355.10211 $[M + H]^+$	355.1029	353.08220 $[M - H]^-$	353.0873
2	Isochlorogenic acid B	$C_{25}H_{24}O_{12}$	30.61	517.13403 $[M + H]^+$	517.1346	515.11975 $[M - H]^-$	515.1190
3	Isochlorogenic acid A	$C_{25}H_{24}O_{12}$	32.46	517.13409 $[M + H]^+$ 499.12347 $[M + H - H_2O]^+$	517.1346	515.11975 $[M - H]^-$	515.1190
4	Isochlorogenic acid C	$C_{25}H_{24}O_{12}$	35.94	517.13391 $[M + H]^+$	517.1346	515.11987 $[M - H]^-$	515.1190

2.2. Active Ingredients and Target Screening of Yinchen

To further elucidate the material basis of Yinchen's potential neuroprotective effects, we conducted a network pharmacological analysis. According to the database queries, 53, 69, and 48 monomeric components were obtained from the TCMSP, TCM Database@Taiwan, and the Chinese Natural Products Chemical Component Database, respectively. After screening and deduplication according to the Lipinski rules and ADMET criteria, 99 active ingredients were finally obtained. Therefore, a total of 103 candidate compounds were collectively identified through the integration of HPLC-HRESIMS/UV analyses (four compounds) with three database searches. The SwissTargetPrediction platform was further used to predict the targets of the active ingredients under the set screening conditions. A total of 4674 targets were obtained, and 829 targets of Yinchen were finally obtained after deleting the duplicates.

2.3. Potential Targets of Yinchen in the Treatment of IS

The GeneCards and DisGeNET databases were further used to retrieve the disease targets of IS, and 4558 (880 with relevance >4) and 1159 (126 with correlation score $\geq$0.1) were obtained, respectively. After deleting duplicates, 923 disease targets of IS were finally obtained. The data were uploaded to the Venny2.1 online platform to obtain 198 intersecting targets of Yinchen and IS (Figure 2A).

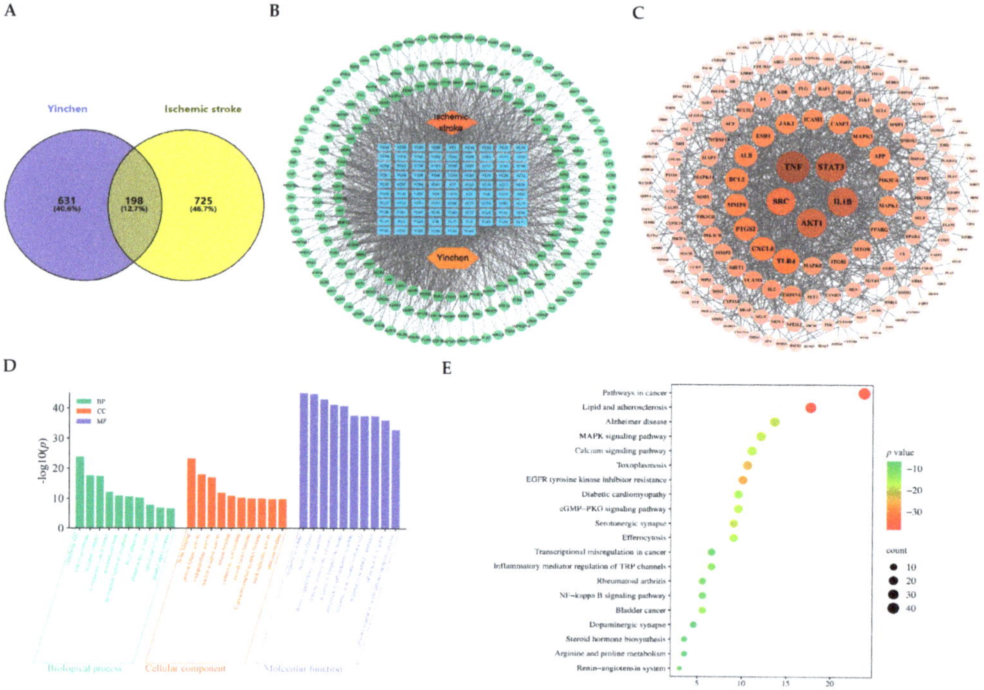

Figure 2. A preliminary screening and network pharmacological analysis of potential therapeutic gene targets of Yinchen against IS. (**A**) A total of 198 common targets of Yinchen and ischemic stroke. (**B**) 'Drug–active ingredient–intersecting target–disease' network (**C**) PPI network plotting of the top five intersecting targets by employing Cytoscape software. (**D**) The top 10 most significantly enriched terms in BP, CC, and MF of GO analysis. The Y-axis represents the enrichment count of the target, and the X-axis represents the GO category of the target gene. (**E**) The top 20 pathways with the most significantly enriched targets were selected. The Y-axis represents the main pathway, and the X-axis represents the gene ratio.

2.4. 'Drug–Active Ingredient–Intersecting Target–Disease' Network

Next, Cytoscape 3.10.1 software was used to construct Yinchen's 'drug–component–target–disease' network. In the network, the red nodes represent the disease, the orange nodes represent the drug, the blue nodes represent the active ingredients in Yinchen, the green nodes represent the intersecting targets, and the edges represent the interactions between the components and the targets. One component often corresponds to multiple targets, and one target may also correspond to multiple components. The network of 'Yinchen–component–target–IS' contains 287 nodes and 1720 edges (Figure 2B).

2.5. Protein–Protein Interaction Network of Intersecting Targets

To further obtain the core targets of Yinchen against IS, the STRING database and Cytoscape 3.10.1 software were used to perform protein–protein interaction (PPI) analysis on 198 intersection targets of Yinchen and IS. In total, 182 interaction targets and 925 PPI relationships were obtained. The size and color of nodes in the network reflect the closeness of the interactions between proteins. The higher the value obtained, the larger the circle and the darker the color, indicating that the target was more important in the network. The top five intersecting targets were TNF, the signal transducer and activator of transcription 3 (STAT3), IL1B, serine/threonine protein kinase 1 (AKT1), and src proto-oncogene, non-receptor tyrosine kinase (SRC) (Figure 2C). These may be the core targets of Yinchen for the treatment of IS.

2.6. GO Functional Enrichment Analysis and KEGG Pathway Enrichment Analysis

In order to clarify the biological functions of the intersecting targets of Yinchen and IS, GO function and KEGG pathway enrichment analysis were performed. The results of GO functional enrichment analysis showed that their biological processes mainly involved circulatory system processes, positive regulation of cell migration, responses to lipopolysaccharides, regulation of inflammatory responses, responses to hypoxia, etc. The cell composition mainly involved membrane rafts, the plasma membrane, the cytoplasmic perinuclear area, dendrites, the cytoplasmic vesicle cavity, etc. The molecular functions were mainly focused on heme binding, protein kinase activity, endopeptidase activity, nuclear receptor activity, G protein-coupled receptor binding, etc. The results of KEGG pathway enrichment analysis showed that the main enriched pathways of key targets were the tumor signaling pathway, the processing of lipids and atherosclerosis, the mitogen-activated protein kinase (MAPK) signaling pathway, the calcium signaling pathway, the cyclic guanosine monophosphate–protein kinase G (cGMP-PKG) signaling pathway, the inflammatory mediator regulation of transient receptor potential (TRP) channels, the nuclear factor kappa B (NF-κB) signaling pathway, and so on (Figure 2D,E). Hence, the results demonstrated the inflammation- and IS-associated core targets of the biological processes of Yinchen in the treatment of IS, further suggesting the role of its anti-inflammatory effects in its potential against IS.

2.7. Molecular Docking of Core Components and Targets

Next, the four identified ligands of Yinchen, including isochlorogenic acid C, isochlorogenic acid B, isochlorogenic acid A, and chlorogenic acid, were redocked to the five core targets (TNF, STAT3, IL1B, AKT1, and SRC) of Yinchen in the treatment of IS using the CDOCKER program in Discovery Studio 2019. From Table 2, it can be seen that compared with the mean docking scores of the targets and their respective agonists or antagonists, all four compounds showed higher mean binding scores; ranked by their average docking score against the five targets from highest to lowest, the order was isochlorogenic acid C, isochlorogenic acid B, isochlorogenic acid A, and chlorogenic acid. According to the results of molecular docking, the four compounds identified in Yinchen showed good scores in their interactions with all of the above five core inflammatory and IS-associated targets, and it was thus determined that they deserved to be further tested in an in vitro experimental study. The binding modes of the four compounds at the binding sites of the five targets are depicted in Figure 3.

Table 2. The CDOCKER scores of the four compounds in Yinchen that interacted with the five core targets.

Compound	TNF	STAT3	IL1B	AKT1	SRC	Mean
Isochlorogenic acid C	68.13	53.47	80.03	73.38	50.54	65.11
Isochlorogenic acid B	70.61	48.85	62.73	77.81	52.06	62.41
Isochlorogenic acid A	67.5	53.72	76.29	67.4	43.13	61.61
Chlorogenic acid	58.39	34.88	57.21	52.46	54.05	51.40
Agonist/Antagonist	60.52	42.6	26.08	46.78	52.93	45.78

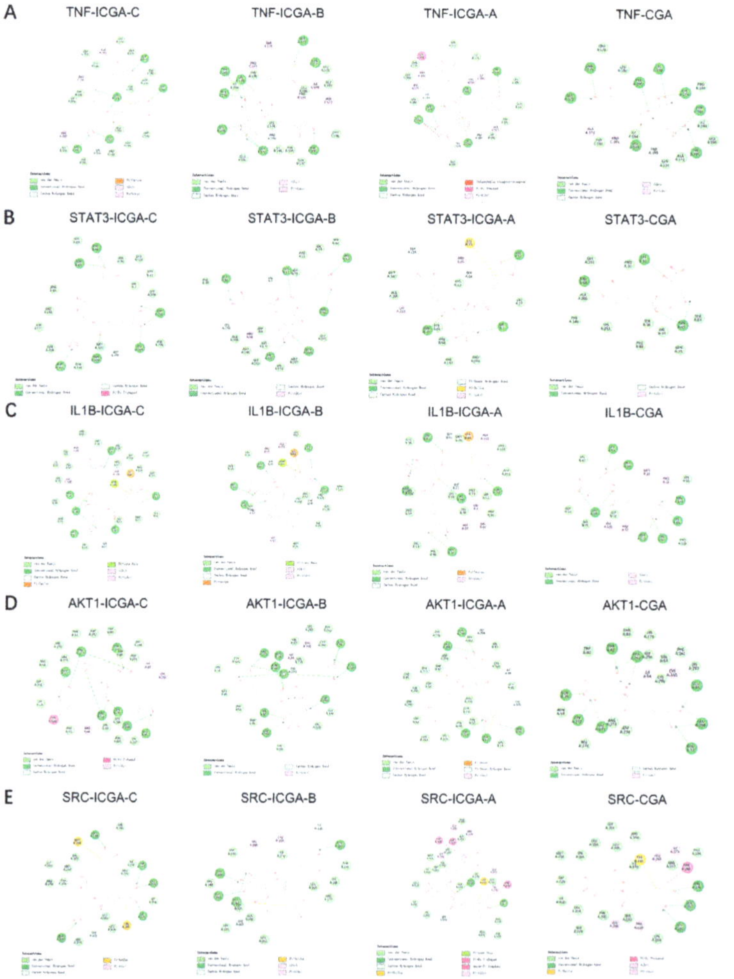

Figure 3. The binding modes of the four compounds (isochlorogenic acid C (ICGA-C), isochlorogenic acid B (ICGA-B), isochlorogenic acid A (ICGA-A), and chlorogenic acid (CGA)) in the ligand-binding sites of (**A**) TNF, (**B**) STAT3, (**C**) IL1B, (**D**) AKT1, and (**E**) SRC.

2.8. Compounds from Yinchen Decrease the Production of NO in LPS-Induced BV2 Cells

After the above network pharmacology and molecular docking analyses, using LPS-induced BV2 microglial cells as an in vitro inflammatory model, we further investigated the anti-inflammatory effects of these four compounds. Dexamethasone (DEX), a representative anti-inflammatory drug, was used as a positive control. LPS is a potent stimulator of microglial activation and NO production, mimicking the inflammatory conditions observed in IS. Results showed that treatment with the five compounds at concentrations of 1, 3, and 10 μM did not significantly decrease BV2 cell viability (Figure 4A). This indicates that the compounds are non-toxic to BV2 cells at the tested concentrations, suggesting that their potential therapeutic effects are unlikely to be compromised by cytotoxicity within this concentration range. BV2 cells were pretreated with different concentrations of these five compounds (1, 3, and 10 μM) for 24 h. The levels of NO in the cell supernatants were measured using the Griess reagent assay, a standard method for quantifying NO production. Furthermore, the four compounds significantly inhibited the production of NO in LPS-stimulated BV2 microglial cells in a dose-dependent manner. DEX was also found to decrease the NO release of LPS-induced BV2 cells starting at a concentration of 1 μM. But the four compounds exhibited greater inhibitory effects on the production of NO at a concentration of 10 μM than DEX (positive control) (Figure 4B). The results give a preliminary verification of the compounds' anti-inflammatory effects in vitro.

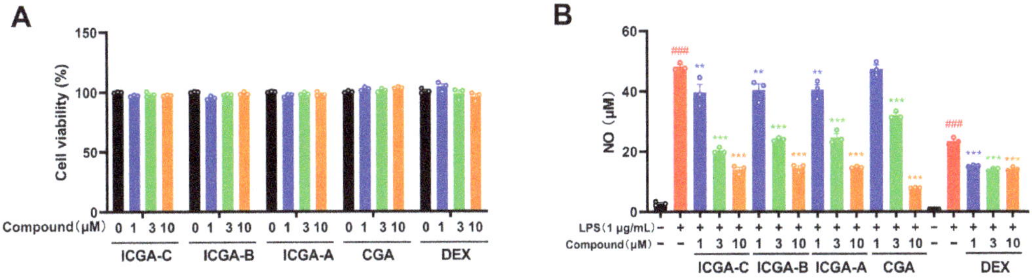

Figure 4. Effects of compounds in Yinchen on cell viability and NO levels in BV2 cells treated with LPS. (**A**) Effects of different concentrations of the four compounds (isochlorogenic acid C (ICGA-C), isochlorogenic acid B (ICGA-B), isochlorogenic acid A (ICGA-A), chlorogenic acid (CGA)) and DEX (1, 3, and 10 μM) on BV2 cell viability. (**B**) The inhibitory effects of the four compounds and DEX at different concentrations (1, 3, and 10 μM) on the NO level of LPS-induced BV2 cells. Data are expressed as mean ± SEM (n = 3). ### $p < 0.001$ vs. the Control group; ** $p < 0.01$ and *** $p < 0.001$ vs. the LPS group.

2.9. Compounds in Yinchen Attenuate the Release of Pro-Inflammatory Cytokines in LPS-Induced BV2 Cells

After confirming that the four compounds from Yinchen showing high scores with all the above five core targets had the effect of reducing NO production, we further investigated whether the compounds had the ability to inhibit the release of pro-inflammatory factors, including TNF-α, IL-1β, IL-6, and MCP-1. Through real-time quantitative reverse transcription PCR (RT-qPCR), it was found that all four compounds had the effect of inhibiting the release of pro-inflammatory factors, compared with the LPS group. Also, these pro-inflammatory factors' down-regulation was observed to behave in a dose-dependent (1, 3, and 10 μM) manner (Figure 5).

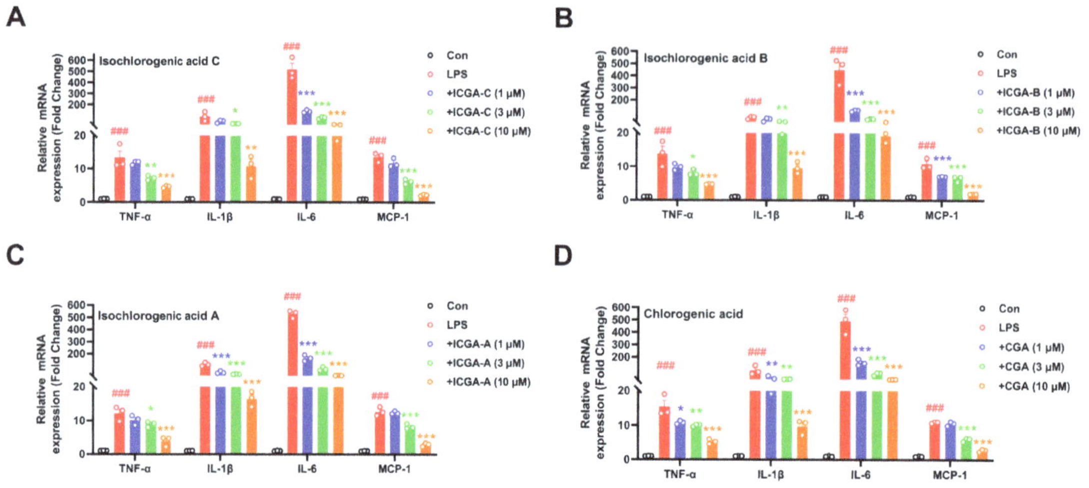

Figure 5. The effects of the four compounds (isochlorogenic acid C (ICGA-C), isochlorogenic acid B (ICGA-B), isochlorogenic acid A (ICGA-A), and chlorogenic acid (CGA)) on the mRNA expression of the pro-inflammatory factors in LPS-induced BV2 cells. (**A**) ICGA-C, (**B**) ICGA-B, (**C**) ICGA-A, (**D**) CGA. Data are expressed as mean ± SEM ($n = 3$). ### $p < 0.001$ vs. the control group; * $p < 0.05$, ** $p < 0.01$ and *** $p < 0.001$ vs. the LPS group.

2.10. ASE Prevents NO Release in LPS-Induced Microglial BV2 Cells

After verifying the anti-inflammatory effects of monomeric active compounds from Yinchen in vitro, we further evaluated the anti-inflammatory effect of ASE in LPS-induced microglial BV2 cells. We first treated BV2 cells with three concentrations of ASE (10, 30, and 100 μg/mL) for 24 h and found that the treatment did not decrease the cell viability (Figure 6A). ASE was found to significantly inhibit the production of NO in LPS-stimulated BV2 microglial cells in a dose-dependent manner (Figure 6B). Specifically, the highest concentration of ASE (100 μg/mL) exhibited the most pronounced inhibitory effect, suggesting that ASE can effectively modulate the inflammatory response in microglial cells. Therefore, in accordance with the anti-inflammatory effects of the four major components in Yinchen, ASE extracted from Yinchen could also inhibit the neuroinflammation in vitro.

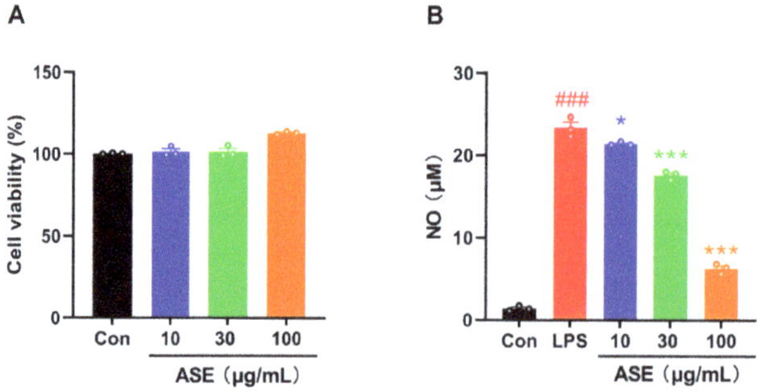

Figure 6. Effects of ASE on cell viability and NO levels in BV2 cells treated with LPS. (**A**) Effects of different concentrations of ASE on BV2 cell viability. (**B**) The inhibitory effect of different concentrations of ASE on the NO levels in LPS-induced BV2 cells. Data are expressed as mean ± SEM ($n = 3$). ### $p < 0.001$ vs. the Control group; * $p < 0.05$ and *** $p < 0.001$ vs. the LPS group.

2.11. ASE Attenuates Neurological Functional Injury After tMCAO

To further investigate the therapeutic effect of ASE against IS in vivo, we established the tMCAO model in Wistar rats. The results showed that the modified neurological severity scores (mNSS) of the tMCAO rats were significantly higher than those of the sham-operated group. However, after treatment, the ASE-treated rats exhibited markedly lower scores than those of the tMCAO rats during the late stage of administration (Figure 7A). Compared with the sham group, the foot-fault rate of tMCAO rats on the wire grid was significantly elevated, while ASE reduced this rate in tMCAO rats (Figure 7B). In the hanging wire test, the scores of tMCAO rats were significantly lower than those of the sham group after reperfusion; following drug administration, the ASE-treated group showed a time-dependent increase, with scores significantly higher than those of the tMCAO group (Figure 7C). Therefore, ASE extracted from Yinchen demonstrated the neurological outcome-improving effect in rats post-stroke, suggesting that Yinchen might have a therapeutic effect against IS.

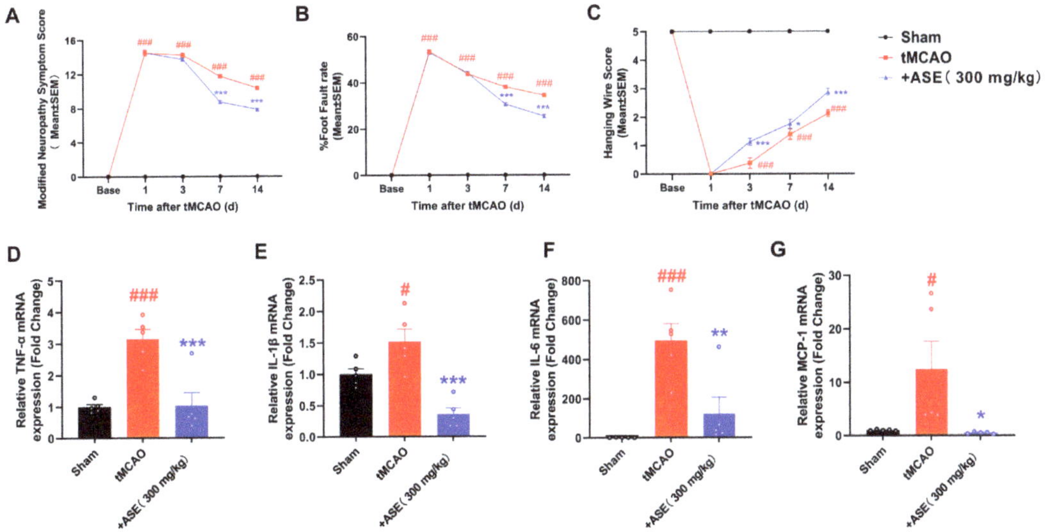

Figure 7. Effects of ASE on tMCAO rats. (**A**) ASE decreased the mNSS of the tMCAO rats. (**B**) ASE decreased the foot fault rate of the tMCAO rats. (**C**) ASE increased the hanging wire score of the tMCAO rats ($n = 8$). (**D–G**) Quantitative evaluation of TNF-α, IL-1β, IL-6, and MCP-1 levels in the ischemic brain ($n = 5$). Data are expressed as mean ± SEM. $^{\#}$ $p < 0.05$ and $^{\#\#\#}$ $p < 0.001$ vs. the Sham group; * $p < 0.05$, ** $p < 0.01$ and *** $p < 0.001$ vs. the tMCAO group.

2.12. ASE Alleviates the Inflammation in the Ischemic Brain of tMCAO Rats

To further investigate the potential mechanism by which ASE acts on tMCAO rats, we measured the expression of pro-inflammatory cytokines (TNF-α, IL-1β, IL-6, and MCP-1) in the ischemic border zone (IBZ) of the brain. As shown in Figure 7D–G, the expression of TNF-α, IL-1β, IL-6, and MCP-1 was significantly higher in the ischemic brain of the tMCAO group compared with the sham group. After the administration of ASE, the levels of these pro-inflammatory cytokines were markedly decreased compared with the tMCAO group, which was consistent with ASE's in vitro anti-neuroinflammatory results. Therefore, ASE could improve neurological function outcomes in tMCAO rats via inhibition of neuroinflammation.

In this study, network pharmacology predicted that 103 compounds of Yinchen had 198 intersecting targets with IS. Also, the top five Yinchen and IS intersecting core targets were TNF, STAT3, IL1B, AKT1, and SRC. Molecular docking results demonstrated that four major active compounds, including isochlorogenic acid C, isochlorogenic acid B, isochlorogenic acid A, and chlorogenic acid, identified by HPLC and MS in ASE, showed good interaction with all the above five core targets. Both the four compounds and ASE were observed to attenuate NO release and suppress the release of the inflammatory factors (TNF-α, IL-1β, IL-6, and MCP-1) in a dose-dependent manner in LPS-induced BV2 microglial cells, and ASE was further found to exert neuroprotective effects against I/R injury and inhibit the production of inflammatory factors in tMCAO rats. These findings suggest that Yinchen has potential as a candidate drug for IS treatment through its anti-inflammatory effects, and four major active compounds identified in Yinchen might constitute the material basis of Yinchen's effect against IS.

3. Discussion

In the present study, we demonstrated that ASE, which is extracted from the TCM component Yinchen, improves neurological outcomes in tMCAO rats by mitigating neuroinflammation. Both ASE and its four characteristic constituents (isochlorogenic acid C, isochlorogenic acid B, isochlorogenic acid A, and chlorogenic acid) exhibited strong binding affinities for the five inflammatory and IS-associated targets (TNF, STAT3, IL1B, AKT1, and SRC) that we identified, and were further found to reduce the production of NO and the generation of pro-inflammatory factors (TNF-α, IL-1β, IL-6, and MCP-1) in LPS-induced BV2 microglial cells. While the traditional formula, Zhengan Xifeng Decoction, which contains Yinchen, has been used to treat IS [17], the specific role and underlying mechanism of Yinchen itself in IS therapy remained unclear. These findings confirmed our hypothesis that Yinchen possesses therapeutic potential for IS. Furthermore, we identified several of its constituents as promising anti-IS candidates, establishing a material basis for Yinchen's efficacy, which is primarily mediated through its potent anti-inflammatory properties both in vivo and in vitro.

Inflammation plays a critical role in the pathogenesis of IS. In the progression of IS, inflammatory cytokines and chemokines are produced, exacerbating neuronal damage and neurovascular injury during stroke [20]. Therefore, combating neuroinflammation is a promising strategy for the treatment of IS. In order to pinpoint the potential key targets of Yinchen for IS treatment, we conducted PPI system analysis. Our results demonstrate that five core genes in Yinchen associated with inflammation and IS, including TNF, STAT3, IL1B, AKT1, and SRC, are significantly related to the treatment of IS. Among them, TNF is an inflammatory cytokine. When brain cells are damaged by ischemia, neurons, microglia, and vascular endothelial cells produce TNF-α. The higher the concentration of serum TNF-α, the larger the volume of cerebral infarction and the more severe the disease is. Therefore, TNF-α is one of the clinical test markers for nerve cell injury after ischemia [21]. As a chemokine, IL-1β can not only transmit information and regulate immune cells and inflammatory factors; it can also transduce the activation and proliferation of T and B lymphocytes. IL-1β promotes the release of neurotoxicity and aggravates brain nerve damage. At the same time, the expression level of inflammation in the body is up-regulated, which further aggravates post-ischemic injury. TNF-α and IL-1β, as the initiating substances in the inflammatory response chain, are involved in the whole process of stroke and can trigger an inflammatory cascade. After infarction, the content of both is higher than normal [22]. Our research also revealed that in the classic tMCAO stroke model, the levels of TNF-α and IL-1β, two of the five core target genes, increased significantly. Su's study demonstrated that Yinchen and a Gancao Decoction significantly reduced the expression levels of IL-1β, IL-6, and TNF-α in the hepatocyte and revealed that hepatocyte necrosis caused by cholestatic liver injury can be alleviated by reducing the release of inflammatory cytokines [23]. Similarly, our research also found that ASE induced an improvement of neurological function and had anti-inflammatory effects in tMCAO rats. It also had the effect of inhibiting the release of pro-inflammatory factors, including TNF-α, IL-6, IL-1β, and MCP-1, and the downregulation of these factors was dose-dependent. Therefore, the effectiveness and accuracy of the five core targets were confirmed through network pharmacology analysis and the subsequent experimental study results, which demonstrated that Yinchen, when used as a single medicinal herb, has potential beneficial effects against IS by attenuating neuroinflammation via modulating the top five Yinchen and IS intersecting core targets. Still, the mechanism by which the top five core targets are regulated by Yinchen remains to be elucidated.

The constituents interacting with the top five Yinchen and IS intersecting core targets may be responsible for Yinchen's effect against IS. Through HPLC-HRESIMS and HPLC-UV analyses, four active compounds, including isochlorogenic acid C, isochlorogenic acid B, isochlorogenic acid A, and chlorogenic acid, were identified in ASE, and all of them showed good scores in their ability to interact with all of the above five core inflammatory and IS-associated targets. As is consistent with ASE, these four compounds can also reduce the levels of NO and the pro-inflammatory factors (TNF-α, IL-1β, IL-6, and MCP-1). This further proves that it is specifically the interaction between TNF and IL1B among the five core targets that enables Yinchen's anti-neuroinflammatory effect. Our results are consistent with those previously reported in the literature, demonstrating that these four compounds exert anti-inflammatory effects in various diseases [24–28]. A renal herb formula with several characteristic components, including isochlorogenic acid C, was found to protect against hyperuricemic nephropathy by inhibiting apoptosis and inflammation [24]. Also, isochlorogenic acid B was observed to alleviate Pb-induced inflammation in the brain, as indicated by decreasing TNF-α and IL-6 levels [25]. Moreover, isochlorogenic acid A was reported to improve liver fibrosis and inflammation by inhibiting toll-like receptor 4 (TLR4)/NF-κB pathways [26]. Although all four compounds have been reported to have anti-inflammatory activities, chlorogenic acid is the only one reported to be able to alleviate IS by inhibiting TLR4-mediated neuroinflammation [27]. Also, the effects of the other three major constituents in Yinchen against IS or their anti-neuroinflammatory role in IS have not been specifically studied yet. Chlorogenic acid was found to primarily restrain the synthesis and release of inflammatory mediators such as TNF-α, NO, cyclooxygenase-2 (COX-2), and PGE2 [28], which was consistent with our experimental results, which showed that it significantly inhibited NO production and reduced TNF-α levels in a dose-dependent manner in LPS-stimulated BV2 microglial cells. Therefore, our preliminary study indicated that the identified ingredients in both Yinchen and ASE exhibited anti-neuroinflammatory effects, and ASE was shown to improve neurological function in tMCAO rats. These findings suggest Yinchen's therapeutic potential for IS, though further research is needed to elucidate its underlying mechanisms and the precise material basis of its effects against neuroinflammation in IS.

In addition to acting on the inflammatory pathways related to TNF-α and IL-1β among the five core targets, KEGG analysis results further demonstrated several signaling pathways related to the potential treatment of IS by Yinchen. The enriched KEGG pathways included the MAPK signaling pathway, the calcium signaling pathways, the cGMP-PKG signaling pathway, the inflammatory mediator for regulation of TRP channels, the NF-κB signaling pathway, etc. Studies have shown that reduced activation of the NF-κB and MAPK signaling pathways can result in decreased expression and activation of the NOD-like receptor family pyrin domain containing 1 (NLRP1) and NLRP3 inflammasomes, as well as increased expression of anti-apoptotic proteins Bcl-2 and Bcl-xL in primary cortical neurons and/or cerebral tissue under in vitro and in vivo ischemic conditions, thus reducing neuronal cell death and brain injury following IS [29]. SRC is one of the five core targets and is found to be strongly associated with the inflammatory process in IS [30]. The pretreatment of agomiR-203a-3p and agomiR-153-3p improved IS-induced neuronal apoptosis by inhibiting the SRC-dependent MAPK signaling pathway, and the inhibition of SRC expression could reduce the level of the expression of NLRP3 inflammasome-related factors [31]. In addition, the serine/threonine protein kinase known as AKT1 is involved in a variety of physiological and pathological processes, including cell differentiation, apoptosis, inflammation, and metabolism following ischemia [32,33]. Once activated, AKT1 triggers a series of signal cascade reactions, which can reduce the death of brain cells, promote the growth of neural cells and vascular endothelial cells, enhance the regeneration and repair of nerve tissue and vessels, and improve neural function after cerebral ischemia [34]. In addition, the involvement of the janus kinase 2 (JAK2)/STAT3 pathway is crucial in the pathological process underlying IS. The increased expression of JAK2/STAT3 observed in individuals suffering from acute IS may contribute to cellular inflammation [35]. Therefore, the role of other signaling pathways in the potential of Yinchen to treat IS is worth further investigation.

Though our study has verified the therapeutic potential of Yinchen against IS and elucidated its material basis through network pharmacology analysis and experimental study, it has certain limitations. Firstly, due to the inherent limitations of network pharmacology in comprehensively mapping bioactive entities, certain compounds and their corresponding target genes might be absent from public databases. Secondly, in this study, we established the classic tMCAO rat model of IS and preliminarily confirmed the neuroprotective effect of ASE and its inhibitory effects on pro-inflammatory cytokines in rat ischemic brain tissues. There is still a lack of evidence for its clinical application. Thirdly, though network pharmacology and our preliminary results have demonstrated the critical role of the identified inflammatory core targets and biological processes in enabling Yinchen's effect against IS, the mechanisms for how Yinchen or its characteristic components specifically modulate these pathways were not investigated in this study. Our future research will still need to evaluate the potential therapeutic mechanisms of Yinchen against IS both in vivo and in vitro.

4. Materials and Methods

4.1. Preparation of the ASE

The aerial parts of *Artemisia scoparia* Waldst. et Kit. were harvested in July 2014 from Urumqi, Xinjiang Uygur Autonomous Region, China. An authenticated voucher specimen (No. 20141227) has been archived at the Xinjiang Institute of Materia Medica, with botanical verification conducted by Associate Professor Jiang He from the same institution. Ten kilograms of dried plant material underwent mechanical fragmentation followed by triple aqueous extraction (150 L of water per cycle, 1 h of reflux per extraction). After filtration and vacuum concentration to a relative density of 1.2–1.25 (60 °C measurement), the condensate underwent tenfold aqueous dilution. The diluted solution underwent 12 h adsorption pretreatment before chromatographic separation through a D101 macroporous resin column, using 70% ethanol as eluent. The collected fractions were concentrated under reduced pressure to achieve identical density parameters (1.2–1.25 at 60 °C), followed by vacuum desiccation at 60 °C to yield 74 g of ASE [16].

4.2. HPLC-UV (DAD) Analysis and UV Spectra of the Major Peaks of the ASE

A quality control analysis of ASE, isochlorogenic acid C, isochlorogenic acid B, isochlorogenic acid A, and chlorogenic acid was performed using HPLC-DAD. Analytical HPLC was performed on a Thermo Ultimate 3000 instrument (Thermo, Waltham,

MA, USA) using a Nano Chrom 120 C18 column (250 × 4.6 mm, 5 μm) with a flow rate of 1.0 mL/min, and the gradient program of MeCN/0.1% H_3PO_4 in H_2O was 10:90 (t = 0 min), 15:85 (t = 10 min), 20:80 (t = 30 min), 30:70 (t = 35 min), 35:65 (t = 50 min), 40:60 (t = 55 min), 55:45 (t = 60 min), 65:35 (t = 65 min), and 90:10 (t = 70 min).

4.3. High-Resolution Mass Measurements of Constituents in the ASE

HPLC-UV analyses were performed using a Dionex Ultimate 300 UPLC system (Thermo, Waltham, MA, USA) coupled with a Thermo QExactive Focus (Thermo, Waltham, MA, USA). HPLC separation was carried out on Nano Chrom 120 C18 column (250 × 4.6 mm, 5 μm) with a flow rate of 1.0 mL/min, and the gradient program of MeCN/0.1% formic acid in H_2O was 10:90 (t = 0 min), 15:85 (t = 10 min), 20:80 (t = 30 min), 30:70 (t = 35 min), 35:65 (t = 50 min), 40:60 (t = 55 min), 55:45 (t = 60 min), 65:35 (t = 65 min), and 90:10 (t = 70 min). The ESI mass spectrometer was equipped with a binary pump, a DAD, a vacuum degasser, an autosampler, and a column heater–cooler (Thermo, Waltham, MA, USA). The MS conditions were set as follows: Spray voltage: 3.3 kV (+), 2.8 kV (−), sheath gas flow rate: 35 PSI, aux gas flow rate: 10Arb, capillary temperature: 32 °C, flow rate: 1.0 mL/min, split ratio: 1:2.

4.4. Screening of Effective Components and Prediction of Targets

The chemical constituents and 3D structural formulas of Yinchen were obtained by using TCMSP (https://tcmsp-e.com, accessed on 22 January 2024), TCM Database@Taiwan (http://tcm.cmu.edu.tw, accessed on 22 January 2024), and the Chinese Natural Products Chemical Component Database (https://www.pharmdata.ac.cn/, accessed on 22 January 2024). The results were combined, and the duplicate values were deleted. According to Lipinski's Rules, that is, relative molecular mass <500, number of hydrogen bond donors <5, number of hydrogen bond acceptors <10, oil–water partition coefficient <5, and number of rotatable bonds ≤10, the chemical constituents of Yinchen were analyzed by Discovery studio 2019, and the ADMET descriptors module was used to evaluate the chemical constituents. The effective components with good water solubility and high intestinal bioavailability were selected for subsequent analysis. The structural formulas of the screened active ingredients were imported into the SwissTargetPrediction database (http://swisstargetprediction.ch/, accessed on 25 January 2024) for target prediction, and the UniProt database (https://www.uniprot.org/, accessed on 25 January 2024) was used to standardize the obtained targets.

4.5. Construction of Drug-Disease Intersecting Targets

'Ischemic Stroke' was used as the keyword to search and screen in the GeneCards (https://www.genecards.org/, accessed on 28 January 2024) and DisGeNET (https://www.disgenet.org/, accessed on 28 January 2024) disease–gene databases. The results were combined, the duplicate values were deleted, and the UniProt database was used to standardize the obtained targets. Venny 2.1.0 (https://bioinfogp.cnb.csic.es/tools/venny/, accessed on 30 January 2024) was used to obtain the intersection between the targets of active ingredients in Yinchen and the disease targets, and the intersection was visualized by a Venn diagram.

4.6. Network Construction of 'Drug–Active Ingredient–Intersecting Target–Disease'

The obtained relevant data were imported into the software Cytoscape 3.10.1 to construct the 'drug-effective component–intersecting target–disease' network of Yinchen. The 'nodes' represented the components and targets, and the 'edges' represented the relationship between the two. The Network Analyzer analysis tool was used to analyze the characteristics of the network.

4.7. Construction of Protein–Protein Interaction Network

The intersecting targets of Yinchen and IS were imported into the STRING database (https://cn.string-db.org/, accessed on 2 February 2024) to create a visual PPI network. The data were imported into Cytoscape 3.10.1 software, and the network was topologically analyzed by the Network Analyzer. The selection of the top five core interaction targets was based on sorting the node degrees from largest to smallest.

4.8. GO and KEGG Pathway Enrichment Analysis

The Metascape database (https://metascape.org/gp/index.html, accessed on 27 August 2024) was used for GO function analysis and KEGG pathway enrichment analysis, and the intersection targets of Yinchen and IS were uploaded to obtain relevant data. The top ten analysis results were selected, and the corresponding data were imported into the Wei Sheng Xin (http://www.bioinformatics.com.cn/, accessed on 27 August 2024) online mapping tool for visualization. The GO functional analysis bar chart included three parts: biological process, cell component, and molecular function, as well as the bubble diagram of the KEGG enrichment analysis.

4.9. Molecular Docking

Molecular docking was performed on the first five core intersection targets and the effective components, which were identified by HPLC-MS of Yinchen. The 3D structure of the proteins corresponding to the top five core targets was downloaded from the protein database PDB (Protein Data Bank) (https://www.rcsb.org/, accessed on 1 June 2025) as a protein receptor library. The 3D structures corresponding to the four identified active ingredients of Yinchen were downloaded from the PubChem database (https://pubchem.ncbi.nlm.nih.gov/, accessed on 1 June 2025). The Prepare Protein tool in Discovery Studio 2019 was used to pretreat the protein by removing water and hydrogenation, and the active center was defined by the Define and Edit Binding Site tool. The location and size of the active center were referred to the position of the protein ligand obtained from the PDB database. The CDOCKER function was then used to perform molecular docking and calculate the -CDOCKER interaction energy. The higher the docking score, the stronger the binding ability of the small ligand molecule to the receptor protein was. The docking scores of the components and targets were statistically analyzed. The agonists or antagonists of the five targets were retrieved from the IUPHAR database (https://www.guidetopharmacology.org, accessed on 1 June 2025), and the docking scores were used to assess the potential activity of the metabolites in Yinchen. The following agonists and antagonists were used for molecular docking: TNF (antagonist: SPD-304); STAT3 (antagonist: S3I-201); IL1B (antagonist: Diacerein); AKT1 (agonist: SC79); and SRC (antagonist: KX2-391).

4.10. Drugs and Reagents

Isochlorogenic acid A, isochlorogenic acid B, isochlorogenic acid C, and dexamethasone were purchased from Shanghai Yuanye Bio-Technology Co., Ltd. (Shanghai, China); chlorogenic acid was purchased from Jiangsu Aikon Biopharmaceutical R&D Co., Ltd. (Heowns, Tianjin, China). The reagents were dissolved in DMSO (Aladdin, Beijing, China) and diluted in saline. Cell viability was evaluated using a CellTiter 96® AQueous One Solution Cell Proliferation Assay (MTS assay, Promega, Madison, WI, USA). The Griess reagent assay kit was purchased from Applygen Gene Technology Co., Ltd. (Beijing, China). RT-qPCR was performed with specific primers and SYBR® Premix Ex TaqTII (TakaRa Clontech, Dalian, China).

4.11. Cell Culture

The BV2 microglial cell line was obtained from the Cell Resource Center, Institute of Basic Medical Sciences, Chinese Academy of Medical Sciences & Peking Union Medical College (Beijing, China). The cells were maintained in Dulbecco's modified Eagle medium (DMEM) (gibco, New York, NY, USA) supplemented with 10% fetal bovine serum (FBS) (PAN, Brisbane, Australia) at 37 °C in a humidified atmosphere of 5% CO_2.

4.12. Cell Viability Assay

BV2 cells with a density of 2.5×10^4 cells per well were seeded in 96-well plates, cultured at 37 °C overnight, and then incubated with ASE (10, 30, and 100 μg/mL) or compounds (1, 3, and 10 μM) for another 24 h. Subsequently, the cells were incubated with MTS reagent at 37 °C for 4 h, and then the absorbance was measured at 490 nm on a microplate reader [36]. Cell viability was calculated using the following formula: $(OD_{\text{Experimental group}} - OD_{\text{Blank}})/(OD_{\text{Control group}} - OD_{\text{Blank}}) \times 100\%$.

4.13. NO Assay

BV2 cells were seeded in 96-well plates at a density of 2.5×10^4 cells per well and incubated for 24 h. The cells were pretreated with compounds at the following stated concentrations (1, 3, and 10 μM) or ASE at the following specified concentrations (10, 30, and 100 μg/mL) for 2 h, followed by stimulation with LPS at 1 μg/mL for 24 h. After the incubation period, 50 μL of cell supernatant was collected, and NO levels were measured using a Griess reagent assay kit. The absorbance was then detected at 540 nm with a microplate reader. The nitrate concentration was calculated according to a standard curve generated from known concentrations of sodium nitrite [37].

4.14. Real-Time Quantitative Reverse Transcription RT-qPCR

Total RNA was extracted from the cells or the rat IBZ brain tissues using the trizol method and was reverse transcribed using the HiScript III All-in-One RT SuperMix Perfect for qPCR (Vazyme, Nanjing, China). A qPCR (2 × AceQ Universal SYBR qPCR Master Mix, Vazyme, Nanjing, China) was subsequently performed using the CFX96 Touch Real-Time PCR Detection System (Bio-Rad, Hercules, CA, USA). Reactions were performed following the manufacturer's instructions. The primer sequences were based on previously published primer sequences [36]. The gene expression levels were quantified using the $2^{-\Delta\Delta Cq}$ method and normalized to the internal reference gene β-actin [36].

4.15. Animals

Male adult Wistar rats (weighing 280–320 g) obtained from Beijing Vital River Laboratory Animal Technology Co., Ltd. (Beijing, China) were used in this study. Animals were housed under standard conditions (temperature 24 ± 1 °C; humidity 50–60%; a 12 h light/dark cycle) and had free access to food and water. The Animal Ethics Committee of the Chinese Academy of Medical Sciences and Peking Union Medical College approved the animal protocols before the start of any protocol-specified procedures (IMM-S-25-0038).

4.16. tMCAO

Rats were fasted overnight and housed at 25 °C with free access to water. They were anesthetized with 4% isoflurane in 70% N_2O/30% O_2 and then maintained at 3% isoflurane. Rectal temperature was kept at 37 ± 0.5 °C using a feedback-controlled heating pad. After making a skin incision midway between the left orbit and the external auditory canal, the left common carotid artery, external carotid artery (ECA), and internal carotid artery (ICA) were exposed. A 0.38 mm diameter of silicone-coated monofilament suture was inserted into the ECA and advanced into the ICA until slight resistance was felt, thereby occluding the origin of the middle cerebral artery. After 1.5 h of occlusion, the filament was gently withdrawn to restore blood flow; successful reperfusion was confirmed by immediate hyperemic flushing of the ICA [38]. The incision was closed, and animals were allowed to recover in a warmed cage. Sham-operated rats (sham group) underwent an identical procedure except for the occlusion step.

4.17. ASE Administration

The rats were randomly assigned into 3 experimental groups of 8 rats each, as follows: sham group, tMCAO group, and ASE + tMCAO group (300 mg/kg) were given an intragastric administration (i.g.) of ASE as an aqueous suspension in 0.5% sodium carboxymethyl cellulose (CMC-Na) starting 24 h after tMCAO and repeated daily for a total of 14 days, and the sham and tMCAO groups were given an equivalent volume of 0.5% CMC-Na.

4.18. Behavioral Tests

Three behavioral tests were used to assess neurological deficits after tMCAO: mNSS, the foot-fault test, and the hanging wire test. The mNSS is an integrated assessment that includes tests of motor function, sensory function, reflexes, and balance. It was evaluated using a scale from 0 to 18, with 0 representing normal function and 18 indicating the most severe impairment [39]. A modified foot-fault test was employed to measure forelimb placement dysfunction. The total number of steps (movement of each forelimb) that the rat used to cross the grid and the total number of foot faults for the left forelimb were recorded [40]. The hanging wire test was used to evaluate both limb strength and balance after stroke [41]. These tests were evaluated on days 1, 3, 7, and 14 after the performance of tMCAO. All surviving animals were euthanized 14 days after tMCAO.

4.19. Statistical Analysis

Data are presented as the mean ± SEM. Statistical analyses were performed using one-way analysis of variance (ANOVA) followed by Dunnett's multiple-comparisons test or two-way ANOVA followed by Tukey's multiple-comparisons test. The number of samples per cell group and the number of animals per group are specified in the figure legends. GraphPad Prism 9.0 software (GraphPad Software Inc., La Jolla, CA, USA) was used for all statistical analyses. A p-value < 0.05 was established as the criterion for statistical significance. Post hoc power analysis for the statistical test power of this study was conducted using G*Power 3.1.9.7 software (Heinrich Heine University, Düsseldorf, Germany). The analysis was based on the actual sample size, the predefined significance level ($\alpha = 0.05$), and the effect size observed in the experiment. The test power $(1-\beta)$ for all intergroup comparisons was 1.0.

5. Conclusions

In this study, network pharmacology and molecular docking technology were used to systematically analyze the action of Yinchen in the treatment of IS, revealing a process characterized by multi-component, multi-target, and multi-pathway action. Among Yinchen and IS's intersecting targets, TNF, STAT3, IL1B, AKT1, and SRC were the top five core targets. Through HPLC-HRESIMS and HPLC-UV analyses, four compounds, including isochlorogenic acid C, isochlorogenic acid B, isochlorogenic acid A, and chlorogenic acid, were identified in ASE, which was extracted from Yinchen. These four major representative compounds showed good interaction with all of the above five core targets through molecular docking. Also, they were found to reduce the production of NO as well as the generation of inflammatory factors (TNF-α, IL-1β, IL-6, and MCP-1) in LPS-induced BV2 microglial cells dose-dependently. ASE also demonstrated anti-neuroinflammatory activity in an in vitro experiment. In vivo, ASE showed neurological functional injury attenuation and neuroinflammation alleviation effects in tMCAO rats. In conclusion, our results suggest that Yinchen has the potential to be a candidate drug for IS treatment through its anti-inflammatory effects.

Considering the limited treatment window and the post-stroke inflammatory cascade, ASE and other active components could be explored as an adjunctive therapy to current standards of care. Its role in mitigating secondary neuronal damage through neuroinflammation inhibition may help improve long-term neurological outcomes in stroke patients. This study provides a scientific foundation for the modern application of the traditional herb Yinchen, suggesting its potential utility beyond hepatobiliary disorders and bringing it into the realm of cerebrovascular diseases.

Supplementary Materials: The following supporting information can be downloaded at https://www.mdpi.com/article/10.3390/ph18121852/s1. Table S1. The UV spectra, molecular formula, and structures of the major peaks of ASE detected by online HPLC-UV (DAD) and HPLC-HRESIMS. Figure S1. HPLC-UV (DAD) profiles of the ASE monitored at 210, 254, and 330 nm. Figure S2. HPLC-UV (DAD) profile and the UV spectrum of the marker compound chlorogenic acid (CGA) monitored at 330 nm. Figure S3. HPLC-UV (DAD) profile and the UV spectrum of the marker compound isochlorogenic acid B (ICGA-B, ICGB) monitored at 330 nm. Figure S4. HPLC-UV (DAD) profile and the UV spectrum of the marker compound isochlorogenic acid A (ICGA-A, ICGA) monitored at 330 nm. Figure S5. HPLC-UV (DAD) profile and the UV spectrum of the marker compound isochlorogenic acid C (ICGA-C, ICGC) monitored at 330 nm.

Author Contributions: M.G.: conceptualization, methodology, data curation, investigation, writing—original draft, writing—review and editing. Y.M.: conceptualization, methodology, investigation, visualization, writing—original draft, writing—review and editing, L.W.: investigation. R.G.: investigation, writing—review and editing. Y.W. and G.M.: investigation. G.D.: resources, writing—review and editing. L.L.: conceptualization, project administration, writing—review and editing, supervision. All authors have read and agreed to the published version of the manuscript.

Funding: This research was funded by grants from the Non-profit Central Research Institute Fund of Chinese Academy of Medical Sciences (2023-RW350-01), National Natural Science Foundation of China (82373885), and CAMS Innovation Fund for Medical Sciences (CIFMS) (2021-I2M-1-016).

Institutional Review Board Statement: The animal study protocol was approved by the Animal Ethics Committee of the Chinese Academy of Medical Sciences and Peking Union Medical College (IMM-S-25-0038, 7 April 2025).

Informed Consent Statement: Not applicable.

Data Availability Statement: The original contributions presented in this study are included in the article/Supplementary Material. Further inquiries can be directed to the corresponding author.

Conflicts of Interest: The authors declare no conflicts of interest.

Abbreviations

The following abbreviations are used in this manuscript:

ANOVA	analysis of variance
ASE	*Artemisia scoparia* extract
BBB	blood–brain barrier
cGMP-PKG	cyclic guanosine monophosphate-protein kinase G
CMC-Na	sodium carboxylmethyl cellulose
CGA	Chlorogenic acid
COX-2	cyclooxygenase-2
DAD	Diode array detector

DAMPs	damage-associated molecular patterns
DMEM	Dulbecco's modified Eagle's medium
ECA	external carotid artery
ET-1	endothelin-1
FBS	fetal bovine serum
GO	Gene Ontology
HREIMS	High Resolution Electrospray Ionization Mass Spectrometry
HPLC	high-performance liquid chromatography
IBZ	ischemic border zone
ICGA-A	Isochlorogenic acid A
ICGA-B	Isochlorogenic acid B
ICGA-C	Isochlorogenic acid C
ICA	internal carotid artery
IL-1β	interleukin-1β
IL-6	interleukin-6
IS	Ischemic stroke
JAK2	janus kinase 2
KEGG	Kyoto Encyclopedia of Genes and Genomes
LPS	Lipopolysaccharide
MAPK	mitogen-activated protein kinase
MCP-1	monocyte chemotactic protein-1
MMP-2	matrix metalloproteinase-2
mNSS	Modified Neurological Severity Score
NF-κB	nuclear factor kappa B
NLRP	NOD-like receptor family pyrin domain
NO	nitric oxide
NSS	neurological severity score
PDB	Protein Data Bank
PGE2	prostaglandin E2
PPI	Protein–protein interaction
qRT-PCR	Quantitative real-time PCR
RMSD	root mean square deviation
ROS	reactive oxygen species
r-tPA	recombinant tissue plasminogen activator
SRC	Src proto-oncogene, non-receptor tyrosine kinase
STAT3	signal transducer and activator of transcription 3
TCM	Traditional Chinese medicine
TLR4	toll-like receptor 4
tMCAO	Transient Middle Cerebral Artery Occlusion
TNF-α	tumor necrosis factor-α
TRP	transient receptor potential

References

1. Hilkens, N.A.; Casolla, B.; Leung, T.W.; de Leeuw, F.E. Stroke. *Lancet* **2024**, *403*, 2820–2836. [CrossRef]
2. Hu, X.; De Silva, T.M.; Chen, J.; Faraci, F.M. Cerebral Vascular Disease and Neurovascular Injury in Ischemic Stroke. *Circ. Res.* **2017**, *120*, 449–471. [CrossRef]
3. Nie, X.; Leng, X.; Miao, Z.; Fisher, M.; Liu, L. Clinically Ineffective Reperfusion After Endovascular Therapy in Acute Ischemic Stroke. *Stroke* **2023**, *54*, 873–881. [CrossRef] [PubMed]
4. Powers, W.J.; Rabinstein, A.A.; Ackerson, T.; Adeoye, O.M.; Bambakidis, N.C.; Becker, K.; Biller, J.; Brown, M.; Demaerschalk, B.M.; Hoh, B.; et al. Guidelines for the early management of patients with acute ischemic stroke: 2019 update to the 2018 guidelines for the early management of acute ischemic stroke: A guideline for healthcare professionals from the American heart association/American stroke association. *Stroke* **2019**, *50*, e344–e418.

5. Zeng, J.; Bao, T.; Yang, K.; Zhu, X.; Wang, S.; Xiang, W.; Ge, A.; Zeng, L.; Ge, J. The mechanism of microglia-mediated immune inflammation in ischemic stroke and the role of natural botanical components in regulating microglia: A review. *Front. Immunol.* **2023**, *13*, 1047550. [CrossRef]
6. Yin, H.; Brian, D.; Weber, R.Z.; Lyden, P.D.; Rust, R. "Time Is Brain"—For Cell Therapies. *Adv. Sci.* **2025**, *18*, e19579. [CrossRef]
7. Kumari, S.; Dhapola, R.; Sharma, P.; Nagar, P.; Medhi, B.; HariKrishnaReddy, D. The impact of cytokines in neuroinflammation-mediated stroke. *Cytokine Growth Factor Rev.* **2024**, *78*, 105–119. [CrossRef]
8. DeLong, J.H.; Ohashi, S.N.; O'Connor, K.C.; Sansing, L.H. Inflammatory Responses After Ischemic Stroke. *Semin. Immunopathol.* **2022**, *44*, 625–648. [CrossRef]
9. Zietz, A.; Gorey, S.; Kelly, P.J.; Katan, M.; McCabe, J.J. Targeting inflammation to reduce recurrent stroke. *Int. J. Stroke* **2024**, *19*, 379–387. [CrossRef] [PubMed]
10. Tirandi, A.; Sgura, C.; Carbone, F.; Montecucco, F.; Liberale, L. Inflammatory biomarkers of ischemic stroke. *Intern. Emerg. Med.* **2023**, *18*, 723–732. [CrossRef] [PubMed]
11. Liberale, L.; Diaz-Cañestro, C.; Bonetti, N.R.; Paneni, F.; Akhmedov, A.; Beer, J.H.; Montecucco, F.; Lüscher, T.F.; Camici, G.G. Post-ischemic administration of the murine Canakinumab-surrogate antibody improves outcome in experimental stroke. *Eur. Heart J.* **2018**, *39*, 3511–3517. [CrossRef] [PubMed]
12. Coveney, S.; Murphy, S.; Belton, O.; Cassidy, T.; Crowe, M.; Dolan, E.; de Gaetano, M.; Harbison, J.; Horgan, G.; Marnane, M.; et al. Inflammatory cytokines, high-sensitivity C-reactive protein, and risk of one-year vascular events, death, and poor functional outcome after stroke and transient ischemic attack. *Int. J. Stroke* **2022**, *17*, 163–171. [CrossRef]
13. Soldatos, A.; Toro, C.; Hoffmann, P.; Romeo, T.; Deuitch, N.; Brofferio, A.; Aksentijevich, I.; Kastner, D.L.; Ombrello, A.K. TNF-Blockade for Primary Stroke Prevention in Adenosine Deaminase 2 Deficiency: A Case Series. *Neurol. Neuroimmunol. Neuroinflamm.* **2023**, *10*, e200073. [CrossRef]
14. Ding, J.; Wang, L.; He, C.; Zhao, J.; Si, L.; Huang, H. Artemisia scoparia: Traditional uses, active constituents and pharmacological effects. *J. Ethnopharmacol.* **2021**, *273*, 113960. [CrossRef]
15. Wei, C.; Qiu, J.; Wu, Y.; Chen, Z.; Yu, Z.; Huang, Z.; Yang, K.; Hu, H.; Liu, F. Promising traditional Chinese medicine for the treatment of cholestatic liver disease process (cholestasis, hepatitis, liver fibrosis, liver cirrhosis). *J. Ethnopharmacol.* **2022**, *297*, 115550. [CrossRef] [PubMed]
16. Wang, X.; Huang, H.; Ma, X.; Wang, L.; Liu, C.; Hou, B.; Yang, S.; Zhang, L.; Du, G. Anti-inflammatory effects and mechanism of the total flavonoids from Artemisia scoparia Waldst. et kit. in vitro and in vivo. *Biomed. Pharmacother.* **2018**, *104*, 390–403. [PubMed]
17. Zhu, J.B.; Wang, Y.H.; Hu, Z.D.; Li, J. Research progress on pathogenesis of ischemic stroke and traditional Chinese medicine commonly used for treatment of ischemic stroke. *China J. Chin. Mater. Medica* **2019**, *44*, 422–432.
18. Zhao, L.; Zhang, H.; Li, N.; Chen, J.; Xu, H.; Wang, Y.; Liang, Q. Network pharmacology, a promising approach to reveal the pharmacology mechanism of Chinese medicine formula. *J. Ethnopharmacol.* **2023**, *309*, 116306. [CrossRef]
19. Crampon, K.; Giorkallos, A.; Deldossi, M.; Baud, S.; Steffenel, L.A. Machine-learning methods for ligand–protein molecular docking. *Drug Discov. Today* **2022**, *27*, 151–164. [CrossRef]
20. Qin, C.; Yang, S.; Chu, Y.-H.; Zhang, H.; Pang, X.-W.; Chen, L.; Zhou, L.-Q.; Chen, M.; Tian, D.-S.; Wang, W. Signaling pathways involved in ischemic stroke: Molecular mechanisms and therapeutic interventions. *Signal Transduct. Target. Ther.* **2022**, *7*, 215. [CrossRef]
21. Băcilă, C.-I.; Vlădoiu, M.-G.; Văleanu, M.; Moga, D.-F.; Pumnea, P.-M. The Role of IL-6 and TNF-Alpha Biomarkers in Predicting Disability Outcomes in Acute Ischemic Stroke Patients. *Life* **2025**, *15*, 47. [CrossRef]
22. Yang, J.; Ran, M.; Li, H.; Lin, Y.; Ma, K.; Yang, Y.; Fu, X.; Yang, S. New insight into neurological degeneration: Inflammatory cytokines and blood–brain barrier. *Front. Mol. Neurosci.* **2022**, *15*, 1013933. [CrossRef] [PubMed]
23. Su, H.; Wang, Q.; Li, Y.; Jin, J.; Tan, B.; Yan, D.; Zou, B.; Song, G.; Weng, F.; Qiu, F. Effect of Different Ratios of Yinchen and Gancao Decoction on ANIT-Treated Cholestatic Liver Injury in Mice and Its Potential Underlying Mechanism. *Front. Pharmacol.* **2021**, *12*, 611610. [CrossRef] [PubMed]
24. Tang, G.Y.; Li, S.; Xu, Y.; Zhang, C.; Xu, X.Y.; Xu, L.; Wang, N.; Feng, Y. Renal herb formula protects against hyperuricemic nephropathy by inhibiting apoptosis and inflammation. *Phytomedicine* **2023**, *116*, 154812. [CrossRef]
25. Shi, J.-X.; Cheng, C.; Ruan, H.-N.; Li, J.; Liu, C.-M. Isochlorogenic acid B alleviates lead-induced anxiety, depression and neuroinflammation in mice by the BDNF pathway. *Neurotoxicology* **2023**, *98*, 1–8. [CrossRef] [PubMed]
26. Liu, X.; Huang, K.; Zhang, R.J.; Mei, D.; Zhang, B. Isochlorogenic Acid A Attenuates the Progression of Liver Fibrosis Through Regulating HMGB1/TLR4/NF-κB Signaling Pathway. *Front. Pharmacol.* **2020**, *11*, 582. [CrossRef]
27. Wu, W.; Xu, L.; Sun, L.; Xue, J.; Wang, F.; Guo, H.; Lei, N.; Liu, D.; Liu, Y.; Liang, D.; et al. Ethanol extract of Periploca forrestii Schltr. and chlorogenic acid alleviate ischemic stroke by inhibiting TLR4-mediated neuroinflammation. *Phytomedicine* **2025**, *145*, 157026. [CrossRef]

28. Huang, J.; Xie, M.; He, L.; Song, X.; Cao, T. Chlorogenic acid: A review on its mechanisms of anti-inflammation, disease treatment, and related delivery systems. *Front. Pharmacol.* **2023**, *14*, 1218015. [CrossRef]
29. Fann, D.Y.-W.; Lim, Y.-A.; Cheng, Y.-L.; Lok, K.-Z.; Chunduri, P.; Baik, S.-H.; Drummond, G.R.; Dheen, S.T.; Sobey, C.G.; Jo, D.-G.; et al. Evidence that NF-κB and MAPK Signaling Promotes NLRP Inflammasome Activation in Neurons Following Ischemic Stroke. *Mol. Neurobiol.* **2018**, *55*, 1082–1096. [CrossRef]
30. Okutani, D.; Lodyga, M.; Han, B.; Liu, M. Src protein tyrosine kinase family and acute inflammatory responses. *Am. J. Physiol. Lung Cell Mol. Physiol.* **2006**, *291*, L129–L141. [CrossRef]
31. Li, Y.; Peng, B.; Li, Y.; Huang, A.; Peng, Y.; Yu, Q.; Li, Y. MiR-203a-3p/153-3p improves cognitive impairments induced by ischemia/reperfusion via blockade of SRC-mediated MAPK signaling pathway in ischemic stroke. *Chem. Biol. Interact.* **2022**, *358*, 109900.
32. Zhao, E.Y.; Efendizade, A.; Cai, L.; Ding, Y. The role of Akt (protein kinase B) and protein kinase C in ischemia-reperfusion injury. *Neurol. Res.* **2016**, *38*, 301–308. [CrossRef] [PubMed]
33. Samakova, A.; Gazova, A.; Sabova, N.; Valaskova, S.; Jurikova, M.; Kyselovic, J. The PI3k/Akt Pathway Is Associated With Angiogenesis, Oxidative Stress and Survival of Mesenchymal Stem Cells in Pathophysiologic Condition in Ischemia. *Physiol. Res.* **2019**, *68* (Suppl. 2), S131–S138. [PubMed]
34. Huang, N.; Li, S.; Xie, Y.; Han, Q.; Xu, X.-M.; Sheng, Z.-H. Reprogramming an energetic AKT-PAK5 axis boosts axon energy supply and facilitates neuron survival and regeneration after injury and ischemia. *Curr. Biol.* **2021**, *31*, 3098–3114.e7. [CrossRef]
35. Zhong, Y.; Yin, B.; Ye, Y.; Dekhel, O.Y.A.T.; Xiong, X.; Jian, Z.; Gu, L. The bidirectional role of the JAK2/STAT3 signaling pathway and related mechanisms in cerebral ischemia-reperfusion injury. *Exp. Neurol.* **2021**, *341*, 113690. [CrossRef] [PubMed]
36. Shen, Y.; Yang, R.; Zhao, J.; Chen, M.; Chen, S.; Ji, B.; Chen, H.; Liu, D.; Li, L.; Du, G. The histone deacetylase inhibitor belinostat ameliorates experimental autoimmune encephalomyelitis in mice by inhibiting TLR2/MyD88 and HDAC3/NF-κB p65-mediated neuroinflammation. *Pharmacol. Res.* **2022**, *176*, 105969. [CrossRef]
37. Becker, A.J.; Ückert, S.; Tsikas, D.; Noack, H.; Stief, C.G.; Frölich, J.C.; Wolf, G.; Jonas, U. Determination of nitric oxide metabolites by means of the Griess assay and gas chromatography–mass spectrometry in the cavernous and systemic blood of healthy males and patients with erectile dysfunction during different functional conditions of the penis. *Urol. Res.* **2000**, *28*, 364–369. [CrossRef]
38. Yang, R.; Shen, Y.-J.; Chen, M.; Zhao, J.-Y.; Chen, S.-H.; Zhang, W.; Song, J.-K.; Li, L.; Du, G.-H. Quercetin attenuates ischemia reperfusion injury by protecting the blood-brain barrier through Sirt1 in MCAO rats. *J. Asian Nat. Prod. Res.* **2022**, *24*, 278–289. [CrossRef]
39. Zhu, H.; Hu, S.; Li, Y.; Sun, Y.; Xiong, X.; Hu, X.; Chen, J.; Qiu, S. Interleukins and Ischemic Stroke. *Front. Immunol.* **2022**, *13*, 828447. [CrossRef]
40. Chen, J.; Li, Y.; Wang, L.; Zhang, Z.; Lu, D.; Lu, M.; Chopp, M. Therapeutic benefit of intravenous administration of bone marrow stromal cells after cerebral ischemia in rats. *Stroke* **2001**, *32*, 1005–1011. [CrossRef]
41. Zhang, R.; Wang, Y.; Zhang, L.; Zhang, Z.; Tsang, W.; Lu, M.; Zhang, L.; Chopp, M. Sildenafil (Viagra) induces neurogenesis and promotes functional recovery after stroke in rats. *Stroke* **2002**, *33*, 2675–2680. [CrossRef] [PubMed]

pharmaceuticals

MDPI

Article

Therapeutic Potential of *Gynostemma pentaphyllum* (Thunb.) Makino Against COVID-19 Identified Through Network Pharmacology

Min Ho Kim [1,2,†], Jin Ah Won [1,†], Jun Sang Yu [1,3], Su Min Kim [1], Dong Keun Lee [4], Xiang-Lan Piao [5,*] and Hye Hyun Yoo [1,*]

1 Pharmacomicrobiomics Research Center, College of Pharmacy, Hanyang University, Ansan 15588, Republic of Korea; mhk2066@hanyang.ac.kr (M.H.K.); jennywon97@hanyang.ac.kr (J.A.W.); yujs0804@jejunu.ac.kr (J.S.Y.); ksm990201@naver.com (S.M.K.)
2 New Drug Development Center, Daegu-Gyeongbuk Medical Innovation Foundation, Daegu 41061, Republic of Korea
3 College of Pharmacy, Jeju National University, Jeju 63243, Republic of Korea
4 GENECT, Konkuk University Campus Town, Seoul 05073, Republic of Korea; pydk42@gmail.com
5 Key Laboratory of Ethnomedicine, Ministry of Education, Minzu University of China, Beijing 100081, China
* Correspondence: xlpiao@muc.edu.cn (X.-L.P.); yoohh@hanyang.ac.kr (H.H.Y.)
† These authors contributed equally to this work.

Abstract: Background/Objectives: The ongoing challenges posed by COVID-19 have highlighted the need for multi-target therapeutic strategies addressing both acute immune responses and systemic complications. *Gynostemma pentaphyllum* (Thunb.) Makino, a traditional herbal medicine rich in flavonoids and saponins, exhibits diverse pharmacological activities, including immunomodulatory and cardiovascular effects. In this study, we investigated the potential of *G. pentaphyllum* as a complementary treatment for COVID-19 using a network pharmacology approach combined with molecular docking analysis. **Methods:** To delve into the therapeutic mechanisms of *G. pentaphyllum*, we identified 59 active compounds and predicted 408 protein targets, of which 19 overlapped with COVID-19-associated genes, including *IL1B, IL6, TNF, ACE*, and *REN*. GO and KEGG enrichment analyses were conducted to determine relevant biological processes and pathways, focusing on cytokine signaling, inflammatory responses, and the renin–angiotensin system. Network analyses evaluated interactions of flavonoids and triterpenoid saponins with immunological, inflammatory, renin–angiotensin system, and host entry pathways. Molecular docking was performed to validate the binding affinities of key compounds to their predicted targets. **Results:** The compound–target–pathway network revealed class-specific patterns: flavonoids primarily mapped to immuno-inflammatory nodes, whereas triterpenoid saponins were enriched for renin–angiotensin system/host-entry–related targets. Docking energies spanned −6.1 to −11.9 kcal/mol, with six compound–target pairs ≤ −10.0 kcal/mol. Notably, NOS2–rutin (−11.9 kcal/mol), NOS2–gypenoside LI (−11.6 kcal/mol), and ACE–gypenoside LI (−11.3 kcal/mol) showed the strongest affinities. **Conclusions:** These findings provide evidence that *G. pentaphyllum* exerts therapeutic effects through the complementary actions of flavonoid and saponin components, each modulating distinct molecular pathways. This dual mechanistic potential underscores the value of *G. pentaphyllum* as a versatile therapeutic for COVID-19 therapy.

Keywords: *Gynostemma pentaphyllum*; flavonoids; triterpenoid saponins; network pharmacology; molecular docking; COVID-19

1. Introduction

Coronavirus disease 2019 (COVID-19), caused by the severe acute respiratory syndrome coronavirus 2 (SARS-CoV-2), continues to pose a major threat to global public health [1]. While vaccines and antiviral agents have mitigated the severity of acute infection in many regions, the emergence of viral variants and the growing incidence of post-acute sequelae—collectively referred to as long COVID—highlight the limitations of current therapeutic options [2,3]. Long COVID, characterized by persistent symptoms such as fatigue, cognitive impairment, and inflammation-related disorders, presents a new clinical challenge that requires novel and integrative treatment approaches [4]. In this context, traditional herbal medicine—long used in the management of respiratory and systemic inflammatory conditions—offers a valuable reservoir of bioactive compounds with potential antiviral, anti-inflammatory, and immunomodulatory properties [5].

Gynostemma pentaphyllum (Thunb.) Makino, a widely used herb in East Asian traditional medicine, has been reported to exhibit a broad spectrum of pharmacological activities, including anti-inflammatory, antioxidant, antitumor, hepatoprotective, and immunomodulatory effects [6]. These therapeutic properties are primarily attributed to two major classes of bioactive compounds: flavonoids and saponins [7]. Among these, specific compounds such as quercetin, ombuin, kaempferol, and gypenoside XVII have been shown in previous studies to inhibit pro-inflammatory cytokines, regulate immune responses, and interfere with viral replication pathways—activities that are particularly relevant to the treatment of COVID-19 [8–11]. Based on these characteristics, *G. pentaphyllum* extracts may hold potential as a complementary therapeutic agent against COVID-19. However, to date, no studies have systematically examined the efficacy or underlying mechanisms of *G. pentaphyllum* in this context.

Network pharmacology has emerged as a powerful in silico strategy for investigating the multi-component, multi-target nature of herbal medicines [12]. By integrating bioinformatics tools, chemical-target prediction, disease gene annotation, pathway enrichment analysis, and protein–protein interaction (PPI) networks, network pharmacology enables researchers to comprehensively map the complex interactions between natural compounds and disease-related targets [13]. This approach has been increasingly adopted in natural product research to uncover molecular mechanisms, identify therapeutic targets, and guide rational drug development [14].

Despite extensive pharmacological investigations into *G. pentaphyllum*, prior network-pharmacology studies have predominantly addressed non-viral indications without directly interrogating coronavirus-related processes or the renin–angiotensin system (RAS). As summarized in previous *G. pentaphyllum* network-pharmacology reports, these works mapped *G. pentaphyllum* constituents to PI3K–Akt, NF-κB, MAPK, JAK–STAT, and cancer-associated modules across liver, metabolic, inflammatory, and oncologic settings but did not evaluate COVID-19-specific immune dysregulation. To our knowledge, no in silico systems study has systematically examined *G. pentaphyllum* against COVID-19 pathophysiology using an integrated network-pharmacology-docking workflow.

In this study, we aimed to explore the therapeutic potential of *G. pentaphyllum* extract as a candidate treatment for COVID-19. To support this, we investigated the putative molecular targets and pathways associated with its bioactive compounds using a network pharmacology approach. Furthermore, molecular docking analysis was employed to assess the binding affinities between representative *G. pentaphyllum*-derived compounds and key COVID-19-related target proteins, thereby providing mechanistic insights into its possible mode of action. Through this integrative approach, we aim to provide a scientific rationale for the potential development of *G. pentaphyllum* extract as a complementary therapeutic agent for COVID-19.

2. Results

2.1. Network Pharmacology Analysis

To investigate the potential therapeutic mechanisms of *G. pentaphyllum* in the treatment of COVID-19, we performed a network pharmacology analysis comprising compound screening, target prediction, disease-related gene identification, and network construction (Figure 1). A total of 59 active compounds were initially identified from *G. pentaphyllum* using the KNApSAcK and PubChem databases. Oral bioavailability and drug-likeness of these compounds were calculated using the SwissADME platform (Table S3). From these compounds, 408 putative protein targets were predicted. In parallel, 143 COVID-19-related targets were retrieved from the MalaCards database, which aggregates disease-related genes from multiple biomedical sources. A set of 19 overlapping targets between *G. pentaphyllum*-derived compounds and COVID-19-associated genes was identified, suggesting potential therapeutic relevance.

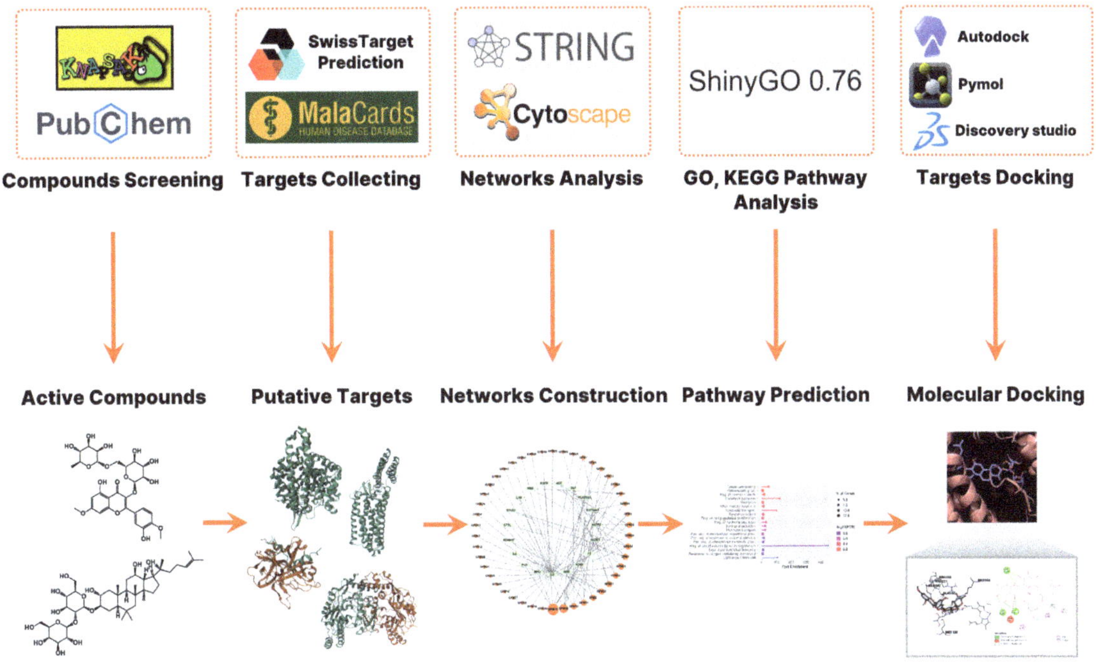

Figure 1. Network pharmacology for identifying mechanisms of *G. pentaphyllum* in treating COVID-19.

To visualize these interactions, we constructed a compound–target (CT) network using Cytoscape 3.10.1 (Figure 2). The network consisted of two types of nodes: orange circular nodes representing active compounds, and green rectangular nodes representing their corresponding protein targets. The size of each compound node reflected the number of targets associated with that compound. Notably, three flavonoids—ombuin, ombuoside, rutin—and three triterpenoids—damulin B, gypensapogenin E, gypenoside LI—demonstrated high degrees of connectivity in the compound–target network. These compounds interacted with multiple key target proteins, suggesting their central roles in mediating the pharmacological effects of *G. pentaphyllum*.

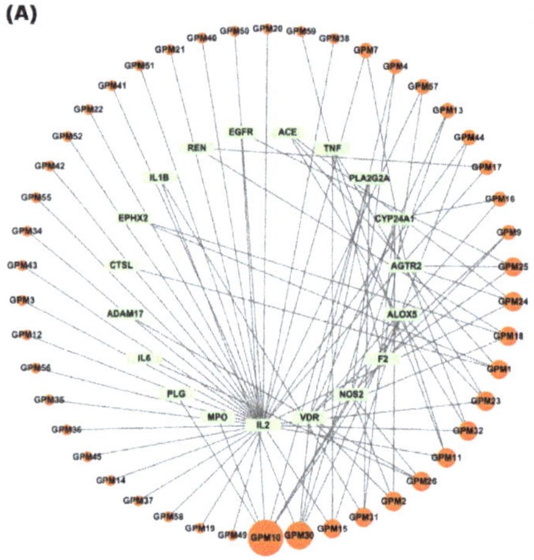

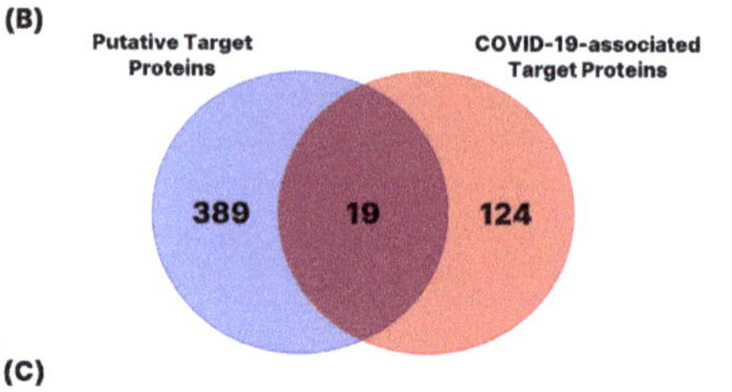

(C)

Code	Compound	Degree	Betweenness	Closeness	Type
GPM10	Ombuin	7	0.2505	0.3092	Flavones
GPM30	Gypensapogenin E	5	0.1364	0.2977	Triterpenoids
GPM24	Damulin B	3	0.0490	0.3216	Triterpenoids
GPM15	Ombuoside	3	0.0807	0.3743	Flavonoid glycosides
GPM23	Rutin	3	0.0807	0.3743	Flavonoid glycosides
GPM32	Gypenoside LI	3	0.04901	0.3216	Triterpenoids

Figure 2. Network pharmacology-based identification of candidate targets and active components of *G. pentaphyllum* against COVID-19. (**A**) Construction of Compound-Target network. Different active compounds (orange circular nodes) are displayed around the periphery, with node size reflecting the number of predicted targets. Putative target proteins (green rectangular nodes) are positioned inside the circle defined by the active compounds. (**B**) Venn diagram showed the overlap between the putative target proteins of *G. pentaphyllum* and COVID-19-associated targets. (**C**) Major active compounds of *G. pentaphyllum* related to COVID-19.

2.2. Protein–Protein Interaction

To further investigate the biological relevance of the 19 overlapping targets between *G. pentaphyllum* compounds and COVID-19-associated genes, a protein–protein interaction (PPI) network was constructed using the STRING database and visualized through Cytoscape 3.10.1 (Figure 3). The resulting network revealed several highly connected hub proteins, including IL1B, IL6, TNF, ACE, and REN, which are central regulators of inflammatory and cardiovascular pathways known to play key roles in COVID-19 pathogenesis. The size of each node represented its degree of connectivity, with IL6 and TNF exhibiting the highest degrees, highlighting their importance within the interaction network.

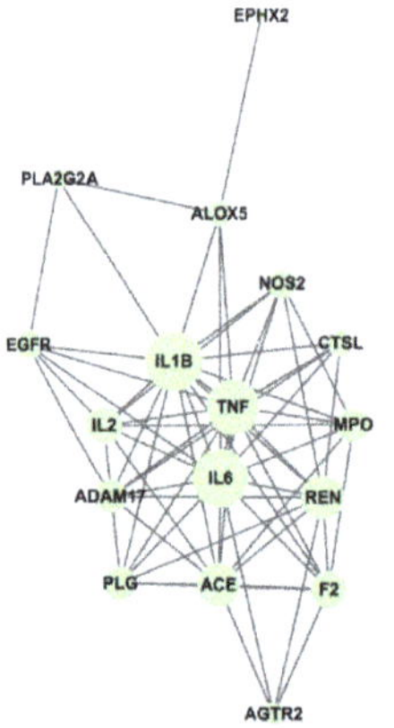

Target	Degree
IL1B	14
IL6	14
TNF	13
ACE	10
REN	10
IL2	8
F2	8

Figure 3. The Protein–Protein Interaction (PPI) network. The top 17 intersecting target proteins were shown in circular nodes with different sizes. The size of the nodes expressed the interaction degree on the network.

2.3. GO and KEGG Pathway Enrichment Analysis

To elucidate the biological functions and signaling pathways associated with the 19 overlapping targets between *G. pentaphyllum* compounds and COVID-19-related genes, we performed Gene Ontology (GO) and Kyoto Encyclopedia of Genes and Genomes (KEGG) pathway enrichment analyses using the ShinyGO 0.77 platform (Figure 4).

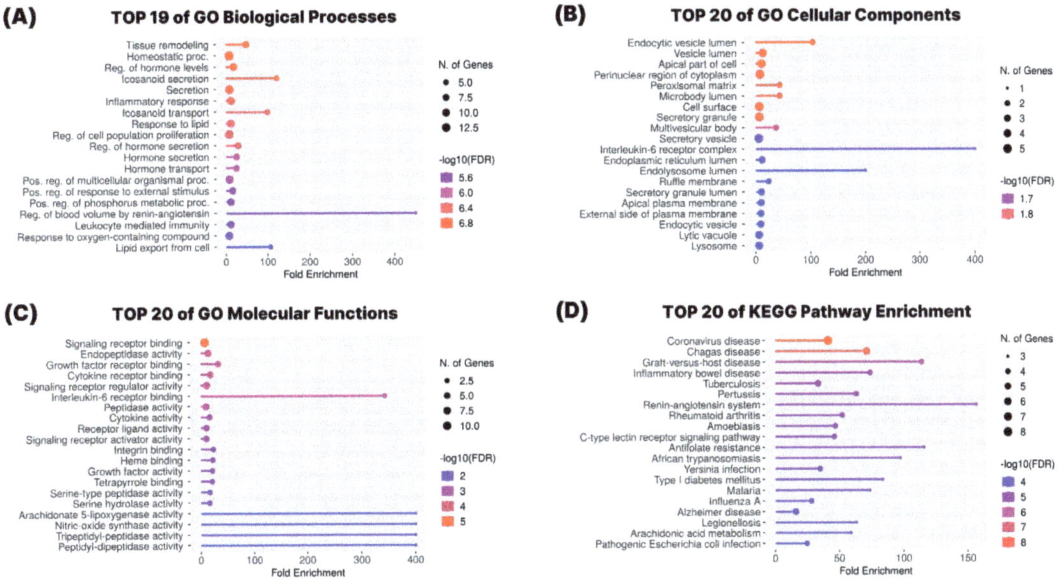

Figure 4. GO and KEGG Pathway Enrichment Analysis. (**A**) Biological process, (**B**) cellular components, and (**C**) molecular functions of Gene Ontology (GO) analysis. (**D**) Kyoto Encyclopedia of Genes and Genomes (KEGG) pathway enrichment analysis.

The GO enrichment analysis was conducted across three functional categories: biological process (BP), cellular component (CC), and molecular function (MF). In the biological process category (Figure 4A), the targets were mainly associated with immune and inflammatory regulation, with significant enrichment in terms such as inflammatory response, regulation of cytokine production, response to lipopolysaccharide, and immune effector process. These findings indicate that *G. pentaphyllum*-related targets play crucial roles in modulating host defense mechanisms relevant to COVID-19. In the cellular component category (Figure 4B), enriched terms included external side of plasma membrane, membrane raft, and secretory granule membrane, suggesting that many of these targets are membrane-associated or secreted proteins, consistent with their involvement in cytokine signaling and immune cell interactions. Regarding molecular function (Figure 4C), the most prominent terms included cytokine activity, receptor binding, and enzyme binding, reinforcing the targets' involvement in immune signaling pathways.

KEGG pathway enrichment analysis further revealed that the 19 targets are significantly involved in pathways central to COVID-19 pathology (Figure 4D). These included the cytokine–cytokine receptor interaction, TNF signaling pathway, IL-17 signaling pathway, NF-κB signaling pathway, and the renin–angiotensin system. These pathways are closely associated with hyperinflammation, cytokine storm, and cardiovascular complications frequently observed in severe COVID-19 cases. The enrichment of these pathways suggests that *G. pentaphyllum* may act through the modulation of both inflammatory signaling and the renin–angiotensin axis to exert potential therapeutic effects.

2.4. Compound–Target–Pathway (CTP) Network

To further elucidate the mechanistic landscape of *G. pentaphyllum*, a compound–target–pathway (CTP) network was constructed, as illustrated in Figure 5. This network visually demonstrates the multi-level interactions among active compounds, their predicted protein targets, and the associated biological pathways. Notably, the bioactive compounds identified from *G. pentaphyllum* clustered into two major phytochemical classes: flavonoids and triterpenoids. These two classes showed distinct interaction profiles within the network, suggesting different modes of action. Flavonoid-type compounds (e.g., GPM10, GPM15, GPM23) were predominantly associated with inflammation-related targets such as TNF, NOS2, EGFR, and IL2, and enriched in signaling pathways related to immune modulation and infection control, including cytokine signaling, tuberculosis, and influenza pathways. In contrast, triterpenoid-type compounds (e.g., GPM24, GPM30, GPM32) interacted with a separate subset of targets including ACE, AGTR2, VDR, and were more involved in cardiovascular and renin–angiotensin system-related pathways, as well as metabolic and viral disease modules. This division of target specificity highlights a dual mechanism of action: flavonoids may primarily exert immunomodulatory and anti-inflammatory effects, while triterpenoids appear to contribute to cardiovascular regulation and viral entry interference. The presence of both compound classes in *G. pentaphyllum* underscores its potential as a broad-spectrum therapeutic candidate that targets COVID-19 pathophysiology through complementary mechanisms.

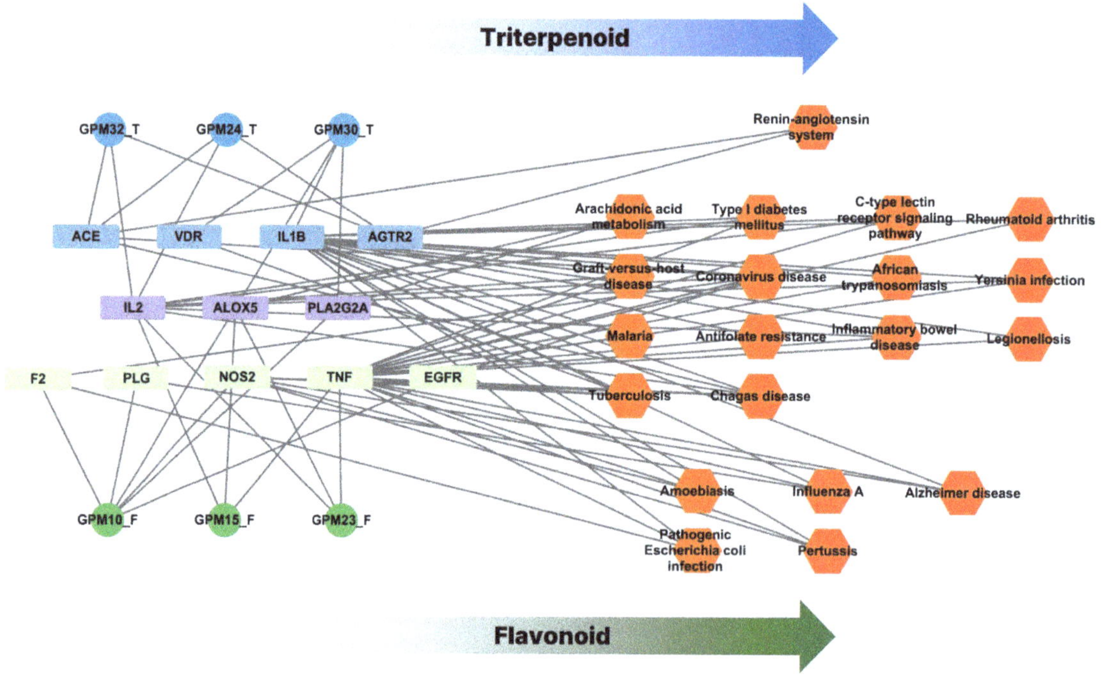

Figure 5. The compound-target-pathway (CTP) network. The compound–target–pathway (CTP) network constructed for *G. pentaphyllum*. Circular nodes represent active compounds, rectangular nodes represent predicted protein targets, and hexagonal nodes represent KEGG pathways. Targets predominantly linked to triterpenoid compounds are shown in blue, flavonoid-related targets in green, and shared targets in purple.

2.5. Molecular Docking Analysis

To validate the interaction between bioactive compounds of *G. pentaphyllum* and key protein targets related to COVID-19, molecular docking simulations were performed against 12 representative host or viral proteins. Docking results for seven major compounds are summarized in Table 1. Docking simulations revealed binding energies ranging from −6.1 to −11.9 kcal/mol, supporting that the majority of key compounds and protein targets identified through network pharmacology exhibit substantial mutual binding potential relevant to COVID-19 pathophysiology. The docking protocol was validated, as the heavy-atom root-mean-square deviation (RMSD) values between the redocked and crystallographic poses were ≤2.0 Å (or within a comparable range).

Table 1. Docking affinities between major compounds and targets associated with active compounds of *G. pentaphyllum* and COVID-19. All docking simulations were performed in duplicate (n = 2), and RMSD values between runs were calculated.

		Targets (kcal/mol) [RMSD] (Å)														
Type	Compounds (Code)	ACE [0.730]	AGTR2 [0.127]	ALOX5 [1.902]	EGFR [0.925]	F2 [0.919]	IL1B [0.885]	IL2 [2.137]	NOS2 [1.377]	PLA2G2A [N.C.]	PLG [0.599]	TNF [2.298]	VDR [0.790]	Mpro [2.173]	RdRp [0.340]	Spike Protein [0.356]
Triterpenoid	Damulin B (GPM24)	−10.3 ± 0.0	−9.5 ± 0.5	−9.2 ± 0.0	−8.2 ± 0.2	−7.9 ± 0.1	−6.5 ± 0.1	−6.5 ± 0.5	−8.8 ± 0.1	−6.5 ± 0.2	−6.1 ± 0.2	−8.1 ± 0.0	−7.6 ± 0.0	−7.3 ± 0.0	−11.4 ± 0.0	−6.8 ± 0.6
	Gypenoside LI (GPM32)	−10.2 ± 0.0	−9.5 ± 0.0	−9.5 ± 0.0	−8.1 ± 0.0	−7.7 ± 0.1	−6.4 ± 0.0	−6.5 ± 0.0	−9.5 ± 0.0	−6.8 ± 0.1	−6.4 ± 0.1	−7.7 ± 0.1	−7.3 ± 0.1	−7.4 ± 0.1	−10.7 ± 0.0	−6.9 ± 0.4
	Gypensapogenin E (GPM30)	−10.0 ± 0.0	−9.9 ± 0.0	−10.6 ± 0.8	−8.3 ± 0.0	−7.8 ± 0.0	−6.6 ± 0.0	−7.5 ± 0.3	−8.7 ± 0.1	−7.0 ± 0.0	−6.6 ± 0.2	−8.7 ± 0.3	−7.6 ± 0.3	−8.0 ± 0.4	−9.5 ± 0.1	−7.2 ± 0.1
Flavonoid	Ombuin (GPM10)	−8.5 ± 0.0	−7.9 ± 0.1	−8.7 ± 0.0	−8.0 ± 0.0	−7.3 ± 0.0	−8.2 ± 0.0	−6.1 ± 0.0	−8.2 ± 0.0	−6.4 ± 0.0	−6.3 ± 0.0	−7.5 ± 0.0	−8.6 ± 0.0	−7.0 ± 0.0	−8.4 ± 0.0	−6.7 ± 0.1
	Ombuoside (GPM15)	−10.1 ± 0.0	−9.3 ± 0.1	−9.5 ± 0.0	−8.1 ± 0.0	−8.6 ± 0.0	−6.5 ± 0.0	−6.4 ± 0.4	−9.7 ± 0.0	−6.5 ± 0.3	−7.2 ± 0.1	−8.2 ± 0.0	−7.5 ± 0.0	−7.7 ± 0	−10.4 ± 0.0	−7.3 ± 0.1
	Rutin (GPM23)	−9.8 ± 0.0	−10.0 ± 0.0	−9.3 ± 0.1	−9.2 ± 0.0	−9.0 ± 0	−7.8 ± 0.0	−6.8 ± 0.0	−9.8 ± 0.0	−7.2 ± 0.0	−6.5 ± 0.5	−7.8 ± 0.3	−7.9 ± 0.1	−7.7 ± 0.1	−10.7 ± 0.0	−7.7 ± 0.0
Reference	Lisinopril (ACE inhibitor)	−7.7 ± 0.1	−7.1 ± 0.2	−7.2 ± 0.1	−6.4 ± 0.0	−6.7 ± 0.1	−6.3 ± 0.0	−5.5 ± 0.0	−7.8 ± 0.3	−5.8 ± 0.1	−5.1 ± 0.4	−7.4 ± 0.1	−6.8 ± 1.0	−6.0 ± 0.1	−7.6 ± 0.3	−5.9 ± 0.1
	Remdesivir (RdRp inhibitor)	−6.0 ± 0.0	−5.2 ± 0.0	−6.2 ± 0.1	−5.1 ± 0.0	−5.6 ± 0.3	−5.4 ± 0.1	−4.7 ± 0.2	−6.3 ± 0.1	−4.8 ± 0.0	−5.1 ± 0.1	−5.1 ± 0.0	−6.2 ± 0.2	−5.7 ± 0.0	−6.7 ± 0.0	−5.1 ± 0.1

Notably, flavonoid-type compounds such as rutin (GPM23), ombuin (GPM10), and ombuoside (GPM15) generally exhibited strong affinities toward immune-related targets including NOS2, PLG, and TNF, with docking scores often exceeding −9.0 kcal/mol. On the other hand, triterpenoid-type compounds such as gypensapogenin E (GPM30), damulin B (GPM24), and gypenoside LI (GPM32) preferentially targeted host cell entry and cardiovascular-related proteins such as ACE, AGTR2, and VDR, with several docking scores below −10.0 kcal/mol.

To visually represent the docking interactions, representative binding models of ombuoside (GPM15, flavonoid) and gypenoside LI (GPM32, triterpenoid) were selected and illustrated. As shown in Figure 6A, ombuoside demonstrated a strong binding affinity to NOS2 (−11.0 kcal/mol), a key enzyme in pro-inflammatory signaling. The docking pose revealed multiple conventional hydrogen bonds and π–π stacking interactions with residues such as GLY202, CYS200, TYR489, and TRP194. These interactions stabilize the ligand within the active site pocket, supporting its potential role in immunomodulation and inflammation suppression. Docking and inhibition studies on diverse iNOS ligands have repeatedly shown that Cys200, Gly202, Trp194 and Tyr489 make key contacts stabilizing inhibitors in the substrate access channel and are associated with reduced NO production [15–17]. Thus, the engagement of these residues by ombuoside supports a plausible mechanism in which tight binding in the heme-proximal pocket hinders L-arginine oxidation and thereby attenuates NO-mediated inflammatory responses. Figure 6B presents the docking of gypenoside LI with ACE (−11.3 kcal/mol), a central component of the renin–

angiotensin system and viral entry mechanism. The triterpenoid scaffold of gypenoside LI formed extensive hydrogen bonds and hydrophobic contacts with residues such as ARG124, PHE570, MET223, and PRO407, suggesting interference with ACE activity and possible inhibition of SARS-CoV-2 spike protein binding. Met223 and Phe570 belong to the S1/S2 subsites that line the substrate-binding channel around the catalytic HEXXH zinc-binding motif, whereas Arg124 and Pro407 are positioned along the neighboring substrate-access channel; residues in these regions are known to govern the binding and potency of ACE inhibitors [18–21]. In particular, Pro407 lies in the hinge region between the two subdomains, where ligand-induced interactions can modulate active-site geometry and catalytic efficiency [22], while Phe570 provides an aromatic platform that frequently participates in π–π/π–alkyl contacts with high-affinity inhibitors [19,21]. Therefore, the observed interactions of gypenoside LI with these functionally important residues support its potential to interfere with ACE activity and reduce downstream angiotensin II–mediated signaling.

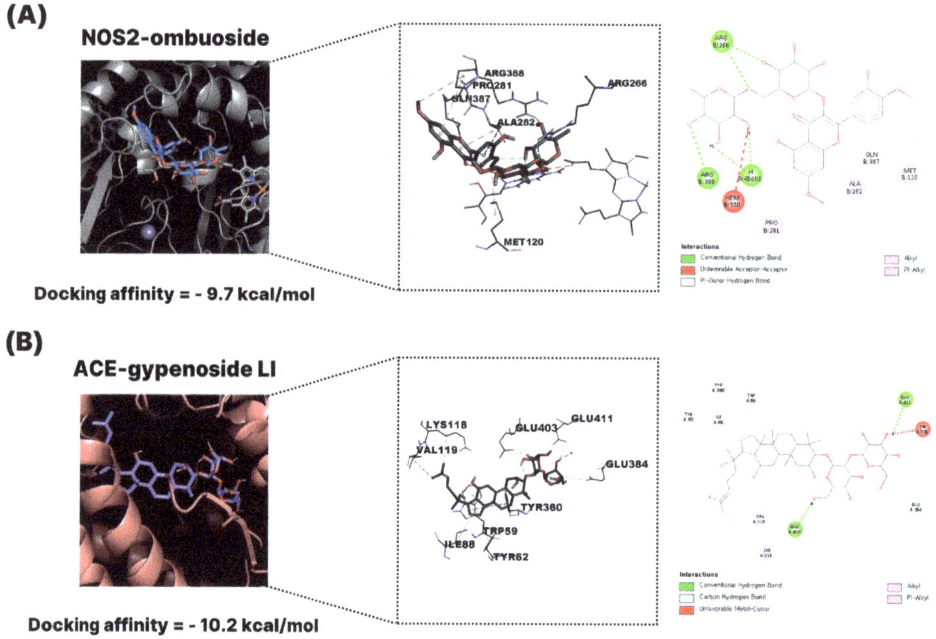

Figure 6. Representative molecular docking diagrams of *G. pentaphyllum* active compounds and key targets associated with COVID-19 using AutoDock Vina (version 1.1.2). (**A**) Docking model of ombuoside (GPM15, flavonoid) with NOS2. (**B**) Docking model of gypenoside LI (GPM32, triterpenoid) with ACE. The visualization includes the overall protein–ligand complex, binding site interactions (3D), and 2D interaction mapping.

2.6. Three-Dimensional Quantitative Structure-Activity Relationship (3D-QSAR) Analysis

To further validate the predictive accuracy of the molecular docking results, a three-dimensional quantitative structure-activity relationship (3D-QSAR) study was conducted using 24 triterpenoids with known ACE inhibitory activities. All molecules were successfully aligned using the O3A algorithm with coherent aglycone scaffold superposition (Figure S1A). The CoMFA model with three principal components (PC = 3) achieved $r^2 = 0.943$ on the training set and $q^2 = 0.582$ (SDEP = 0.463) under leave-one-out cross-validation (Figure S1B). Y-scrambling validation with 100 permutations yielded a q^2 distribution centered at -0.389 (maximum = 0.299), with 0 out of 100 permutations exceeding the observed q^2 value ($p < 0.01$), confirming the statistical robustness of the model (Figure S1C). Using this validated model, gypenoside LI was predicted to have $pIC_{50} = 4.98$ ($IC_{50} \approx 10.5$ μM). The CoMFA stdev × coeff contour maps revealed key structural features associated with ACE inhibitory activity (Figure S1D). In the steric field, green contours (favorable bulk regions) were predominantly located near the aglycone lateral face and central ring junction, while yellow contours (unfavorable bulk regions) flanked the sugar termini. In the electrostatic field, blue contours (regions where positive potential is favorable) aligned with glycosidic oxygen atoms, whereas red contours (regions where negative potential is favorable) appeared in opposing positions, suggesting a polarized binding environment. When gypenoside LI was overlaid onto these contour maps, its aglycone core occupied green steric regions while its hydroxyl-rich sugar chains were positioned near red electrostatic regions, consistent with the predicted moderate-to-good potency.

2.7. Molecular Dynamics (MD) Simulation Analysis

To assess the structural stability of the docked protein-ligand complexes over physiologically relevant timescales, 50 ns molecular dynamics simulations were performed for ACE-gypenoside LI and NOS2-ombuoside complexes. For the ACE-gypenoside LI complex, the protein backbone RMSD stabilized at 0.16–0.22 nm after initial equilibration, while the ligand RMSD plateaued at 0.25–0.30 nm without large fluctuations, indicating a stable binding mode (Figure S2A). RMSF analysis revealed that most residues exhibited low positional fluctuations (<0.15 nm), with elevated fluctuations observed only in flexible loop regions and the C-terminus (Figure S2B). The radius of gyration remained constant at 2.38–2.40 nm throughout the trajectory, confirming that the overall protein structure was preserved (Figure S2C). Similarly, the NOS2-ombuoside complex displayed stable protein backbone dynamics, although the ligand RMSD stabilized at a higher value of 0.7–0.9 nm, suggesting greater conformational flexibility within the binding pocket (Figure S3). MM-GBSA binding free energy calculations yielded $\Delta G\_bind = -32.56 \pm 6.84$ kcal/mol for the ACE-gypenoside LI complex and $\Delta G\_bind = -26.57 \pm 4.90$ kcal/mol for the NOS2-ombuoside complex, both indicating thermodynamically favorable binding (Figures S2 and S3). The ACE complex exhibited approximately 6 kcal/mol stronger binding affinity compared to the NOS2 complex, primarily attributable to more favorable van der Waals interactions (-61.69 vs. -41.47 kcal/mol) and non-polar solvation contributions (-9.20 vs. -4.97 kcal/mol). Binding free energy values converged to stable means after the equilibration phase in both systems.

3. Discussion

This study identified *G. pentaphyllum* as a potential multi-target agent for the treatment of COVID-19. Among the active compounds in *G. pentaphyllum*, ombuin and quercetin were highlighted for their strong associations with key inflammatory and cardiovascular targets. Five core targets—IL1B, IL6, TNF, ACE, and REN—were identified as central to *G. pentaphyllum*'s potential therapeutic action. These targets are critically involved in immune dysregulation and the renin–angiotensin system, both of which are central to COVID-19 pathophysiology [23,24]. Enrichment analyses confirmed that *G. pentaphyllum*'s predicted targets are involved in cytokine signaling and inflammatory pathways. Additionally, molecular docking supported the potential of ombuin to interact strongly with all five targets. Collectively, these findings suggest that *G. pentaphyllum* may exert therapeutic effects in COVID-19 through coordinated modulation of immune and cardiovascular pathways. Previous network pharmacology studies on *G. pentaphyllum* have primarily focused on metabolic, inflammatory, and oncological diseases [25–59], and, to date, coronavirus-related signaling or RAS-associated pathways have not been analyzed. In particular, our analysis newly identified targets such as NOS2, F2, and REN, which are mechanistically relevant to COVID-19 pathogenesis (Table 2).

Table 2. KEGG pathways of diseases associated with *G. pentaphyllum* analyzed through network pharmacology.

Category	Disease	Pathways	Key Target	Refs.
Liver	NAFLD and NASH	Apoptosis; Non-alcoholic fatty liver disease; PI3K-Akt signaling pathway; Lipid and atherosclerosis	AKT1, GSK3B	[25]
	Hepatic fibrosis	Proteoglycans in cancer; PI3K–Akt signaling pathway; EGFR tyrosine kinase inhibitor resistance; EGFR signaling pathway	AKT1, IL6, STAT3, EGFR	[26,27]
	Liver injury	Apoptosis signaling pathway	STAT3, HIF1A, PTGS2, EGFR, PPARG, MTOR, AKT1, ESR1, TNF	[28]
	Metabolism-associated fatty liver disease	NF-κB signaling pathway; PI3K-Akt signaling pathway; TNF signaling pathway; HIF-1 signaling pathway	TNF, IL6, PTGS2, TP53, CCL2, VEGFA	[29]
	Non-alcoholic fatty liver disease	HIF-1 signaling pathway; AGE-RAGE signaling pathway in diabetic complications; Chagas disease; Beta-oxidation pathway	IL6, PTGS2, NFKB1, CDK6, SERPINE1, ADRB2, PCNA, TOP2A, TYMS, PPARA	[30,31]
Heart	Heart failure	PI3K/Akt signaling pathway; MAPK signaling pathway; Ras signaling pathway	MAPK, EGFR, PI3KCA, MCL1	[32]
Lung	Non-small-cell lung cancer	Chemical carcinogenesis receptor activation; Lipid and atherosclerosis; Human cytomegalovirus infection; Pyrimidine metabolism; Pantothenate and CoA biosynthesis	MMP9, STAT3, TYMS, MYC, ESR1, HIF1A	[33,34]
	Acute lung injury	TNF-α signaling pathway; NF-κB signaling pathway	CXCL2, CXCL1, CXCL10, CCL2, TNFAIP3, SOCS3, IFIT2, TLR2, IL1, IL6, IRF7,	[35]
	Lung cancer	MAPK14/STAT3 signaling pathway	STAT3, MAPK14, EGFR, TYMS	[36]
Brain/nervous system	Alzheimer's disease	Amoebiasis; African trypanosomiasis; Cytokine-cytokine receptor interaction	EGFR, IL1B, IL6, NOS3, PON1	[37]
	Depression	HIF-1 signaling pathway; PI3K-Akt signaling pathway; TNF signaling pathway	SIRT1	[38]
	Glioma	EGFR tyrosine kinase inhibitor resistance; Prolactin signaling pathway; VEGF signaling pathway	STAT3, HSP90AA1, IL6, ESR1, PIK3CA, MTOR, PTPN11, MAPK3, BCL2L1, PTGS2	[39]
Cancer	Breast cancer	PI3K-Akt signaling pathway; Breast cancer pathway; EGFR tyrosine kinase inhibitor resistance	ALB, EGFR, ESR1, AR, PGR, HSP90AA1	[40]
	Osteosarcoma	PI3K-Akt signaling pathway; MAPK signaling pathway; Cellular senescence	CCND1, RELA, TNF	[41]
	Esophageal cancer	PI3K-Akt signaling pathway; MAPK signaling pathway; IL-17 signaling pathway	AKT1, TP53, VEGFA	[42]
	Cervical intraepithelial neoplasia	Cancer; Fluid shear stress and atherosclerosis; Lipid and atherosclerosis	IL6, IL1B, TNF, TP53, PTGS2	[43]
	Renal cell carcinoma	Cancer; Prolactin signaling pathway; PI3K-Akt signaling pathway, Ras/MAPK pathways	VEGFA, PIK3CA, JAK2, CCND1, MAPK3, EGFR, CASP3, HRAS, STAT3, SRSC	[44,45]
	Anaplastic thyroid cancer	Cancer; PI3K-Akt signaling pathway; Proteoglycans in cancer	HSP90AA1, SRC, CASP3	[46]
	Bladder cancer	PI3K-Akt signaling pathway; Pathway in cancer; Proteoglycans in cancer	VEGFA, STAT3, PI3KCA	[47]
	Gastric cancer	Glycerophospholipid metabolism; Alanine, aspartate and glutamate metabolism; Central carbon metabolism in cancer; PD-L1 checkpoint in cancer; T-cell receptor signaling pathway; Th17 differentiation	ALB, EGFR, HSP90AA1, MMP9, ESR1, IGF1, PPARG, ANXA5	[48,49]
	Ophthalmopathy	JAK–STAT signaling pathway	STAT1, STAT3, STAT4	[50]
	Retinitis Pigmentosa	Cancer; HIF-1 signaling pathway; TNF signaling pathway; PI3K-Akt signaling pathway	FGF2, IL6, MAPK14, MMP2, MMP9, SLC2A1	[51]
	Pancreatic cancer	Cancer; AGE-RAGE signaling pathway in diabetic complications; hepatitis C; IL-17 signaling pathway; Platinum drug resistance	MET, SPP1, ADRA1A, HMOX1, CCL2, ICAM1, VCAM1, BCL2, PRKCB, NCF1,	[52]

Table 2. *Cont.*

Category	Disease	Pathways	Key Target	Refs.
Metabolic/ Endocrine	Type II Diabetes	Insulin resistance; PI3K-Akt signaling pathway; FOXO signaling pathway	STAT3, PIK3CA, AKT1, EGFR, VEGFA, INSR	[53]
	Hyperlipidemia	Lipid metabolism and atherosclerosis; TNF signaling pathway; PI3K-Akt signaling pathway	NCOA2, NR3C2, PGR, PPARG, IL6, PPARG, VEGFA	[54]
	Diabetic cataracts	AGE-RAGE signaling pathway in diabetic complications; Fluid shear stress and atherosclerosis; Pathways in cancer	IL6, IL1B, TNF, CASP3, MMP9, AKT1, TGFB1, HIF1A, PTGS2, JUN	[55]
	Glucose metabolic disorders	AGE-RAGE signaling pathway	SRC, PIK3CA, HRAS, AKT1	[56]
	Obesity	AGE-RAGE signaling pathway; glycerolipid metabolism; lipid and atherosclerosis metabolism; Cholesterol metabolism	HMGCR, ACE, LIPC, LIPG, PPARA, PPARD, PPARG	[57]
Immune/ Inflammatory	Acute Pharyngitis	Cancer; PI3K-Akt signaling pathway; JAK–STAT signaling pathway	EGFR, STAT3, MAPK3, SRC, AKT1	[58]
	Diarrhea	Cancer; PI3K-Akt pathway; MAPK pathway	AKT1, STAT3, SRC, ESR1, EGFR, HSP90AA1	[59]
Respiratory system	COVID-19	Coronavirus disease; renin–angiotensin system	NOS2, F2, REN *, IL1B, IL6, TNF, ACE, EGFR	This study

* Underlined targets indicate those newly identified in the present study.

Among the 19 intersecting targets identified between *G. pentaphyllum* compounds and COVID-19-associated genes, several key nodes—*IL1B, IL6, TNF, ACE,* and *REN*—emerged as central in both the protein–protein interaction and compound–target networks. These targets are well-recognized mediators in COVID-19 pathophysiology [60]. *IL1B, IL6,* and *TNF* are pro-inflammatory cytokines that contribute to the cytokine storm observed in severe COVID-19 cases, leading to acute respiratory distress and systemic inflammation [23]. On the other hand, *ACE* (angiotensin-converting enzyme) and *REN* (renin) are components of the renin–angiotensin system (RAS), which plays a dual role in both viral entry and vascular homeostasis [24,61]. SARS-CoV-2 is known to use *ACE2* as a receptor, and dysregulation of the RAS has been linked to increased disease severity [62]. The convergence of these two mechanistic axes—cytokine regulation and RAS modulation—supports the rationale for developing *G. pentaphyllum* as a multi-target therapeutic candidate for COVID-19.

An important feature of *G. pentaphyllum* is its distinctive phytochemical profile, comprising both flavonoids and triterpenoid saponins—two classes of compounds that are rarely co-enriched in a single medicinal plant [10]. In this study, flavonoids and triterpenoid saponins emerged as the representative active compounds based on network topology and docking affinity. These two compound types exhibited clearly differentiated target profiles and functional pathways. Flavonoids were primarily associated with immunological targets (e.g., *NOS2, TNF, IL2*), suggesting roles in anti-inflammatory and cytokine-modulating activities [63]. In contrast, triterpenoids interacted more strongly with targets related to the renin–angiotensin system (e.g., *ACE, AGTR2*), implicating its potential in regulating vascular homeostasis and interfering with viral entry processes [64]. This dual engagement of immune and cardiovascular axes supports a multi-faceted pharmacological action, whereby *G. pentaphyllum* may simultaneously modulate systemic inflammation and protect vascular integrity—two hallmarks of COVID-19 severity [65]. The presence of both compound types within a single extract positions *G. pentaphyllum* as a unique candidate for broad-spectrum antiviral intervention. However, the therapeutic relevance of these compounds is contingent upon their actual concentrations in *G. pentaphyllum* preparations and their bioavailability in vivo. A summary of available quantitative data on major phytochemical components and published pharmacokinetic profiles is provided in Supplementary Information to support further dose-feasibility assessment [66–80] (Tables S1 and S2). Additionally, the co-occurrence of flavonoids and triterpenoids in *G. pentaphyllum* may provide synergistic therapeutic benefits, as recent studies have demonstrated that these phytochemical classes can produce enhanced anti-inflammatory and antimicrobial effects when combined [64,81].

While this study focused on the acute phase of SARS-CoV-2 infection, the identified pharmacological actions of *G. pentaphyllum* may also have relevance for post-acute sequelae of COVID-19, often referred to as long COVID. Persistent inflammation, endothelial dysfunction, and renin–angiotensin system imbalance are key features shared between acute COVID-19 and long-term complications [2]. Persistent endothelial dysfunction and elevated inflammatory markers (IL-6, TNF-α) have been documented in long COVID patients for at least 6 months post-infection [82,83]. Importantly, natural polyphenol-rich compounds have shown clinical efficacy in reducing these inflammatory biomarkers and improving vascular function in post-COVID patients [84–86]. The dual-targeting capacity of *G. pentaphyllum*, via flavonoid-mediated cytokine regulation and triterpenoid-mediated vascular and hormonal modulation, offers a potentially valuable therapeutic strategy for addressing both acute symptoms and longer-term pathological changes. Additionally, the multi-target nature of *G. pentaphyllum* could prove beneficial in the face of emerging SARS-CoV-2 variants or related respiratory viral infections, where treatment approaches that act on host-based pathways rather than viral proteins may retain efficacy [87]. These findings support further preclinical validation and provide a rationale for considering *G. pentaphyllum* in broader antiviral and immunoregulatory contexts.

The reliability of our molecular docking predictions was further supported by complementary in silico validation approaches. 3D-QSAR analysis of 24 triterpenoid saponins demonstrated robust predictive performance ($q^2 = 0.58$, $r^2 = 0.94$), with gypenoside LI occupying sterically and electrostatically favorable regions around the ACE active site, consistent with strong inhibitory activity (Figure S1 and Table S4). Additionally, 100 ns MD simulations demonstrated stable protein-ligand interactions for both ACE–gypenoside LI and NOS2–ombuoside complexes, with minimal conformational drift (protein RMSD < 0.2 nm, ligand RMSD < 0.15 nm). MM-GBSA free energy calculations confirmed thermodynamically favorable binding throughout the trajectory, with ΔG_bind values of -32.6 ± 6.8 kcal/mol for ACE–gypenoside LI and -26.6 ± 4.9 kcal/mol for NOS2–ombuoside (Figures S2 and S3). These multi-layered computational validations strengthen confidence in the predicted interactions as plausible therapeutic targets worthy of experimental validation.

Despite the promising findings, this study has several limitations. First, all predictions were derived from in silico analyses, including network pharmacology and molecular docking, without experimental validation. Although these computational methods provide valuable insights into compound–target interactions and pathway associations, their predictions must be interpreted with caution until confirmed by in vitro and in vivo studies and supported by gene or protein expression analyses to verify coordinated modulation of immune and cardiovascular signaling. Second, the pharmacokinetics, bioavailability, and synergistic interactions of the active compounds within the complex *G. pentaphyllum* extract remain to be experimentally characterized, and the therapeutic feasibility in relation to effective dose ranges has not been evaluated. Moreover, variability in extraction solvents and plant parts across previous studies may influence phytochemical composition and affect translational relevance. Third, the study focused on molecular targets broadly associated with COVID-19 but did not distinguish between different clinical stages or viral variants, which may involve distinct pathological processes. Therefore, direct experimental evidence confirming the COVID-19-specific relevance of the identified targets is still needed. Future research should focus on experimental validation in relevant cellular and animal models, and assess the therapeutic efficacy of *G. pentaphyllum* in both acute and long-term manifestations of COVID-19 [88]. These efforts will be essential for translating computational predictions into clinically meaningful outcomes.

4. Materials and Methods

4.1. Screening for Active Compounds, Putative Target Proteins and COVID-19 Associated Genes

In this study, the active compounds of *G. pentaphyllum* Makino and their putative target proteins were retrieved from the KNApSAcK and PubChem databases [89]. To identify the chemical constituents of the herb, the keyword "*Gynostemma pentaphyllum*" was used in the KNApSAcK search interface, which serves as a unique repository encompassing a wide range of medicinal plants and their bioactive components. Putative target proteins for each active compound were predicted using the SwissTargetPrediction web tool (http://www.swisstargetprediction.ch/, accessed on 2 February 2024) [90], which utilizes the SMILES notation of chemical structures to estimate target affinity. Predicted targets with a probability score of zero were excluded from further analysis. Genes associated with COVID-19 were obtained from the MalaCards database (https://www.malacards.org/, accessed on 22 March 2024), a comprehensive disease-centric resource modeled after the GeneCards platform [91]. The keywords employed for gene retrieval included: "COVID-19," "Severe COVID-19," "Severe Acute Respiratory Syndrome," "Critical COVID-19," "Adult Respiratory Distress Syndrome," and "Long COVID."

4.2. Network Construction

The overlapping targets were identified by intersecting putative compound-related target proteins with COVID-19-associated genes. These common targets were considered potential therapeutic targets for COVID-19. The compound–target interaction network was visualized using Cytoscape (version 3.10.1) [92], and key bioactive compounds were identified based on network topology parameters, such as degree, betweenness, and closeness centrality. Additionally, a protein–protein interaction (PPI) network of the common targets was identified using the STRING web tool (https://string-db.org/, accessed on 29 March 2024) and filtered with an interaction score of less than 0.5 [92]. Targets were prioritized based on their degree values, which indicate their relative importance within the network.

4.3. Gene Ontology (GO) Analysis and Kyoto Encyclopedia of Genes and Genomes (KEGG) Pathway Enrichment Analysis

To further elucidate the pathogenesis of COVID-19 and clarify the underlying mechanism of action of *G. pentaphyllum*, the intersecting genes were subjected to functional enrichment analysis using ShinyGO web tool (https://bioinformatics.sdstate.edu/go77/, accessed on 30 March 2024) [93]. This analysis included Gene Ontology (GO) enrichment, which encompasses biological processes, cellular components, and molecular functions, as well as Kyoto Encyclopedia of Genes and Genomes (KEGG) pathway enrichment.

4.4. Molecular Docking

Molecular docking studies were performed to evaluate the binding affinity and interaction patterns between the bioactive compounds of *G. pentaphyllum* and their key protein targets associated with COVID-19. SDF files of the compounds were obtained from the PubChem database and converted to PDB files using PyMOL, and subsequently to PDBQT files using AutoDockTools 1.5.7. The grid box size was defined as $60 \times 60 \times 60$ Å for all targets with a grid spacing of 0.375 Å. The x, y, and z coordinates for each protein are summarized in Table S5. It was run at a 'num_modes' of 10 and an 'energy_range' of 4. Energy minimization was performed using ChemBio3D Ultra 12.0 with the MMFF94 force field until the root-mean-square (RMS) gradient reached a value of 0.01 kcal/mol·Å. The compounds without 3D structures were converted using Avogadro2 (version 1.102.1) [94].

The three-dimensional (3D) structure of the major proteins was retrieved from the Protein Data Bank (PDB) with the following PDB IDs: ACE (1O86), AGTR2 (5UNG), ALOX5 (3V99), EGFR (2ITX), F2 (1PPB), IL1β (8C3U), IL2 (1M48), NOS2 (2NSI), PLA2G2A (3U8I), PLG (1CEB), TNF (2AZ5), VDR (1DB1), Mpro (6LU7), RdRp (6M71), and Spike protein (6WPT). Selected proteins had water molecules removed, hydrogen atoms added, and Kollman charges assigned using AutoDockTools [95]. Molecular docking was performed using AutoDock Vina, and the results were visualized using Discovery Studio Client [95]. The docking protocol was validated by re-docking the co-crystallized ligands into their native binding sites, and comparing the resulting poses with the corresponding experimental structures using RMSD analysis calculated with Discovery Studio Client.

4.5. Three-Dimensional Quantitative Structure-Activity Relationship (3D-QSAR)

Twenty-four triterpenoids with known ACE inhibitory activity were collected from literature sources [96], and their IC_{50} values were converted to pIC_{50} ($-\log_{10} IC_{50}$). Three-dimensional structures were generated, energy-minimized using the MMFF94 force field, and aligned to Protopanaxatriol using RDKit's O3A algorithm. Comparative Molecular Field Analysis (CoMFA) was performed using Open3DQSAR v2.3 with a 2.0 Å grid ($23 \times 18 \times 16$ nodes) to calculate steric (Lennard-Jones) and electrostatic (Gasteiger charges) fields. After field processing (cutoff $\pm$ 30, zero level 0.05, sdcut 2.0) and Block Unscaled Weighting, partial least squares (PLS) regression was performed with three principal components (PC = 3) determined by leave-one-out cross-validation (LOO-CV). Model robustness was validated by Y-scrambling (100 permutations). Standard-deviation $\times$ coefficient contour maps were visualized in PyMOL 3.1.6 with green/yellow (steric favorable/unfavorable) and blue/red (electrostatic positive/negative favorable) isosurfaces.

4.6. Molecular Dynamics (MD) Simulation

Molecular dynamics simulations were performed using GROMACS 2025.3 with CUDA support. Two protein-ligand complexes (ACE-Gypenoside LI and NOS2-Ombuoside) were prepared with complete protein coordinates, cofactors (heme and tetrahydrobiopterin for NOS2), and explicit hydrogens. Systems were parameterized using a biomolecular force field, solvated in periodic cubic boxes with explicit water, and neutralized with counterions. After energy minimization (steepest descent with positional restraints) and equilibration (NVT pre-equilibration and restrained thermalization/pressure equilibration), production simulations were conducted for 50 ns using the Verlet cutoff scheme, PME for long-range electrostatics, LINCS constraints for hydrogen bonds, and a 2-fs time step. Binding free energies were estimated using MM-GBSA (gmx_MMPBSA, igb = 5, gbsa = 2) on 200 snapshots from the final 50 ns, calculating gas-phase van der Waals (ΔE_vdW) and electrostatic (ΔE_elec) interactions, as well as polar (ΔG_polar) and non-polar (ΔG_non-polar) solvation contributions.

5. Conclusions

This study demonstrated the potential of *G. pentaphyllum* extract as a complementary therapeutic candidate for COVID-19 through an integrative in silico approach. Through network pharmacology and molecular docking, 59 curated compounds and 19 COVID-19–overlapping targets were identified. Furthermore, we found six flavonoids and triterpenoid saponins as key active compounds, each exhibiting distinct target profiles—flavonoids being primarily linked to immunological and inflammatory pathways (*IL1B, IL6, TNF, NOS2*), and triterpenoids to the renin–angiotensin system and host entry regulation (*ACE, REN, AGTR2*). These dual mechanistic pathways reflect the multi-target nature of the extract and its relevance to COVID-19 pathogenesis. To translate these findings, future studies should validate target engagement experimentally and assess whether representative flavonoid and saponin fractions show complementary or synergistic effects. Establishing exposure–activity relationships through quantitative profiling and pharmacokinetic evaluation will also be essential. Overall, the findings in this study provide a preliminary mechanistic basis that supports a hypothesis for further experimental validation of *G. pentaphyllum* as a multi-target herbal candidate with potential relevance to both acute and persistent manifestations of COVID-19 by modulating immuno-inflammatory signaling and RAS/host-entry–related proteins.

Supplementary Materials: The following supporting information can be downloaded at: https://www.mdpi.com/article/10.3390/ph18121851/s1, Figure S1. Validation of 3D-QSAR CoMFA model and contour analysis for ACE inhibitors. Figure S2. Molecular dynamics simulation validation of ACE-Gypenoside LI complexes. Figure S3. Molecular dynamics simulation validation of NOS2-Ombuoside complexes. Table S1. Content of components determined in *G. pentaphyllum* from literature. Table S2. Pharmacokinetic parameters of *G. pentaphyllum* extracts and major components following oral administration in animal models. Table S3. The oral bioavailability (OB) and drug-likeness (DL) of major components from *G. pentaphyllum* extracts. Table S4. Statistical parameters and computational settings for 3D-QSAR and molecular dynamics validation. Table S5. The grid box centers of target proteins used in molecular docking simulations.

Author Contributions: Conceptualization, J.S.Y., X.-L.P. and H.H.Y.; Methodology, M.H.K., J.A.W. and J.S.Y.; Validation, J.S.Y.; Formal Analysis, M.H.K., J.A.W., S.M.K. and D.K.L.; Investigation, M.H.K., J.A.W. and S.M.K.; Data Curation, M.H.K. and J.A.W.; Writing—Original Draft, M.H.K. and J.A.W.; Writing—Review and Editing, J.A.W., J.S.Y., X.-L.P. and H.H.Y.; Visualization, M.H.K. and J.A.W.; Supervision, X.-L.P. and H.H.Y.; Funding Acquisition, H.H.Y. All authors have read and agreed to the published version of the manuscript.

Funding: This research was supported by the National Research Foundation of Korea (NRF) grant funded by the Korea government (MSIT) (RS-2023-00217123).

Institutional Review Board Statement: Not applicable.

Informed Consent Statement: Not applicable.

Data Availability Statement: The original contributions presented in this study are included in the article/Supplementary Material. Further inquiries can be directed to the corresponding authors.

Conflicts of Interest: The authors declare no conflicts of interest.

References

1. Davis, H.E.; McCorkell, L.; Vogel, J.M.; Topol, E.J. Long COVID: Major Findings, Mechanisms and Recommendations. *Nat. Rev. Microbiol.* **2023**, *21*, 133–146. [CrossRef] [PubMed]
2. Parotto, M.; Gyöngyösi, M.; Howe, K.; Myatra, S.N.; Ranzani, O.; Shankar-Hari, M.; Herridge, M.S. Post-Acute Sequelae of COVID-19: Understanding and Addressing the Burden of Multisystem Manifestations. *Lancet Respir. Med.* **2023**, *11*, 739–754. [CrossRef]
3. Xie, Y.; Choi, T.; Al-Aly, Z. Postacute Sequelae of SARS-CoV-2 Infection in the Pre-Delta, Delta, and Omicron Eras. *N. Engl. J. Med.* **2024**, *391*, 515–525. [CrossRef]
4. Cai, M.; Xie, Y.; Topol, E.J.; Al-Aly, Z. Three-Year Outcomes of Post-Acute Sequelae of COVID-19. *Nat. Med.* **2024**, *30*, 1564–1573. [CrossRef]
5. Zheng, S.; Xue, T.; Wang, B.; Guo, H.; Liu, Q. Application of Network Pharmacology in the Study of the Mechanism of Action of Traditional Chinese Medicine in the Treatment of COVID-19. *Front. Pharmacol.* **2022**, *13*, 926901. [CrossRef]
6. Ahmed, A.; Saleem, M.A.; Saeed, F.; Afzaal, M.; Imran, A.; Nadeem, M.; Ambreen, S.; Imran, M.; Hussain, M.; Al Jbawi, E. *Gynostemma pentaphyllum* an Immortal Herb with Promising Therapeutic Potential: A Comprehensive Review on Its Phytochemistry and Pharmacological Perspective. *Int. J. Food Prop.* **2023**, *26*, 808–832. [CrossRef]

7. Wang, B.; Li, M.; Gao, H.; Sun, X.; Gao, B.; Zhang, Y.; Yu, L. Chemical Composition of Tetraploid *Gynostemma pentaphyllum* Gypenosides and Their Suppression on Inflammatory Response by NF-κB/MAPKs/AP-1 Signaling Pathways. *Food Sci. Nutr.* **2020**, *8*, 1197–1207. [CrossRef]
8. Zhou, K.; Zhang, Y.; Zhou, Y.; Xu, M.; Yu, S. Production of Gypenoside XVII from Ginsenoside Rb1 by Enzymatic Transformation and Their Anti-Inflammatory Activity In Vitro and In Vivo. *Molecules* **2023**, *28*, 7001. [CrossRef]
9. Saeedi-Boroujeni, A.; Mahmoudian-Sani, M.-R. Anti-Inflammatory Potential of Quercetin in COVID-19 Treatment. *J. Inflamm.* **2021**, *18*, 3. [CrossRef] [PubMed]
10. Li, Y.; Lin, W.; Huang, J.; Xie, Y.; Ma, W. Anti-Cancer Effects of *Gynostemma pentaphyllum* (*Thunb.*) *Makino* (*Jiaogulan*). *Chin. Med.* **2016**, *11*, 43. [CrossRef]
11. Khazdair, M.R.; Anaeigoudari, A.; Agbor, G.A. Anti-Viral and Anti-Inflammatory Effects of Kaempferol and Quercetin and COVID-2019: A Scoping Review. *Asian Pac. J. Trop. Biomed.* **2021**, *11*, 327. [CrossRef]
12. Li, L.; Yang, L.; Yang, L.; He, C.; He, Y.; Chen, L.; Dong, Q.; Zhang, H.; Chen, S.; Li, P. Network Pharmacology: A Bright Guiding Light on the Way to Explore the Personalized Precise Medication of Traditional Chinese Medicine. *Chin. Med.* **2023**, *18*, 146. [CrossRef]
13. Su, W.; Chen, P.; Yang, Z.; Zhong, N.; Ma, Q.; Zeng, X.; Zhang, J.; Wang, Y.; Li, P. Network Pharmacology Integrated Molecular Docking Reveals the Potential of Hypericum Japonicum Thunb. Ex Murray against COVID-19. *Biotechnol. Biotechnol. Equip.* **2021**, *35*, 453–461. [CrossRef]
14. Jain, N.K.; Tailang, M.; Chandrasekaran, B.; Khazaleh, N.; Thangavel, N.; Makeen, H.A.; Albratty, M.; Najmi, A.; Alhazmi, H.A.; Zoghebi, K.; et al. Integrating Network Pharmacology with Molecular Docking to Rationalize the Ethnomedicinal Use of *Alchornea laxiflora* (*Benth.*) Pax & K. Hoffm. for Efficient Treatment of Depression. *Front. Pharmacol.* **2024**, *15*, 1290398. [CrossRef] [PubMed]
15. Arrari, F.; Ortiz-Flores, R.-M.; Lhamyani, S.; Garcia-Fuentes, E.; Jabri, M.-A.; Sebai, H.; Bermudez-Silva, F.-J. Protective Effects of Spirulina Against Lipid Micelles and Lipopolysaccharide-Induced Intestinal Epithelium Disruption in Caco-2 Cells: In Silico Molecular Docking Analysis of Phycocyanobilin. *Nutrients* **2024**, *16*, 4074. [CrossRef]
16. Hussain, M.S.; Azam, F.; Eldarrat, H.A.; Alkskas, I.; Mayoof, J.A.; Dammona, J.M.; Ismail, H.; Ali, M.; Arif, M.; Haque, A. Anti-Inflammatory, Analgesic and Molecular Docking Studies of Lanostanoic Acid 3-*O*-α-D-Glycopyranoside Isolated from *Helichrysum stoechas*. *Arab. J. Chem.* **2020**, *13*, 9196–9206. [CrossRef]
17. Nguyen, N.T.; Dai, V.V.; Meervelt, L.V.; Thao, D.T.; Thong, N.M. 4-(1-Methylamino)Ethylidene-1,5-Disubstituted Pyrrolidine-2,3-Diones: Synthesis, Anti-Inflammatory Effect and in Silico Approaches. *Beilstein J. Org. Chem.* **2025**, *21*, 817–829. [CrossRef] [PubMed]
18. Harrison, C.; Acharya, K.R. ACE for All—A Molecular Perspective. *J. Cell Commun. Signal.* **2014**, *8*, 195–210. [CrossRef]
19. Fadahunsi, O.S.; Olorunnisola, O.S.; Adegbola, P.I.; Subair, T.I.; Elegbeleye, O.E. Angiotensin Converting Enzyme Inhibitors from Medicinal Plants: A Molecular Docking and Dynamic Simulation Approach. *Silico Pharmacol.* **2022**, *10*, 20. [CrossRef]
20. Heo, S.-Y.; Kang, N.; Kim, E.-A.; Kim, J.; Lee, S.-H.; Ahn, G.; Oh, J.H.; Shin, A.Y.; Kim, D.; Heo, S.-J. Purification and Molecular Docking Study on the Angiotensin I-Converting Enzyme (ACE)-Inhibitory Peptide Isolated from Hydrolysates of the Deep-Sea Mussel Gigantidas Vrijenhoeki. *Mar. Drugs* **2023**, *21*, 458. [CrossRef]
21. Oyebamiji, A.K.; Akintelu, S.A.; Akintayo, E.T.; Akintayo, C.O.; Aworinde, H.O.; Adekunle, O.D. Dataset on Substituents Effect on Biological Activities of Linear RGD-Containing Peptides as Potential Anti-Angiotensin Converting Enzyme. *Data Brief* **2023**, *50*, 109478. [CrossRef]
22. Guy, J.L.; Jackson, R.M.; Jensen, H.A.; Hooper, N.M.; Turner, A.J. Identification of Critical Active-Site Residues in Angiotensin-Converting Enzyme-2 (ACE2) by Site-Directed Mutagenesis. *FEBS J.* **2005**, *272*, 3512–3520. [CrossRef]
23. Schultheiß, C.; Willscher, E.; Paschold, L.; Gottschick, C.; Klee, B.; Henkes, S.-S.; Bosurgi, L.; Dutzmann, J.; Sedding, D.; Frese, T.; et al. The IL-1β, IL-6, and TNF Cytokine Triad Is Associated with Post-Acute Sequelae of COVID-19. *Cell Rep. Med.* **2022**, *3*, 100663. [CrossRef]
24. Ni, W.; Yang, X.; Yang, D.; Bao, J.; Li, R.; Xiao, Y.; Hou, C.; Wang, H.; Liu, J.; Yang, D.; et al. Role of Angiotensin-Converting Enzyme 2 (ACE2) in COVID-19. *Crit. Care* **2020**, *24*, 422. [CrossRef]
25. Wang, C.; Wang, P.; Chen, W.; Bai, Y. Mechanisms of *Gynostemma pentaphyllum* against Non-Alcoholic Fibre Liver Disease Based on Network Pharmacology and Molecular Docking. *J. Cell. Mol. Med.* **2022**, *26*, 3760–3771. [CrossRef]
26. Zhang, Y.; Shi, G.; Luo, Z.; Wang, J.; Wu, S.; Zhang, X.; Zhao, Y. Activity Components from *Gynostemma pentaphyllum* for Preventing Hepatic Fibrosis and of Its Molecular Targets by Network Pharmacology Approach. *Molecules* **2021**, *26*, 3006. [CrossRef] [PubMed]
27. Qi, J.; Ping, D.; Sun, X.; Huang, K.; Peng, Y.; Liu, C. A Herbal Product Inhibits Carbon Tetrachloride-Induced Liver Fibrosis by Suppressing the Epidermal Growth Factor Receptor Signaling Pathway. *J. Ethnopharmacol.* **2023**, *311*, 116419. [CrossRef]
28. Hu, L.; Zhao, X.; He, X.; Guo, Y.; Cheng, H.; Chen, S.; Zhou, G.; Wang, J.; Lu, Y. *Gynostemma pentaphyllum* Ameliorates CCl4-Induced Liver Injury via PDK1/Bcl-2 Pathway with Comprehensive Analysis of Network Pharmacology and Transcriptomics. *Chin. Med.* **2024**, *19*, 70. [CrossRef] [PubMed]

29. Li, S.; Li, S.-L.; Liu, J.-K.; Wang, Z.; Yuan, P.-P. Mechanism of *Gynostemma pentaphyllum* in treatment of metabolism associated fatty liver disease based on network pharmacology and molecular docking. *Zhongguo Zhong Yao Za Zhi* **2021**, *46*, 5080–5087. [CrossRef] [PubMed]
30. Li, X.; Lai, H.; Wang, X. Integrating Transcriptomics, Network Analysis, and Single-Cell RNA Sequencing to Identify and Validate Key Target Genes of Gynostemma in the Treatment of Non-Alcoholic Fatty Liver Disease. *Eur. J. Pharm. Sci.* **2025**, *212*, 107214. [CrossRef]
31. Hong, M.; Cai, Z.; Song, L.; Liu, Y.; Wang, Q.; Feng, X. *Gynostemma pentaphyllum* Attenuates the Progression of Nonalcoholic Fatty Liver Disease in Mice: A Biomedical Investigation Integrated with In Silico Assay. *Evid.-Based Complement. Altern. Med. ECAM* **2018**, *2018*, 8384631. [CrossRef]
32. Zheng, Y.; Wei, W.; Wang, Y.; Li, T.; Wei, Y.; Gao, S. Gypenosides Exert Cardioprotective Effects by Promoting Mitophagy and Activating PI3K/Akt/GSK-3β/Mcl-1 Signaling. *PeerJ* **2024**, *12*, e17538. [CrossRef]
33. Liang, R.; Wu, J.; Lin, R.; Ran, L.; Shu, B.; Deng, H. Molecular Mechanisms of *Gynostemma pentaphyllum* in Prevention and Treatment of Non-Small-Cell Lung Cancer. *Evid.-Based Complement. Altern. Med. ECAM* **2022**, *2022*, 9938936. [CrossRef] [PubMed]
34. Qi, Y.-S.; Xie, J.-B.; Xie, P.; Duan, Y.; Ling, Y.-Q.; Gu, Y.-L.; Piao, X.-L. Uncovering the Anti-NSCLC Effects and Mechanisms of Gypenosides by Metabolomics and Network Pharmacology Analysis. *J. Ethnopharmacol.* **2021**, *281*, 114506. [CrossRef]
35. Tu, Q.; Zhu, Y.; Yuan, Y.; Guo, L.; Liu, L.; Yao, L.; Zou, Y.; Li, J.; Chen, F. Gypenosides Inhibit Inflammatory Response and Apoptosis of Endothelial and Epithelial Cells in LPS-Induced ALI: A Study Based on Bioinformatic Analysis and in Vivo/Vitro Experiments. *Drug Des. Devel. Ther.* **2021**, *15*, 289–303. [CrossRef] [PubMed]
36. Qi, Y.-S.; Xiao, M.-Y.; Xie, P.; Xie, J.-B.; Guo, M.; Li, F.-F.; Piao, X.-L. Comprehensive Serum Metabolomics and Network Analysis to Reveal the Mechanism of Gypenosides in Treating Lung Cancer and Enhancing the Pharmacological Effects of Cisplatin. *Front. Pharmacol.* **2022**, *13*, 1070948. [CrossRef]
37. Wang, J.; Shi, J.; Jia, N.; Sun, Q. Network Pharmacology Analysis Reveals Neuroprotection of *Gynostemma pentaphyllum (Thunb.)* Makino in Alzheimer' Disease. *BMC Complement. Med. Ther.* **2022**, *22*, 57. [CrossRef] [PubMed]
38. Liu, Y.; Li, Y.; Li, J.; Rao, H.; Sun, J.; Xiu, J.; Wu, N. Gypenosides Alleviate Oxidative Stress in the Hippocampus, Promote Mitophagy, and Mitigate Depressive-like Behaviors Induced by CUMS via SIRT1. *J. Ethnopharmacol.* **2025**, *337*, 118823. [CrossRef]
39. Liu, H.-Y.; Ji, Y.-L.; Du, H.; Chen, S.-H.; Wang, D.-P.; Lv, Q.-L. Bacoside a Inhibits the Growth of Glioma by Promoting Apoptosis and Autophagy in U251 and U87 Cells. *Naunyn. Schmiedebergs Arch. Pharmacol.* **2024**, *397*, 2105–2120. [CrossRef]
40. Wang, W.-X.; He, X.-Y.; Yi, D.-Y.; Tan, X.-Y.; Wu, L.-J.; Li, N.; Feng, B.-B. Uncovering the Molecular Mechanism of *Gynostemma pentaphyllum (Thunb.)* Makino against Breast Cancer Using Network Pharmacology and Molecular Docking. *Medicine* **2022**, *101*, e32165. [CrossRef]
41. Zhang, Y.; Ji, P.; Xiao, X.; Wang, J.; Wan, Z.; Cao, H.; Kong, L.; Jin, Y. Network Pharmacology, Molecular Docking, and Molecular Dynamics Simulations Shed Light on the Mechanism behind *Gynostemma pentaphyllum*'s Efficacy against Osteosarcoma. *Medicine* **2024**, *103*, e39454. [CrossRef]
42. Guo, J.; Wu, Z.; Chang, X.; Huang, M.; Wang, Y.; Liu, R.; Li, J. Network Pharmacology Analysis and In Vitro Validation of the Active Ingredients and Potential Mechanisms of *Gynostemma pentaphyllum* Against Esophageal Cancer. *Comb. Chem. High Throughput Screen.* **2025**, *28*, 500–513. [CrossRef]
43. Wang, H.; Chen, Y.; Lin, T. Based on Network Pharmacology and Molecular Docking Technology to Explore the Pharmacodynamic Components and Mechanism of Gynostemmae Pentaphylli Herba Reversing Cervical Intraepithelial Neoplasia. *BMC Complement. Med. Ther.* **2025**, *25*, 112. [CrossRef]
44. Liu, H.; Li, X.; Duan, Y.; Xie, J.-B.; Piao, X.-L. Mechanism of Gypenosides of *Gynostemma pentaphyllum* Inducing Apoptosis of Renal Cell Carcinoma by PI3K/AKT/mTOR Pathway. *J. Ethnopharmacol.* **2021**, *271*, 113907. [CrossRef]
45. Liu, H.; Li, X.; Xie, J.; Lv, C.; Lian, F.; Zhang, S.; Duan, Y.; Zeng, Y.; Piao, X. Gypenoside L and Gypenoside LI Inhibit Proliferation in Renal Cell Carcinoma via Regulation of the MAPK and Arachidonic Acid Metabolism Pathways. *Front. Pharmacol.* **2022**, *13*, 820639. [CrossRef]
46. Liu, M.; Liao, H.; Peng, Q.; Huang, J.; Liu, W.; Dai, M.; Li, Z.; Xie, Y.; Liu, J.; Ying, Y.; et al. Comprehensive Network Pharmacology and Experimentation to Unveil the Therapeutic Efficacy and Mechanisms of Gypenoside LI in Anaplastic Thyroid Cancer. *BMC Cancer* **2025**, *25*, 870. [CrossRef]
47. Li, X.; Liu, H.; Lv, C.; Du, J.; Lian, F.; Zhang, S.; Wang, Z.; Zeng, Y. Gypenoside-Induced Apoptosis via the PI3K/AKT/mTOR Signaling Pathway in Bladder Cancer. *BioMed Res. Int.* **2022**, *2022*, 9304552. [CrossRef]
48. Pan, L.; Lan, B.; Li, S.; Jin, Y.; Cui, M.; Xia, Y.; Wei, S.; Huang, H. Gypenoside Inhibits Gastric Cancer Proliferation by Suppressing Glycolysis via the Hippo Pathway. *Sci. Rep.* **2024**, *14*, 19003. [CrossRef] [PubMed]
49. Wu, H.; Lai, W.; Wang, Q.; Zhou, Q.; Zhang, R.; Zhao, Y. Gypenoside Induces Apoptosis by Inhibiting the PI3K/AKT/mTOR Pathway and Enhances T-Cell Antitumor Immunity by Inhibiting PD-L1 in Gastric Cancer. *Front. Pharmacol.* **2024**, *15*, 1243353. [CrossRef] [PubMed]

50. Li, K.; Li, H.; Xu, W.; Liu, W.; Du, Y.; He, J.-F.; Ma, C. Research on the Potential Mechanism of Gypenosides on Treating Thyroid-Associated Ophthalmopathy Based on Network Pharmacology. *Med. Sci. Monit. Int. Med. J. Exp. Clin. Res.* **2019**, *25*, 4923–4932. [CrossRef] [PubMed]
51. Li, X.; Alhasani, R.H.; Cao, Y.; Zhou, X.; He, Z.; Zeng, Z.; Strang, N.; Shu, X. Gypenosides Alleviate Cone Cell Death in a Zebrafish Model of Retinitis Pigmentosa. *Antioxidants* **2021**, *10*, 1050. [CrossRef]
52. Yang, P.; Xu, P.; Cheng, C.; Jiao, J.; Wu, Y.; Dong, S.; Xie, J.; Zhu, X. Integrating Network Pharmacology and Experimental Models to Investigate the Efficacy of QYHJ on Pancreatic Cancer. *J. Ethnopharmacol.* **2022**, *297*, 115516. [CrossRef]
53. Yang, S.; Zhao, M.; Lu, M.; Feng, Y.; Zhang, X.; Wang, D.; Jiang, W. Network Pharmacology Analysis, Molecular Docking Integrated Experimental Verification Reveal the Mechanism of *Gynostemma pentaphyllum* in the Treatment of Type II Diabetes by Regulating the IRS1/PI3K/Akt Signaling Pathway. *Curr. Issues Mol. Biol.* **2024**, *46*, 5561–5581. [CrossRef] [PubMed]
54. Shen, Z.; Gao, X.; Huang, D.; Xu, X.; Shen, J. The Potential of *Gynostemma pentaphyllum* in the Treatment of Hyperlipidemia and Its Interaction with the LOX1-PI3K-AKT-eNOS Pathway. *Food Sci. Nutr.* **2024**, *12*, 8000–8012. [CrossRef] [PubMed]
55. Pei, A.; Ma, Y.; Gao, M.; Zhao, Q. Protective Efficacy and Mechanism of Gypenosides against Diabetic Cataracts via the Ferroptosis Pathway: A Study Based on Network Pharmacology. *Eur. J. Pharmacol.* **2025**, *1007*, 178175. [CrossRef]
56. Xie, J.-B.; Xie, P.; Guo, M.; Li, F.-F.; Xiao, M.-Y.; Qi, Y.-S.; Pei, W.-J.; Luo, H.-T.; Gu, Y.-L.; Piao, X.-L. Protective Effect of Heat-Processed *Gynostemma pentaphyllum* on High Fat Diet-Induced Glucose Metabolic Disorders Mice. *Front. Pharmacol.* **2023**, *14*, 1215150. [CrossRef]
57. Xie, P.; Guo, M.; Xie, J.-B.; Xiao, M.-Y.; Qi, Y.-S.; Duan, Y.; Li, F.-F.; Piao, X.-L. Effects of Heat-Processed *Gynostemma pentaphyllum* on High-Fat Diet-Fed Mice of Obesity and Functional Analysis on Network Pharmacology and Molecular Docking Strategy. *J. Ethnopharmacol.* **2022**, *294*, 115335. [CrossRef] [PubMed]
58. Ding, Y.; Wang, X.; Feng, Y.; Zhang, X.; Li, C.; Ge, Y.; Yang, Y.; Su, J.; Chu, X. Exploring the Effects of the Anti-Diarrheal Formula on Intestinal Oxidative Stress Based on Network Pharmacology, Molecular Docking, and Microbiomics. *Fitoterapia* **2025**, *185*, 106742. [CrossRef]
59. Yang, L.; Xie, X.; Tu, Z.; Fu, J.; Xu, D.; Zhou, Y. The Signal Pathways and Treatment of Cytokine Storm in COVID-19. *Signal Transduct. Target. Ther.* **2021**, *6*, 255. [CrossRef]
60. Gheblawi, M.; Wang, K.; Viveiros, A.; Nguyen, Q.; Zhong, J.-C.; Turner, A.J.; Raizada, M.K.; Grant, M.B.; Oudit, G.Y. Angiotensin-Converting Enzyme 2: SARS-CoV-2 Receptor and Regulator of the Renin-Angiotensin System. *Circ. Res.* **2020**, *126*, 1456–1474. [CrossRef]
61. Jackson, C.B.; Farzan, M.; Chen, B.; Choe, H. Mechanisms of SARS-CoV-2 Entry into Cells. *Nat. Rev. Mol. Cell Biol.* **2022**, *23*, 3–20. [CrossRef] [PubMed]
62. Alzaabi, M.M.; Hamdy, R.; Ashmawy, N.S.; Hamoda, A.M.; Alkhayat, F.; Khademi, N.N.; Al Joud, S.M.A.; El-Keblawy, A.A.; Soliman, S.S.M. Flavonoids Are Promising Safe Therapy against COVID-19. *Phytochem. Rev.* **2022**, *21*, 291–312. [CrossRef]
63. Choudhary, S.; Nehul, S.; Singh, A.; Panda, P.K.; Kumar, P.; Sharma, G.K.; Tomar, S. Unraveling Antiviral Efficacy of Multifunctional Immunomodulatory Triterpenoids against SARS-COV-2 Targeting Main Protease and Papain-like Protease. *IUBMB Life* **2024**, *76*, 228–241. [CrossRef]
64. Liskova, A.; Samec, M.; Koklesova, L.; Samuel, S.M.; Zhai, K.; Al-Ishaq, R.K.; Abotaleb, M.; Nosal, V.; Kajo, K.; Ashrafizadeh, M.; et al. Flavonoids against the SARS-CoV-2 Induced Inflammatory Storm. *Biomed. Pharmacother.* **2021**, *138*, 111430. [CrossRef] [PubMed]
65. Li, X.-C.; Li, F.-F.; Pei, W.-J.; Yang, J.; Gu, Y.-L.; Piao, X.-L. The Content and Principle of the Rare Ginsenosides Produced from *Gynostemma pentaphyllum* after Heat Treatment. *Molecules* **2023**, *28*, 6415. [CrossRef]
66. Wu, Q.; Jang, M.; Piao, X.-L. Determination by UPLC-MS of Four Dammarane-Type Saponins from Heat-Processed *Gynostemma pentaphyllum*. *Biosci. Biotechnol. Biochem.* **2014**, *78*, 311–316. [CrossRef]
67. Xie, P.; Xie, J.-B.; Xiao, M.-Y.; Guo, M.; Qi, Y.-S.; Li, F.-F.; Piao, X.-L. Liver Lipidomics Analysis Reveals the Anti-Obesity and Lipid-Lowering Effects of Gypnosides from Heat-Processed *Gynostemma pentaphyllum* in High-Fat Diet Fed Mice. *Phytomedicine* **2023**, *115*, 154834. [CrossRef]
68. Wang, Y.-R.; Xing, S.-F.; Lin, M.; Gu, Y.-L.; Piao, X.-L. Determination of Flavonoids from *Gynostemma pentaphyllum* Using Ultra-Performance Liquid Chromatography with Triple Quadrupole Tandem Mass Spectrometry and an Evaluation of Their Antioxidant Activity in Vitro. *J. Liq. Chromatogr. Relat. Technol.* **2018**, *41*, 437–444. [CrossRef]
69. Jo, H.-G.; Baek, C.Y.; Hwang, Y.; Baek, E.; Park, C.; Song, H.S.; Lee, D. Investigating the Anti-Inflammatory, Analgesic, and Chondroprotective Effects of *Gynostemma pentaphyllum (Thunb.)* Makino in Osteoarthritis: An In Vitro and In Vivo Study. *Int. J. Mol. Sci.* **2024**, *25*, 9594. [CrossRef]
70. Cao, H.; Xiao, G.; Li, D.; Chen, X.; Chen, W.; Chen, Z. *Gynostemma pentaphyllum* Promotes Skeletal Muscle Recovery via Its Inhibition of PXR-IL-6 Expression. *Phytomedicine Plus* **2022**, *2*, 100305. [CrossRef]
71. Kao, T.H.; Huang, S.C.; Inbaraj, B.S.; Chen, B.H. Determination of Flavonoids and Saponins in *Gynostemma pentaphyllum (Thunb.)* Makino by Liquid Chromatography–Mass Spectrometry. *Anal. Chim. Acta* **2008**, *626*, 200–211. [CrossRef] [PubMed]

72. Huang, S.C.; Hung, C.F.; Wu, W.B.; Chen, B.H. Determination of Chlorophylls and Their Derivatives in *Gynostemma pentaphyllum* Makino by Liquid Chromatography–Mass Spectrometry. *J. Pharm. Biomed. Anal.* **2008**, *48*, 105–112. [CrossRef]
73. Liu, L.; Huang, Y.; Wang, Q.; Wang, Z.; Pan, K.; Zhang, J.; Peng, Y.; Wang, G.; Yin, Z.; Sun, J. Simultaneous Determination of 13 Representative Saponins from the Total Saponins of *Gynostemma pentaphyllum* in Rat Plasma Using LC-MS/MS for Pharmacokinetic Study. *J. Pharm. Biomed. Anal.* **2025**, *264*, 116970. [CrossRef]
74. Zhang, L.; Lin, Y.; Guan, H.; Hu, L.; Pan, G. Simultaneous Determination of Gypenoside LVI, Gypenoside XLVI, 2α-OH-Protopanaxadiol and Their Two Metabolites in Rat Plasma by LC–MS/MS and Its Application to Pharmacokinetic Studies. *J. Chromatogr. B* **2015**, *1005*, 9–16. [CrossRef]
75. Guo, S.; Sui, C.; Ma, Y. Development of a Targeted Method for Quantification of Gypenoside XLIX in Rat Plasma, Using SPE and LC–MS/MS. *Biomed. Chromatogr.* **2017**, *31*, e3898. [CrossRef]
76. He, Y.; Liang, Q.; Luo, L.; He, Y.; Huang, X.; Wen, C. Determination of Gypenoside A and Gypenoside XLIX in Rat Plasma by UPLC-MS/MS and Applied to the Pharmacokinetics and Bioavailability. *Int. J. Anal. Chem.* **2022**, *2022*, 6734408. [CrossRef]
77. Li, H.; Yang, A.; Yang, M.; Zhou, F.; Zhang, R.; Zheng, Z.; Wang, X. Pharmacokinetic Studies of Gypenoside XLVI in Rat Plasma Using UPLC-MS/MS Method. *Curr. Pharm. Anal.* **2024**, *20*, 143–151. [CrossRef]
78. Wang, H.; Chen, C.; Xue, M.; Zhang, Y.; Chen, K.; Sun, B.; Wang, P.; Tong, X.; Yu, X.; Li, H.; et al. Identification and Mechanism of Hepatoprotective Saponins and Endogenous Metabolites in the Sweet Variant of *Gynostemma pentaphyllum*. *Bioorganic Chem.* **2025**, *165*, 108996. [CrossRef] [PubMed]
79. Yang, Q.; Zang, H.; Xing, T.; Zhang, S.; Li, C.; Zhang, Y.; Dong, Y.; Hu, X.; Yu, J.; Wen, J.; et al. Gypenoside XLIX Protects against Acute Kidney Injury by Suppressing IGFBP7/IGF1R-Mediated Programmed Cell Death and Inflammation. *Phytomedicine* **2021**, *85*, 153541. [CrossRef]
80. Dejani, N.N.; Elshabrawy, H.A.; da Silva Maia Bezerra Filho, C.; de Sousa, D.P. Anticoronavirus and Immunomodulatory Phenolic Compounds: Opportunities and Pharmacotherapeutic Perspectives. *Biomolecules* **2021**, *11*, 1254. [CrossRef]
81. Wrońska, N.; Szlaur, M.; Zawadzka, K.; Lisowska, K. The Synergistic Effect of Triterpenoids and Flavonoids—New Approaches for Treating Bacterial Infections? *Molecules* **2022**, *27*, 847. [CrossRef]
82. Wu, X.; Xiang, M.; Jing, H.; Wang, C.; Novakovic, V.A.; Shi, J. Damage to Endothelial Barriers and Its Contribution to Long COVID. *Angiogenesis* **2024**, *27*, 5–22. [CrossRef] [PubMed]
83. Aljadah, M.; Khan, N.; Beyer, A.M.; Chen, Y.; Blanker, A.; Widlansky, M.E. Clinical Implications of COVID-19-Related Endothelial Dysfunction. *JACC Adv.* **2024**, *3*, 101070. [CrossRef] [PubMed]
84. Samarelli, F.; Graziano, G.; Gambacorta, N.; Graps, E.A.; Leonetti, F.; Nicolotti, O.; Altomare, C.D. Small Molecules for the Treatment of Long-COVID-Related Vascular Damage and Abnormal Blood Clotting: A Patent-Based Appraisal. *Viruses* **2024**, *16*, 450. [CrossRef]
85. Noce, A.; Marrone, G.; Di Lauro, M.; Vita, C.; Montalto, G.; Giorgino, G.; Chiaramonte, C.; D'Agostini, C.; Bernardini, S.; Pieri, M. Potential Anti-Inflammatory and Anti-Fatigue Effects of an Oral Food Supplement in Long COVID Patients. *Pharmaceuticals* **2024**, *17*, 463. [CrossRef]
86. Chatterjee, D.; Maparu, K. Long COVID Syndrome: Exploring Therapies for Managing and Overcoming Persistent Symptoms. *Inflammopharmacology* **2025**, *33*, 4097–4113. [CrossRef]
87. Peluso, M.J.; Deeks, S.G. Mechanisms of Long COVID and the Path toward Therapeutics. *Cell* **2024**, *187*, 5500–5529. [CrossRef] [PubMed]
88. Oktavianawati, I.; Santoso, M.; Bakar, M.F.A.; Kim, Y.-U.; Fatmawati, S. Recent Progress on Drugs Discovery Study for Treatment of COVID-19: Repurposing Existing Drugs and Current Natural Bioactive Molecules. *Appl. Biol. Chem.* **2023**, *66*, 89. [CrossRef]
89. Afendi, F.M.; Okada, T.; Yamazaki, M.; Hirai-Morita, A.; Nakamura, Y.; Nakamura, K.; Ikeda, S.; Takahashi, H.; Altaf-Ul-Amin, M.; Darusman, L.K.; et al. KNApSAcK Family Databases: Integrated Metabolite–Plant Species Databases for Multifaceted Plant Research. *Plant Cell Physiol.* **2012**, *53*, e1. [CrossRef]
90. Beyerstedt, S.; Casaro, E.B.; Rangel, É.B. COVID-19: Angiotensin-Converting Enzyme 2 (ACE2) Expression and Tissue Susceptibility to SARS-CoV-2 Infection. *Eur. J. Clin. Microbiol. Infect. Dis.* **2021**, *40*, 905–919. [CrossRef]
91. Espe, S. Malacards: The Human Disease Database. *J. Med. Libr. Assoc.* **2018**, *106*, 140–141. [CrossRef]
92. Leyva-López, N.; Gutierrez-Grijalva, E.P.; Ambriz-Perez, D.L.; Heredia, J.B. Flavonoids as Cytokine Modulators: A Possible Therapy for Inflammation-Related Diseases. *Int. J. Mol. Sci.* **2016**, *17*, 921. [CrossRef]
93. Ge, S.X.; Jung, D.; Yao, R. ShinyGO: A Graphical Gene-Set Enrichment Tool for Animals and Plants. *Bioinformatics* **2020**, *36*, 2628–2629. [CrossRef] [PubMed]
94. Hanwell, M.D.; Curtis, D.E.; Lonie, D.C.; Vandermeersch, T.; Zurek, E.; Hutchison, G.R. Avogadro: An Advanced Semantic Chemical Editor, Visualization, and Analysis Platform. *J. Cheminformatics* **2012**, *4*, 17. [CrossRef]

95. Seo, J.I.; Yu, J.S.; Zhang, Y.; Yoo, H.H. Evaluating Flavonoids as Potential Aromatase Inhibitors for Breast Cancer Treatment: In Vitro Studies and in Silico Predictions. *Chem. Biol. Interact.* **2024**, *392*, 110927. [CrossRef]
96. Ali, M.Y.; Zaib, S.; Jannat, S.; Khan, I. Inhibition of Angiotensin-I Converting Enzyme by Ginsenosides: Structure–Activity Relationships and Inhibitory Mechanism. *J. Agric. Food Chem.* **2021**, *69*, 6073–6086. [CrossRef] [PubMed]

pharmaceuticals

Article

The Hepatoprotective Properties of the Revised Formulation of Dahuang Xiaoshi Tang, an Ancient Chinese Herbal Decoction, Are Probed by Integrated Metabolomics and Network Pharmacology

Xiangpeng Kong [1], Xiaoyang Wang [2], Haiqin Ren [3], Yajun Yao [4], Hui Zhang [5], Huifeng Li [1], Huifang Li [1], Yangang Cheng [1], Zhuqing Song [1], Miaorong Pei [1,*] and Karl Wah Keung Tsim [2,*]

[1] College of Traditional Chinese Medicine and Food Engineering, Shanxi University of Chinese Medicine, Jinzhong 030619, China; kong_xiangpeng@sxtcm.edu.cn (X.K.); lihuifeng2046@163.com (H.L.); lihuifangzy@sxtcm.edu.cn (H.L.); chengyg1992@163.com (Y.C.); 19581931302@163.com (Z.S.)

[2] Division of Life Science, Center for Chinese Medicine, The Hong Kong University of Science and Technology, Clear Water Bay, Hong Kong, China; xwangfr@connect.ust.hk

[3] College of Pharmacy, Harbin University of Commerce, Harbin 150076, China; haiqinren@163.com

[4] Department of Chinese Medicine, Shanxi Pharmaceutical Vocational College, Taiyuan 030031, China; yaoyajun0601@163.com

[5] School of Pharmacy, Faculty of Medicine, Macau University of Science and Technology, Macau SAR, China; 3240002660@student.must.edu.mo

* Correspondence: peimr602@163.com (M.P.); botsim@ust.hk (K.W.K.T.); Tel.: +86-0351-3179-903 (M.P.); +852-2358-7332 (K.W.K.T.)

Abstract: Background: Dahuang Xiaoshi Tang (DXT), an ancient Chinese herbal remedy dating back to 220 AD, as documented initially in "Treatise on Febrile and Miscellaneous Diseases," is used to treat damp-heat jaundice with interior sthenia syndrome. In DXT, anthraquinones and alkaloids form insoluble complexes, reducing its effectiveness. A revised herbal extract, DXT-M, was developed, and its hepatoprotective properties were demonstrated in animal models using pharmacodynamic, metabolomic, network pharmacological, and toxicological approaches. **Methods**: The α-naphthalene isothiocyanate was utilised to establish the acute liver injury rat model. The assays of glutamate pyruvate transaminase, glutamic oxalacetic transaminase, alkaline phosphatase, bilirubin, total bile acid, complement 3 (C3) and C4, interleukin-2 (IL-2) and IL-6, tumour necrosis factor α (TNF-α), and pathological morphology were used to evaluate the hepatoprotection of DXT in comparison to DXT-M. The ^{1}H-NMR-based serum and urine metabolomics were performed to identify potential biomarkers and metabolic pathways of DXT-M in treating hepatitis. The intrinsic regulatory mechanisms of DXT in liver protection, as well as the combination of network toxicology, were elucidated. Statistical analyses included RM two-way ANOVA with Geisser–Greenhouse correction and Dunnett's post hoc test for longitudinal data, and one-way ANOVA with Dunnett's post hoc test for group comparisons. Data were shown as mean ± SD. **Results**: Liver-injured animals exhibited weight loss, ruffled fur, and liver damage, accompanied by elevated liver function indicators. DXT-M effectively improved these symptoms, repaired liver damage, restored liver function, and regulated immune status by modulating complement 3. Metabonomics and other analyses indicated the CYP/GST-ROS axis is key to its hepatoprotective effects. DXT-M outperformed DXT in efficacy. **Conclusions**: DXT-M demonstrated significant effectiveness in restoring liver pathological damage, correcting abnormal biochemical indicators of liver function, and regulating complement factors. The pathway of CYP/GST-ROS served as the shared regulatory axis and transformation site for DXT-M's liver protective effects. These findings suggest that DXT-M has potential as a treatment for acute liver injury, highlighting the need for further research into its underlying molecular mechanisms as well as its complete material basis. This study's main limitation is its focus on acute models; future research should include other liver diseases and clinical observation to evaluate its full potential.

Keywords: Dahuang Xiaoshi Tang; liver injury; metabolomics; network pharmacology; network toxicology; hepatoprotection

1. Introduction

As a vital organ, the liver performs essential functions including metabolism, detoxification, and immune regulation. Liver diseases—from acute injury to chronic conditions such as hepatitis, fibrosis, and cancer—pose significant global health burdens, causing millions of deaths annually and representing a leading cause of disability worldwide [1,2]. Acute Liver Injury (ALI) is a severe clinical syndrome marked by rapid hepatocyte necrosis, inflammatory pathway activation, and metabolic dysfunction, which can progress to fatal liver failure [3,4]. Elevated alanine aminotransferase (ALT), often triggered by hepatotoxic agents, viral infections, or autoimmune reactions, is a standard indicator of ALI [5,6]. The underlying mechanisms involve direct cytotoxicity leading to necrosis or apoptosis of hepatic and biliary epithelial cells, oxidative stress with glutathione depletion, immune activation and pro-inflammatory cytokine release, and dysregulated metabolic pathways—especially those related to energy metabolism and the tricarboxylic acid cycle [7,8]. Although advances have been made in understanding ALI pathogenesis, treatment remains limited, relying mainly on supportive measures and removal of causative factors [6,9]. Thus, there is a pressing need for effective multitarget pharmacological interventions. In this context, Traditional Chinese Medicine (TCM), characterised by multi-component formulations, presents a promising therapeutic paradigm [10,11]. By harmonising the "Yin–Yang" equilibrium within the body and enhancing the immune system, TCM exhibits preventive and therapeutic capabilities in disease management [12,13]. However, the accurate elucidation of the pharmacological basis of TCM is challenging due to variations in the types and quantities of chemical components, which mutually influence one another, thereby presenting difficulties in evaluating its efficacy and researching its mechanism of action [14,15]. The inconsistent quality of TCM raw materials, stemming from their diverse variety, origin, and variations in planting, collecting, and processing, poses a challenge in ensuring the stability and controllability of the herbal extracts, which introduce numerous uncertainties in clinical efficacy [16–18]. By employing extraction and refining preparative methods in TCM chemistry, the identification of active chemical constituents in refined TCM components has become relatively transparent, ensuring the stability, controllability, and clinical effectiveness of TCM components [19].

In TCM mixtures with hepatoprotective activity, many herbs contain carboxyl acids and phenolic compounds, exhibiting varying acidity levels. These herbs, which include specific constituents, are commonly referred to as acidic herbs, such as Rhei Radix Et Rhizoma (RRR) and Glycyrrhizae Radix Et Rhizoma [20–22]. Similarly, there is also a substantial presence of herbs containing alkaloids. These herbs, which possess varying degrees of alkalinity, are also referred to as alkaline herbs, such as Phellodendri Chinensis Cortex (PCC), Coptidis Rhizoma, and Aconiti Lateralis Radix Praeparata [23–25]. The paired herb of acidic and alkaline herbs in the same formula is known as acid–alkaline paired herbal medicine [26,27]. During the decocting process of TCM mixtures containing paired acid–alkaline herbs, such as those with anthraquinone and acid saponin, the acid components can combine with alkaloids to form insoluble complexes [28]. This phenomenon leads to the loss of active ingredients, ultimately affecting clinical effectiveness. The herbal prescription known as Dahuang Xiaoshi Tang (DXT), described in "Treatise on Febrile and Miscellaneous Diseases" (<<Shanghan Zabing Lun>> in China at 220 AD), is composed of Rhei Radix et Rhizoma (RRR), Phellodendri Chinensis Cortex (PCC), Gardeniae Fructus (GF), and Natrii Sulfas (NS). It is commonly used to treat damp-heat jaundice accompanied by interior sthenia syndrome, and different types of hepatitis caused by dampness and heat [29,30]. Its therapeutic potential against damp-heat jaundice is attributed to the integrated actions of key bioactive constituents, including anthraquinones from RRR [31–34], alkaloids such as berberine from PCC [35,36], and iridoid glycosides like geniposide from GF [37,38]. Interestingly, DXT is a classic example of a herbal formula featuring paired acid–alkaline herbs, specifically RRR-PCC [39]. During the decoction process of DXT, the anthraquinones in RRR readily bind with the alkaloids in PCC, forming an insoluble macromolecular complex that precipitates [40], resulting in the depletion of its active constituents and a decrease in the therapeutic effectiveness of DXT.

To address the reduction of active ingredients caused by the co-decoction of acidic and alkaline ingredients in DXT, a re-formulation approach was adopted to study the hepatoprotective efficacy and related mechanisms of DXT. Here, extracts from individual herbs, i.e., RRR, PCC, and GF, of DXT were prepared and combined according to an optimised proportion [41]. This revised preparation of DXT was named DXT-M. Based on the critical role of the liver in metabolic regulation, we speculate that DXT-M can improve acute liver injury by repairing endogenous metabolic disorders, immune imbalance and pathological damage. The proposed mechanisms of DXT-M in countering the pathogenesis of acute liver injury were summarised in Figure 1. In this study, we systematically evaluated the hepatoprotective effects of DXT-M in an ANIT-induced rat model of ALI through integrated pharmacological, metabolomic, network pharmacological, and toxicological analyses [42]. This study systematically assesses the hepatoprotective effects of the reformed DXT-M preparation. The primary objectives were to confirm DXT-M's superior efficacy over traditional DXT, identify metabolic biomarkers and pathways affected by DXT-M using ^{1}H-NMR-based metabolomics, and explore mechanisms and potential hepatotoxic risks through a "compound–target–pathway" network. This multi-omics approach seeks to provide a scientific basis for developing DXT-M as a treatment for acute liver injury.

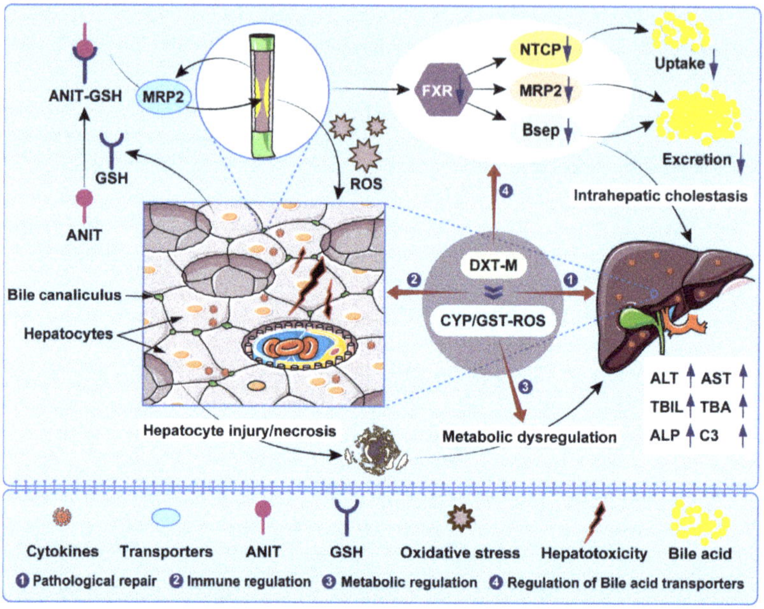

Figure 1. The proposed mechanisms of DXT-M in acute liver injury [41,43,44]. The blue arrows: upward indicated an increase or rise, while downward signified a decrease or reduction.

2. Results

2.1. Chemical Analysis of DXT Herbal Extract

As illustrated in Supplementary Figure S1A, the HPLC chromatographic peaks of refined extracts deriving from RRR, PCC, and GF exhibited greater peak clarity than the crude herbal extract, while retaining the principal components. In alignment with the previous reports [22,45–47], representative anthraquinone substances were detected in crude and refined RRR extracts [31–34]. Similarly, berberine, a predominant alkaloid, was identified in both crude and refined extracts of PCC [35,36], and geniposide, a prevalent iridoid glycoside, was found in both crude and refined extracts of GF [37,38]. The structures of representative phytochemicals in the constituent herbs of DXT were presented in Supplementary Figure S1B. These compounds are representative of the major bioactive classes (anthraquinones, alkaloids, and iridoid glycosides) that underpin the pharmacological profile of DXT (Supplementary Table S1). Consequently, the material basis of the refined extract of each herb in DXT-M, achieved by eliminating impurities and retaining essential constituents, was more clearly defined than that of the crude extracts. This refinement enhances quality, stability and controllability, providing a foundation for subsequent efficacy determination.

2.2. Effect of DXT and DXT-M on Animals with Liver Damage

Qualitative observations (data not presented) revealed that, compared to the control group, animals with a-naphthylisothiocyanate (ANIT)-induced liver injury showed reduced activity, feeding, and body weight, and exhibited recumbency, yellow urine, and perianal soiling. After receiving therapeutic agents, these symptoms improved to different extents. The DXT and low-dose DXT-M groups showed increased vigour, while the medium and high-dose DXT-M groups significantly improved recumbency, perianal soiling, and yellow urine, as well as vigour. As depicted in Figure 2A, all groups gained weight consistently before liver injury. However, on the sixth day, the animals with liver injury experienced significant weight loss compared to the controls. DXT-treated groups showed less weight reduction, with the medium-dose DXT-M group showing recovery. By the seventh day, all groups experienced weight loss. The model group showed a marked reduction compared to the control group, and, except for the high-dose DXT-M group, the body weight decline rate in the other treatment groups was significantly mitigated relative to the model group.

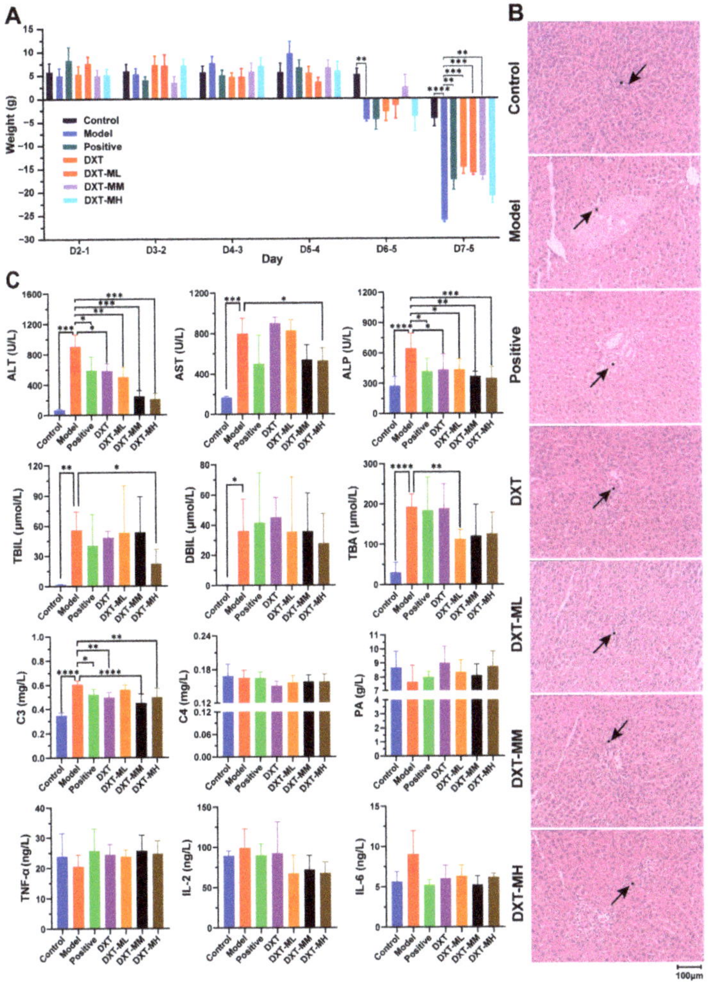

Figure 2. Effects of DXT and DXT-M on animals with liver damage. (**A**) Therapeutic effects of DXT and DXT-M on sequential body weight changes in ANIT-induced liver injury rats. X-axis: consecutive day differences (ΔDn = Dn − Dn-1, where Dn is body weight on day n); Y-axis: data are expressed as mean ± SEM. Statistical analysis was performed using Geisser–Greenhouse corrected RM two-way ANOVA followed by Dunnett's post hoc test (** $p < 0.01$, *** $p < 0.001$, and **** $p < 0.0001$ vs. ANIT model group). (**B**) Representative *H&E*-stained liver sections from experimental groups (100× magnification). The black arrows symbolise the biliary duct. Scale bar: 100 μm. (**C**) Effects of DXT and DXT-M on serum levels of liver function markers (ALT, AST, ALP), bilirubin (TBIL), total bile acids (TBA), complement components (C3, C4), and inflammatory cytokines (TNF-α, IL-2, IL-6) in ANIT-induced liver injury rats. Data are expressed as mean ± SD (n = 6 per group). Statistical significance determined by one-way ANOVA with Dunnett's post hoc test (* $p < 0.05$, ** $p < 0.01$, *** $p < 0.001$, and **** $p < 0.0001$ vs. ANIT model group).

The histopathological analysis in Figure 2B showed that normal animals had well-structured liver lobules, intact hepatocytes, clear bile ducts, and no vein dilation or edema. In contrast, liver-injured animals displayed disrupted lobules, hepatocyte necrosis, portal inflammation, narrowed bile ducts, and dilated veins with stasis and edema. Treatment with DXT and various doses of DXT-M improved these tissue injuries to varying extents. In the decoction groups, hepatocyte necrosis decreased, and the bile duct structure improved, although the lumens were incomplete. In groups receiving different DXT-M doses, hepatocytes showed minimal necrosis, normal portal structure, reduced inflammation, clear bile ducts with intact epithelium, and normal veins. Figure 2C demonstrated that liver injury significantly raised liver function indices (ALT, AST, ALP, TBIL, TBA) compared to controls. Treatments varied in effectiveness, with ursodeoxycholic acid and DXT notably reducing ALT and ALP. Furthermore, DXT-M exhibited a favourable dose-dependent modulation of ALT and ALP, surpassing the efficacy of DXT. High-dose DXT-M significantly decreased AST and TBIL, while low-dose DXT-M lowered TBA. Liver-injured animals had higher complement C3 levels, which ursodeoxycholic acid, DXT, and medium/high doses of DXT-M normalised.

2.3. *Regulation of DXT-M on Endogenous Metabolites of Animals with Liver Damage*

2.3.1. Metabolites Identification of Serum and Urine in 1H-NMR Spectrum

Here, the chemical shifts of peaks and coupled split peaks in the ^{1}H-NMR spectra of serum (δ0.6–4.2) and urine (δ0.52–4.56 and δ6.0–9.4) from animals in each group were analysed. From the serum ^{1}H-NMR spectra, eight differential metabolites were identified, including amino acids such as threonine, glutamic acid, taurine, glutamine, and their derivatives, as well as lipid metabolites and carbohydrate substances like glucose and myo-inositol. In the urine ^{1}H-NMR spectra, eleven differential metabolites were identified, encompassing amino acids such as phenylalanine, glycine, homoserine, lysine, and alanine; organic acids such as oxoglutaric acid, citric acid, and aminoadipic acid; gut-host co-metabolites such as phenylacetylglycine and hippuric acid; and nitrogen-containing substances such as methylamine. The typical ^{1}H-NMR spectra for serum and urine from each group of animals were depicted in Supplementary Figure S2, with the identification results of metabolites for each group provided in Supplementary Table S2.

2.3.2. Chemometric Analysis of Serum and Urine 1H-NMR Data

PCA analysis of serum and urine metabolomic data in Figure 3(A1,A2) revealed distinct group separations: the control group on the left negative axis, the model group on the right positive axis, and the DXT-M group in between, suggesting its potential to balance metabolites in liver-injured animals. OPLS-DA in Figure 3(B1,B2) further classified these groups, showing significant differences with high R^2Y and Q^2 values for serum (0.985 and 0.903) and urine (0.976 and 0.945), indicating strong model interpretation and predictivity. Figure 3(C1,C2) showed that permutation tests (200 iterations) for serum and urine consistently resulted in lower left R^2 and Q^2 values compared to the original values on the right. Figure 3(D1,D2) S-plots identified key metabolites in a liver injury model, with variable importance indicated by *VIP* values. Hierarchical clustering in Figure 3E separated control and model groups. Following the intervention with DXT-M, the clustering pattern of the model group showed a tendency to revert to that of the control group. In comparison to the control group, the model group exhibited significantly elevated concentrations of metabolites, including oxoglutaric acid, glutamine, taurine, glucose, ethanol, myo-inositol, phenylacetylglycine, homoserine, hippuric acid, citric acid, and methylamine. In the DXT-M-treated group, the levels of these metabolites showed a trend similar to that observed in the control group. Similarly, the model group displayed significantly reduced levels of threonine, glutamic acid, lipid, lysine, phenylalanine, glycine, alanine, and aminoadipic acid compared to the control group. The levels of these metabolites in the DXT-M-treated group also exhibited a trend toward normalisation.

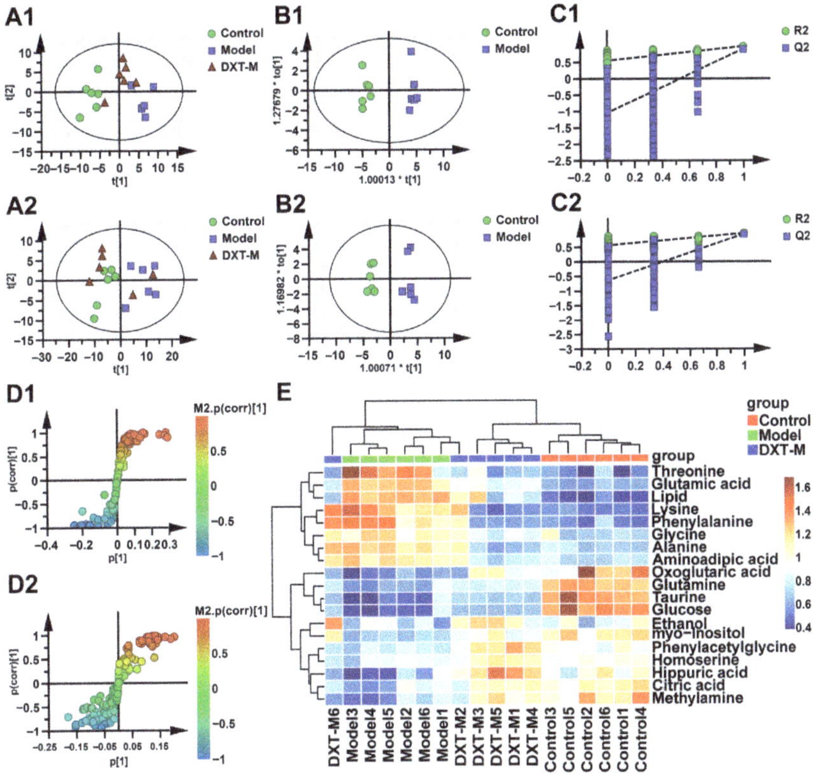

Figure 3. Multivariate analysis of serum and urine metabolomics. (**A1–D1**) Serum analysis: (**A1**) PCA score plots of Control, Model, and DXT-M treated groups; (**B1**) OPLS-DA model between Control vs. Model; (**C1**) Permutation test (200 iterations); (**D1**) s-Plot with $|p(corr)| \geq 0.5$ highlighting key metabolites. (**A2–D2**) Corresponding urine analyses. *t*[1] and *t*[2] indicate the first and second principal components, respectively. The asterisk (*) at the axis labels (t[1], t[2]) denotes scaled scores in the OPLS-DA model. (**E**) Hierarchical clustering heatmap of significantly altered metabolites (red: upregulation; blue: downregulation; $p < 0.05$, $VIP > 1.0$). Heatmap columns: C1–C6 (Control), M1–M6 (Model), DXT-M1–6 (DXT-M).

2.3.3. Endogenous Screening and Correlation Analysis with Biochemical Indicators

A univariate *t*-test was used to assess the significance of metabolites across the control, model, and DXT-M groups, identifying key metabolites via S-plot, *VIP* values ($VIP > 1$), and *t*-test ($p \leq 0.05$). As shown in Figure 4A and Supplementary Table S2, 8 metabolites were identified as potential biomarkers in the serum. Compared to controls, taurine, glucose, myo-inositol, and glutamine levels decreased, except for ethanol, but were adjusted after DXT-M treatment. Threonine, glutamic acid, and lipid levels increased but normalised post-treatment. Similarly, 11 significant urinary biomarkers were identified. In liver-injured animals, urine levels of alanine, lysine, aminoadipic acid, phenylalanine, and glycine rose significantly compared to the control group. Treatment with DXT-M reduced these metabolites, with all except glycine showing significant changes. Conversely, oxoglutaric acid, citric acid, methylamine, phenylacetylglycine, homoserine, and hippuric acid levels decreased, with substantial reductions in all but phenylacetylglycine and homoserine. DXT-M treatment significantly increased the levels of these 11 metabolites.

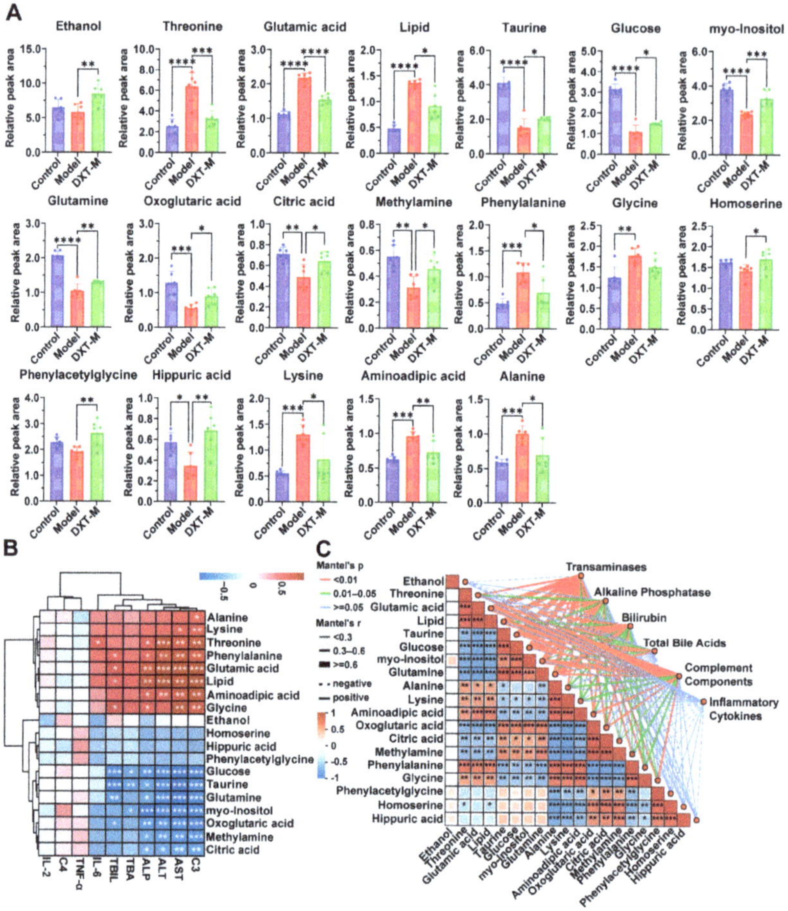

Figure 4. Metabolomic alterations and their pathophysiological correlations. (**A**) Relative peak areas of differential metabolites in serum and urine metabolomics across experimental groups. Data are presented as mean ± SD (n = 6 per group). Statistical significance was determined by one-way ANOVA followed by Dunnett's post hoc test (* $p < 0.05$, ** $p < 0.01$, *** $p < 0.001$, and **** $p < 0.0001$ vs. ANIT model group). (**B**) Hierarchical cluster heatmap (complete linkage, Euclidean distance) of Spearman's rank correlations between differential metabolites and clinical indices. $|r| \geq 0.6$, and Benjamini–Hochberg FDR-adjusted $p < 0.05$. Analysed parameters include liver enzymes (ALT, AST, ALP), bilirubin (TBIL), total bile acids (TBA), complement components (C3, C4), and inflammatory cytokines (TNF-α, IL-2, IL-6). The color gradient indicates the strength of correlation (red: positive correlation, $r > 0.6$; blue: negative correlation, $r < -0.6$), with the intensity proportional to the magnitude of the coefficient. (**C**) Mantel test correlation matrix between clinical indices (transaminases, alkaline phosphatase, bilirubin, total bile acids, complement components, and inflammatory cytokines) and differential metabolites. Edge thickness reflects Mantel's r statistic with 999 permutations ($p < 0.05$ by Benjamini–Hochberg FDR correction).

The association between biochemical indicators and potential metabolites was analysed using Spearman correlation and the Mantel test, with the results shown in Figure 4B,C. Figure 4B revealed that alanine, lysine, threonine, phenylalanine, glutamic acid, lipid, aminoadipic acid, and glycine positively correlate with C3, AST, ALT, ALP, TBIL, TBA, and IL-6, while glucose, taurine, glutamine, myo-inositol, oxoglutaric acid, methylamine, and citric acid showed negative correlations. C3, AST, ALT, ALP, TBIL, TBA, and IL-6 clustered together, separated from TNF-α, C4, and IL-2. The heatmap in Figure 4C highlighted significant correlations: transaminases with taurine, glucose, glutamine, α-ketoglutaric acid, and amino adipic acid; alkaline phosphatase with inositol and glutamic acid; and bilirubin with taurine, glucose, and glutamine. Total bile acids were only correlated with taurine and glucose. Complement components negatively correlated with lipids, glutamic acid, inositol, and threonine. These results, consistent with Figure 4B, suggested that biochemical changes were associated with variations in metabolite levels. The Mantel test showed significant spatial correlations among metabolites. Threonine, glutamic acid, and lipids positively correlated with alanine, lysine, and aminoadipic acid, but negatively with taurine, glucose, myo-inositol, and glutamine. TCA cycle metabolites, oxoglutaric and citric acid, were synergistic with methylamine, positively correlating with homoserine and hippuric acid, and negatively with phenylalanine. Phenylacetylglycine and homoserine also showed synergy, positively correlating with hippuric acid and negatively with alanine.

2.3.4. Analysis of the Metabolic Pathway

Key metabolites in serum and urine regulated by DXT-M were analysed using MetaboAnalyst 5.0 to investigate their corresponding metabolic pathways. Pathways with an impact value ≥ 0.01 and p-value ≥ 1 were considered relevant to DXT-M's liver protection. Serum metabolites enriched pathways like arginine biosynthesis, galactose metabolism, alanine, aspartate and glutamate metabolism, taurine and hypotaurine metabolism (Figure 5(A1)), while urine metabolites enriched pathways such as the alanine, aspartate and glutamate metabolism, phennylalanine metabolism, TCA cycle, glyoxylate and dicarboxylate metabolism, lysine degradation, phenylalanine metabolism, phenylalanine, tyrosine and tryptophan biosynthesis (Figure 5(A2)). In addition, it is worth noting that alanine, aspartate and glutamate metabolism were the common metabolic pathways enriched in both serum and urine, indicating their critical role in managing liver dysfunction by DXT-M. In addition, a KEGG-based metabolic network diagram depicted in Figure 5B highlighted the involvement of metabolites like hippuric acid, methylamine, taurine, and others in pathways related to taurine and hypotaurine metabolism, alanine, aspartate and glutamate metabolism, lysine degradation, galactose metabolism, the tricarboxylic acid (TCA) cycle, and biosynthesis of phenylalanine, tyrosine, tryptophan, and arginine.

2.4. *Integrated Analysis of Hepatoprotective Mechanisms*

2.4.1. Screening Results of Potential Targets

Using the TCMSP database, the chemical constituents of DXT-M were analysed, identifying 322 unique targets after merging duplicates (Figure 6(A1)). An OMIM search for "hepatitis" found 171 targets, while GeneCards provided 790 targets with high relevance scores. Additional targets were sourced from TTD (83), DisGeNET (248), and DRUGBANK (79), resulting in a comprehensive database of 1017 disease targets (Figure 6(A2)). The Venny platform identified 122 overlapping targets between DXT-M and hepatitis (Figure 6(A3)). These were further analysed using the Metscape plug-in v3.1.3 in Cytoscape v3.8.2, revealing 37 targets in the metabolite–reaction–enzyme–gene network.

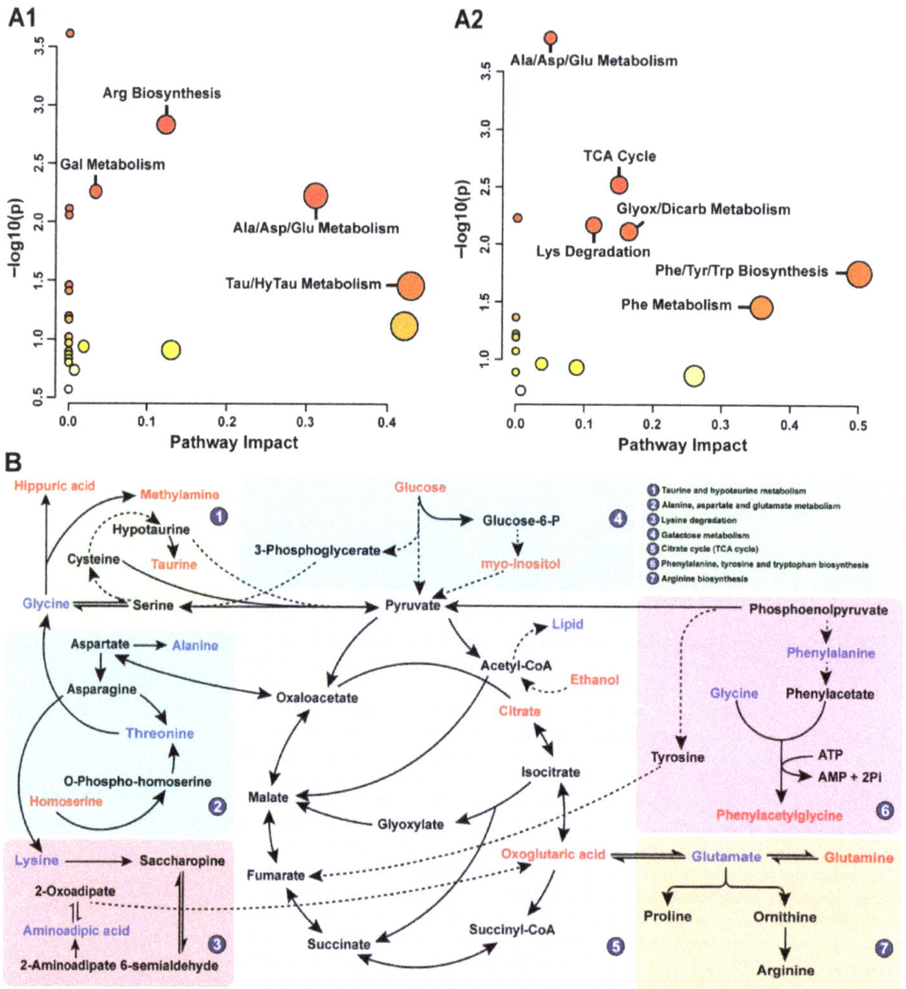

Figure 5. Metabolic pathway enrichment and interaction network of differential metabolites. (**A1**) Serum and (**A2**) urine metabolomics pathway enrichment analysis. Bubble colour intensity represents −log10(p) values (red: higher significance); bubble size indicates pathway impact value (larger size = greater regulatory effect). (**B**) Interaction network between annotated differential metabolites and metabolic pathways. Metabolites in red were significantly upregulated by DXT-M treatment, while those in blue were downregulated. Solid lines: direct interactions; dashed lines: indirect interactions. Key enriched pathways: ① Taurine and hypotaurine metabolism, ② Alanine, aspartate and glutamate metabolism, ③ Lysine degradation, ④ Galactose metabolism, ⑤ Citrate cycle (tricarboxylic acid cycle, TCA cycle), ⑥ Phenylalanine, tyrosine and tryptophan biosynthesis, ⑦ Arginine biosynthesis.

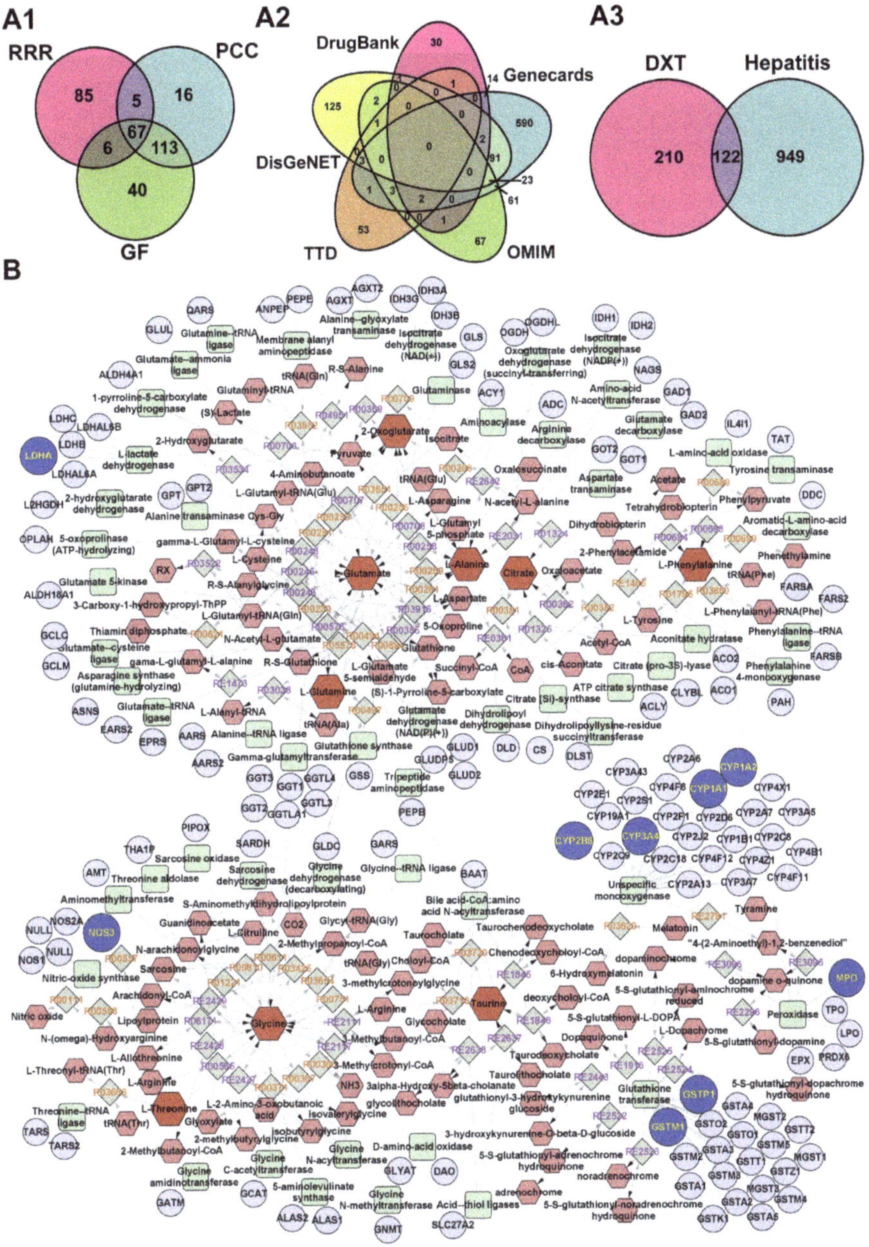

Figure 6. Venn analysis and compound–reaction–enzyme–gene (CREG) network of DXT-M in hepatitis treatment. (**A1**) Venn diagram of potential targets for DXT-M from TCMSP database. (**A2**) Hepatitis-related targets collected from DrugBank, DisGeNET, GeneCards, TTD, and OMIM databases. (**A3**) Intersection targets between DXT-M and hepatitis. (**B**) CREG network integrating DXT-M and hepatitis shared targets with differential metabolites from serum/urine metabolomics. Node types: red hexagons (compounds), gray diamonds (reactions), green squares (enzymes), blue circles (genes). Darker colors highlight key nodes: deep red (significantly altered metabolites), deep blue (DXT-M and hepatitis intersection targets).

2.4.2. Compound-Reaction-Enzyme-Gene Network

As illustrated in Figure 6B, the advanced integrated analysis conducted by Metscape has successfully generated networks comprising compounds, reactions, enzymes, and genes across multiple metabolic pathways, including bile acid biosynthesis, various amino acid metabolisms, glycolysis, gluconeogenesis, and the TCA cycle, among others. The target enzyme LDHA is involved in glycolysis and gluconeogenesis by interacting with endogenous metabolites such as ethanol and glucose. Targets such as MPO and GSTM1 are implicated in the regulation of tyrosine metabolism through phenylalanine. GSTM1, GSTP1, NOS3, and other enzymes modulated the urea cycle and associated amino acid metabolisms through endogenous metabolites. Enzymes such as GPT and ODC1 also influence these metabolic processes via distinct endogenous metabolites. Furthermore, GSTM1, CYP1A1, and other enzymes regulate tryptophan metabolism through enzyme-mediated regulation of metabolites. Glycine and taurine are potentially involved in bile acid biosynthesis through indirect target regulation, while glycine, alanine, and threonine participate in their respective amino acid metabolisms. Citrate and 2-oxoglutarate are likely involved in the TCA cycle. These metabolites and targets are interconnected through shared or key regulatory nodes, forming an integrated molecular network characterised by hierarchical synergy. This network shows coordination between phenotypic effects and intrinsic mechanisms.

2.4.3. Target Interaction Analysis

The 122 potential targets of DXT-M for hepatitis treatment, as outlined in Section 2.4.1, were imported into the STRING database with the species parameter set to 'human' and the screening criterion established at a high-confidence threshold of 0.700 for PPI analysis. Subsequently, the data were imported into Cytoscape v3.8.2 software to construct a PPI network and perform topological analysis, as depicted in Figure 7(A1). Utilising this framework, the MCODE plug-in was employed to identify three core sub-networks within the PPI network, illustrated in Figure 7(A2–A4). Analysis of the core sub-networks in Figure 7(A2,A3) reveals that the key targets with higher degree values essentially correspond to the principal targets within the PPI network of the 122 potential DXT-M targets for hepatitis treatment. Furthermore, examination of the core sub-network in Figure 7(A4) indicates that nodes such as GSTP1, GSTM1, CYP1A1, CYP1A2, CYP2B6, and CYP3A4 exhibit a significant degree of overlap with the integrated targets identified in Section 2.4.2. Consequently, based on the degree values of each target in Figure 7(A1), and in conjunction with the representative component targets of DXT-M and the integrated targets from Section 2.4.2, a total of 19 targets were selected (see Supplementary Table S3).

2.4.4. Hepatoprotective Targets Enrichment Analysis

Nineteen potential targets were analysed with the DAVID database for GO and KEGG enrichment, focusing on FDR-adjusted *p*-values ($p < 0.05$) and Count values. This identified 14 BP terms (Count ≥ 4), 1 CC term, and 8 MF terms (Count ≥ 3), as shown in Figure 7(B1). BP terms included xenobiotic metabolism, cell proliferation, and apoptosis regulation, among others. The CC term was about the endoplasmic reticulum membrane, and MF terms covered enzyme, heme binding, etc. Correlation analysis (Figure 7(B2)) revealed a regulatory network centred on the CYP450 enzyme family (CYP1A2, CYP1A1, CYP3A4, CYP2B6), which is involved in xenobiotic metabolism and other activities. CYP1A2, CYP1A1, and CYP3A4 also participate in long-chain fatty acid biosynthesis. PTGS2, MPO, etc., are associated with oxidative stress responses and affect apoptosis and cell proliferation, contributing to the MAPK/ERK cascade. Protein interaction analysis revealed that CYP enzymes interacted with JUN, among others, and some responded to lipopolysaccharide. KEGG pathway analysis (Figure 7C) revealed that CYP1A2, among others, was enriched in xenobiotic metabolism. CYP3A4 was involved in all metabolism pathways, and CYP2B6 was linked to lipid metabolism and atherosclerosis. HRAS, among others, was central in cancer pathways. NOS3, etc., controlled cardiovascular disease pathways, and HRAS, etc., played a key role in hormone signalling networks.

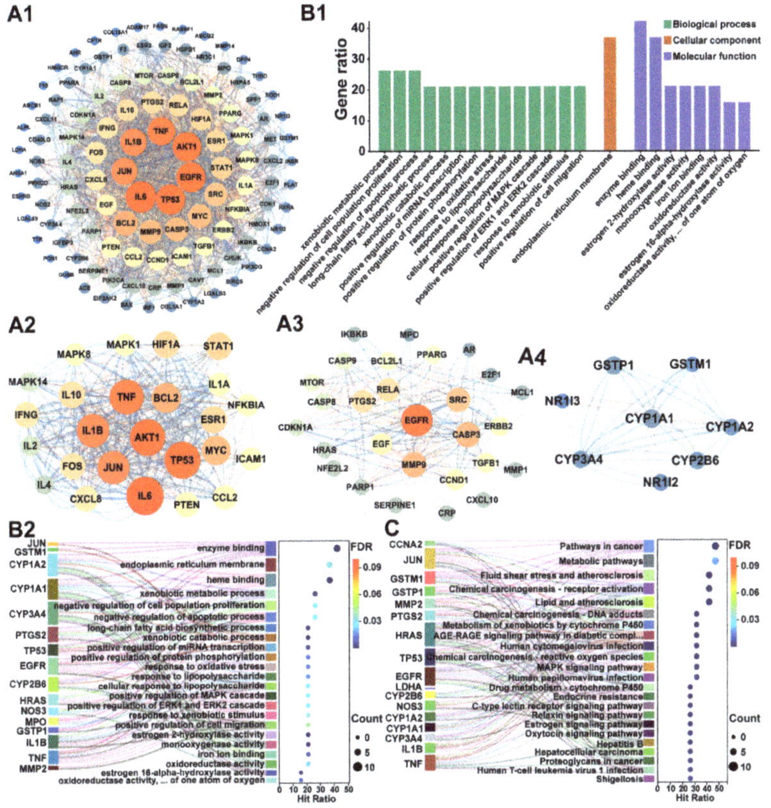

Figure 7. Network pharmacological analysis of DXT-M in hepatitis intervention. (**A1–A4**) Protein–protein interaction (PPI) network analysis showing: (**A1**) Global PPI network of 122 intersection targets. (**A2–A4**) Topologically significant subnetworks identified via MCODE plug-in in Cytoscape (v3.8.2); Cluster 1 (Score: 18.083, 25 nodes), Cluster 2 (Score: 9.481, 28 nodes), Cluster 3 (Score: 6.571, 8 nodes), with node colour/size indicating degree centrality and edge thickness reflecting STRING combined scores. (**B1**,**B2**) Functional enrichment analysis including: (**B1**) Significantly enriched GO terms (FDR-adjusted $p < 0.05$) displayed as a clustered bar plot; (**B2**) Sankey-bubble plot displaying left DXT-M targets, middle GO terms, and right enrichment bubbles. (**C**) KEGG pathway enrichment Sankey-bubble plot. The layout follows the same scheme as (**B2**), with the right column showing enriched KEGG pathways. The GO term "oxidoreductase activity, . . . of one atom of oxygen" refers to "oxidoreductase activity, acting on paired donors, with incorporation or reduction of molecular oxygen, reduced flavin or flavoprotein as one donor, and incorporation of one atom of oxygen". The KEGG pathway "AGE-RAGE signalling pathway in diabetic compl" refers to the AGE-RAGE signalling pathway in diabetic complications.

2.5. Network Toxicology Analysis

2.5.1. Target Screening and Interaction Analysis

The Comparative Toxicogenomics Database identified 419 targets linked to drug-induced liver injury. After combining with 322 DXT-M targets, a Venn diagram showed

44 overlapping targets (Figure 8A). These were analysed using the STRING database and Cytoscape v3.8.2 to create a PPI network, as shown in Figure 8(B1). The MCODE plug-in identified core subnetworks of DXT-M liver injury targets, depicted in Figure 8(B2–B4). Key targets, such as CYP3A4, CYP1A2, CYP2B6, CYP1A1, GSTP1, and GSTM1, appear in both the PPI network and core subnetworks, and are crucial for DXT-M's role in modulating metabolism, as detailed in Section 2.4.2. Concurrently, TNF, IL1B, CCL2, MMP9, HMOX1, PPARA, and IFNG were key nodes in the PPI network and core subnetwork. Consequently, 14 core liver toxicity targets of DXT-M were identified for further analysis (Supplementary Table S4).

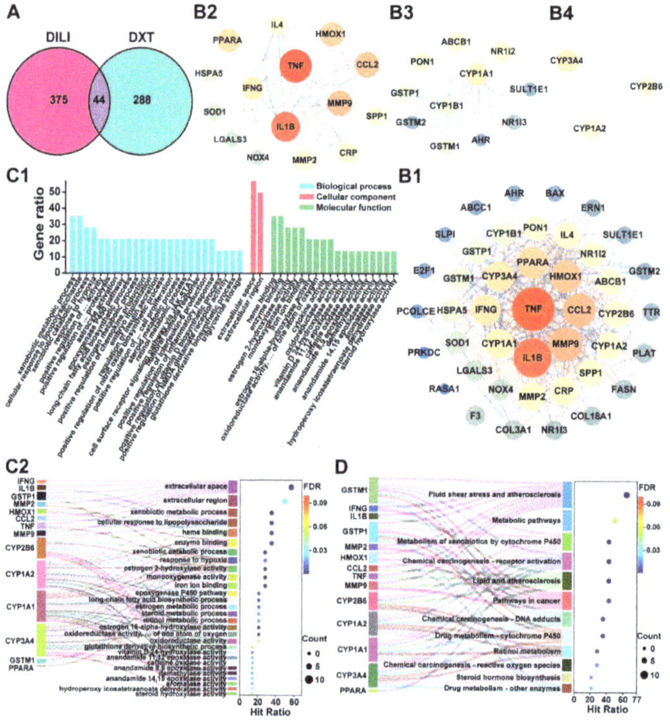

Figure 8. Network toxicological of DXT-M associated drug-induced liver injury (DILI) risk. (**A**) Venn diagram of overlapping targets between DXT-M and known DILI-related targets. (**B1–B4**) PPI network analysis: (**B1**) Global PPI network of 44 intersection targets; (**B2–B4**) Topologically significant modules identified via MCODE in Cytoscape (v3.8.2)-Cluster 1 (Score: 12.714, 15 nodes), Cluster 2 (Score: 6.6, 11 nodes), Cluster 3 (Score:3.0, 3 nodes), with node properties scaled by degree centrality and edge weights reflecting STRING confidence scores. (**C1**,**C2**) Functional annotation: (**C1**) Significantly enriched GO terms (FDR-adjusted $p < 0.05$) categorised by biological processes, cellular components and molecular functions; The GO term "positive regulation of ... proteolysis" refers to the complete term: "positive regulation of membrane protein ectodomain proteolysis". (**C2**) Sankey-bubble plot visualising target–GO term relationships with bubble size representing target count and colour indicating FDR *p*-value. (**D**) KEGG pathway enrichment Sankey-bubble plot. The GO term "positive regulation of ... activity" refers to "positive regulation of calcidiol 1-monooxygenase activity"; The GO term "positive regulation of ... proteolysis" refers to "positive regulation of membrane protein ectodomain proteolysis"; The GO term "positive regulation of ... cell proliferation" refers to "positive regulation of vascular associated smooth muscle cell proliferation"; The GO term "oxidoreductase activity, ... of one atom of oxygen" refers to "oxidoreductase activity, acting on paired donors, with incorporation or reduction of molecular oxygen, reduced flavin or flavoprotein as one donor, and incorporation of one atom of oxygen".

2.5.2. Toxicity-RelatedTargets Enrichment Analysis

The 14 toxic targets of DXT-M from Section 2.5.1 were analysed using the DAVID database for GO and KEGG pathway enrichment analysis. With FDR-adjusted *p*-value ($p < 0.05$), 14 BP, 2 CC, and 19 MF terms were identified (Figure 8(C1)). Key BP terms included xenobiotic, lipid, and metabolism, as well as cellular stress and immune responses. Other BP terms involved signalling and enzymatic activities, highlighting vascular and inflammatory regulation. The CC terms, extracellular space and region, linked targets to the extracellular compartment. Enriched MF terms mainly involved enzymatic catalytic functions, especially oxidoreductase activities, and binding functions. Similar to DXT-M pharmacodynamic targets, CYP is central to DXT-M toxicity targets and GO entries. Figure 8(C2) showed that toxicity targets were enriched in xenobiotic metabolism (CYP1A2, CYP1A1, CYP3A4, CYP2B6, GSTM1, GSTP1), extracellular localisation (IFNG, IL1B, TNF, MMP9), and heme/iron-dependent catalysis, with key activities contributing to stress responses and lipid/steroid metabolism. Figure 8D indicated that KEGG pathway enrichment analysis identified key drug toxicity targets, including CYP1A2, CYP3A4, GSTM1, and GSTP1, mainly in drug metabolism pathways. HMOX1 was linked to fluid shear and oxidative stress pathways. IL1B, TNF, etc., were associated with inflammation and cancer-related pathways. PPARA was involved in the regulation of chemical carcinogenesis and inflammatory response pathways.

2.6. *Target–Component Fitting Validation*

Receptor proteins like EGFR, TP53, and TNF were sourced from the PDB, while GSTP1, CCL2, and IFNG were obtained from UniProt. DXT-M drugs contain anthraquinones, iridoid glycosides, and alkaloids, forming a chemical library of bioactive constituents. Active sites of targets, including EGFR and TP53, were identified using co-crystallised ligands, while proteins without such ligands were used MOE's Site Finder for pocket identification. HRAS interactions were examined through full-protein docking. Binding Z-scores are in Supplementary Table S5 and Figure 9A, with interaction diagrams in Figure 9B–I and PLIF analysis in Supplementary Figure S3. In the ligand–target fitting score clustering diagram (Figure 9A), DXT-M active ingredients were grouped into anthraquinones from RRR, iridoid glycosides from GF, and alkaloids from PCC. One target cluster included PTGS2, CYP1A2, CYP1A1, and PPARA, while others formed a separate cluster. Anthraquinones in RRR showed high affinity for the first cluster but lower scores. Geniposide, crocin from GF, and palmatine in PCC had high affinity with 23 targets, whereas berberine and berberrubine in PCC had weaker affinity. Anthraquinones in RRR mainly targeted PTGS2, CYP1A2, CYP1A1, and PPARA. β-sitosterol from RRR, PCC, and GF bound well to most targets, except for PTGS2, CYP1A2, CYP1A1, and PPARA. Quercetin showed weak affinity for all targets. The 3D interaction analysis revealed key binding residues: LDHA (Arg168, Glu191, His192, Asp194), MPO (Asp94, His95, Asp98, Thr100), NOS3 (Cys184, Trp156), CYP1A1 (Asn255, Phe258, Asp313, Ala317), CYP1A2 (Thr124, Phe260, Gly316, Ala317, Asp320), CYP3A4 (Arg105, Arg212, Arg372, Glu374, Arg375), GSTM1 (Tyr7, Trp8, Ser73), and GSTP1 (Arg14, Leu53, Tyr109).

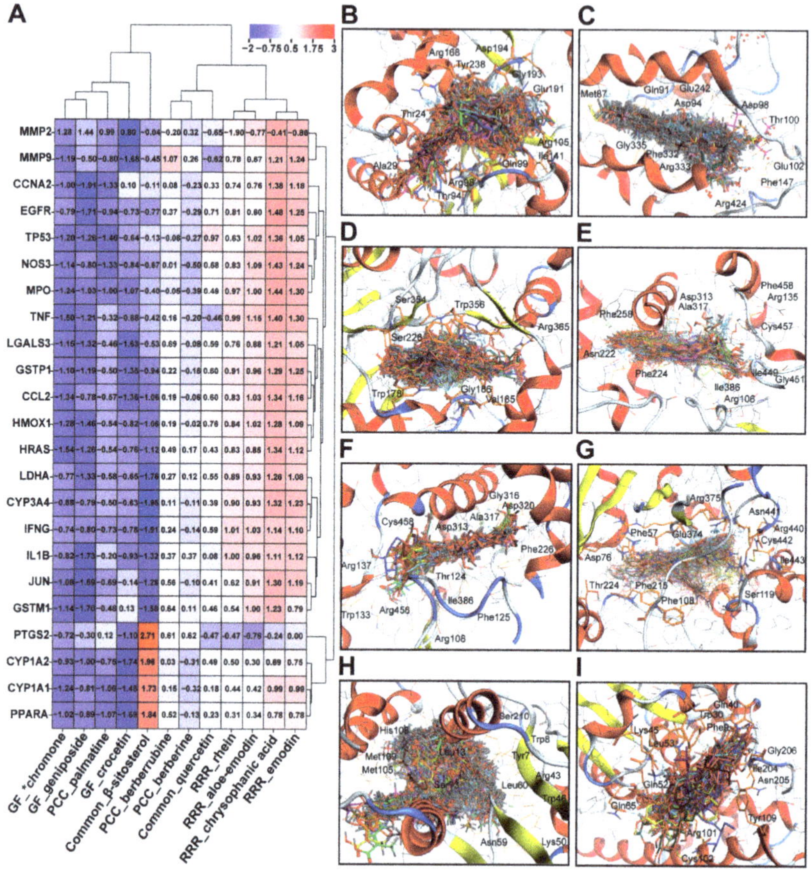

Figure 9. Fitting validation of DXT-M representative compounds with core targets. (**A**) Hierarchically clustered heatmap (complete linkage, Euclidean distance) of docking scores between 12 representative DXT-M compounds and 23 integrated targets (network pharmacology–toxicology screening). Data were column-wise Z-score normalised (blue: strong binding affinity; red: weak affinity). (**B–I**) Ligand–receptor binding conformations: Ligands shown as stick models (colored by atom type), proteins as molecular surfaces (electrostatic potential). PDB IDs: LDHA (5W8J), MPO (4C1M), NOS3 (7TSG), CYP1A1 (4I8V), CYP1A2 (2HI4), CYP3A4 (6MA8), GSTM1 (8VOU), and GSTP1 (AF-P09211-F1).

2.7. The Component–Target–Pathway Association Analysis

After integrating and deduplicating DXT-M's targets, 24 unique targets were identified. Enrichment analysis via the DAVID Database revealed 25 significant pathways, excluding LDHA. Figure 10 illustrates the hepatoprotective and hepatotoxic relevance of DXT-M through shared targets, including GSTM1, IL1B, GSTP1, MMP2, TNF, CYP2B6, CYP1A1, CYP1A2, and CYP3A4. These targets may function through common pathways related to metabolism, cytochrome P450, xenobiotic metabolism, retinol metabolism, steroid hormone biosynthesis, vascular issues, atherosclerosis, and cancer, including hepatocellular carcinoma and chemical carcinogenesis. DXT-M's liver-protective effects may involve targets such as JUN, NOS3, and TP53, which function through relaxin, estrogen, and HIF-1 signalling pathways, and may also influence cancer-related pathways, including prostate cancer and VEGF signalling. In contrast, its liver toxicity is linked to targets like IFNG and HMOX1, mainly through the diabetic cardiomyopathy pathway, potentially increasing risks due to overlapping pathways.

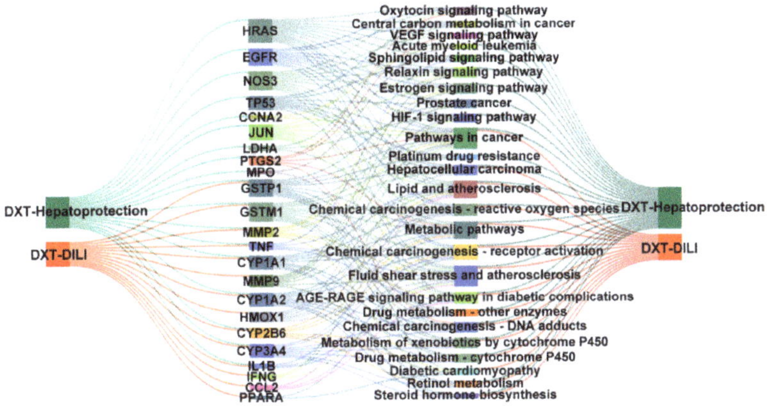

Figure 10. Systems pharmacology network of DXT-M dual effects on liver injury.

3. Discussion

3.1. Metabolic Reprogramming Underlies DXT-M's Hepatoprotective Mechanisms

TCM's holistic approach and syndrome differentiation are fundamental to its diagnostic and therapeutic efficacy, and the metabolomic profile identified in this study objectively reflected the disease phenotype, aligning with the holistic principles of TCM [48,49]. Prescriptions like DXT, formulated through component-based compatibility and refined constituent retention, demonstrate enhanced pharmacological precision. DXT-M significantly improved hepatoprotective indicators—notably body weight, serum enzymes (ALT, AST), bilirubin, bile acids, and complement C3—while repairing liver damage with a clear dose–response relationship, outperforming traditional decoction [43,44,50]. While precision medicine advances target identification, its single-target paradigm often fails to address the complex heterogeneity of diseases [51]. TCM syndrome, reflecting systemic regulatory imbalance, aligns with metabolomics profiling of endogenous biomarkers. This study identified 19 serum/urine biomarkers, with liver injury exhibiting dysregulation in metabolites, including glutamic acid, alanine, taurine, and hippuric acid—many of which are linked to TCA cycle-driven dysmetabolism of glucose, lipids, and amino acids [52,53]. The correlation network delineated in Figure 5B provides a mechanistic roadmap linking these metabolic alterations modulated by DXT-M to the observed phenotypic recovery. Several key correlations warrant elaboration. First, the strong negative correlations between taurine, glucose, glutamine, and critical liver injury indices (ALT, AST, TBIL, TBA) are highly informative. As a key hepatoprotective agent, taurine alleviates cholestasis by conjugating bile acids (reducing TBIL/TBA) [54,55] and mitigates hepatocyte damage via antioxidant activity (lowering ALT/AST) [56–58]. In addition, taurine supports fat and cholesterol metabolism [59,60]; its depletion during liver injury impairs these functions, a deficit that DXT-M treatment effectively counteracts.

The negative correlation of glucose and glutamine with these enzymes underscores the critical role of energy metabolism in liver repair. DXT-M's restoration of glucose and glutamine levels likely replenishes the tricarboxylic acid (TCA) cycle, providing essential energy and biosynthetic precursors for hepatocyte regeneration, which in turn normalises transaminase levels. Furthermore, the positive correlations of amino acids such as alanine, lysine, and threonine with the same panel of injury markers underscore their potential as biomarkers of disrupted nitrogen metabolism. In a damaged liver, impaired transamination and ureagenesis lead to the accumulation of these amino acids in the bloodstream [61,62]. Therefore, the reduction of these amino acids following DXT-M treatment reflects a restoration of hepatic aminotransferase function and ammonia detoxification capacity. Finally, the close clustering of complement C3 with traditional liver function tests (ALT, AST, ALP) and its significant correlation with specific metabolites reveals an intriguing interface between innate immunity and metabolism in this injury model. The complement system is a known mediator of inflammatory liver injury. The correlation pattern suggests that the metabolic stress signalled by perturbations in lipids and glutamate may be linked to complement activation [63,64]. DXT-M's ability to concurrently normalise complement C3 levels and correct these metabolic disturbances points to its dual anti-inflammatory and metabolic-regulatory actions, which collectively contribute to its overall hepatoprotective efficacy.

The analysis revealed that in ANIT-induced acute liver injury models, there was a significant decrease in glucose levels, a marked increase in lipid levels, and the occurrence of recumbency and rapid weight loss. These findings indicate a disruption in energy and substance metabolism. Previous research has established that glucose is crucial to the body's energy metabolism, as it produces pyruvate [65]. Pyruvate is then subjected to aerobic oxidation, resulting in the production of carbon dioxide and water, or anaerobic fermentation in yeast, leading to the formation of lactic acid or ethanol, thereby generating ATP to support the body's essential functions [66]. The tricarboxylic acid (TCA) cycle, a crucial step in aerobic oxidation, is closely linked to the body's energy metabolism [67–69]. In addition, in animals with liver injury, there was a marked reduction in the levels of citrate and α-ketoglutarate within the TCA cycle pathway compared to healthy controls. This diminution in TCA cycle intermediates resulted in impaired energy metabolism. Conversely, administration of DXT-M significantly increased the endogenous biomarkers of citric acid and α-ketoglutarate levels within the TCA cycle. Additionally, DXT-M effectively modulated the dysregulated glucose and lipid metabolism in liver-injured animals, thereby ameliorating their abnormal physiological indicators. Consequently, DXT-M is proposed as a potential therapeutic intervention for enhancing energy metabolism in liver-damaged animals by modulating the TCA cycle and regulating glucose metabolism.

The TCA cycle is a crucial intermediary pathway connecting various nutrients, including sugars, lipids, and proteins [70–72]. It facilitates the renewal and metabolism of amino acids through processes such as amino acid transamination, deamination, and α-ketoglutaric acid metabolism [73,74]. Following acute liver injury induced by ANIT, transaminases such as ALT and AST are released into the bloodstream, resulting in an abnormal elevation of serum ALT and AST levels. In the presence of aminotransferase, the TCA cycle intermediate α-ketoglutaric acid accepts amino groups to form glutamic acid, thereby expediting the depletion of α-ketoglutaric acid intermediates and diminishing energy metabolism within the TCA cycle. Furthermore, a reciprocal transformation and equilibrium dynamic exist between glutamate and glutamine, facilitated by the enzymatic activities of glutamine synthetase and glutaminase [75,76]. Glutamine serves as a detoxification agent for ammonia and plays a crucial role in the storage and transportation of ammonia [77–79]. In liver injury, hepatocytes sustain damage, disrupting the metabolism of glutamine and glutamate [75]. ANIT-induced liver injury leads to a substantial increase in glutamate levels and a significant decrease in glutamine levels. However, treatment with DXT-M effectively restores the balance of glutamate and glutamine metabolism, indicating its potential in liver detoxification through regulating glutamate-glutamine equilibrium. In instances of liver injury, aside from the previously mentioned impairments in glucose metabolism and the tricarboxylic acid (TCA) cycle, there is also a potential for disruptions in protein and lipid metabolism, as well as other substances [80–82].

The liver plays a crucial role in metabolism, detoxification, and immune regulation [83,84]. According to the Zangxiang theory in TCM, the liver aids in blood storage and relief functions [85]. The liver's ability to store and circulate blood aids nutrient transformation and distribution in the body [86]. However, when pathogens invade, this function is disrupted, causing depression, impaired fluid and qi flow, reduced physical activity, and weakened nourishment [87]. Contemporary studies have demonstrated that inadequate warmth and nourishment provided by the body's qi and blood can result in symptoms such as stagnation of qi, deficiency of qi, and stasis of blood, often accompanied by varying degrees of abnormal metabolism of substances and energy, primarily caused by disruptions in the TCA cycle [88–90]. The study found that animals with liver injury showed signs like recumbency and weight loss, along with abnormal liver function and energy metabolism issues related to the TCA cycle. These findings support the Zangxiang theory's view of liver dysfunction. After administering DXT-M, these abnormalities improved, indicating that DXT-M has the potential to correct metabolic imbalances in liver injury by affecting TCA cycle biomarkers. The research highlights the metabolic profile of liver injury caused by ANIT and explains how DXT-M provides liver protection. In summary, the coordinated normalisation of this interconnected metabolite–clinical index network, as deciphered from Figure 6B, substantiates the multitarget and system-level therapeutic mechanism of DXT-M.

3.2. Bidirectional Regulation Network of DXT-M's Hepatoprotection and Hepatotoxicity

Integrated metabolomics and network pharmacology revealed that DXT-M could modulate endogenous metabolites via specific targets, influencing hepatic energy metabolism and hepatoprotection. DXT-M components regulated ethanol and sugars through LDHA, impacting glycolysis and hepatic energy balance [91,92]. It could also modulate metabolites, such as phenylalanine, via targets (MPO, GSTM1, GSTP1, CYP450s, e.g., CYP3A4, CYP1A2), affecting tyrosine metabolism and linking to antioxidant/detoxification effects [93–95]. Furthermore, DXT-M components could influence glutamic acid, glycine, and 2-ketoglutaric acid through specific targets (GSTM1, GSTP1, NOS3), thereby regulating the urea cycle and arginine/proline/glutamic acid pathways, and maintaining a balance in nitrogen metabolism and supporting liver detoxification/repair [96–98]. DXT-M also modulated tryptophan metabolism via targets (GSTM1, GSTP1, CYP1A1, CYP1A2, CYP2B6, CYP3A4), affecting inflammatory factors [99,100]. Additionally, DXT-M and its components interact with bile acid receptors (BSEP, MRP2, and NSTP) and regulate conjugation molecules (glycine and taurine), thereby influencing bile acid biosynthesis and enterohepatic circulation, which contributes to hepatoprotection [41,43,101]. Key enzymes identified (CYP, GST, NOS3) significantly mediate DXT-M's regulation of hepatic energy metabolism and oxidative stress through pathways including pyruvate-aspartate-glutamate metabolism, taurine metabolism, and the TCA cycle.

According to TCM principles, DXT, a prescription for damp-heat jaundice, exerts hepatoprotective effects when applied in conjunction with syndrome differentiation; however, its intrinsic properties can cause adverse effects if misused [30,102,103]. Network toxicology identified overlapping targets of hepatic drug-metabolising enzymes (CYP, GST) in DXT-M's hepatoprotective (metabolomics-network pharmacology) and hepatotoxic mechanisms. Core pathway enrichment revealed 14 shared pathways (e.g., detoxification, energy metabolism, inflammation) and distinct hepatoprotection-specific pathways [104,105]. Crucially, the CYP450-GST (detoxification)-ROS (inflammation) axis (targets: CYP2B6, CYP1A1, CYP1A2, CYP3A4, GSTM1, GSTP1, IL1B, MMP2, TNF) represented the common intersection. CYP450 and GST facilitate xenobiotic detoxification via Phase I/II metabolism, but can also generate toxic metabolites that saturate GST capacity, leading to ROS accumulation, oxidative stress, inflammation (TNF-α, IL-1β), mitochondrial dysfunction, and disrupted TCA cycle energy metabolism, ultimately causing hepatotoxicity [106–109]. The GST/ROS balance determines the outcome of detoxification versus toxicity. DXT-M can ameliorate

TCA cycle dysregulation (linked to hepatoprotection) and act via targets (e.g., NOS3, JUN, TP53) in specific pathways to promote vascular remodelling and mitochondrial function.

3.3. Translational Implications and Future Perspectives

The observed correlation between metabolic reprogramming patterns and pharmacodynamic improvements underscored the hepatoprotective efficacy of DXT-M in acute liver injury, suggesting its significant potential as a candidate for managing this condition. Integrated analyses of network pharmacology and toxicology revealed that key enzymes mediating the hepatoprotective effects of DXT-M, such as CYP450s and GSTs, may also serve as potential targets for its toxicity, indicating a dual-faceted mechanism inherent to its composition [109–111]. Future research should prioritise the experimental validation of this regulatory network using targeted approaches, such as siRNA or pharmacological inhibitors. Building upon this foundation, a promising future direction is the development of a more refined, multi-component formulation based on the representative bioactive compounds of DXT-M's constituent herbs (e.g., anthraquinones, berberine, and geniposide). This strategy will help identify the core synergistic combination responsible for the observed efficacy and further elucidate the precise molecular mechanisms. Additionally, clinical translation will necessitate careful patient stratification and monitoring of metabolic enzyme activities to ensure safe application within a personalised medicine framework [112]. Given the identified overlap between efficacy and toxicity targets, the clinical translation of DXT-M as a multitarget therapeutic agent necessitates a personalised medicine approach [113]. Future clinical applications should involve careful patient stratification, and monitoring liver function and drug-metabolising enzyme activity (e.g., CYP3A4) would be crucial to mitigate potential herb–drug interactions or toxicity in susceptible individuals. Well-designed clinical trials are crucial for translating preclinical findings into safe and effective patient care.

Several limitations warrant consideration in interpreting these findings. The use of a single animal model (ANIT-induced acute liver injury) may not fully recapitulate the complexity of human liver diseases, and the absence of pharmacokinetic data for key active components limits understanding of their in vivo behaviour [114]. Most importantly, as these findings are derived solely from preclinical experiments, future research should incorporate clinical data through retrospective analyses of patient cases to validate the relevance of the identified metabolic profiles and molecular targets in human populations [115,116]. Such clinical correlation will be essential for translating these systemic insights into safe and effective therapeutic strategies.

4. Materials and Methods

4.1. Materials and Reagents

Rhei Radix Et Rhizoma (RRR; the dried root and rhizome of *Rheum palmatum* L.), Phellodendri Chinensis Cortex (PCC; the dried cortex of *Phellodendrn chinense* Schneid), Gardeniae Fructus (GF; the dried ripe fruit of *Gardenia jasminoides* Ellis.), Natrii Sulfas (NS; the kind of sulfate crystal mineral drug mainly containing $Na_2SO_4 \cdot 10H_2O$), were purchased from Shanxi Wanmin Pharmacy (Taiyuan, China). Aloe-emodin, rhein, emodin, chrysophanol, physcion, berberine, and geniposide were purchased from the National Institutes for Food and Drug Control (Beijing, China). α-naphthalene isothiocyanate (ANIT) was purchased from ALFA Aesar Chemical (Tianjin, China), and Ursodeoxycholic acid tablets were purchased from Shanghai Xinyi Pharmaceutical (Beijing, China). 3-Trimethylsilyl-propionate-d_4 sodium (TPS) and deuteriumoxide (D_2O) were purchased from Beijing Bailingwei Technology (Beijing, China). Glutamate pyruvate transaminase (ALT/GPT), glutamic oxalacetic transaminase (AST/GOT), alkaline phosphatase (ALP), total bilirubin (TBIL), indirect bilirubin (DBIL) and total bile acid (TBA) kits were purchased from Siemens Healthineers (Shanghai, China). Prealbumin (PA), Complement C3 (C3) and C4 kits were purchased from Ningbo Meikang Bioengineering (Ningbo, China). Interleukin-2 (IL-2), Interleukin-6 (IL-6) and tumour necrosis factor α (TNF-α) kits were purchased from Shanghai Bioengineering (Shanghai, China).

4.2. Herbal Refined Extracts Preparation

DXT was prepared by boiling a mixture of RRR (12 g), PCC (12 g), GF (9 g), and NS (12 g) according to the original prescription ratio using 10 volumes of water per extraction for two cycles, with the combined filtrate concentrated to 0.5 g crude drug per mL [29]; DXT-M was formulated from refined extracts of RRR, PCC, and GF combined with native NS in the optimised ratio of RRR refined extract 0.8478 g, PCC refined extract 0.3150 g, GF refined extract 0.9990 g, and NS 4 g [41]. The individual refined extracts were prepared as follows: RRR (1000 g) was extracted three times with water (1:10, *w*/*v*, 30 min each), and the combined filtrates were concentrated to 0.75 g/mL (equivalent to 0.75 g crude drug per mL) before purification on an AB-8 macroporous resin column (loaded at 0.94 g crude drug per mL resin), where the column was washed with water until the effluent became clear and then eluted with 95% ethanol until the eluate was colorless, with the ethanol eluate concentrated under reduced pressure to a thick extract and dried at low temperature to yield 94.2 g of refined extract; PCC (1000 g) was refluxed three times with 75% ethanol (1:10, *w*/*v*, 1.5 h each), and after ethanol recovery, the combined filtrate was concentrated to 0.5 g/mL (equivalent to 0.5 g crude drug per mL) and processed on an AB-8 resin column (loaded at 1 g crude drug per mL resin) with water wash until clear effluent followed by elution with 50% ethanol until the resin bed became colorless, with the ethanol eluate concentrated under reduced pressure to a thick extract and dried at low temperature to yield 52.5 g of refined extract; GF (1000 g) was decocted twice with water (1:12, *w*/*v*, 1 h each), and the combined filtrate was concentrated to 0.5 g/mL (equivalent to 0.5 g crude drug per mL) before separation on an HPD-100 resin column (loaded at 1.5 g crude drug per mL resin) using water wash until clear effluent and subsequent elution with 75% ethanol until the eluate became colorless, with the ethanol eluate concentrated under reduced pressure to a thick extract and dried at low temperature to yield 74.0 g of refined extract [45,47].

4.3. Qualitative Analysis of RRR, PCC and GF

0.1 g of RRR, PCC, and GF dried herbal extracts were each dissolved in methanol in 10 mL flasks and then filtered through a 0.22 μm membrane. 0.76 mg aloe-emodin, 0.41 mg rhein, 0.92 mg emodin, 1.17 mg physcion, and 0.51 mg chrysophanol were dissolved separately in methanol to a total volume of 10 mL. Mix 2 mL of each to form a mixed reference solution of anthraquinones. Reference solutions were also prepared by dissolving 1.00 mg of berberine and 0.30 mg of geniposide in methanol to a final volume of 10 mL, separately. The chemical constituents of RRR, PCC, GF extracts and their reference substances were analysed using Agilent 1260 HPLC (Santa Clara, CA, USA). The YMC-Pack ODS-AD Column (Kyoto, Japan) was used for RRR and GF, while a Phenomenex Gemini-NX Column (Torrance, CA, USA) was used for PCC. Elution details and detection wavelengths are in Table 1. NS, primarily sodium sulfate decahydrate ($Na_2SO_4 \cdot 10H_2O$), was not further analysed due to its known composition [117,118].

Table 1. Elutions and detection wavelengths for DXT and DXT-M compositions.

Time/Min	A (Acetonitrile + 0.0375% TFA)	B (Water + 0.0375% TFA)	Detective Wavelengths	Compositions
0	0	100%	380 nm	RRR
15	15%	85%		
35	30%	70%		
40	35%	65%		
50	40%	60%		
55	60%	40%		
60	100%	0		
65	100%	0		
0	0	100%	345 nm	PCC
7	20%	80%		
12	25%	75%		
18	80%	20%		
25	80%	20%		
0	0	100%	238 nm	GF
30	25%	75%		
50	40%	60%		

4.4. Animals Feeding

Equal numbers of male and female Wistar rats (200 ± 20 g) were provided by the Experimental Animal Center, Academy of Military Medical Sciences (Beijing, China, SCXK (Army) 2012-0004). They were fed standard food and water for 7 days under a 12 h light/dark cycle at 20 ± 2 °C and 40 ± 5% humidity to acclimate. Throughout the study, every effort was made to minimise animal suffering and stress. All procedures were performed by personnel trained in rodent handling, using gentle restraint to minimise the duration of any discomfort. The housing conditions were strictly maintained to ensure animal well-being. Experiments were conducted in accordance with the guidelines of the Animal Ethics Committee of Shanxi University of Chinese Medicine, ensuring minimal animal suffering (Approval number: AWE2025093635).

4.5. Animal Grouping, Modelling and Administration Procedure

Wistar rats (n = 6 per group, balanced by sex) were randomly divided into seven groups: control, model, positive (ursodeoxycholic acid), DXT, low, medium, and high doses of DXT-M (5.4, 10, and 20 times the human equivalent dose). After a 7-day adaptation period, the control and model groups received a daily 0.5% sodium carboxymethylcellulose (CMCNa) solution (1 mL/100 g) for 7 days. Other groups received an equal volume of drug solution with 0.5% CMCNa solution. On day five, 2 h post-administration, control rats received olive oil (1 mL/100 g), while others got ANIT (60 mg/kg in olive oil) to induce acute jaundiced liver injury. Daily body weight and biological signs were monitored. The flowchart of the animal experiment is depicted in Figure 11.

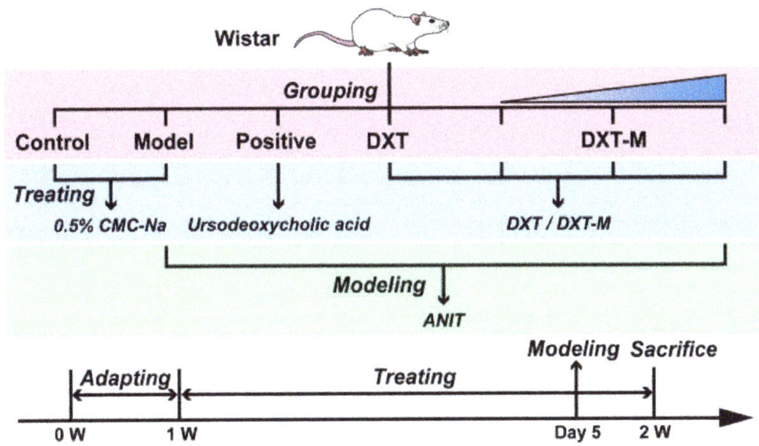

Figure 11. Schematic illustration of the animal experimental procedure and timeline.

4.6. Biological Samples Collection and Preparation

After administration on day 6, animals from the control, model, and medium dose DXT-M groups were placed in metabolic cages to collect urine over a 24 h period. The urine was centrifuged at 3000 rpm for 15 min, and the supernatant was stored at −80 °C. On day 7, two hours post-administration, animals were deeply anesthetised with isoflurane to ensure complete loss of consciousness before blood collection and subsequent euthanasia. Euthanasia was confirmed by the absence of pedal reflex. The blood was left at room temperature for 30 min, then centrifuged at 3000 rpm for 15 min at 4 °C to obtain serum, which was stored at −80 °C.

4.7. Biochemical and Pathological Test

Serum biochemical indicators were evaluated using kits, while liver function and metabolism markers (ALT, AST, ALP, TBIL, DBIL, TBA) were assessed through chemical colourimetric analysis. PA and Complement levels (C3, C4) were measured via immunoturbidimetry, and TNF-α, IL-2, and IL-6 levels were determined using ELISA. After humane euthanasia, rat livers were fixed in formalin, paraffin-embedded, *H&E*-stained, and examined under a 100× magnification Olympus DP80 Microscope (Tokyo, Japan).

4.8. Metabolomics Study Based on ^{1}H NMR Analysis

The serum and urine samples were thawed on ice for NMR analysis. 350 μL of serum was mixed with 250 μL of D_2O, vortexed, and then centrifuged. The supernatant was subsequently placed in an NMR tube. 500 μL of urine was combined with 200 μL of PBS buffer, vortexed, and then centrifuged. The supernatant was subsequently transferred to an NMR tube. ^{1}H-NMR spectra were obtained using a 600 MHz Bruker spectrometer with standard parameters. Data were processed with MestReNova, and the spectra were segmented, normalised, and analysed using principal component analysis (PCA) and orthogonal partial least squares discriminant analysis (OPLS-DA) in SIMCA-P. Metabolites with variable importance plot (*VIP*) > 1 and $p < 0.05$ were deemed significant, and hierarchical clustering visualised metabolite patterns.

4.9. Integrated Analysis Workflow

4.9.1. Procedure for Target Screening

Compounds from RRR, PCC and GF were selected from the TCMSP Database based on oral bioavailability (OB) ≥ 30% and drug-likeness (DL) ≥ 0.18. Protein targets were converted to gene names via Uniprot to form a DXT-M target database. Search for hepatitis-related targets using "hepatitis" in OMIM, GeneCards, TTD, and DisGeNET, and include clinical drug targets from DRUGBANK. Combine and remove duplicates to create a comprehensive database of hepatitis targets. Use Venny 2.1.0 to visualise overlaps between DXT-M and hepatitis targets post-deduplication.

4.9.2. Construction of the Integrated Network

Intersection targets from Section 4.9.1 were imported into Cytoscape v3.8.2 using the Metscape plug-in to explore potential targets in the metabolite–reaction–enzyme–gene network. Targets regulated in this network, as well as differential metabolites from Section 4.8, were also imported into Metscape. Consequently, compound–reaction–enzyme–gene networks linked to metabolite enrichment pathways were constructed.

4.9.3. Target Screening, Target Interaction, and Enrichment Analysis

Potential targets were added to the STRING Database to create a PPI network, analysed using Cytoscape v3.8.2. The MCODE plug-in identified the core subnetwork, highlighting key targets. These targets, along with those from item 2.9.2, underwent GO and KEGG enrichment analysis via the DAVID Database with $p < 0.05$. For further analysis, GO entries and KEGG pathways were selected based on p values. Results were visualised on WeiShengXin, and Sankey diagrams were generated using CNSknowall to connect core targets with GO items or KEGG pathways.

4.10. Network Toxicology Workflow

The Comparative Toxicogenomics Database was used to filter genes linked to drug-induced liver injury to create a hepatotoxicity target database. Venny 2.1.0 identified overlapping targets with the DXT-M component database, forming the DXT-M hepatotoxicity target database. STRING analysed these targets' PPI, and Cytoscape v3.8.2 with MCODE identified core subnetworks. Key targets were identified through network topology and analysed for GO and KEGG pathways using the DAVID Database.

4.11. Target–Component Fitting Procedures

3D protein structures were sourced from the Protein Data Bank and UniProt, then refined with MOE software v2018.10. Key constituents of DXT-M were optimised via energy minimisation. Potential protein binding sites were identified using endogenous ligands or site finders. Rigid docking of DXT-M's chemical constituents with target amino acids was facilitated by the London dG and GBVI/WSA dG scoring methods. Ligand–receptor affinities were evaluated using fitting scores, protein–ligand interaction fingerprints (PLIF), and 3D interaction analyses.

4.12. Bidirectional Regulatory Network of DXT-M in Hepatoprotection and Hepatotoxicity

The core hepatoprotective and hepatotoxicity targets of DXT-M were merged, deduplicated, and analysed for KEGG pathway enrichment using the DAVID Database. The bidirectional regulatory network of DXT-M's liver effects was visualised as a Sankey diagram on the CNSknowall platform.

4.13. Statistical Analysis

Statistical analyses were conducted using GraphPad Prism (v10.1.2), R (v4.2.1) and DPS software (21.05) [119]. Data normality was checked with the Shapiro–Wilk test. For normal data, Repeated measures (RM) two-way ANOVA with the Geisser–Greenhouse correction and Dunnett's post hoc test were used to analyse body weight and longitudinal data, while one-way ANOVA with Dunnett's post hoc test was used to compare serum markers, cytokines, and metabolites. Results were shown as mean ± standard deviation (SD). Hierarchical clustering heatmaps used Euclidean distance and complete linkage. Spearman's rank correlation assessed metabolite and clinical index correlations.

5. Conclusions

This study systematically elucidated the multidimensional "phenotype–metabolism–target" mechanism of DXT-M in combating liver injury. This was achieved by integrating animal experiments, untargeted metabolomics, and network pharmacology–toxicology analysis. The findings revealed that DXT-M significantly ameliorated ANIT-induced acute liver injury phenotypes, normalised liver function parameters such as transaminase, bilirubin, and bile acid levels, and restored the status of the complement system, while also repairing hepatic pathological damage. DXT-M achieved this by modulating a network of metabolites (including citrate, taurine, glutamate, alanine, and others), which interact with targets of hepatic drug-metabolising enzymes, NOS3, and LDHA, thereby correcting endogenous metabolic disorders through intrinsic target molecules. Notably, CYP/GST acted as a bidirectional regulatory switch between hepatoprotection (detoxification) and ROS (hepatotoxicity), while NOS3/TP53 function as synergistic hepatoprotective targets, as confirmed by molecular docking studies showing high residual affinity. The bidirectional regulation mechanism of DXT-M's hepatoprotective and hepatotoxic effects requires further elucidation. Future studies should focus on further validating this regulatory network, elucidating the complete material basis, and conducting clinical retrospective analyses to translate these findings into safe and effective therapies.

Supplementary Materials: The following supporting information can be downloaded at: https://www.mdpi.com/article/10.3390/ph18101534/s1, Figure S1: HPLC chromatograms of DXT and DXT-M compositions. Figure S2: Representative ^{1}H-NMR spectra of control, model, and DXT-M treated groups. Figure S3: Protein–ligand interaction fingerprints (PLIF) of DXT-M target binding modes. Table S1: Gradient elution conditions and detection methods for DXT&DXT-M compositions. Table S2: Differential metabolites identified in serum and urine metabolomics analysis. Table S3: Topological analysis of core target proteins in network pharmacology. Table S4: Topological analysis of core target proteins in network toxicology. Table S5: Fitness scores of DXT-M representative components with core targets.

Author Contributions: Conceptualisation, X.K.; methodology, H.R.; software, X.K.; validation, Y.C. and Z.S.; formal analysis, X.W., H.R. and Y.C.; investigation, H.R., Y.Y., H.Z. and H.L. (Huifang Li); resources, Y.Y. and H.L. (Huifeng Li); data curation, H.Z., H.L. (Huifeng Li) and H.L. (Huifang Li); writing—original draft preparation, X.K. and X.W.; writing—review and editing, K.W.K.T.; visualisation, H.R., X.W., Y.Y. and Z.S.; supervision, K.W.K.T. and M.P.; project administration, M.P.; funding acquisition, M.P. and X.K. All authors have read and agreed to the published version of the manuscript.

Funding: This research was funded by National Natural Science Foundation of China (81273660, 81573688, 81903913), Shanxi Provincial Department of Science and Technology Basic Research Program (20210302124292, 202303021221157), Shanxi Provincial Health Commission Project (2022081), Shanxi Provincial Higher Education Science and Technology Innovation Project (2021L361), Shanxi Provincial Higher Education Teaching Reform Project (J20241079), Shanxi University of Chinese Medicine Scientific and Technological Innovation Capacity Cultivation Program Project (2022PY-TH-10, 2024PY-CXY-008).

Institutional Review Board Statement: The animal study protocol was approved by the Animal Ethics Committee of Shanxi University of Chinese Medicine (Approval number: AWE202509363, retrospective approval date 1 September 2025).

Informed Consent Statement: Not applicable.

Data Availability Statement: Data presented in this study is contained within the article. Further inquiries can be directed to the corresponding authors.

Acknowledgments: This work was financially supported by the Branch of Chinese Medicine Chemistry, College of Chinese Medicine and Food Engineering, Shanxi University of Chinese Medicine. Thanks are given to the Home for Researchers (www.home-for-researchers.com) for drawing the cover image. We would like to express our gratitude to Yujiang Guo from the Third Clinical Medical College of Shanxi University of Chinese Medicine for the data collection.

Conflicts of Interest: The authors declare no conflicts of interest.

Abbreviations

DXT	Dahuang Xiaoshi Tang
RRR	Rhei Radix Et Rhizoma
PCC	Phellodendri Chinensis Cortex
GF	Gardeniae Fructus
NS	Natrii Sulfas
ANIT	α-Naphthalene isothiocyanate
ALT/GPT	Glutamate pyruvate transaminase
AST/GOT	Glutamic oxalacetic transaminase
ALP	Alkaline phosphatase
TBIL	Total bilirubin
DBIL	Indirect bilirubin
TBA	Total bile acid
C3	Complement 3
C4	Complement 4
PA	Prealbumin
IL-2	Interleukin-2
IL-6	Interleukin-6
TNF-α	Tumour necrosis factor α
TCM	Traditional Chinese medicine
HPLC	High Performance Liquid Chromatography
HE	Hematoxylin-eosin
PCA	Principal component analysis
OPLS-DA	Orthogonal partial least squares-discriminant analysis
VIP	Variable importance plot
PPI	Protein–protein interaction
GO	Gene Ontology
BP	Biological Process
CC	Cellular Component
MF	Molecular Function
TCA	Tricarboxylic acid cycle
GSH	Glutathione
CYP450	Cytochrome P450
GST	Glutathione S-transferase

References

1. Devarbhavi, H.; Asrani, S.K.; Arab, J.P.; Nartey, Y.A.; Pose, E.; Kamath, P.S. Global Burden of Liver Disease: 2023 Update. *J. Hepatol.* **2023**, *79*, 516–537. [CrossRef]
2. Gan, C.; Yuan, Y.; Shen, H.; Gao, J.; Kong, X.; Che, Z.; Guo, Y.; Wang, H.; Dong, E.; Xiao, J. Liver Diseases: Epidemiology, Causes, Trends and Predictions. *Signal Transduct. Target. Ther.* **2025**, *10*, 33. [CrossRef]
3. Maiwall, R.; Kulkarni, A.V.; Arab, J.P.; Piano, S. Acute liver failure. *Lancet* **2024**, *404*, 789–802. [CrossRef]
4. Hassan, G.S.; Flores Molina, M.; Shoukry, N.H. The Multifaceted Role of Macrophages During Acute Liver Injury. *Front. Immunol.* **2023**, *14*, 1237042. [CrossRef]

5. Koch, D.G.; Speiser, J.L.; Durkalski, V.; Fontana, R.J.; Davern, T.; McGuire, B.; Stravitz, R.T.; Larson, A.M.; Liou, I.; Fix, O.; et al. The Natural History of Severe Acute Liver Injury. *Am. J. Gastroenterol.* **2017**, *112*, 1389–1396. [CrossRef]
6. Tujios, S.; Stravitz, R.T.; Lee, W.M. Management of Acute Liver Failure: Update 2022. *Semin. Liver Dis.* **2022**, *42*, 362–378. [CrossRef] [PubMed]
7. Lefkowitch, J.H. The Pathology of Acute Liver Failure. *Adv. Anat. Pathol.* **2016**, *23*, 144–158. [CrossRef]
8. Zhang, J.; Wang, X.; Peng, Y.; Wei, J.; Luo, Y.; Luan, F.; Li, H.; Zhou, Y.; Wang, C.; Yu, K. Combined Metabolomic and Proteomic Analysis of Sepsis Related Acute Liver Injury and Its Pathogenesis Research. *Int. Immunopharmacol.* **2024**, *130*, 111666. [CrossRef] [PubMed]
9. Stine, J.G.; Lewis, J.H. Current and Future Directions in the Treatment and Prevention of Drug-Induced Liver Injury: A Systematic Review. *Expert. Rev. Gastroenterol. Hepatol.* **2016**, *10*, 517–536. [CrossRef]
10. Huo, X.; Gu, Y.; Zhang, Y. The Discovery of Multitarget Compounds with Anti-Inflammation Activity from Traditional Chinese Medicine by TCM-Target Effects Relationship Spectrum. *J. Ethnopharmacol.* **2022**, *293*, 115289. [CrossRef] [PubMed]
11. Ren, J.; Yang, L.; Qiu, S.; Zhang, A.; Wang, X. Efficacy Evaluation, Active Ingredients, and Multitarget Exploration of Herbal Medicine. *Trends Endocrinol. Metab.* **2023**, *34*, 146–157. [CrossRef]
12. Huang, Y.; Yao, P.; Leung, K.W.; Wang, H.; Kong, X.; Wang, L.; Dong, T.T.; Chen, Y.; Tsim, K.W. The Yin-Yang Property of Chinese Medicinal Herbs Relates to Chemical Composition but not Anti-Oxidative Activity: An Illustration using Spleen-Meridian Herbs. *Front. Pharmacol.* **2018**, *9*, 1304. [CrossRef]
13. Zhang, H.; Wang, Z. Yin-Yang and Zheng: Exported from Chinese Medicine. *Chin. J. Integr. Med.* **2014**, *20*, 250–255. [CrossRef]
14. Liu, Y.; Li, X.; Chen, C.; Ding, N.; Ma, S.; Yang, M. Exploration of Compatibility Rules and Discovery of Active Ingredients in TCM Formulas by Network Pharmacology. *Chin. Herb. Med.* **2024**, *16*, 572–588. [CrossRef]
15. Wang, Q.; Zhao, Y.; Qin, X.; Tian, J. Deciphering Relationship between Depression and Microbial Molecules Based on Multi-Omics: A Case Study of Chaigui Granules. *Chin. Herb. Med.* **2024**, *16*, 612–621. [CrossRef]
16. Chen, Z.; Vong, C.; Zhang, T.; Yao, C.; Wang, Y.; Luo, H. Quality Evaluation Methods of Chinese Medicine Based on Scientific Supervision: Recent Research Progress and Prospects. *Chin. Med.* **2023**, *18*, 126. [CrossRef] [PubMed]
17. Song, X.; Li, Y.; Shi, Y.; Jin, L.; Chen, J. Quality Control of Traditional Chinese Medicines: A Review. *Chin. J. Nat. Med.* **2013**, *11*, 596–607. [CrossRef]
18. Wang, Y.; Jiao, J.; Wu, Z.; Zheng, Q.; Yang, M. Quality Process Control System of Chinese Medicine Preparation Based on "Holistic View". *China J. Chin. Mater. Med.* **2018**, *43*, 197–203.
19. Dong, B.; Ma, P.; Chen, X.; Peng, Y.; Peng, C.; Li, X. Drug-Polysaccharide/Herb Interactions and Compatibility Rationality of Sijunzi Decoction Based on Comprehensive Pharmacokinetic Screening for Multi-Components in Rats with Spleen Deficiency Syndrome. *J. Ethnopharmacol.* **2023**, *302*, 115871. [CrossRef]
20. Ji, X.; Liu, N.; Huang, S.; Zhang, C. A Comprehensive Review of Licorice: The Preparation, Chemical Composition, Bioactivities and Its Applications. *Am. J. Chin. Med.* **2024**, *52*, 667–716. [CrossRef] [PubMed]
21. Mohtashami, L.; Amiri, M.S.; Ayati, Z.; Ramezani, M.; Jamialahmadi, T.; Emami, S.A.; Sahebkar, A. Ethnobotanical Uses, Phytochemistry and Pharmacology of Different Rheum Species (Polygonaceae): A Review. *Adv. Exp. Med. Biol.* **2021**, *1308*, 309–352.
22. Ta, W.; Yang, X.; Wang, J.; Han, C.; Hua, R.; Lu, W. Comparison of Intestinal Absorption Characteristics between Rhubarb Traditional Chinese Medicine Preparation and Activity Ingredients Using in Situ and in Vitro Model. *Chin. Herb. Med.* **2022**, *15*, 117–122. [CrossRef]
23. Jain, S.; Tripathi, S.; Tripathi, P.K. Antioxidant and Antiarthritic Potential of Berberine: In Vitro and In Vivo Studies. *Chin. Herb. Med.* **2023**, *15*, 549–555. [CrossRef]
24. Kong, X.; Liu, E.Y.; Chen, Z.; Xu, M.L.; Yu, A.X.; Wu, Q.; Xia, Y.; Duan, R.; Dong, T.T.; Tsim, K.W. Synergistic Inhibition of Acetylcholinesterase by Alkaloids Derived from Stephaniae Tetrandrae Radix, Coptidis Rhizoma and Phellodendri Chinensis Cortex. *Molecules* **2019**, *24*, 4567. [CrossRef] [PubMed]
25. Shi, Y.; Zhao, Y.; Qian, J.; Dong, Z.; Wen, G.; Zhao, D.; Kennelly, E.J. Aconitum Diterpenoid Alkaloid Profiling to Distinguish between the Official Traditional Chinese Medicine (TCM) Fuzi and Adulterant Species Using LC-qToF-MS with Chemometrics. *J. Nat. Prod.* **2021**, *84*, 570–587. [CrossRef]
26. Guo, Y.; Gao, T.; Li, C.; Wei, Y.; Shao, S.; Sun, S.; Yang, Y.; Lv, S. Release characteristics of principal components of acid-base drug pair Glycyrrhizae Radix et Rhizoma-Strychni Semen compatibility decoction in sedimentary phase. *Chin. Tradit. Herb. Drugs* **2022**, *53*, 3000–3005.
27. Pei, M.; Duan, X.; Pei, X.; Xuan, Y.; Wang, X.; Zhao, L.; Zhang, S.; Liu, B.; Wang, S. Research on compatibility chemistry of acid-alkaline pair medicines in formulas of traditional Chinese medicine. *China J. Chin. Mater. Med.* **2009**, *34*, 1989–1993.
28. Pei, M.; Xuan, Y.; Duan, X.; Pei, X. Studies on chemical structure of complexes compounds formed by acid and alkaline components of pair medicines in decoction. *China J. Chin. Mater. Med.* **2009**, *34*, 3054–3059.

29. Kong, X.; Li, H.; Pei, M.; Cao, Y. The potency study of Dahuang Xiaoshi Tang on rat jaundice model with damp-heat pathogen. Pharmacol. *Clin. Chin. Mater. Med.* **2012**, *28*, 9–12.
30. Wang, C.; Wu, B. Summary of modern application of zhongjing formula. *Inner Mongolia J. Tradit. Chin. Med.* **2019**, *38*, 146–147.
31. Tan, P.; Zhang, H.; Zhang, D.; Wu, S.; Niu, M.; Wang, J.; Xiao, X. Quality Evaluation of Rhubarb Dispensing Granules Based on Multi-Component Simultaneous Quantitative Analysis and Bioassay. *China J. Chin. Mater. Med.* **2017**, *42*, 2683–2690.
32. Wang, Y.; Zhang, J.; Xu, Z.; Zhang, G.; Lv, H.; Wang, X.; Xu, G.; Li, X.; Yang, Z.; Wang, H.; et al. Identification and Action Mechanism of Lipid Regulating Components from Rhei Radix et Rhizoma. *J. Ethnopharmacol.* **2022**, *292*, 115179. [CrossRef]
33. Lv, H.; Niu, J.; Pan, W.; Wang, Y.; Wang, L.; Wang, M.; Shi, Y.; Zhang, G.; Al Hamyari, B.; Wang, S.; et al. Stool-Softening Effect and Action Mechanism of Free Anthraquinones Extracted from *Rheum palmatum* L. on Water Deficit-Induced Constipation in Rats. *J. Ethnopharmacol.* **2024**, *319*, 117336. [CrossRef]
34. Wu, C.; Bian, Y.; Lu, B.; Wang, D.; Azami, N.; Wei, G.; Ma, F.; Sun, M. Rhubarb Free Anthraquinones Improved Mice Nonalcoholic Fatty Liver Disease by Inhibiting Nlrp3 Inflammasome. *J. Transl. Med.* **2022**, *20*, 294. [CrossRef]
35. Cao, X.; Sun, L.; Li, D.; You, G.; Wang, M.; Ren, X. Quality Evaluation of Phellodendri Chinensis Cortex by Fingerprint—Chemical Pattern Recognition. *Molecules* **2018**, *23*, 2307. [CrossRef]
36. Jia, R.; Hou, Y.; Zhang, L.; Li, B.; Zhu, J. Effects of Berberine on Lipid Metabolism, Antioxidant Status, and Immune Response in Liver of Tilapia (*Oreochromis niloticus*) under a High-Fat Diet Feeding. *Antioxidants* **2024**, *13*, 548. [CrossRef]
37. Zhang, L.; Ai, Y.; Chen, Y.; Li, C.; Li, P.; Chen, J.; Jiang, L.; Pan, Y.; Sun, A.; Yang, Y.; et al. Elucidation of Geniposide and Crocin Accumulation and Their Biosysnthsis-Related Key Enzymes during Gardenia jasminoides Fruit Growth. *Plants* **2023**, *12*, 2209. [CrossRef]
38. Shan, M.; Yu, S.; Yan, H.; Guo, S.; Xiao, W.; Wang, Z.; Zhang, L.; Ding, A.; Wu, Q.; Li, S. A Review on the Phytochemistry, Pharmacology, Pharmacokinetics and Toxicology of Geniposide, a Natural Product. *Molecules* **2017**, *22*, 1689. [CrossRef] [PubMed]
39. Kong, X.; Pei, M.; Deng, L.; Zhao, L. Exploring the monarch-minister compatibility in Dahuang Xiaoshi Tang's composition. *Chin. Tradit. Pat. Med.* **2014**, *36*, 175–177.
40. Pei, M.; Duan, X.; Pei, X. Compatibility chemistry of acid-alkaline pair medicine of Dahuang and Huangbai in Dahuang Xiaoshi decoction. *China J. Chin. Mater. Med.* **2009**, *34*, 2312–2315.
41. Kong, X.; Yao, Y.; Ren, H.; Pei, M.; Li, H. Compatibility Optimisation of Dahuang Xiaoshi Decoction Components Based on Liver Protection and Evaluation of Its Efficacy. *Her. Med.* **2024**, *43*, 874–884.
42. Zhao, W.; Wang, B.; Li, S. Network Pharmacology for Traditional Chinese Medicine in Era of Artificial Intelligence. *Chin. Herb. Med.* **2024**, *16*, 558–560. [CrossRef]
43. Xue, H.; Fang, S.; Zheng, M.; Wu, J.; Li, H.; Zhang, M.; Li, Y.; Wang, T.; Shi, R.; Ma, Y. Da-Huang-Xiao-Shi Decoction Protects against3, 5-Diethoxycarbonyl-1,4-Dihydroxychollidine-Induced Chronic Cholestasis by Upregulating Bile Acid Metabolic Enzymes and Efflux Transporters. *J. Ethnopharmacol.* **2021**, *269*, 113706. [CrossRef] [PubMed]
44. Zhu, G.; Feng, F. Uplc-Ms-Based Metabonomic Analysis of Intervention Effects of Da-Huang-Xiao-Shi Decoction on Anit-Induced Cholestasis. *J. Ethnopharmacol.* **2019**, *238*, 111860. [CrossRef]
45. Kong, X.; Yao, Y.; Li, H.; Zhang, S.; Qi, Y.; Pei, M. Optimization of macroporous adsorption resin purification process for Gardeniae Fructus components. *Chin. Tradit. Pat. Med.* **2022**, *44*, 894–898.
46. Kong, X.; Yao, Y.; Li, H.; Pei, M. Determination of anthraquinone constituents in refined component of Rhei Radix et Rhizoma by QAMS. *West China J. Pharm. Sci.* **2021**, *36*, 419–422.
47. Yao, Y.; Kong, X.; Li, H.; Dang, T.; Pei, M. The purification technology research for the components of the Phellodendri Chinensis Cortex in macroporous adsorptionby total alkaloid as index. *Guangdong Chem. Ind.* **2022**, *49*, 38–40+86.
48. Li, D.; Guo, H.; Niu, L.; Yin, Q.; Zhang, Y.; Zhuang, P. Clinical Value-Oriented Research Paradigm about Inheritance and Innovation Development of Tcm Dominant Diseases. *Chin. Herb. Med.* **2023**, *15*, 476–484. [CrossRef]
49. Zhang, Y. Awareness and Ability of Paradigm Shift are Needed for Research on Dominant Diseases of Tcm. *Chin. Herb. Med.* **2023**, *15*, 475. [CrossRef]
50. Wang, W.; Jiang, S.; Xu, C.; Tang, L.; Liang, Y.; Zhao, Y.; Zhu, G. Transcriptome and Gut Microbiota Profiling Analysis of ANIT-Induced Cholestasis and the Effects of Da-Huang-Xiao-Shi Decoction Intervention. *Microbiol. Spectr.* **2022**, *10*, e0324222. [CrossRef] [PubMed]
51. Liu, X.; Luo, X.; Jiang, C.; Zhao, H. Difficulties and Challenges in the Development of Precision Medicine. *Clin. Genet.* **2019**, *95*, 569–574. [CrossRef] [PubMed]
52. Liao, W.; Jin, Q.; Liu, J.; Ruan, Y.; Li, X.; Shen, Y.; Zhang, Z.; Wang, Y.; Wu, S.; Zhang, J.; et al. Mahuang Decoction Antagonizes Acute Liver Failure via Modulating Tricarboxylic Acid Cycle and Amino Acids Metabolism. *Front. Pharmacol.* **2021**, *12*, 599180. [CrossRef]
53. Sookoian, S.; Castaño, G.O.; Scian, R.; Fernández Gianotti, T.; Dopazo, H.; Rohr, C.; Gaj, G.; San Martino, J.; Sevic, I.; Flichman, D.; et al. Serum Aminotransferases in Nonalcoholic Fatty Liver Disease are a Signature of Liver Metabolic Perturbations at the Amino Acid and Krebs Cycle Level. *Am. J. Clin. Nutr.* **2016**, *103*, 422–434. [CrossRef] [PubMed]

54. Tagawa, R.; Kobayashi, M.; Sakurai, M.; Yoshida, M.; Kaneko, H.; Mizunoe, Y.; Nozaki, Y.; Okita, N.; Sudo, Y.; Higami, Y. Long-Term Dietary Taurine Lowers Plasma Levels of Cholesterol and Bile Acids. *Int. J. Mol. Sci.* **2022**, *23*, 1793. [CrossRef]
55. Wang, Y.; Mei, X.; Yuan, J.; Lai, X.; Xu, D. Taurine Zinc Solid Dispersions Enhance Bile-Incubated L02 Cell Viability and Improve Liver Function by Inhibiting Erk2 and Jnk Phosphorylation during Cholestasis. *Toxicology* **2016**, *366–367*, 10–19. [CrossRef]
56. Liu, Y.; Li, F.; Zhang, L.; Wu, J.; Wang, Y.; Yu, H. Taurine Alleviates Lipopolysaccharide-Induced Liver Injury by Anti-Inflammation and Antioxidants in Rats. *Mol. Med. Rep.* **2017**, *16*, 6512–6517. [CrossRef]
57. Miyazaki, T.; Matsuzaki, Y. Taurine and Liver Diseases: A Focus on the Heterogeneous Protective Properties of Taurine. *Amino Acids* **2014**, *46*, 101–110. [CrossRef]
58. González-Contreras, J.; Villalobos Gámez, J.L.; Gómez-Sánchez, A.I.; García-Almeida, J.M.; Enguix Armanda, A.; Rius Díaz, F.; Lucena González, M.I. Cholestasis Induced by Total Parenteral Nutrition: Effects of the Addition of Taurine (Tauramin®) on Hepatic Function Parameters; Possible Synergistic Action of Structured Lipids (SMOFlipid®). *Nutr. Hosp.* **2012**, *27*, 1900–1907.
59. Bonfleur, M.L.; Borck, P.C.; Ribeiro, R.A.; Caetano, L.C.; Soares, G.M.; Carneiro, E.M.; Balbo, S.L. Improvement in the Expression of Hepatic Genes Involved in Fatty Acid Metabolism in Obese Rats Supplemented with Taurine. *Life Sci.* **2015**, *135*, 15–21. [CrossRef] [PubMed]
60. Siregar, A.S.; Nyiramana, M.M.; Kim, E.J.; Shin, E.J.; Woo, M.S.; Kim, J.M.; Park, S.H.; Hahm, J.R.; Choi, Y.J.; Kang, D. Oyster Broth Concentrate and Its Major Component Taurine Alleviate Acute Alcohol-Induced Liver Damage. *Food Sci. Nutr.* **2022**, *10*, 2390–2399. [CrossRef]
61. Sookoian, S.; Pirola, C.J. The Nonalcoholic Steatohepatitis Metabotype: Imbalance of Circulating Amino Acids and Transamination Reactions Reflect Impaired Mitochondrial Function. *Hepatology* **2018**, *67*, 1177–1178. [CrossRef]
62. Harada, S.; Takebayashi, T.; Kurihara, A.; Akiyama, M.; Suzuki, A.; Hatakeyama, Y.; Sugiyama, D.; Kuwabara, K.; Takeuchi, A.; Okamura, T.; et al. Metabolomic Profiling Reveals Novel Biomarkers of Alcohol Intake and Alcohol-Induced Liver Injury in Community-Dwelling Men. *Environ. Health Prev. Med.* **2016**, *21*, 18–26. [CrossRef]
63. Zhong, F.; Hu, Z.; Jiang, K.; Lei, B.; Wu, Z.; Yuan, G.; Luo, H.; Dong, C.; Tang, B.; Zheng, C.; et al. Complement C3 Activation Regulates the Production of Trna-Derived Fragments Gly-Trfs and Promotes Alcohol-Induced Liver Injury and Steatosis. *Cell Res.* **2019**, *29*, 548–561. [CrossRef]
64. Zuo, T.; Gong, B.; Gao, Y.; Yuan, L. An in Vitro Study on the Stimulatory Effects of Extracellular Glutamate on Astrocytes. *Mol. Biol. Rep.* **2023**, *50*, 6611–6617. [CrossRef] [PubMed]
65. Liu, G.; Li, Y.; Liao, N.; Shang, X.; Xu, F.; Yin, D.; Shao, D.; Jiang, C.; Shi, J. Energy Metabolic Mechanisms for High Altitude Sickness: Downregulation of Glycolysis and Upregulation of the Lactic Acid/Amino Acid-Pyruvate-Tca Pathways and Fatty Acid Oxidation. *Sci. Total Environ.* **2023**, *894*, 164998. [CrossRef]
66. Zangari, J.; Petrelli, F.; Maillot, B.; Martinou, J. The Multifaceted Pyruvate Metabolism: Role of the Mitochondrial Pyruvate Carrier. *Biomolecules* **2020**, *10*, 1068. [CrossRef] [PubMed]
67. Fan, Y.; Liu, S.; Chen, X.; Feng, M.; Song, F.; Gao, X. Toxicological Effects of Nux Vomica in Rats Urine and Serum by Means of Clinical Chemistry, Histopathology and (1)H Nmr-Based Metabonomics Approach. *J. Ethnopharmacol.* **2018**, *210*, 242–253. [CrossRef]
68. Hara, Y.; Kume, S.; Kataoka, Y.; Watanabe, N. Changes in Tca Cycle and Tca Cycle-Related Metabolites in Plasma upon Citric Acid Administration in Rats. *Heliyon* **2021**, *7*, e08501. [CrossRef] [PubMed]
69. Liang, Q.; Wang, B.; Pang, L.; Wang, Y.; Zheng, M.; Wang, Q.; Yan, J.; Xu, J. Application Of Citrate As a Tricarboxylic Acid (Tca) Cycle Intermediate, Prevents Diabetic-Induced Heart Damages In Mice. *Iran. J. Basic Med. Sci.* **2016**, *19*, 43–48.
70. Guasch-Ferré, M.; Santos, J.L.; Martínez-González, M.A.; Clish, C.B.; Razquin, C.; Wang, D.; Liang, L.; Li, J.; Dennis, C.; Corella, D.; et al. Glycolysis/Gluconeogenesis- and Tricarboxylic Acid Cycle-Related Metabolites, Mediterranean Diet, and Type 2 Diabetes. *Am. J. Clin. Nutr.* **2020**, *111*, 835–844. [CrossRef]
71. Liu, S.; Dai, Z.; Cooper, D.E.; Kirsch, D.G.; Locasale, J.W. Quantitative Analysis of the Physiological Contributions of Glucose to the TCA Cycle. *Cell Metab.* **2020**, *32*, 619–628.e21. [CrossRef]
72. Zou, K.; Hinkley, J.M.; Park, S.; Zheng, D.; Jones, T.E.; Pories, W.J.; Hornby, P.J.; Lenhard, J.; Dohm, G.L.; Houmard, J.A. Altered Tricarboxylic Acid Cycle Flux In Primary Myotubes From Severely Obese Humans. *Int. J. Obes.* **2019**, *43*, 895–905. [CrossRef]
73. Chitalia, V. α-Ketoglutarate—A New Currency of Longevity. *Sci. Transl. Med.* **2014**, *6*, 244ec117. [CrossRef]
74. Maus, A.; Peters, G.J. Glutamate and α-ketoglutarate: Key players in glioma metabolism. *Amino Acids* **2017**, *49*, 21–32. [CrossRef]
75. Limón, I.D.; Angulo-Cruz, I.; Sánchez-Abdon, L.; Patricio-Martínez, A. Disturbance of the Glutamate-Glutamine Cycle, Secondary to Hepatic Damage, Compromises Memory Function. *Front. Neurosci.* **2021**, *15*, 578922. [CrossRef] [PubMed]
76. Sonnewald, U.; Schousboe, A. Introduction to the Glutamate-Glutamine Cycle. *Adv. Neurobiol.* **2016**, *13*, 1–7. [PubMed]
77. Hakvoort, T.B.; He, Y.; Kulik, W.; Vermeulen, J.L.; Duijst, S.; Ruijter, J.M.; Runge, J.H.; Deutz, N.E.; Koehler, S.E.; Lamers, W.H. Pivotal Role of Glutamine Synthetase in Ammonia Detoxification. *Hepatology* **2017**, *65*, 281–293. [CrossRef] [PubMed]
78. Schemitt, E.G.; Hartmann, R.M.; Colares, J.R.; Licks, F.; Salvi, J.O.; Marroni, C.A.; Marroni, N.P. Protective Action of Glutamine in Rats with Severe Acute Liver Failure. *World J. Hepatol.* **2019**, *11*, 273–286. [CrossRef]

79. Xu, F.; Dai, C.; Peng, S.; Zhao, Y.; Jia, C.; Xu, Y. Preconditioning with Glutamine Protects Against Ischemia/Reperfusion-Induced Hepatic Injury in Rats with Obstructive Jaundice. *Pharmacology* **2014**, *93*, 155–165. [CrossRef]
80. Cai, S.; Boyer, J.L. The Role of Bile Acids in Cholestatic Liver Injury. *Ann. Transl. Med.* **2021**, *9*, 737. [CrossRef] [PubMed]
81. Kakazu, E.; Kondo, Y.; Kogure, T.; Ninomiya, M.; Kimura, O.; Ueno, Y.; Shimosegawa, T. Plasma Amino Acids Imbalance in Cirrhotic Patients Disturbs the Tricarboxylic Acid Cycle of Dendritic Cell. *Sci. Rep.* **2013**, *3*, 3459. [CrossRef]
82. Shu, Y.; He, D.; Li, W.; Wang, M.; Zhao, S.; Liu, L.; Cao, Z.; Liu, R.; Huang, Y.; Li, H.; et al. Hepatoprotective Effect of *Citrus aurantium* L. Against APAP-Induced Liver Injury by Regulating Liver Lipid Metabolism and Apoptosis. *Int. J. Biol. Sci.* **2020**, *16*, 752–765. [CrossRef]
83. Lorente, S.; Hautefeuille, M.; Sanchez-Cedillo, A. the Liver, a Functionalized Vascular Structure. *Sci. Rep.* **2020**, *10*, 16194. [CrossRef] [PubMed]
84. Paulusma, C.C.; Lamers, W.H.; Broer, S.; van de Graaf, S. Amino Acid Metabolism, Transport and Signalling in the Liver Revisited. *Biochem. Pharmacol.* **2022**, *201*, 115074. [CrossRef] [PubMed]
85. Zhang, Y.; Fang, X. Hepatocardiac or Cardiohepatic Interaction: From Traditional Chinese Medicine to Western Medicine. *Evid.-Based Complement. Altern. Med.* **2021**, *2021*, 6655335. [CrossRef] [PubMed]
86. Trefts, E.; Gannon, M.; Wasserman, D.H. The Liver. *Curr. Biol.* **2017**, *27*, R1147–R1151. [CrossRef]
87. Zhang, J.; Liu, Y.; Xu, Y. Soothing Liver-Qi Stagnation Method for Cancer-Related Depression: A Protocol for Systematic Review and Meta-Analysis. *Medicine* **2020**, *99*, e22797. [CrossRef]
88. Han, J.; Li, Q.; Pan, C.; Sun, K.; Fan, J. Effects and Mechanisms of Qishenyiqi Pills and Major Ingredients on Myocardial Microcirculatory Disturbance, Cardiac Injury and Fibrosis Induced by Ischemia-Reperfusion. *Pharmacol. Res.* **2019**, *147*, 104386. [CrossRef]
89. Wang, D.; Li, Q.; Pan, C.; Yan, L.; Sun, K.; Wang, X.; Anwaier, G.; Liao, Q.; Xie, T.; Fan, J.; et al. Yu-Ping-Feng Formula Ameliorates Alveolar-Capillary Barrier Injury Induced by Exhausted-Exercise Via Regulation of Cytoskeleton. *Front. Pharmacol.* **2022**, *13*, 891802. [CrossRef]
90. Wu, G.; Zhong, J.; Zheng, N.; Wang, C.; Jin, H.; Ge, G.; Han, J.; Gao, Y.; Sheng, L.; Zhang, W.; et al. Investigation of Modulating Effect of Qingfei Paidu Decoction on Host Metabolism and Gut Microbiome in Rats. *China J. Chin. Mater. Med.* **2020**, *45*, 3726–3739.
91. Ooi, A.T.; Gomperts, B.N. Molecular Pathways: Targeting Cellular Energy Metabolism in Cancer Via Inhibition of Slc2A1 and Ldha. *Clin. Cancer Res.* **2015**, *21*, 2440–2444. [CrossRef] [PubMed]
92. Yao, S.; Chai, H.; Tao, T.; Zhang, L.; Yang, X.; Li, X.; Yi, Z.; Wang, Y.; An, J.; Wen, G.; et al. Role of Lactate and Lactate Metabolism in Liver Diseases (Review). *Int. J. Mol. Med.* **2024**, *54*, 59. [CrossRef]
93. Hillis, A.L.; Tamir, T.; Perry, G.E.; Asara, J.M.; Johnson, J.L.; Yaron, T.M.; Cantley, L.C.; White, F.M.; Toker, A. Parallel Phosphoproteomics and Metabolomics Map the Global Metabolic Tyrosine Phosphoproteome. *Proc. Natl. Acad. Sci. USA* **2024**, *121*, e2413837121. [CrossRef] [PubMed]
94. Pu, X.; Gao, Y.; Li, R.; Li, W.; Tian, Y.; Zhang, Z.; Xu, F. Biomarker Discovery for Cytochrome P450 1A2 Activity Assessment in Rats, Based on Metabolomics. *Metabolites* **2019**, *9*, 77. [CrossRef]
95. Xu, T.; Pan, Y.; Ding, Q.; Cao, F.; Chang, K.; Qiu, J.; Zhuge, H.; Hao, L.; Wei, H.; Si, C.; et al. The Micro-743a-3p-Gstm1 Pathway Is an Endogenous Protective Mechanism against Alcohol-Related Liver Disease in Mice. *Cell. Mol. Biol. Lett.* **2024**, *29*, 35. [CrossRef]
96. Brosnan, J.T. Glutamate, at The Interface Between Amino Acid and Carbohydrate Metabolism. *J. Nutr.* **2000**, *130*, 988S–990S. [CrossRef]
97. Morris, S.M., Jr. Regulation of Enzymes of The Urea Cycle and Arginine Metabolism. *Annu. Rev. Nutr.* **2002**, *22*, 87–105. [CrossRef]
98. Russell, T.M.; Richardson, D.R. Glutathione-S-Transferases as Potential Targets for Modulation of Nitric Oxide-Mediated Vasodilation. *Biomolecules* **2022**, *12*, 1292. [CrossRef]
99. Dong, F.; Annalora, A.J.; Murray, I.A.; Tian, Y.; Marcus, C.B.; Patterson, A.D.; Perdew, G.H. Endogenous Tryptophan-Derived Ah Receptor Ligands are Dissociated from Cyp1A1/1B1-Dependent Negative-Feedback. *Int. J. Tryptophan Res.* **2023**, *16*, 11786469231182508. [CrossRef]
100. Haduch, A.; Bromek, E.; Kuban, W.; Daniel, W.A. The Engagement of Cytochrome P450 Enzymes in Tryptophan Metabolism. *Metabolites* **2023**, *13*, 629. [CrossRef] [PubMed]
101. Di Ciaula, A.; Garruti, G.; Lunardi Baccetto, R.; Molina-Molina, E.; Bonfrate, L.; Wang, D.Q.; Portincasa, P. Bile Acid Physiology. *Ann. Hepatol.* **2017**, *16*, s4–s14. [CrossRef] [PubMed]
102. Tu, C.; Niu, M.; Li, C.; Liu, Z.; He, Q.; Li, R.; Zhang, Y.; Xiao, X.; Wang, J. Network Pharmacology Oriented Study Reveals Inflammatory State-Dependent Dietary Supplement Hepatotoxicity Responses in Normal and Diseased Rats. *Food Funct.* **2019**, *10*, 3477–3490. [CrossRef]
103. Wang, L.; Chen, S.; Liu, S.; Biu, A.M.; Han, Y.; Jin, X.; Liang, C.; Liu, Y.; Li, J.; Fang, S.; et al. A Comprehensive Review of Ethnopharmacology, Chemical Constituents, Pharmacological Effects, Pharmacokinetics, Toxicology, and Quality Control of Gardeniae Fructus. *J. Ethnopharmacol.* **2024**, *320*, 117397. [CrossRef]

104. Liang, J.; Wei, X.; Hou, W.; Wang, H.; Ma, R.; Gao, Y.; Du, Y.; Zhang, Q. Liver Metabolomics Reveals Potential Mechanism of Jieduan-Niwan Formula Against Acute-On-Chronic Liver Failure (Aclf) by Improving Mitochondrial Damage and Tca Cycle. *Chin. Med.* **2023**, *18*, 157. [CrossRef] [PubMed]
105. Zhang, I.W.; Curto, A.; López-Vicario, C.; Casulleras, M.; Duran-Güell, M.; Flores-Costa, R.; Colsch, B.; Aguilar, F.; Aransay, A.M.; Lozano, J.J.; et al. Mitochondrial Dysfunction Governs Immunometabolism in Leukocytes of Patients with Acute-on-Chronic Liver Failure. *J. Hepatol.* **2022**, *76*, 93–106.
106. Allameh, A.; Niayesh-Mehr, R.; Aliarab, A.; Sebastiani, G.; Pantopoulos, K. Oxidative Stress in Liver Pathophysiology and Disease. *Antioxidants* **2023**, *12*, 1653. [CrossRef]
107. Gao, A.; Ni, Y.; Chen, C.; Xin, W.; Wang, Y.; Zhang, W. Covalent Binding of Geniposide Metabolites to Hepatic Proteins: A Potential Mechanism for Its Hepatotoxicity. *Chem-Biol. Interact.* **2025**, *408*, 111411. [CrossRef]
108. Zhao, M.; Ma, J.; Li, M.; Zhang, Y.; Jiang, B.; Zhao, X.; Huai, C.; Shen, L.; Zhang, N.; He, L.; et al. Cytochrome P450 Enzymes and Drug Metabolism in Humans. *Int. J. Mol. Sci.* **2021**, *22*, 12808. [CrossRef] [PubMed]
109. Zhao, Y.; Huang, H.; Lv, N.; Huang, C.; Chen, H.; Xing, H.; Guo, C.; Li, N.; Zhao, D.; Chen, X.; et al. Glutathione S-Transferases Mediate in Vitro and in Vivo Inactivation of Genipin: Implications for an Underlying Detoxification Mechanism. *J. Agric. Food Chem.* **2023**, *71*, 2399–2410. [CrossRef]
110. Brewer, C.T.; Chen, T. Hepatotoxicity of Herbal Supplements Mediated by Modulation of Cytochrome P450. *Int. J. Mol. Sci.* **2017**, *18*, 2353. [CrossRef]
111. Zuo, H.; Huang, H.; Lin, Y.; Cai, X.; Kong, X.; Luo, D.; Zhou, Y.; Huang, H. Enzyme Activity of Natural Products on Cytochrome P450. *Molecules* **2022**, *27*, 515. [CrossRef] [PubMed]
112. Ma, Y.; Mu, J.; Gou, X.; Wu, X. Precision Medication Based on the Evaluation of Drug Metabolizing Enzyme and Transporter Functions. *Precis. Clin. Med.* **2025**, *8*, pbaf004. [CrossRef]
113. Sadee, W.; Wang, D.; Hartmann, K.; Toland, A.E. Pharmacogenomics: Driving Personalised Medicine. *Pharmacol. Rev.* **2023**, *75*, 789–814. [CrossRef] [PubMed]
114. Feng, G.; Bi, J.; Jin, W.; Wang, Q.; Dan, Z.; Fan, B. Effect of Rhei Radix et Rhizoma and Eupolyphaga Steleophaga on Liver Protection Mechanism Based on Pharmacokinetics and Metabonomics. *Chin. Herb. Med.* **2024**, *16*, 121–131. [CrossRef]
115. Li, C.; Li, Y.; Bai, Z.; Wang, J.; Li, G.; Xiao, X. Herb Induced Liver Injury by Xianling Gubao Tablets: A Case Assessed for Causality Using Updated Rucam and Integrated Evidence Chain. *Chin. Herb. Med.* **2024**, *16*, 301–309. [CrossRef] [PubMed]
116. Monnerie, S.; Comte, B.; Ziegler, D.; Morais, J.A.; Pujos-Guillot, E.; Gaudreau, P. Metabolomic and Lipidomic Signatures of Metabolic Syndrome and Its Physiological Components in Adults: A Systematic Review. *Sci. Rep.* **2020**, *10*, 669. [CrossRef]
117. Tao, L.; Fu, J.; Wang, F.; Song, Y.; Li, Y.; Zhang, J.; Wang, Z. The Application of Mirabilite in Traditional Chinese Medicine and Its Chemical Constituents, Processing Methods, Pharmacology, Toxicology and Clinical Research. *Front. Pharmacol.* **2023**, *14*, 1293097. [CrossRef]
118. Gan, S.; Shi, X.; Han, T.; Wu, C. Determination of Sodium Sulfate in Medicinal Mirabilite by Ion Chromatography. *China Pharm.* **2012**, *21*, 39–40.
119. Tang, Q.; Zhang, C. Data Processing System (Dps) Software with Experimental Design, Statistical Analysis and Data Mining Developed for Use in Entomological Research. *Insect. Sci.* **2013**, *20*, 254–260. [CrossRef]

pharmaceuticals

MDPI

Article

Schisandrin B Alleviates Lipid Metabolism Disorders and Apoptosis of MAFLD via Modulation of PPARγ-PCK1 and Caspase-3 Signaling Pathways

Meng Gao, Feilong Liu, Xiyuan Feng, Mengyang Wang, Zhihong Zhang, He Li , Chunmei Wang and Jinghui Sun *

School of Pharmacy, Beihua University, Jilin 132013, China; s9912062636@163.com (M.G.); m18831442942@163.com (F.L.); 18004369287@163.com (X.F.); 15643584357@163.com (M.W.); zhzhang518@163.com (Z.Z.); yitonglh@126.com (H.L.); wangcm74@126.com (C.W.)

* Correspondence: sunjinghui2008@126.com

Abstract: Objectives: This study focuses on the regulatory mechanism of Schisandrin B (Sch B) on the lipid metabolism and apoptosis of AML-12 liver cells, with a particular emphasis on its potential therapeutic effect and mechanism of action in preventing and treating metabolic-associated fatty liver disease (MAFLD) by activating the PPARγ signaling pathway. **Methods**: An MAFLD cell model was established by inducing AML-12 cells with a mixture of oleic acid (OA) and palmitic acid (PA) (2:1). AML-12 cells were divided into a control group, a model group, and 20 μM and 40 μM Sch B groups. The cells were lysed and prepared into the cell suspension, then the cell suspension was centrifuged to obtain its supernatant, and the levels of total cholesterol (TC), triglycerides (TG), alanine aminotransferase (ALT), and aspartate aminotransferase (AST) in the supernatant were detected according to the instructions of the kits. Effects of Sch B on the pathological changes of AML-12 cells were observed by Oil Red O staining. The key targets were screened through network pharmacology, and relevant targets were verified through molecular docking simulation. The activity of PPARγ was detected using a dual luciferase reporter plasmid, and the level of cell apoptosis was detected using the Annexin V-FITC/PI double staining method. The Western blot method was used to analyze the expression of genes related to lipid metabolism and apoptosis pathways. **Results**: Sch B could regulate lipid metabolism disorders in OA+PA-induced MAFLD cell model. The activation of PPARγ-PCK1/Aspase is a key step in the action of Sch B, which can effectively block fatty acid synthesis, improve fatty acid oxidation, and reduce lipid droplet aggregation in liver cells, thereby alleviating lipid metabolism abnormalities in the MAFLD cell model and inhibiting cell apoptosis. **Conclusions**: This finding may lay an important theoretical foundation and open a new research direction for the deep development and application of *Schisandra chinensis*.

Keywords: Schisandrin B; peroxisome proliferator-activated receptor gamma; metabolic-associated fatty liver disease

1. Introduction

Metabolic-associated fatty liver disease (MAFLD), formerly known as nonalcoholic fatty liver disease (NAFLD), is one of the most common chronic liver diseases in the world, and it has become the second major cause of end-stage liver disease in recent decades [1]. MAFLD is closely related to obesity, metabolic syndrome, type II diabetes, and so on [2]. MAFLD can not only lead to non-alcoholic fatty liver disease, cirrhosis, and even hepatocellular carcinoma, but also increase the mortality rate of liver-related diseases [3]. As of 2020, the global morbidity of MAFLD has reached 25% [4]. Due to the lack of approved specific drugs for treating MAFLD, dietary control and exercise are still the preferred treatment methods recommended by most scientific associations. However, these methods are not always sustainable and reliable.

Schisandrin B (Sch B) is an active lignan component in *Schisandra chinensis*, a plant in Magnoliaceae, and is widely used due to its prevention and treatment of liver diseases, and blood lipid-lowering and antioxidation effects [5–7]. Previous studies have confirmed that Sch B has a significant alleviating effect on MAFLD animal models, but its underlying mechanism is still unclear [8–10]. Peroxisome proliferator-activated receptor (PPAR), a member of the nuclear receptor family, plays a crucial role in maintaining metabolic homeostasis. Currently, there are three subtypes of PPAR, namely PPARα, PPARβ/δ, and PPARγ. PPAR can serve as a sensor for fatty acids, regulating various pathways involved in lipid and glucose metabolism, as well as energy metabolism [11,12]. Its role in liver injury has been repeatedly confirmed, and it is also an effective target for treating a variety of metabolic diseases, including type II diabetes and hyperlipidemia [13–16]. At present, it has been confirmed that Sch B has a definite liver protection and anti-inflammatory potential, and it can alleviate liver fibrosis induced by carbon tetrachloride through various regulatory mechanisms [17]. In addition, Sch B can effectively inhibit the inflammatory response of microglia induced by lipopolysaccharide (LPS) by activating the PPAR-γ signaling pathway [18]. However, there is still a lack of research on the specific role and molecular mechanism of Sch B in MAFLD, so this research gap provides us with new research directions to explore the potential value of Sch B in MAFLD treatment and explore its new regulatory targets.

Our team discovered through network pharmacology and molecular docking technology that the key target of *Schisandra chinensis* for treating MAFLD was PPARγ [19], which was verified in a high-fat diet-induced C57BL/6 mouse model. It was found that SchB could alleviate MAFLD in mice by regulating the PPARγ signaling pathway and gut microbiota [20]. On this basis, experiments around two innovative points were conducted in this study. On the one hand, AML-12 mouse liver cell lines were used for in vitro verification, which served as a key supplement to previous in vivo studies on a high-fat diet-induced mouse model to explore not only the protective and therapeutic effects of Sch B on the cells, but also the molecular mechanisms of action of Sch B at the cellular level. On the other hand, the focus of mechanism research could be further expanded from PPARγ to PCK1 and Caspase-3, and the core targets of Sch B therapy for MAFLD could be screened out through network pharmacology; then, molecular docking simulations, luciferase reporter plasmid experiments, and Western blot were used to verify whether Sch B would regulate lipid metabolism disorders through PPARγ, and simultaneously, flow cytometry was used to detect its effect on cell apoptosis, so as to clarify the multidimensional regulatory role of Sch B in the pathogenesis of MAFLD. This "in vitro–in vivo" progressive progress can not only provide a more comprehensive insight into the therapeutic potential of Sch B, but also a theoretical basis for further research, development, and application of Sch B.

2. Results

2.1. *Effects of Different Induction Times on MAFLD Cell Model*

An MAFLD cell model was established by inducing AML-12 cells with oleic acid (OA) and palmitic acid (PA) at a ratio of 2:1 for 12 h and 24 h, respectively. As shown in Figure 1, compared with that in the control group, the lipid droplet content in cells induced by OA+PA for 12 h and 24 h increased significantly ($p < 0.001$), while the lipid droplet content of those induced for 24 h was significantly higher than that for 12 h ($p < 0.001$), indicating that OA+PA could significantly increase the steatosis of AML-12, so the cells induced for 24 h were used to establish the MAFLD cell model in subsequent experiments.

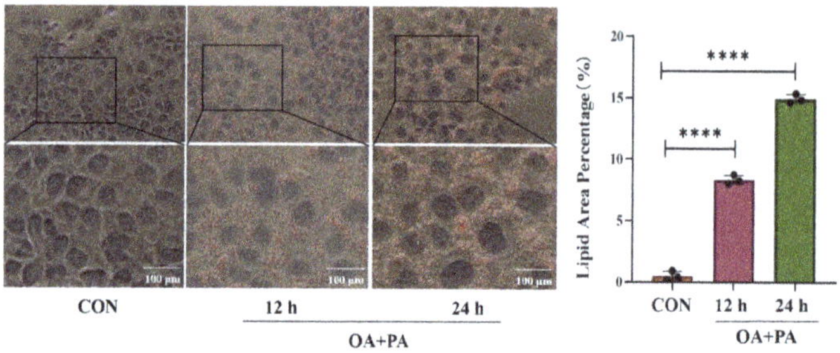

Figure 1. Effects of the induction at different times on MAFLD cell model (mean ± *S.E.*, $n = 3$). **** $p < 0.0001$ vs. MOD.

2.2. Effects of Sch B on AML-12 Cell Activities

The cell survival results showed that compared with those in the CON group, the OD values of cells in the DMSO group were significantly reduced ($p < 0.01$), and compared with those in the DMSO group, the OD values of cells in the 20 μM and 40 μM Sch B groups were significantly increased ($p < 0.05$), indicating that the inhibitory effect and toxicity of Sch B at these two concentrations on AML-12 cells were lower, so 20 and 40 μM SchB were selected for culturing AML-12 cells for 12 h in subsequent experiments (Figure 2).

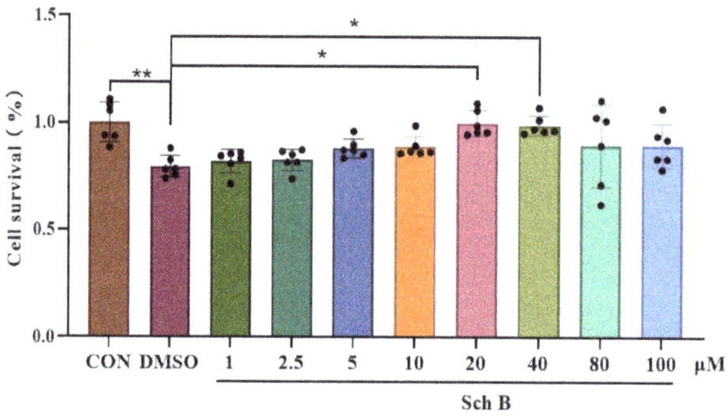

Figure 2. Effects of Sch B on AML-12 cell activities (mean ± *S.E.*, $n = 6$). * $p < 0.05$; ** $p < 0.01$.

2.3. Histomorphological Results of AML-12 Cells by Oil Red Staining

AML-12 cells were induced by OA+PA for 24 h to establish an MAFLD model, then 20 μM and 40 μM Sch B was added into the culture medium, respectively, and 12 h later, the cells were stained by Oil Red O staining. As shown in Figure 3, under a light microscope, the nuclei of AML-12 cells in the CON group were stained blue, and no red neutral fat color was observed, and those in the MOD group were stained blue, with an obvious red wrapping around the nucleus (vs. CON, $p < 0.01$), indicating that OA+PA could induce a large amount of neutral fat deposition in the cytoplasm, leading to cellular steatosis. Compared with those in the MOD group, the nuclei of AML12 cells in the 20 μM Sch B group showed only less red wrapping around the nucleus (vs. MOD, $p < 0.05$), while those in the 40 μM Sch B group exhibited much less red wrapping (vs. MOD, $p < 0.01$), indicating that the decrease in the concentration of Sch B could reduce the OAPA-induced lipid deposition in the cytoplasm, and the increase in the concentration of Sch B could alleviate the lipid deposition.

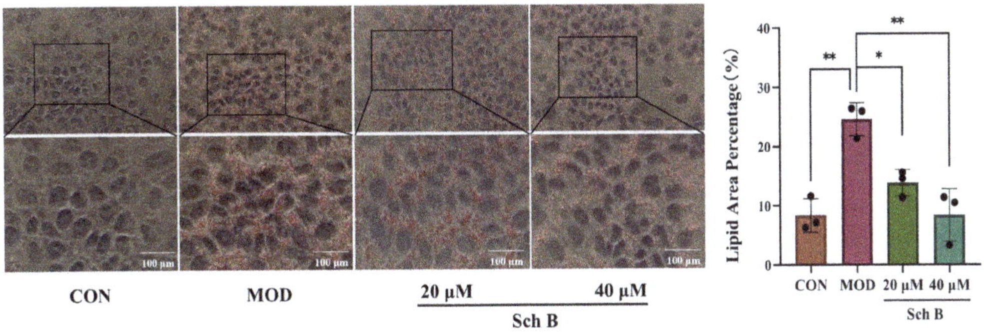

Figure 3. Histomorphological results of AML-12 cells stained with Oil Red (×100). (mean ± *S.E.*, $n = 3$). * $p < 0.05$; ** $p < 0.01$.

2.4. Effects of Sch B on TG, TC, ALT, and AST Levels in AML Cells

As shown in Figure 4, the levels of TG, TC, ALT, and AST in the MOD group were significantly higher than those in the CON group ($p < 0.001$), and compared with those in the MOD group, the levels of TG, TC, ALT, and AST in the 20 and 40 μM Sch B groups were significantly lower ($p < 0.01$).

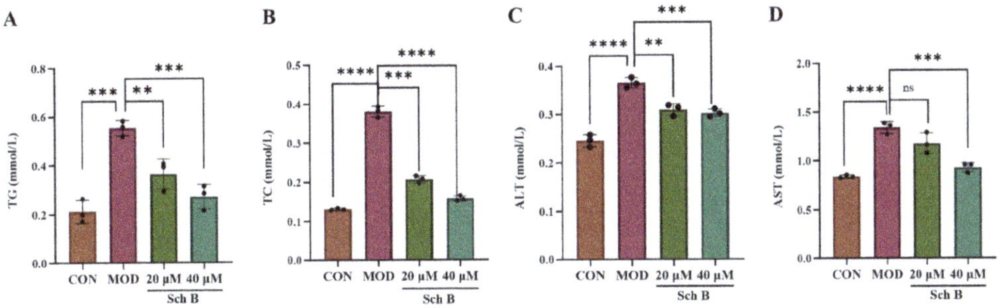

Figure 4. (**A–D**) Effects of Sch B on TG, TC, ALT, and AST levels in AML-12 cells (mean ± *S.E.*, $n = 3$). ns (not significant); ** $p < 0.01$; *** $p < 0.001$; **** $p < 0.0001$.

2.5. Network Pharmacology Prediction

2.5.1. Acquisition of Intersecting Targets

The Sch B targets were predicted through the SwissTarget Prediction database, the CHEMBL database, and the PharmMapper database, and it was found that there were 286 targets of Sch B. With the keyword "metabolic-associated fat liver disease", MAFLD-related targets were retrieved in the Genecards and OMIM databases. Using the Genecards database with a relevance score > 45 as the conditional card value, 1775 disease targets were obtained after they were merged and deduplicated. The target genes of Sch B and MAFLD were intersected, and then 75 intersection target genes were obtained, which were considered the interaction target genes for the drug treatment of MAFLD (Figure 5A). The "network. xlsx" and "type. xlsx" files were constructed using Sch B target data, and the files were imported into Cytoscape 3.9.1 to obtain a drug-disease target map (Figure 5B).

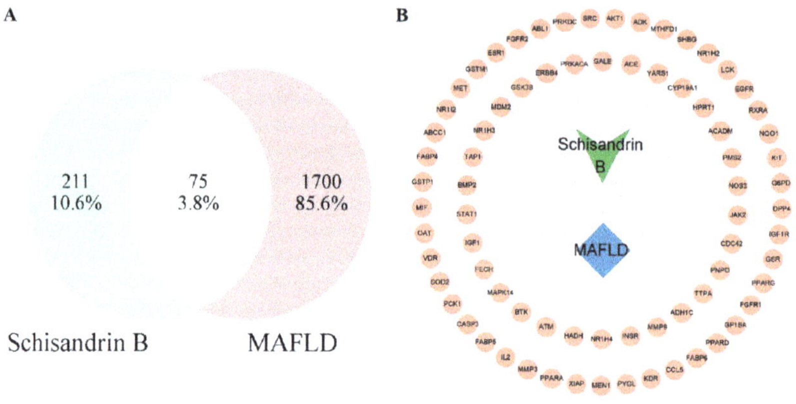

Figure 5. Venn diagram (**A**) and drug-disease target map (**B**) of Sch B and MAFLD-related targets.

2.5.2. Construction and Analysis of Protein–Protein Interaction Network (PPI)

The intersection gene file was imported into the STRING database to obtain a PPI. The centralized analysis and evaluation were conducted on all target gene information using Cytoscape 3.9.1. The median values of betweenness centrality (BC), compact centrality (CC), and degree centrality (DC) were set to be greater than or equal to the median for screening. The results showed that the median value of BC was 71.1232, that of CC was 0.0072, and that of DC was 16.4383, indicating that there were 14 nodes and 78 edges in the network. The top six screened targets were AKT1, ESR1, PPARG, CASP3, EGFR, and IGF1. Three core targets, PPARG, PCK-1, and CASP3, were identified through screening based on lipid metabolism and apoptosis (Figure 6).

2.5.3. Gene Ontology (GO) Enrichment Analysis

The intersection targets were imported into the David database for enrichment analysis, and 405 GO entries were identified, of which 290 were related to biological processes (BP), mainly including peptidyl-tyrosine phosphorylation, platelet-derived growth factor receptor-beta signaling pathway, and vascular endothelial growth factor receptor-1 signaling pathway; 31 were related to cellular composition (CC), including receptor complex, RNA polymerase II transcription regulator complex, and postsynapse; 84 were related to molecular function (MF), including nuclear receptor activity, brain-derived neurotrophic factor receptor activity, and macrophage colony-stimulating factor receptor activity. The top 10 GO inputs of BP, CC, and MF were selected for plotting (Figure 7).

2.5.4. Kyoto Encyclopedia of Genes and Genomes (KEGG) Pathway Enrichment Analysis

A total of 94 pathways were identified through KEGG pathway analysis, and 20 pathways were selected based on *p*-values. The top 20 KEGG pathways were plotted on a bubble plot (Figure 8), with Fold Enrichment values on the horizontal axis. The number of genes enriched in the corresponding pathways was represented by the size of the bubbles, and the depth of color represented significance, through which the significant enrichment information could be observed intuitively. Based on the three core targets of PPARG, PCK-1, and Caspase-3, the pathways involved in lipid metabolism and apoptosis mainly include the PPAR signaling pathway, lipid and atherosclerosis, and non-alcoholic fatty liver disease.

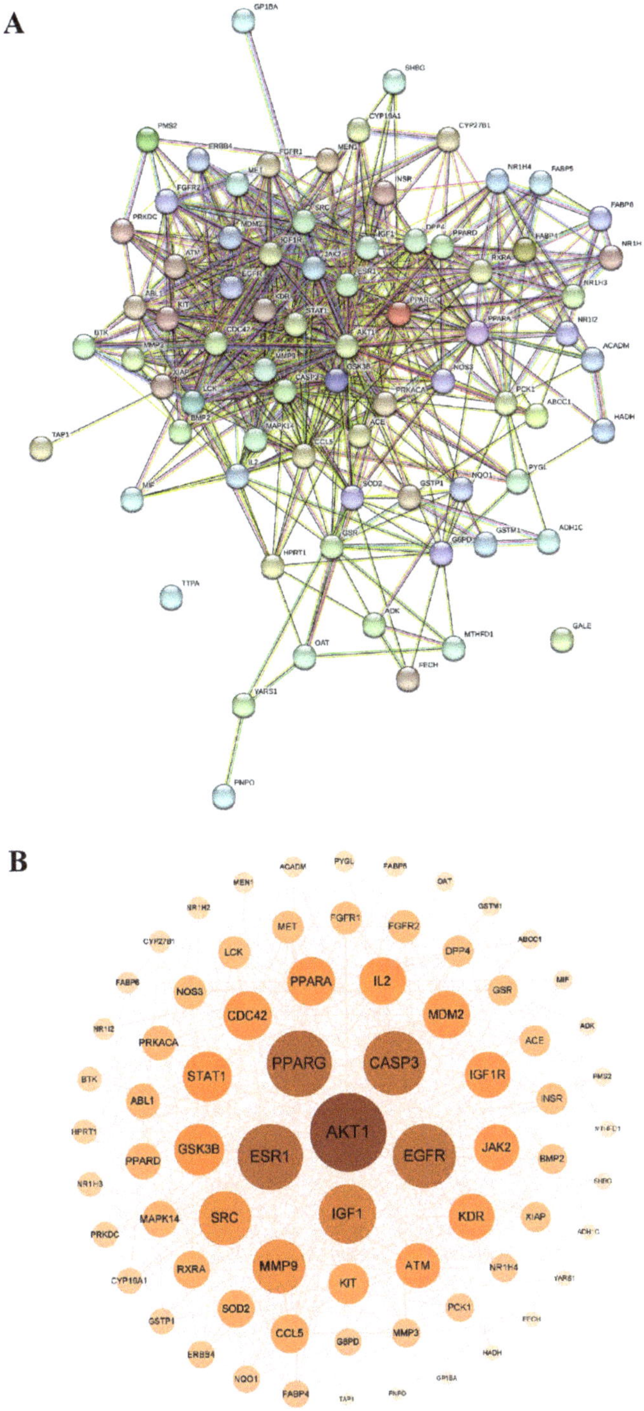

Figure 6. Protein–protein interaction network diagram. (**A**) Intersection target PPI network diagram; (**B**) core target network diagram.

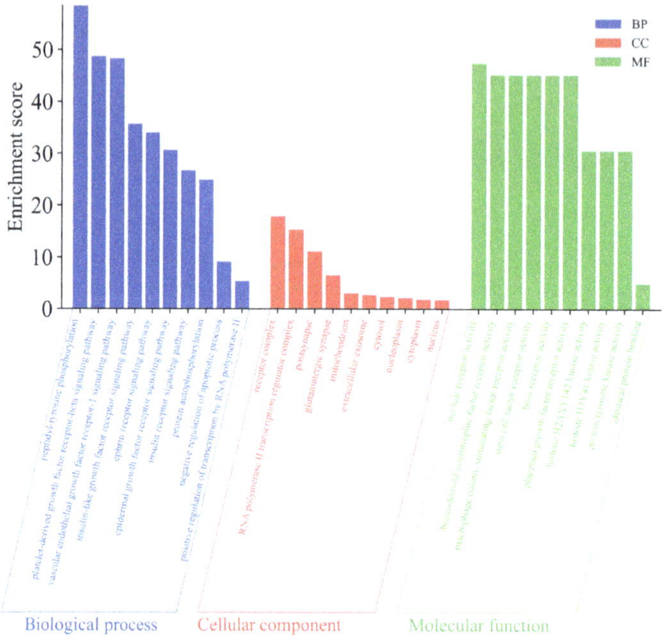

Figure 7. GO enrichment analysis bar chart.

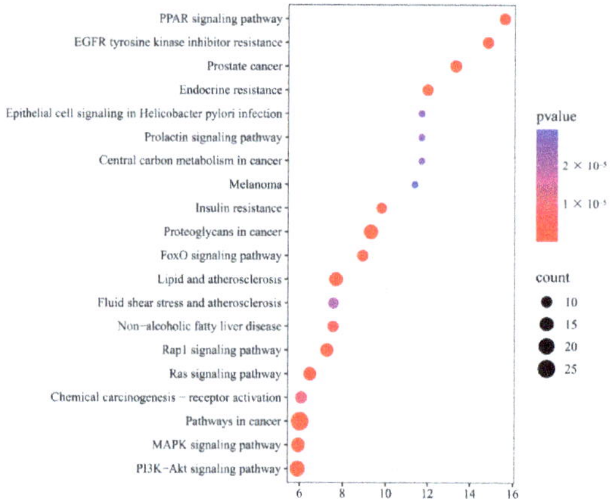

Figure 8. KEGG pathway enrichment bubble plot.

2.6. Molecular Docking Simulation Results

Molecular docking of Sch B with related core targets was performed using AutoDock Vina software (V1.2.7), and an energy matrix graph was plotted (the core components and core target values of Molecular docking are detailed in Supplementary Figure S1). The binding energy < −5.0 kJ/mol represents a good binding, and the visualization was achieved using PyMoL. The docking results showed that the binding energies of PCK-1, AKT1, ESR1, PPARG, CASP3, EGFR, and IGF1 were all < −5.0 kJ/mol (Figure 9A). Select lipid metabolism and apoptosis-related targets PPARG, PCK-1, and CASP3 were selected for visualization display (Figure 9B).

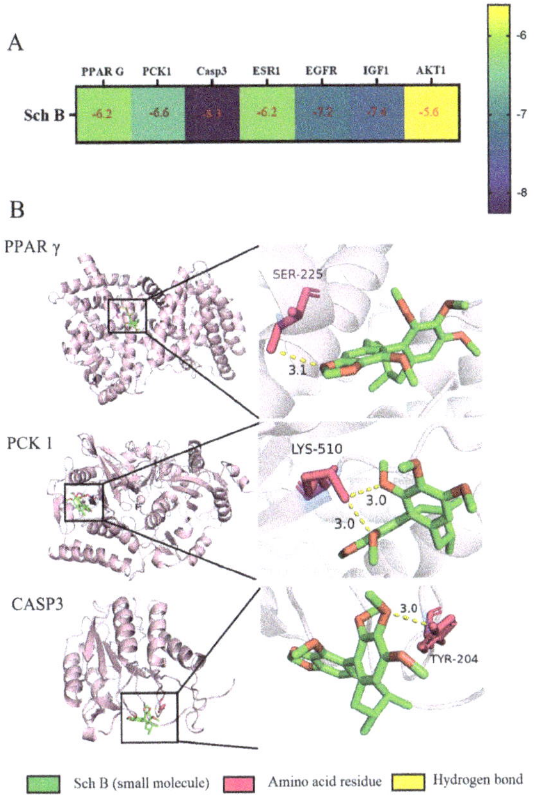

Figure 9. Molecular docking results of core targets. (**A**) Docking score. (**B**) Molecular docking diagram.

2.7. Expression of PPARγ Protein in MAFLD Cell Model

The protein expression level of PPARγ in the AML-12 cell model of MAFLD mice induced by a high-fat diet (OA+PA) was detected by Western blot (Figure 10). It was found that compared with that in the CON group, the expression level of PPARγ protein in AML-12 cells in the MAFLD model group was significantly reduced ($p < 0.001$), indicating that PPARγ could play a crucial role in the progression of MAFLD.

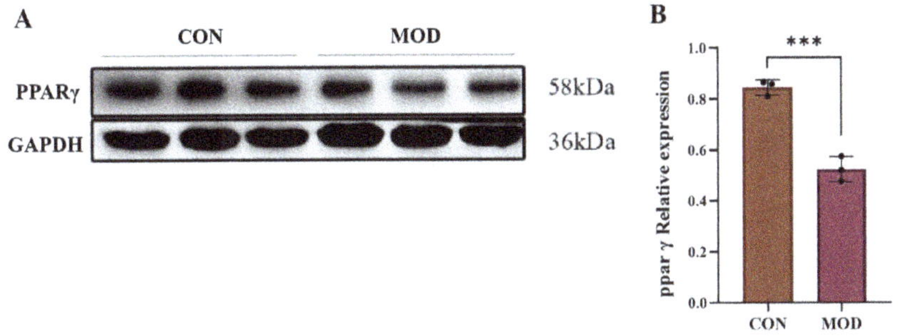

Figure 10. (**A**,**B**) Effect of OA+PA induction on PPARγ protein expression in AML-12 cells (mean ± *S.E.*, $n = 3$). *** $p < 0.001$.

2.8. Detection of PPAR γ Luciferase Reporter Gene

As shown in Figure 11, the transcriptional activity of PPARγ in AML-12 cells decreased after OA+PA induction (CON vs. MOD, $p < 0.01$), while compared with that in the MOD group, the activity of PPARγ increased in the Sch B groups (20 μM Sch B vs. MOD, $p < 0.01$; 40 μM Sch B vs. MOD, $p < 0.001$).

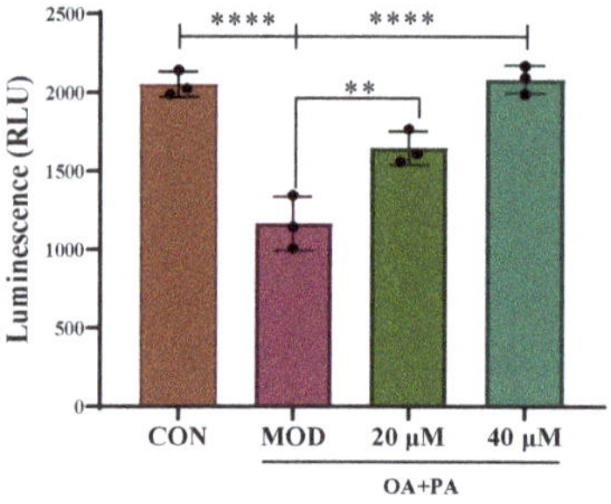

Figure 11. Results of PPARγ luciferase reporter gene (mean ± *S.E.*, $n = 3$). ** $p < 0.01$; **** $p < 0.0001$.

2.9. Effects of Sch B on Expression of PPARγ Pathway-Related Proteins

Proteins involved in the regulation of lipid metabolism and apoptosis were screened by network pharmacology methods, including PPARγ, Caspase-3, and PCK1. The expression of these proteins was detected by Western blot, in which GAPDH was taken as an internal reference. As shown in Figure 12, compared with that in the CON group, the expression of PPARγ and PCK1 in the MOD group was significantly reduced ($p < 0.01$; $p < 0.05$), while the expression of Caspase-3 was significantly increased ($p < 0.05$); compared with that in the MOD group, the expression of PPARγ and PCK1 was significantly increased after Sch B treatment ($p < 0.01$; $p < 0.05$), while the expression of Caspase-3 was significantly decreased ($p < 0.01$).

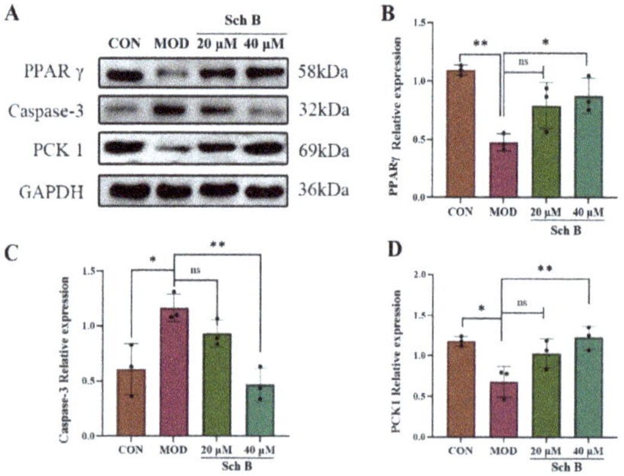

Figure 12. (**A–D**) Effects of Sch B on the expression of PPARγ, PCK1, and Caspase-3 proteins (mean ± *S.E.*, $n = 3$). ns (not significant); * $p < 0.05$; ** $p < 0.01$.

2.10. Effects of Sch B on the Expression of Lipid Metabolism-Related Proteins

2.10.1. Effects of Sch B on the Expression of Lipid Synthesis and Cholesterol Metabolism-Related Proteins

Compared with that in the CON group, the expression of cholesterol metabolism-related protein ABCA1 was significantly reduced in the MOD group ($p < 0.05$), indicating that the cholesterol reverse transport may be hindered and the fatty acid synthesis may be enhanced. Compared with that in the MOD group, the expression of ABCA1 in the Sch B groups was significantly increased ($p < 0.01$), suggesting that Sch B can regulate cholesterol metabolism-related proteins to promote cholesterol reverse transport, and inhibit the fatty acid synthesis. Compared with that in the CON group, the expression of fatty acid synthesis protein ACSL4 was significantly increased in the MOD group ($p < 0.05$), indicating an increase in fatty acid synthesis in the MOD group. Compared with that in the MOD group, the expression of histone was significantly reduced in the 40 μM Sch B group ($p < 0.01$), indicating that the intervention with Sch B could decrease the expression of fatty acid synthesis proteins, leading to a reduction in fatty acid synthesis (Figure 13).

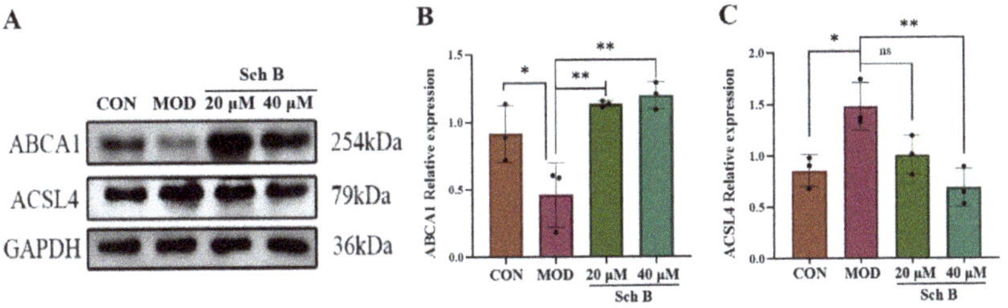

Figure 13. (**A–C**) Effects of Sch B on the expression of ABCA1 and ACSL4 proteins (mean ± *S.E.*, $n = 3$). ns (not significant); * $p < 0.05$; ** $p < 0.01$.

2.10.2. Fatty Acid Oxidation

Compared with those in the CON group, the expression levels of fatty acid oxidation-related proteins CPT1A, CPT2, and ACOX1 were significantly decreased in the MOD group ($p < 0.05$; $p < 0.01$; $p < 0.001$), indicating that the fatty acid β-oxidation process might be inhibited in the MOD group. Compared with those in the MOD group, the expression levels of these three proteins in the 40 μM Sch B group were significantly increased ($p < 0.05$), indicating that Sch B could promote the expression of fatty acid oxidation-related proteins and improve fatty acid oxidation function (Figure 14).

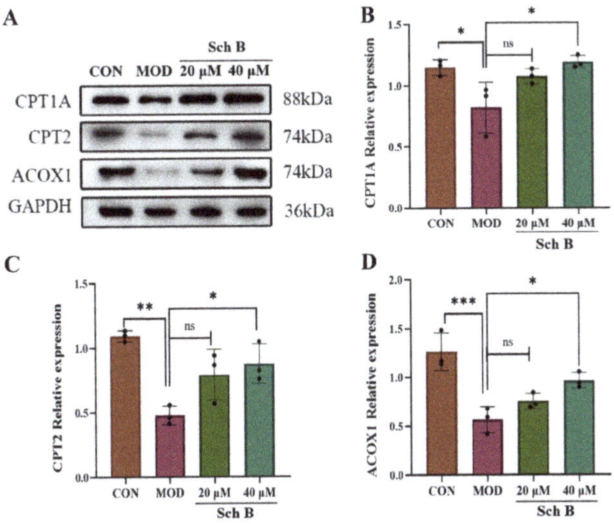

Figure 14. (**A–D**) Effects of Sch B on the expression of CPT1A, CPT2 and ACOX1 proteins (mean ± *S.E.*, $n = 3$). ns (not significant); * $p < 0.05$; ** $p < 0.01$; *** $p < 0.001$.

2.11. Effects of Sch B on Cell Apoptosis

2.11.1. Annexin V-FITC/PI Detection of Cell Apoptosis

As shown in Figure 15, in the flow cytometry plot, the Q1 region (lower right) presents the distribution pattern of early apoptotic cells (EA cells), late apoptotic cells (LA cells) are identified and classified in the Q2 region (upper right), the Q3 region (lower left) exhibits normal cells (N cells), and mechanically damaged cells (Nec cells) are shown in the Q4 region (upper left).

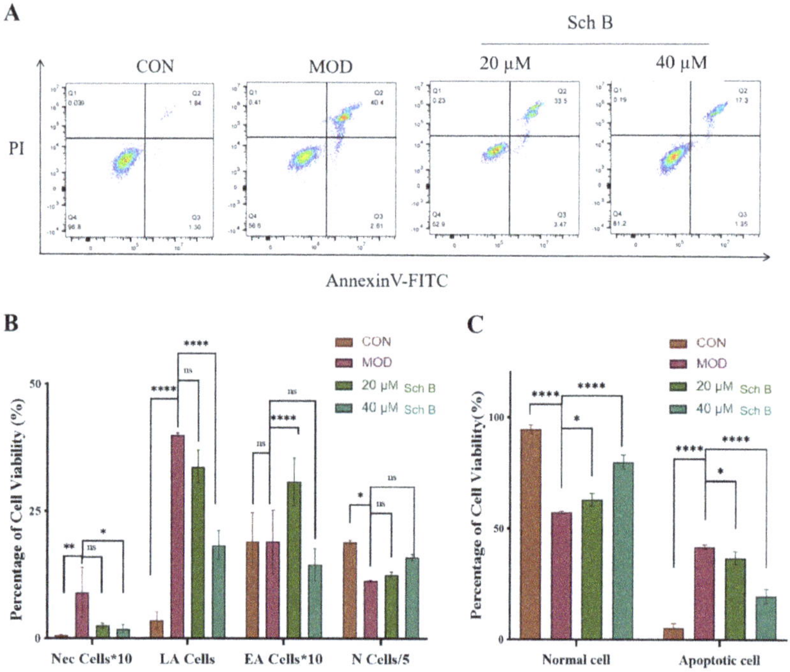

Figure 15. Effects of Sch B on apoptosis (mean ± *S.E.*, $n = 3$). (**A**) Flow cytometry. (**B**) Flow cytometry visualization. (**C**) Comparison of healthy cells and apoptotic cells. ns (not significant); * $p < 0.05$; ** $p < 0.01$; **** $p < 0.0001$.

The results showed that the proportion of late-stage apoptotic cells (LA cells) increased, while the proportion of normal cells (N cells) decreased in the MOD group, indicating the successful establishment of the apoptosis model. After the treatment with Sch B, the apoptosis of LA cells decreased gradually, while N cells rebounded, indicating that Sch B could partially inhibit apoptosis. The apoptotic cells in the 40 μM Sch B group were further reduced, while N cells recovered to near-normal cell levels, demonstrating a dose-dependent protective effect.

2.11.2. Effects of Sch B on Expression of Apoptosis-Related Proteins

As shown in Figure 16, compared with that in the CON group, the relative expression level of pro-apoptotic protein Bax in the MOD group was significantly increased ($p < 0.05$), while the expression level of anti-apoptotic protein Bcl-2 was significantly decreased ($p < 0.01$). After the administration of Schi B, the relative expression levels of Bax and Bcl-2 proteins were significantly reversed compared to the MOD group, indicating that Sch B could significantly inhibit the expression of pro-apoptotic protein Bax and promote the expression of anti-apoptotic protein Bcl-2.

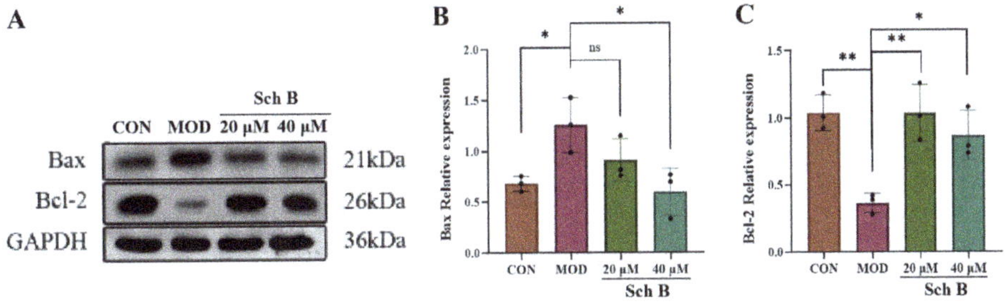

Figure 16. (**A–C**) Effects of Sch B on the expression of apoptosis-related proteins (mean ± *S.E.*, *n* = 3). ns > 0.01; * $p < 0.05$; ** $p < 0.01$.

3. Discussion

From the perspective of cell model construction, oleic acid (OA) and palmitic acid (PA) are the two most commonly used free fatty acids that can simulate the pathological process of lipid accumulation in liver cells [21]. In this study, a mixed-induction MAFLD model of OA and PA (2:1) was used to simulate the pathological process of hepatic steatosis caused by the accumulation of free fatty acids in vivo. The Oil Red O staining results showed that after the induction for 24 h, the lipid droplet content was the highest, and the levels of TC, TG, and liver injury markers ALT and AST increased in AML cells, indicating a successful model construction. After the treatment with 20 μM and 40 μM Sch B, the lipid droplet deposition was dose-dependently reduced, and the levels of TC, TG, ALT, and AST were lowered in AML cells.

In terms of molecular mechanisms, 75 intersecting targets between Sch B and MAFLD was first screened by network pharmacology in this study, and the top 6 targets were further identified as AKT1, ESR1, PPARG, CASP3, EGFR, and IGF1 by constructing a PPI network diagram. Screening was conducted with a focus on lipid metabolism and apoptosis, among which PPARγ, PCK-1, and CASP3 were significantly enriched as core targets. PPARγ is widely expressed in various adipose tissues and participates in lipid metabolism activities, playing an important role in adipocyte differentiation, adipogenesis, lipid metabolism, and glucose metabolism [22]. On the other hand, Pck1, as a key enzyme in gluconeogenesis, plays a crucial regulatory role in liver energy metabolism, and its functional disorders are closely related to various metabolic diseases [23,24]. It is worth noting that our research team found in previous experiments that after the administration of Sch B, the upregulation of PPARγ in C57BL/6 mice could regulate the expression of its downstream protein Pck1 [20]. In addition, the Caspase family plays a crucial role in cell apoptosis [25]. An excessive accumulation of neutral lipids in the body can form lipid droplets, and free fatty acids that have not yet been metabolized in the body can deposit in the liver when the process of fatty acid oxidation is impaired [26]. Moreover, studies have shown that activating autophagy mechanisms can effectively improve lipid deposition in the body and simultaneously inhibit the process of cell apoptosis [27,28]. It was found in the KEGG pathway analysis that the activities of lipid metabolism-related pathways, such as PPAR signaling pathway, lipid and atherosclerosis, and non-alcoholic fatty liver disease, were high, indicating a research direction for subsequent mechanism studies. It was confirmed by the molecular docking simulation that the binding energy of Sch B to three lipid metabolism and apoptosis targets, PPARγ, PCK-1, and CASP3, was less than −5.0 kJ/mol, indicating the tight docking and strong affinity. In addition, the dual luciferase reporter plasmid detection directly confirmed that Sch B could directly activate the activity of PPARγ. Combined with Western blot to verify PPARγ and its downstream lipid metabolism and apoptosis genes, the experiment found that the expression of PPARγ and PCK-1 was significantly reduced and the expression of Caspase-3 was significantly increased in the MOD group. However, after Sch B treatment, the expression of PPARγ and its downstream lipid metabolism regulation-related genes (CPT1A, CPT2, ACOX1, ABCA1, ACSL4, and ABCA1) and apoptosis-related genes (Bax and Bcl-2) were reversed. The flow cytometry also showed that the administration of schisandrin B could alleviate the increase in late-stage apoptotic cells in MAFLD, with a dose-dependent protective effect.

Specifically, activating PPARγ is the "core switch" for Sch B to improve lipid metabolism disorders. On the one hand, PPARγ can reduce lipid synthesis at the source by inhibiting the expression of genes related to lipid synthesis. Acsl4, as a key enzyme regulating unsaturated fatty acid metabolism, is mainly distributed in peroxisomes and endoplasmic reticulum, playing an important catalytic role in fatty acid activation and participating in regulating fatty acid synthesis through transcriptional regulation mechanisms [29,30]. ABCA1 (ATP binding cassette transporter A1) is responsible for transporting intracellular cholesterol and phospholipids to the extracellular environment, which is related to the production of high-density lipoprotein (HDL), and involved in cholesterol reverse transport [31]. PPARγ inhibits lipid synthesis genes and promotes cholesterol reverse transport by activating ABCA1 simultaneously, reducing intracellular cholesterol levels to suppress lipid synthesis and improve lipid accumulation in liver cells. On the other hand, CPT1A, CPT2, and ACOX1 play important catalytic roles in the fatty acid β-oxidation metabolic pathway, among which CPT1A, as the main regulatory enzyme of this metabolic process, functions to transport long-chain fatty acids to the mitochondrial matrix for breakdown metabolism to generate energy [32], CPT2 is responsible for catalyzing the conversion reaction of acylcarnitine to acyl CoA, providing a substrate for subsequent oxidation processes [33], and ACOX1 mainly plays a key role in the oxidative degradation of extremely long-chain fatty acids [34]. PPARγ can directly regulate the expression of downstream fatty acid oxidation key enzymes such as CPT1A, CPT2, and ACOX1 to accelerate the entry of fatty acids into mitochondria for oxidative degradation and reduce lipid accumulation in liver cells. Bcl-2 and Bax proteins can determine the survival or apoptosis of cells. When the Bcl-2 protein is inhibited, its dimer with Bax decreases, leading to cell apoptosis [35]. PPARγ also plays a dominant role in inhibiting cell apoptosis [36]. In the pathological state of MAFLD, lipid accumulation may activate the apoptotic signaling pathway through the autophagy mechanism, and the activation of PPARγ can block the cascade reaction of liver cell apoptosis caused by MAFLD by downregulating Caspase-3 and Bax and upregulating Bcl-2 expression. It is speculated that Sch B may regulate the apoptosis-related proteins Bax and Bcl-2 by activating PPARγ, providing a protective barrier for liver cells and reducing cell death caused by lipid toxicity.

In summary, in this study, the potential targets of Sch B for treating MAFLD were predicted by network pharmacology analysis. The results showed that Sch B may regulate liver lipid metabolism and apoptosis through multiple targets and pathways, thereby exerting its therapeutic effects. It was confirmed that Sch B could specifically activate PPARγ as the core regulatory target to regulate the expression of downstream lipid metabolism and apoptosis-related genes, improving lipid metabolism disorders and inhibit cell apoptosis in OA+PA-induced MAFLD cell models, which may provide more direct and comprehensive experimental evidence for the interaction between Sch B and PPARγ, as well as the core regulatory role of PPARγ. In addition, the team's previous study on Sch B alleviating MAFLD was further expanded in this study, in which a progressive study of "in vivo verification→in vitro mechanism analysis" was conducted. The in vivo efficacy of Sch B in a high-fat diet-induced mouse model had been confirmed previously by our team, while in this study, AML-12 liver cells were used for in vitro experiments to directly observe the effect of Sch B on liver cells. Then, the mechanism dimension of Sch B intervention in

MAFLD was expanded by focusing on PCK1 and Caspase-3, in which PCK1, a key factor in metabolism, could provide a new direction for analyzing the regulation of Sch B on metabolic networks, and simultaneously, the study of Caspase-3-mediated cell apoptosis could answer the core question of how Sch B could protect liver cells from lipid toxicity-induced death. However, this study still has certain limitations. Network pharmacology has suggested multiple potential targets and pathways, but this study mainly focuses on PPARγ and its lipid metabolism and apoptosis-related genes, so the role of other pathways such as growth factor receptor signaling pathway and cancer in Sch B regulation has not been further studied. In the future, more experiments should be conducted to verify the synergistic effect of these pathways with PPARγ.

4. Materials and Methods

4.1. Experimental Drugs and Reagents

Sch B (Chengdu Pufide Biotechnology Co., Ltd., Chengdu, China); ALT, AST, TG, and TC reagent kits (Nanjing Jiancheng Bioengineering Research Institute, Nanjing, China); Modified Oil Red O staining kit (Shanghai Biyun Tian Biotechnology Co., Ltd., Shanghai, China); ECL chromogenic solution (Dalian Meilun Biotechnology Co., Ltd., Dalian, China); BCA protein assay kit, ammonium persulfate, 30% acrylamide, TEMED, 5×SDS loading buffer, glycine HCL-Tris, pancreatic enzymes, and streptomycin (Beijing Dingguo Changsheng Biotechnology Co., Ltd., Beijing, China); Skimmed milk powder (BD, Franklin Lakes, NJ, USA); Fetal bovine serum and DMEM/F12 culture medium (Shanghai Dathir Biotechnology Co., Ltd., Shanghai, China); Dual luciferase reporter gene detection kit (Promega, Madison, WI, USA); Annexin V-FITC/PI dual staining kit (Shanghai Beibo Biotechnology Co., Ltd., Shanghai, China); All antibodies (ABclonal, Wuhan, China).

4.2. Cytology Experiments

4.2.1. AML-12 Cell Culture

AML-12 cells (Mouse cell line, Shanghai Instituteof Biochemistry and Cell Biology, Shanghai, China) were cultured in a complete medium containing DMEM/F12 medium + 10% FBS + 1% penicillin and streptomycin, in a 5% carbon dioxide incubator with a constant humidity and temperature at 37 °C. When the growth density of AML-12 cells reached about 90%, the cell passaging was performed.

4.2.2. Establishment of MAFLD Cell Model

Palmitic acid (PA, 0.9188 g) and oleic acid (OA, 2.0094 g) powders were separately weighed and poured into centrifuge tubes, and then 50 mL of NaOH (100 mM) was added. The PA solution needed to be heated in an 80 °C water bath until the solution was clear. Then, 50 μL of the two solutions were separately added into 950 μL of BSA solution (10%) dropwise in a 55 °C water bath, shaken, and mixed repeatedly, and continued to be shaken and incubated for 10 min in a 55 °C water bath. At this time, the final concentration of PA was 3.3 mM, and that of OA was 6.6 mM. Finally, OA and PA solutions were filtered with a needle tube and a 0.22 mm filter in a super clean bench, and the filtered solutions were subpackaged into centrifuge tubes. AML-12 cells were incubated with the PA and OA solution in the complete culture medium at 37 °C for 24 h, and the cell solutions were stored in a refrigerator at 4 °C in a cell room, in which 100 μL OA and 100 μL PA were added to 1800 μL of complete culture medium.

4.3. CCK-8 Detection of Sch B Activity

An appropriate amount of Sch B was dissolved in DMSO to prepare a 100 mM stock solution. Then, 10 μL of 100 mM stock solution were mixed well with 990 μL of DMSO to prepare 1 mL of the solution at a concentration of 100 μM/L. The prepared 100 μM/L stock solution was diluted according to different concentration ratios, so that the final concentrations of Sch B were 1, 2.5, 5, 10, 20, 40, 80, and 100 μM/L, respectively. At the same time, a blank group and a DMSO control group were set up, and they were kept in a −20 °C refrigerator for packaging. AML-12 cells were inoculated into wells of a 96-well plate in advance, and then the old culture medium was discarded. The plate was washed with PBS, and the newly prepared complete culture medium was added into the well. Then, 1uL of stock solution containing different concentrations of Sch B was separately added into each well, with 6 duplicate wells in each group. The cells continued to be cultured in a cell incubator for 12 h, and then the cells were taken out. Following the instructions of the kit, 20 μL of detection reagent was added to each well, and the cells were incubated in the cell culture incubator for 2 h. OD values of the cell solutions at 450 nm were measured using an Infinite M200TECAN microplate reader (TECAN Group, Männedorf, Switzerland). Sch B concentrations for the subsequent experiments were screened and determined based on the cell survival rate results.

4.4. Detection of TG and TC

The counting of AML cells was performed under an optical microscope, and the cell density of AML cell suspension was adjusted to 1 million cells/mL. The prepared cell suspension was centrifuged at 1000 rpm for 10 min, and the supernatant was discarded to obtain the cell pellet. The cell pellet was dissolved in 0.2 mL of anhydrous ethanol for homogenization and sonicated under ice water bath conditions (power: 300 W for 3~5 s/time, at an interval of 30 s, and repeated 5 times) to prepare the cell homogenate. Then, 2.5 μL of cell homogenate and 250 μL of working solution were added into each well of a 96-well plate, while blank and calibration wells were set up and 3 duplicate wells were set up in each group. The well plate was shaken to mix the solution well, and the cells were incubated at 37 °C for 10 min. The absorbance value of the solution from each well was measured at the 500 nm wavelength using an enzyme-linked immunosorbent assay (ELISA) microplate reader. The contents of TG and TC in each group of cells were calculated based on the absolute OD value (measured well OD value minus control well OD value).

4.5. Determination of ALT and AST

The method used for preparing AML cells was the same as that in Section 4.4, and the wavelength for the measurement by enzyme-linked immunosorbent assay (ELISA) reader was set up at 505 nm for measuring the OD value of each well. The absolute OD values (measured well OD value minus control well OD value) were substituted into the standard curve to obtain the corresponding ALT and AST activity values.

4.6. Cell Oil Red O Staining Detection

AML cells were inoculated into a six-well plate in advance. The complete culture medium was discarded before staining, and the cells were washed three times with PBS, and fixed with 4% paraformaldehyde solution for 30 min. Then, the fixative was discarded, and the cells were washed twice with distilled water. The cells were soaked in 60% isopropanol for 5 min. The isopropanol was discarded, and newly prepared Oil Red O staining solution was added. After soaking for 20 min, the staining solution was discarded. The cells were washed with 60% isopropanol for 3 s, and then the isopropanol was discarded. The cells were rinsed with pure water 3 times until there was no excess staining solution. Mayer hematoxylin staining solution was added to redye the cell nucleus for 1 min, then the Mayer hematoxylin staining solution was discarded, and the cells were washed with water 3 times. After adding Oil Red O buffer, the cells were left standing for 1 min, and the buffer was discarded. Pure water was added to cover the cells, and the cells were observed and photographed under an optical microscope.

4.7. Prediction of Targets by Network Pharmacology Methods

4.7.1. Acquisition of Intersection Targets of Sch B and MAFLD

The smile number of Sch B obtained from the Pubchem Database (https://pubchem.ncbi.nlm.nih.gov/, accessed on 7 April 2025) was imported into the Swiss Target Prediction Database (http://www.swisstargetprediction.ch/, accessed on 9 April 2025), the PharmMapper Database (https://www.lilab-ecust.cn/pharmmapper/submitfile.html, accessed on 9 April 2025), and the CHEMBL Database (https://www.ebi.ac.uk/chembl/, accessed on 10 April 2025) for the prediction of Sch B target genes, and the targets were standardized through the Uniprot Database (http://www.uniprot.org, accessed on 10 April 2025). Using the keyword 'metabolic-associated fatty liver disease', potential MAFLD targets were screened through GeneCards (http://www.Genecards.org/, accessed on 11 April 2025) and OMIM (https://omim.org/, accessed on 12 April 2025) Database and deduplicated. Sch B target and MAFLD targets were imported into the Wei Sheng Xin platform (http://www.bioinformatics.com.cn/, accessed on 13 April 2025), a bioinformatics platform, to obtain intersecting targets.

4.7.2. Construction of Sch B Target Network

The intersection targets of Sch B and MAFLD were obtained through the Wei Sheng Xin Platform, and a Venn diagram was drawn for intuitive display. The interactions among Sch B, intersecting targets, and MAFLD were constructed and visualized using Cytoscape 3.9.1 software.

4.7.3. Construction of Target PPI

PPI for Sch B was constructed through the STRING Database (http://www.string-db.org/, accessed on 15 April 2025). The obtained data were imported into Cytoscape 3.9.1, and the core target information was obtained by the screening based on the values of BC, CC, and DC larger than or equal to the median values.

4.7.4. GO Biological Process Enrichment and KEGG Pathway Analysis

The intersection targets were imported into the David Database for GO (https://davidbioinformatics.nih.gov/, accessed on 18 April 2025) functional enrichment analysis and KEGG pathway enrichment analysis, and the results were visualized on the Wei Sheng Xin Visualization Cloud Platform.

4.8. Molecular Docking and Visualization Analysis

The molecular docking between Sch B and important targets was performed using AutoDock Vina software (V1.2.7), and its binding activity was verified. The 2D structure of Sch B was downloaded from the Pubchem Database and input into Chembio3D to minimize the energy, and then AutodockTools-1.5.7 was used for hydrogenation, calculation, and allocation of charges, and for setting rotation buttons, which were stored in the form of "pdbqt". Uniprot ID was obtained from the Uniprot Database (http://www.uniprot.org/, accessed on 22 April 2025), and the key target proteins were downloaded through the RCSBPDB Database (https://www.rcsb.org/, accessed on 23 April 2025). The proteins were input into PyMoL software (V3.1.6.1) to remove the original ligands and water, and transferred into AutoDocktools (V1.5.7) for hydrogenation, calculation, and allocation of the charges, and for specifying the atomic type, which were stored in the form of "pdbqt". The protein ligand was used as the center of the docking box, and the lattice box covered the proteins and molecules. Other parameters were default values. The interaction mode was studied using PyMOL technology.

4.9. Dual Luciferase Reporter Gene Detection

Following the instructions of luciferase reporter gene detection kit, the PPARγ luciferase reporter plasmid and lipofectamine 3000 mixed with serum-free Opti-MEM was incubated at room temperature for 20 min. This mixture was added to fetal bovine serum DMEM/F12 complete culture medium containing AML-12 cells, and the luciferase reporter gene construct and Renilla luciferase expression vector were co-transfected. Twenty-four hours later, the AML-12 cells were treated with Sch B for one hour, then incubated with OA+PA (1 μM) for two hours, and firefly and renilla luciferase activities were detected using a dual luciferase reporter gene assay kit. The PPARγ transcriptional activity was calculated as (relative light unit firefly luciferase/renilla luciferase) × 100.

4.10. Cell Apoptosis Detection by Annexin V-FITC/PI Dual Staining

Adherent AML-12 cells were digested with trypsin, followed by adding complete culture medium containing serum to terminate the digestion, and the cell suspension was centrifuged to collect the cell pellet. The cells were washed twice with pre-cooled PBS, and the cell suspension was centrifuged at 300 rpm for 5 min, and the supernatant was discarded to collect the cell pellet for preparing the cell suspension. Then, 100 μL of 1×Annexin V binding buffer were injected into the cell suspension, followed by adding 5 μL of Annexin V-FITC to it, which was incubated at room temperature in the dark for 15 min. The cell suspension was added with 5 μL of PI (the final concentration was 1–2 μg/mL), then incubated in the dark for 5 min, and immediately 400 μL of the binding buffer was added. The solution was mixed well for testing on the machine.

4.11. Protein Immunoblot Results

AML-12 cells were digested with trypsin and collected by centrifugation. The cells were washed twice with pre-cooled PBS solution, and lysed with RIPA lysis reagent at 4 °C for 30 min. The lysate was centrifuged at 12,000× *g* and 4 °C for 10 min to obtain the supernatant of cell lysate. The BCA protein quantification method was used to determine the total protein in the supernatant. To the protein supernatant 5 × SDS protein electrophoresis buffer was added, and then the cells were denatured in a boiling water bath for 5 min and stored at −20 °C for use. The proteins were separated by SDS-PAGE electrophoresis and transferred onto PVDF membranes for 2 h. The membranes were blocked with TBST containing 5% skim milk powder (1.5 h). The membranes were incubated with the primary antibodies at 4 °C overnight. Then, they were washed three times with TBST and incubated with the secondary antibody at room temperature for 1 h. A luminescent reagent was added on the membranes for development, and the images were photographed with a gel imager (UVP Chemsolo Auto gel imager, Jena Analytical Instruments, Jena, Germany). The grayscale values of different bands were measured using an Image J analysis software, in which GAPDH (1:50,000) was used as the internal reference. The ratio of each grayscale value to the GAPDH grayscale value was taken as the relative expression level of proteins.

4.12. Statistical Analysis

SigmaPlot 12.5 was used for analysis. The data results are presented in the form of mean ± standard error (mean ± S.E.), and Tukey's tests were used to determine the level of inter-group significance. One way analysis of variance was used to evaluate the differences. Ns means $p > 0.05$, which indicated no statistical significance, whereas $p < 0.05$ indicated a statistical significance. GraphPad Prism 9.5.1 was used for plotting. The grayscale values detected by Western blot were analyzed using Image J software (V1.54g).

5. Conclusions

An in vitro model of AML-12 mouse liver cell metabolism-related fatty liver disease (MAFLD) was constructed using oleic acid (OA) and palmitic acid (PA). The results showed that Schisandrin B has a significant regulatory effect on lipid metabolism disorders in the OA+PA-induced MAFLD cell model. Its mechanism of action mainly relies on the activation of the PPARγ-PCK1/Aspase-3 signaling pathway, which can not only inhibit the generation of fatty acids but also enhance the breakdown metabolism of fatty acids, thereby reducing lipid deposition in liver cells. Through this series of biochemical reactions, the lipid metabolism disorder in the MAFLD cell model could be significantly alleviated, and the process of cell apoptosis could be effectively inhibited (Figure 17). This finding may lay an important theoretical foundation and create a new research direction for the deep development and application of *Schisandra chinensis*.

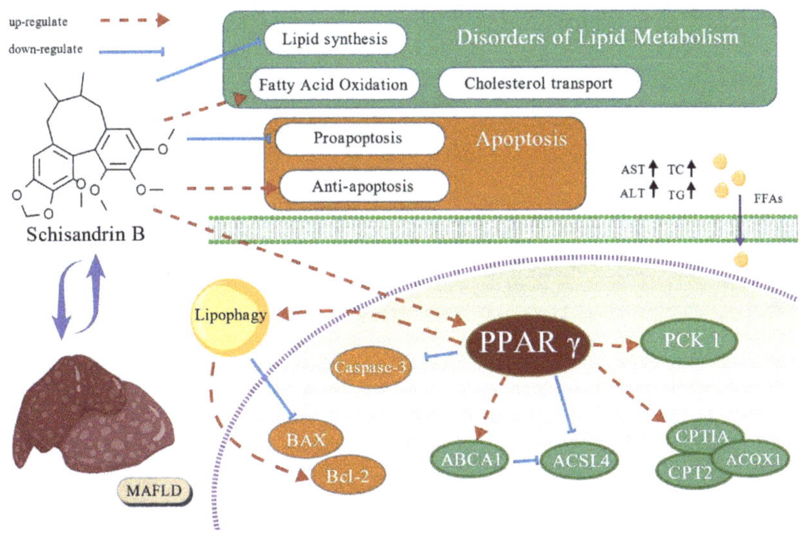

Figure 17. Potential mechanism of Sch B alleviating MAFLD.

Supplementary Materials: The following supporting information can be downloaded at: https://www.mdpi.com/article/10.3390/ph18101441/s1, Figure S1: Core components and core targets in molecular docking.

Author Contributions: Conceptualization, M.G. and J.S.; methodology, M.G., M.W. and J.S.; software, M.G. and J.S.; validation, M.G., F.L., X.F. and J.S.; formal analysis, M.G. and Z.Z.; investigation, M.G., H.L. and J.S.; resources, M.G. and C.W.; data curation, M.G. and J.S.; writing—original draft preparation, M.G. and J.S.; writing—review and editing, H.L., C.W. and J.S.; visualization, M.G. and J.S.; supervision, C.W.; project administration, C.W. and J.S.; funding acquisition, H.L. and J.S. All authors have read and agreed to the published version of the manuscript.

Funding: This research was funded by the National Natural Science Foundation of China (82274081) and by the Science and Technology Development Plan Project of Jilin Province (YDZJ202301ZYTS152).

Institutional Review Board Statement: Not applicable.

Informed Consent Statement: Not applicable.

Data Availability Statement: The original contributions presented in this study are included in the article/Supplementary Material. Further inquiries can be directed to the corresponding authors.

Conflicts of Interest: The authors declare no conflicts of interest.

Abbreviations

The following abbreviations are used in this manuscript:

Sch B	Schisandrin B
MAFLD	Metabolic-associated fatty liver disease
PPAγ	Peroxisome proliferator-activated receptor gamma
OA	Oleic acid
PA	Palmitic acid
TC	Total cholesterol
TG	Triglycerides
ALT	Alanine aminotransferase
AST	Aspartate aminotransferase
PPI	Protein–protein interaction network
BC	Betweenness centrality
CC	Compact centrality
DC	Degree centrality
GO	Gene Ontology
BP	Biological processes
MF	Molecular function
KEGG	Kyoto Encyclopedia of Genes and Genomes

References

1. Li, Y.X.; Zhou, Y.Y.; Wang, L.Y.; Lin, X.Q.; Mao, M.H.; Yin, S.Q.; Zhu, L.; Jiao, Y.F.; Yu, W.F.; Gao, P.; et al. Emerging trends and hotspots in the links between the gut microbiota and MAFLD from 2002 to 2021: A bibliometric analysis. *Front. Endocrinol.* **2022**, *13*, 990953. [CrossRef]
2. Gamboa, C.M.; Wang, Y.J.; Xu, H.T.; Kalemba, K.; Wondisford, F.E.; Sabaawy, H.E. Optimized 3D Culture of Hepatic Cells for Liver Organoid Metabolic Assays. *Cells* **2021**, *10*, 3280. [CrossRef] [PubMed]
3. Doustmohammadian, A.; Nezhadisalami, A.; Tameshke, F.S.; Motamed, N.; Maadi, M.; Farahmand, M.; Sohrabi, M.; Clark, C.C.T.; Ajdarkosh, H.; Faraji, A.H.; et al. A randomized triple-blind controlled clinical trial evaluation of sitagliptin in the treatment of patients with non-alcoholic fatty liver diseases without diabetes. *Front. Med.* **2022**, *9*, 937554. [CrossRef] [PubMed]
4. Mun, J.; Kim, S.; Yoon, H.G.; You, Y.; Kim, O.K.; Choi, K.C.; Lee, Y.H.; Lee, J.; Park, J.; Jun, W. Water Extract of Curcuma longa L. Ameliorates Non-Alcoholic Fatty Liver Disease. *Nutrients* **2019**, *11*, 2536. [CrossRef] [PubMed]
5. Zhang, W.W.; Wang, W.S.; Shen, C.Z.; Wang, X.H.; Pu, Z.C.; Yin, Q. Network pharmacology for systematic understanding of Schisandrin B reduces the epithelial cells injury of colitis through regulating pyroptosis by AMPK/Nrf2/NLRP3 inflammasome. *Aging* **2021**, *13*, 23193–23209. [CrossRef]
6. Zhao, F.; Pan, H.H.; Chen, X.Y.; Miao, S. Study on the Role of Schisandrin B in Ameliorating Hepatic Ischemia-Reperfusion Injury by Modulating Hepatocyte Autophagy. *Iran. J. Pharm. Res.* **2025**, *24*, 157033. [CrossRef]
7. Li, C.; Ji, K.B.; Kim, E.Y.; Choi, H.Y.; Yoon, J.H.; Zhang, X.; Kim, R.E.; Park, K.S.; Liu, H.; Kim, M.K. Schisandrin B mitigates oxidative damage in early porcine embryos exposed to Ochratoxin A via NRF2 pathway activation. *Anim. Reprod. Sci.* **2025**, *279*, 107889. [CrossRef]
8. Yan, L.S.; Zhang, S.F.; Luo, G.; Cheng, B.C.; Zhang, C.; Wang, Y.W.; Qiu, X.Y.; Zhou, X.H.; Wang, Q.G.; Song, X.L.; et al. Schisandrin B mitigates hepatic steatosis and promotes fatty acid oxidation by inducing autophagy through AMPK/mTOR signaling pathway. *Metabolism* **2022**, *131*, 155200. [CrossRef]
9. Ma, R.J.; Zhan, Y.K.; Zhang, Y.M.; Wu, L.G.; Wang, X.; Guo, M. Schisandrin B ameliorates non-alcoholic liver disease through anti-inflammation activation in diabetic mice. *Drug Dev. Res.* **2022**, *83*, 735–744. [CrossRef]
10. Kwan, H.Y.; Niu, X.Y.; Dai, W.L.; Tong, T.J.; Chao, X.J.; Su, T.; Chan, C.L.; Lee, K.C.; Fu, X.Q.; Yi, H.; et al. Lipidomic-based investigation into the regulatory effect of Schisandrin B on palmitic acid level in non-alcoholic steatotic livers. *Sci. Rep.* **2015**, *5*, 9114. [CrossRef]
11. Wagner, N.; Wagner, K.D. The Role of PPARs in Disease. *Cells* **2020**, *9*, 2367. [CrossRef]

12. Chen, H.; Tan, H.B.; Wan, J.; Zeng, Y.; Wang, J.C.; Wang, H.C.; Lu, X.J. PPAR-γ signaling in nonalcoholic fatty liver disease: Pathogenesis and therapeutic targets. *Pharmacol. Ther.* **2023**, *245*, 108391. [CrossRef]
13. Gross, B.; Pawlak, M.; Lefebvre, P.; Staels, B. PPARs in obesity-induced T2DM, dyslipidaemia and NAFLD. *Nat. Rev.* **2017**, *13*, 36–49. [CrossRef] [PubMed]
14. Ji, J.; Wu, L.W.; Feng, J.; Mo, W.H.; Wu, J.Y.; Yu, Q.; Li, S.N.; Zhang, J.; Dai, W.Q.; Xu, X.F.; et al. Cafestol preconditioning attenuates apoptosis and autophagy during hepatic ischemia-reperfusion injury by inhibiting ERK/PPARγ pathway. *Int. Immunopharmacol.* **2020**, *84*, 106529. [CrossRef] [PubMed]
15. Xiang, S.H.; Chen, K.; Xu, L.; Guo, C.Y. Bergenin exerts hepatoprotective effects by inhibiting the release of inflammatory factors, apoptosis and autophagy via the PPAR-γ pathway. *Drug Des. Dev. Ther.* **2020**, *14*, 129–143. [CrossRef] [PubMed]
16. Feng, J.; Dai, W.Q.; Mao, Y.Q.; Wu, L.W.; Li, J.J.; Chen, K.; Yu, Q.; Kong, R.; Li, S.N.; Zhang, J.; et al. Simvastatin re-sensitizes hepatocellular carcinoma cells to sorafenib by inhibiting HIF-1α/PPAR-γ/PKM2-mediated glycolysis. *J. Exp. Clin. Cancer Res.* **2020**, *39*, 24. [CrossRef]
17. Zhang, H.; Chen, Q.S.; Dahan, A.; Xue, J.Y.; Wei, L.W.; Tan, W.F.; Zhang, G.Q. Transcriptomic analyses reveal the molecular mechanisms of schisandrin B alleviates CCl(4)-induced liver fibrosis in rats by RNA-sequencing. *Chem. Biol. Interact.* **2019**, *309*, 108675. [CrossRef]
18. Liu, N.; Zheng, J.X.; Zhuang, Y.S.; Zhou, Z.K.; Zhao, J.H.; Yang, L. Anti-Inflammatory Effects of Schisandrin B on LPS-Stimulated BV2 Microglia via Activating PPAR-γ. *Inflammation* **2017**, *40*, 1006–1011. [CrossRef]
19. Sun, J.H.; Lin, H.; Wang, K.; Zeng, Q.C.; Li, H.; Wang, C.M.; Chen, J.G. Study of Schisandra chinensis in Treating Metabolic Associated Fatty Liver Disease Based on Network Pharmacology and Molecular Docking Technology. *J. Beihua Univ. (Nat. Sci.)* **2022**, *23*, 768–774.
20. Wan, J.C.; Lang, C.J.; Gao, M.; Liu, F.L.; Feng, X.Y.; Li, H.; Wang, C.M.; Sun, J.H. Schisandrin B alleviates metabolic associated fatty liver disease by regulating the PPARγ signaling pathway and gut microbiota in mice. *Front. Pharmacol.* **2025**, *16*, 1583307. [CrossRef]
21. Zhang, M.; Bai, X.; Du, Q.; Xu, J.J.; Wang, D.Q.; Chen, L.; Dong, K.T.; Chen, Z.Y.; Yang, J.H. The Different Mechanisms of Lipid Accumulation in Hepatocytes Induced by Oleic Acid/Palmitic Acid and High-Fat Diet. *Molecules* **2023**, *28*, 6714. [CrossRef]
22. Wang, Y.P.; Nakajima, T.; Gonzalez, F.J.; Tanaka, N. PPARs as Metabolic Regulators in the Liver: Lessons from Liver-Specific PPAR-Null Mice. *Int. J. Mol. Sci.* **2020**, *17*, 2061. [CrossRef]
23. Beale, E.G.; Harvey, B.J.; Forest, C. *PCK1* and *PCK2* as candidate diabetes and obesity genes. *Cell Biochem. Biophys.* **2007**, *48*, 89–95. [CrossRef]
24. Tuo, L.; Xiang, J.; Pan, X.M.; Hu, J.L.; Tang, H.; Liang, L.; Xia, J.; Hu, Y.; Zhang, W.; Huang, A.L.; et al. PCK1 negatively regulates cell cycle progression and hepatoma cell proliferation via the AMPK/p27Kip1 axis. *J. Exp. Clin. Cancer Res.* **2019**, *38*, 50. [CrossRef]
25. Fan, T.J.; Han, L.H.; Cong, R.S.; Liang, J. Caspase family proteases and apoptosis. *Acta Biochim. Biophys. Sin.* **2005**, *37*, 719–727. [CrossRef] [PubMed]
26. Alturaif, S.A.; Alhusaini, A.; Sarawi, W.; Hasan, I.; Alsaab, J.; Ali, R.; Mohammed, R.; Alotaibi, S.S.; Almutairi, F.; Alsaif, S.; et al. Indole-3-Acetic Acid: Promising Protective Agent Against Methotrexate-Induced Liver Injury via Modulation of TLR4/NF-κB/Caspase-3 Pathway. *Pharmaceuticals* **2025**, *18*, 828. [CrossRef] [PubMed]
27. Lam, T.; Harmancey, R.; Vasquez, H.; Gilbert, B.; Patel, N.; Hariharan, V.; Lee, A.; Covey, M.; Taegtmeyer, H. Reversal of intramyocellular lipid accumulation by lipophagy and a p62-mediated pathway. *Cell Death Discov.* **2016**, *2*, 16061. [CrossRef] [PubMed]
28. Yang, J.W.; Zou, Y.; Chen, J.; Cui, C.; Song, J.; Yang, M.M.; Gao, J.; Hu, H.Q.; Xia, L.Q.; Wang, L.M.; et al. Didymin alleviates metabolic dysfunction-associated fatty liver disease (MAFLD) via the stimulation of Sirt1-mediated lipophagy and mitochondrial biogenesis. *J. Transl. Med.* **2023**, *19*, 921. [CrossRef]
29. Kan, C.F.K.; Singh, A.B.; Dong, B.; Shende, V.R.; Liu, J.W. PPARδ activation induces hepatic long-chain acyl-CoA synthetase 4 expression in vivo and in vitro. *Biochim. Biophys. Acta* **2015**, *1851*, 577–587. [CrossRef]
30. Ding, K.Y.; Liu, C.B.; Li, L.; Yang, M.; Jiang, N.; Luo, S.L.; Sun, L. Acyl-CoA synthase ACSL4: An essential target in ferroptosis and fatty acid metabolism. *Chin. Med. J.* **2023**, *136*, 2521–2537. [CrossRef]
31. Gwon, M.H.; Im, Y.S.; Seo, A.R.; Kim, K.Y.; Moon, H.R.; Yun, J.M. Phenethyl Isothiocyanate Protects against High Fat/Cholesterol Diet-Induced Obesity and Atherosclerosis in C57BL/6 Mice. *Nutrients* **2020**, *12*, 3657. [CrossRef]
32. Schlaepfer, I.R.; Joshi, M. CPT1A-mediated Fat Oxidation, Mechanisms, and Therapeutic Potential. *Endocrinology* **2020**, *161*, bqz046. [CrossRef] [PubMed]
33. Wu, M.X.; Tan, J.; Cao, Z.Y.; Cai, Y.W.; Huang, Z.Q.; Chen, Z.T.; He, W.B.; Liu, X.; Jiang, Y.; Gao, Q.Y.; et al. Sirt5 improves cardiomyocytes fatty acid metabolism and ameliorates cardiac lipotoxicity in diabetic cardiomyopathy via CPT2 de-succinylation. *Redox Biol.* **2024**, *73*, 103184. [CrossRef]

34. Chen, X.F.; Tian, M.X.; Sun, R.Q.; Zhang, M.L.; Zhou, L.S.; Jin, L.; Chen, L.L.; Zhou, W.J.; Duan, K.L.; Chen, Y.J.; et al. SIRT5 inhibits peroxisomal ACOX1 to prevent oxidative damage and is downregulated in liver cancer. *EMBO Rep.* **2018**, *19*, e45124. [CrossRef]
35. Lin, K.N.; Zhao, W.; Huang, S.Y.; Li, H. Grape seed proanthocyanidin extract induces apoptosis of HL-60/ADR cells via the Bax/Bcl-2 caspase-3/9 signaling pathway. *Transl. Cancer Res.* **2021**, *10*, 3939–3947. [CrossRef]
36. Li, T.; Zhang, L.; Jin, C.; Xiong, Y.; Cheng, Y.Y.; Chen, K. Pomegranate flower extract bidirectionally regulates the proliferation, differentiation and apoptosis of 3T3-L1 cells through regulation of PPARγ expression mediated by PI3K-AKT signaling pathway. *Biomed. Pharmacother.* **2020**, *131*, 110769. [CrossRef]

pharmaceuticals

Article

Oligomeric Proanthocyanidins Reverse Lenvatinib Resistance in Hepatocellular Carcinoma Through ITGA3-Mediated Pathway

Takayuki Noma [1,2], Yuan Li [1,3], Yuma Wada [2], Yuji Morine [2], Tetsuya Ikemoto [2], Yu Saito [2], Shinichiro Yamada [2], Hiroki Teraoku [2], Mitsuo Shimada [2] and Ajay Goel [1,4,*]

[1] Department of Molecular Diagnostics and Experimental Therapeutics, Beckman Research Institute of City of Hope, Biomedical Research Center, Monrovia, CA 91016, USA; tnoma@coh.org (T.N.); yuali@coh.org (Y.L.)
[2] Department of Surgery, Tokushima University, Tokushima 779-1510, Japan; wada.yuuma@tokushima-u.ac.jp (Y.W.); ymorine@tokushima-u.ac.jp (Y.M.); ikemoto.tetsuya@tokushima-u.ac.jp (T.I.); saito.yu.1001@tokushima-u.ac.jp (Y.S.); yamada.shinichirou@tokushima-u.ac.jp (S.Y.); teraoku.hiroki@tokushima-u.ac.jp (H.T.); mitsuo.shimada@tokushima-u.ac.jp (M.S.)
[3] Department of Clinical Laboratory, Yangpu Hospital, Tongji University School of Medicine, Shanghai 200090, China
[4] City of Hope Comprehensive Cancer Center, Duarte, CA 91010, USA
* Correspondence: ajgoel@coh.org; Tel.: +1-626-218-3452

Abstract: Background: Oligomeric proanthocyanidins (OPCs) are natural polyphenolic compounds with strong antitumor properties and have gained attention as potential agents to overcome drug resistance. Hepatocellular carcinoma (HCC) remains a major cause of cancer deaths worldwide, and although Lenvatinib is widely used, its effectiveness is limited by acquired resistance. This study explores the potential of OPCs to overcome Lenvatinib resistance in HCC. **Methods**: To evaluate the potential of OPCs to overcome Lenvatinib resistance in HCC, we established Lenvatinib-resistant Huh-7 and PLC-PRF-5 cell lines and conducted systematic cell culture experiments to assess their antitumor effects. Furthermore, genome-wide transcriptomic profiling, network pharmacology approaches, and pathway enrichment analysis were performed to identify resistance-associated signaling pathways that could serve as therapeutic targets. **Results**: The combination of OPCs and Lenvatinib demonstrated a significant synergistic anti-proliferative effect in resistant hepatocellular carcinoma cells, with the most synergistic dose combinations showing Bliss synergy scores exceeding 10. Transcriptomic profiling revealed that the adhesion molecule ITGA3 is a key factor in Lenvatinib resistance and contributes to the acquisition of anoikis resistance. The combination treatment suppressed ITGA3–EGFR–AKT signaling, restored anoikis sensitivity, significantly reduced spheroid formation (fold change = 0.10–0.12; $p < 0.001$), and markedly increased apoptosis (fold change = 2.7–5.0; $p < 0.001$). **Conclusions**: This study is the first to demonstrate that OPCs can overcome chemotherapy resistance by targeting the integrin pathway, providing scientific evidence for their potential use as an adjunctive therapy for chemotherapy-resistant HCC.

Keywords: hepatocellular carcinoma; oligomeric proanthocyanidins; lenvatinib resistance; synergistic effect; anoikis; ITGA3

1. Introduction

Hepatocellular carcinoma (HCC) is the major type of primary liver cancer, with approximately 800,000 cases annually, ranking as the third leading cause of cancer-related deaths [1]. More than half of HCC patients are diagnosed at an advanced stage, where systemic therapy remains the primary treatment option. Sorafenib and Lenvatinib, both multi-tyrosine kinase inhibitors (TKIs), were the first systemic agents introduced for the treatment of advanced HCC. Sorafenib was approved as first-line therapy in 2007 [2,3], and in 2018, Lenvatinib was approved as an alternative following the REFLECT trial, which demonstrated its non-inferiority to Sorafenib [4]. More recently, immune checkpoint inhibitors (ICIs), particularly PD-1 inhibitors, have rapidly transformed the treatment landscape for HCC, with the IMbrave150 trial establishing atezolizumab plus bevacizumab as an effective option [5,6]. On the other hand, Lenvatinib has still been reported to be effective for non-viral HCC, including cases related to metabolic disorders and diabetes-associated NASH, which are expected to increase in the future [7–9]. Therefore, its clinical use continues to be relevant and sustained. However, the overall response rate of Lenvatinib remains limited at around 24%, and complex resistance mechanisms, including Epidermal growth factor receptor (EGFR) pathway activation, RNA modifications, autophagy, and ferroptosis, have been reported to contribute to this resistance [10–13]. In recent years, to address Lenvatinib resistance, combination strategies with other molecular targeted agents or ICIs have been regarded as promising approaches [11,14,15]. Nevertheless, challenges such as increased toxicity and high cost remain. Therefore, developing cost-effective and less toxic combination therapies to overcome resistance remains critical for improving HCC treatment.

In this context, several naturally derived plant compounds have garnered increasing attention from researchers and clinicians due to their multi-targeted mechanisms and safer therapeutic profiles compared to conventional chemotherapies and molecular targeted therapies [16–18]. Oligomeric proanthocyanidins (OPCs), a class of polyphenolic compounds, have received significant attention in recent years due to their potential antioxidant and antitumor properties. OPCs are abundantly found in grape seeds and are present in a wide range of plants with purple or red pigmentation. Previous research conducted by our group has revealed that the antitumor activity of OPCs is mediated through several key pathways, including the PI3K-Akt signaling, ferroptosis [19], DNA replication and cell cycle regulation [20], ABC transporters [21], and the Hippo signaling [22]. Furthermore, recent studies have demonstrated the synergistic and cooperative effects of OPCs with other natural compounds and therapies [22]. Based on this evidence, we hypothesize that OPCs might synergistically regulate multiple cancer cell signaling pathways, exhibiting potent antitumor activity in HCC, and potentially overcoming chemotherapy resistance.

In this study, we systematically evaluated for the first time the antitumor effects of OPCs using network pharmacology approaches in HCC using two different HCC cell lines. Additionally, we performed genome-wide transcriptomic profiling analysis to identify the molecular mechanism(s) and key pathways associated with Lenvatinib resistance in HCC. Finally, we validated the mechanism by which OPCs overcome Lenvatinib resistance.

2. Results

2.1. Establishment of Lenvatinib-Resistant HCC Cell Lines and Evaluation of OPCs-Mediated Synergistic Effects

To investigate whether OPCs can help overcome Lenvatinib resistance in HCC, we established Lenvatinib-resistant Huh-7 cells (rHuh-7) and Lenvatinib-resistant PLC-PRF-5 cells (rPLC) by gradually increasing the concentration of Lenvatinib over several months in parental Huh-7 cells (pHuh-7) and PLC-PRF-5 cells (pPLC). Notably, the half-maximal inhibitory concentration (IC_{50}) of Lenvatinib was significantly higher in the resistant cell lines compared to their respective parental controls, with rHuh-7 exhibiting a more than 10-fold increase in resistance vs. pHuh-7 (IC_{50}: 50.3 μM vs. 3.5 μM; Figure 1A), and rPLC showing a 2-fold increase in resistance vs. pPLC cells (IC_{50}: 59.7 μM vs. 23.1 μM; Figure 1E).

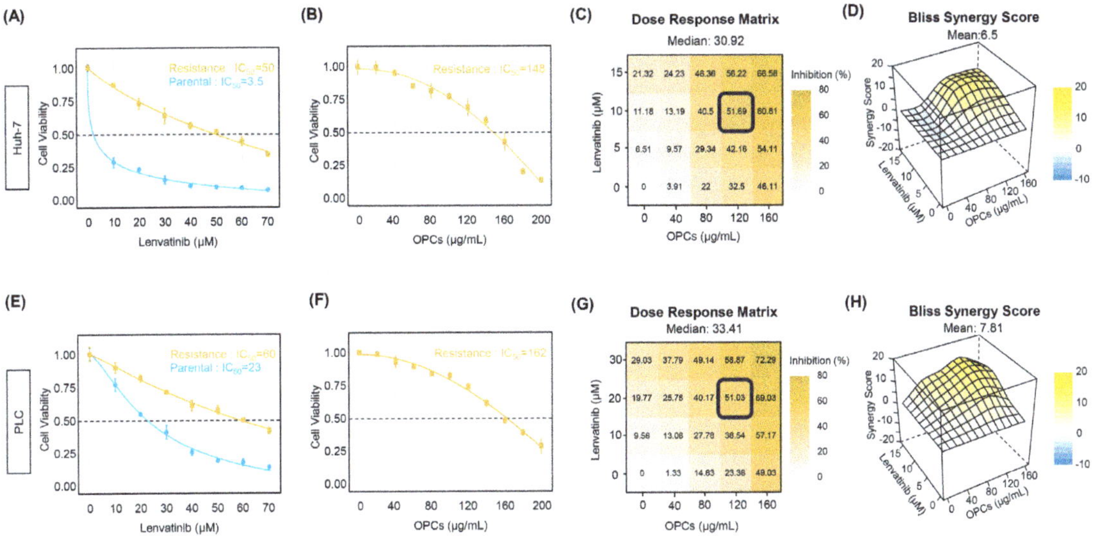

Figure 1. Establishment of Lenvatinib-Resistant HCC Cell Lines and Synergistic Effects of OPCs and Lenvatinib. (**A**,**E**) Dose–response curves of Lenvatinib in parental (pHuh-7 and pPLC) and resistant (rHuh-7 and rPLC) HCC cell lines. The IC_{50} of Lenvatinib increased markedly in resistant cells: rHuh-7 showed a >10-fold increase compared to pHuh-7 (50.3 μM vs. 3.5 μM), and rPLC showed a 2-fold increase compared to pPLC (59.7 μM vs. 23.1 μM). (**B**,**F**) Dose–response curves of OPCs in Lenvatinib-resistant HCC cell lines (rHuh-7 and rPLC). OPCs reduced cell viability in a dose-dependent manner, with IC_{50} values of 147.9 μg/mL for rHuh-7 and 162.0 μg/mL for rPLC. (**C**,**G**) Dose–response matrices showing the percentage reduction in cell viability of rHuh-7 and rPLC cells treated with different combinations of Lenvatinib and OPCs. In rHuh-7 cells, the combination of 10 μM Lenvatinib with 120 μg/mL OPCs reduced cell viability by 51.7%. In rPLC cells, the combination of 20 μM Lenvatinib with 120 μg/mL OPCs reduced viability by 51.0%. (**D**,**H**) Bliss synergy scores for the combinations of Lenvatinib and OPCs in rHuh-7 and rPLC cells. The most synergistic combinations achieved scores of 12.5 in rHuh-7 and 11.6 in rPLC, indicating robust synergistic effects in both cell lines.

Next, we assessed whether OPCs could exert antiproliferative effects in HCC cell lines. OPCs reduced cell viability in a dose-dependent manner, with IC_{50} values of 147.9 μg/mL for rHuh-7 (Figure 1B) and 162.0 μg/mL for rPLC (Figure 1F). Since the goal was to evaluate whether OPCs can overcome Lenvatinib resistance in HCC cells, we planned combinatorial treatments with varying concentrations of Lenvatinib and OPCs in Lenvatinib-resistant HCC cell lines to decipher the synergistic effects of these compounds. Criteria were established to identify the optimal dose ratio of Lenvatinib and OPCs in combination therapy (dose response inhibited by >50% and the highest Bliss synergy score). The concentration of OPCs was set at (0, 40, 80, 120, 160 μg/mL), considering the IC_{50} for OPCs in each cell line. On the other hand, the concentration of Lenvatinib was set to (0, 5, 10, 15 μM) for the rHuh-7 and (0, 10, 20, 30 μM) for the rPLC, considering that the IC_{50} of Lenvatinib in the parental cell lines was different, at 3.5 μM and 23.1 μM, respectively. In rHuh-7 cells, the combination of 10 μM Lenvatinib with 120 μg/mL OPCs inhibited cell growth by 51.7%, compared with 11.2% for Lenvatinib alone and 32.5% for OPCs alone, with a Bliss synergy score of 12.5 (Figure 1C,G). In rPLC cells, the combination of 20 μM Lenvatinib with 120 μg/mL OPCs inhibited growth by 51.0%, compared with 19.8% and 23.4% for single treatments, with a Bliss synergy score of 11.6 (Figure 1D,H). Accordingly, we used 10 μM Lenvatinib plus 120 μg/mL OPCs for rHuh-7, and 20 μM Lenvatinib plus 120 μg/mL OPCs for rPLC in subsequent experiments. These results indicate that OPCs exhibit apparent antitumor activity and demonstrate a significant synergistic effect with Lenvatinib in resistant HCC cells, providing an optimal basis for subsequent combination experiments.

2.2. Evaluation of the Effects of Lenvatinib and OPCs on Cell Migration and Invasion

We next assessed the effects of Lenvatinib and OPCs on colony formation, migration, and invasion in Lenvatinib-resistant HCC cells. Lenvatinib alone had a minimal impact on colony formation in both rHuh-7 and rPLC, whereas OPCs significantly reduced colony-forming ability. Notably, the combination treatment further suppressed colony formation by 82.0% in rHuh-7 and 77.8% in rPLC ($p < 0.01$; Figure 2A). Wound healing assays revealed no difference between control and Lenvatinib-treated cells. In contrast, combination therapy significantly impaired cell migration, as indicated by a log2 fold change (FC) of 0.37 in rHuh-7 and 0.21 in rPLC ($p < 0.01$; Figure 2B). Similarly, in invasion assays, Lenvatinib alone had little effect, while the combination with OPCs significantly reduced invasion (rHuh-7: 0.32, rPLC: 0.08 relative to control; $p < 0.01$; Figure 2C). Together, these results demonstrate that the combination of OPCs and Lenvatinib significantly suppresses malignant potential in Lenvatinib-resistant HCC cells.

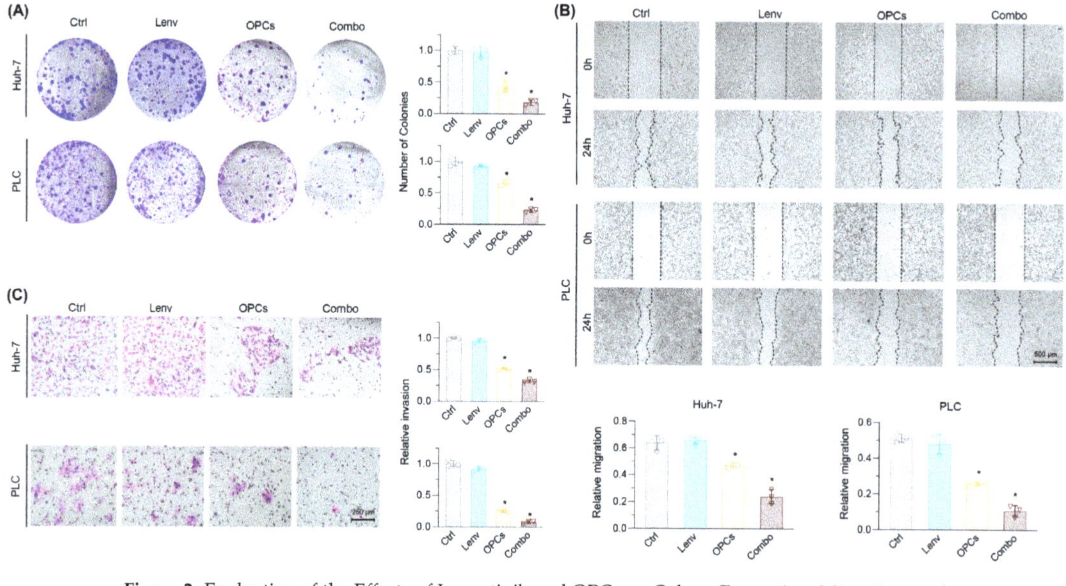

Figure 2. Evaluation of the Effects of Lenvatinib and OPCs on Colony Formation, Migration, and Invasion in rHuh-7 and rPLC Cells. (**A**) Colony formation in Lenvatinib-resistant cell lines (rHuh-7, rPLC) treated with Lenvatinib (Lenv), OPCs, or the combination. Lenvatinib alone had little effect, while OPCs significantly reduced colony formation. The combination treatment further decreased colony formation in both cell lines. (**B**) Wound healing assay showing the impact on cell migration. Lenvatinib alone had no effect, but the combination with OPCs significantly reduced migration in both rHuh-7 and rPLC. (**C**) Invasion assay results. Lenvatinib alone did not affect invasion, but combination treatment with OPCs significantly inhibited invasion in both cell lines. Data represent mean ± SD (* $p < 0.05$ vs. control).

2.3. Combination of OPCs and Lenvatinib Induces Apoptosis and Suppresses Cancer Stemness in Resistance HCC Cell Lines

To evaluate the apoptotic modulation induced by Lenvatinib and OPCs in HCC cell lines, we performed an Annexin V binding assay. The baseline viable cell rates were 94.3% for rHuh-7 and 89.6% for rPLC. As expected, treatment with Lenvatinib did not affect the viability of the resistant cell lines (rHuh-7: 92.5%, rPLC: 88.9%; Figure 3A). In contrast, treatment with OPCs alone and in combination with Lenvatinib significantly reduced the viable cell rates in both rHuh-7 (OPCs: 84.1%, combination: 71.0%) and rPLC (OPCs: 81.2%, combination: 65.9%; Figure 3A). Furthermore, approximately 25% of the cells underwent apoptosis following the combination therapy with OPCs and Lenvatinib. In rHuh-7, the apoptotic cell rates were as follows: control vs. Lenvatinib vs. OPCs vs. combination = 5.6% vs. 7.3% vs. 15.8% vs. 28.2%, respectively, with significant differences observed between the control and OPCs ($p < 0.01$) and between the control and combination treatment ($p < 0.01$). Similarly, in rPLC, the apoptotic cell rates were as follows: control vs. Lenvatinib vs. OPCs vs. combination, 9.0% vs. 10.7% vs. 17.8% vs. 24.4%, respectively, with significant differences between the control and OPCs ($p < 0.01$) and between the control and combination treatment ($p < 0.01$; Figure 3A). In addition, we examined the expression of apoptosis-related proteins to gain further insight into this cell death mechanism. Western blot analysis revealed increased levels of scleaved PARP, cleaved caspase 3, and BAX, supporting that combination therapy is more effective in inducing apoptosis than monotherapy. These data suggest that the combination of Lenvatinib and OPCs induces apoptosis in HCC cells (Figure 3B). These observations provide clear evidence that the combined use of OPCs and Lenvatinib enhances apoptosis in Lenvatinib-resistant HCC cells.

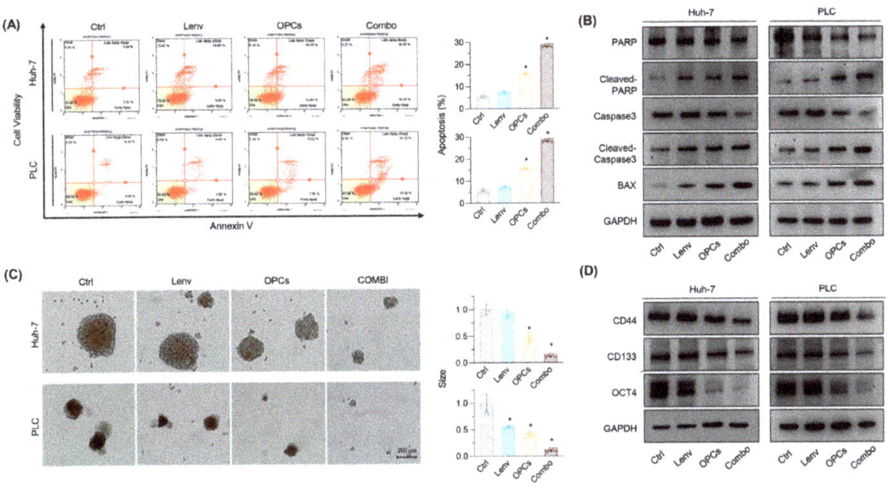

Figure 3. OPCs Induce Apoptosis and Suppress Cancer Stemness in Lenvatinib-Resistant HCC Cells. (**A**) Annexin V assay showing the effects of Lenvatinib (Lenv), OPCs, and their combination on apoptosis in Lenvatinib-resistant cell lines (rHuh-7, rPLC). Combination therapy significantly increased apoptosis in both cell lines compared to control and Lenv alone. (**B**) Western blot analysis of apoptosis-related proteins (PARP, cleaved-PARP, Caspase 3, cleaved-Caspase 3, BAX) in rHuh-7 and rPLC after treatment. Combination therapy demonstrated enhanced expression of apoptosis markers compared to monotherapy. (**C**) Spheroid formation assay in rHuh-7 and rPLC. OPCs and combination treatments significantly reduced the size of spheroids. (**D**) Western blot analysis of cancer stem cell markers (Nanog, CD44, OCT4) in rHuh-7 and rPLC. The combination of OPCs and Lenvatinib significantly reduced stem cell marker expression compared to control and Lenv alone. Data represent mean ± SD (* $p < 0.05$ vs. control).

Next, to determine whether OPCs also affect cancer stemness, we performed spheroid formation assays with cancer spheroids developed from two Lenvatinib-resistant cells. Spheroid size was assessed after the end of treatment; OPCs treatment and Lenvatinib significantly reduced the number and size of spheroids (Figure 3C). In rHuh-7, spheroid size was reduced significantly by OPCs (FC = 0.47; $p < 0.01$), and these effects were even more pronounced by the combination treatment (FC = 0.12; $p < 0.01$). Similar effects were observed in rPLC (OPCs: FC = 0.41; combination: FC = 0.10; $p < 0.01$). Protein expression of the cancer stem markers CD44 and CD133, as well as OCT4, was also assessed in various cancers, including HCC and OPCs. The combination treatment significantly reduced the expression of both markers compared to untreated controls and cells treated with Lenvatinib. The combination of OPCs and Lenvatinib was the most potent inhibitor of protein expression of both stemness markers (Figure 3D). These findings from the cancer spheroid assay highlight that OPCs influence cancer stemness in overcoming Lenvatinib resistance. Overall, our findings demonstrate that OPCs, especially when combined with Lenvatinib, effectively reduce cancer stemness in resistant HCC cells.

2.4. Transcriptome Profiling Identified Involved Pathways and Genes That Could Be Targeted to Overcome Lenvatinib Resistance

A comprehensive genome-wide transcriptomic profiling analysis was performed on parental and Lenvatinib-resistant HCC cells using a public dataset (GSE186191) to identify the most important signaling and regulatory pathways associated with Lenvatinib resistance. This analysis identified 961 upregulated and 974 downregulated genes in Lenvatinib-resistant Huh-7 cells, and 762 upregulated and 419 downregulated genes in Lenvatinib-resistant Hep3B cells ($|\log2 FC| > 1.0$, $p < 0.05$; Figure 4A). A total of 225 genes were found to be commonly altered in both cell lines, and pathway enrichment analysis using the Database for Annotation, Visualization, and Integrated Discovery (DAVID) Bioinformatics Database 2021 (https://david.ncifcrf.gov/, accessed on 22 October 2024) [23] revealed that 10 Kyoto Encyclopedia of Genes and Genomes (KEGG) pathways were preferentially enriched (FC > 2.0, $p < 0.05$; Figure 4B). The extracellular matrix (ECM)-related signaling pathway was identified as the most relevant pathway with the highest enrichment score. Additionally, other related pathways, such as the focal adhesion and PI3K-Akt signaling pathways, which are associated with proliferative signaling, were also enriched. Integrins, components of these pathways, have recently been shown to contribute to cancer malignancy, including chemotherapy resistance, by interacting with proliferative pathways such as the PI3K-AKT pathway and other signaling networks [24–26]. Based on these findings, we hypothesized that the ECM-related signaling pathway may play a crucial role in Lenvatinib resistance in hepatocellular carcinoma. To test this hypothesis, we examined the expression of ITGA3 and ITGB8, key components of this pathway, in our Lenvatinib-resistant cell lines. Both genes were significantly upregulated in resistant cells compared to parental controls (ITGA3: rHuh-7: FC = 2.1, $p = 0.007$; rPLC: FC = 1.7, $p < 0.001$; ITGB8: rHuh-7: FC = 1.6, $p = 0.005$; rPLC: FC = 1.5, $p = 0.004$; Figure 4C). Given its higher fold change, ITGA3 was selected as the primary target for subsequent experiments. Taken together, these findings indicate that ITGA3 is a key ECM-related factor contributing to Lenvatinib resistance in HCC.

To further validate the biological relevance of ITGA3 in clinical HCC, we analyzed ITGA3 expression in paired tumor and non-tumor mucosa specimens ($n = 83$). Quantitative reverse transcription polymerase chain reaction (qRT-PCR) revealed that ITGA3 expression was significantly upregulated in tumor tissues compared to adjacent non-tumor tissues ($p < 0.001$, Figure 4D). We then evaluated the prognostic impact of ITGA3 expression using overall survival (OS) data. Kaplan–Meier survival analysis demonstrated that patients with high ITGA3 expression had significantly poorer OS than those with low ITGA3 expression ($p < 0.001$; HR = 2.73, 95% CI: 1.56–4.78, Figure 4E). These findings support the notion that ITGA3 may serve as a prognostic biomarker and a potential therapeutic target in HCC.

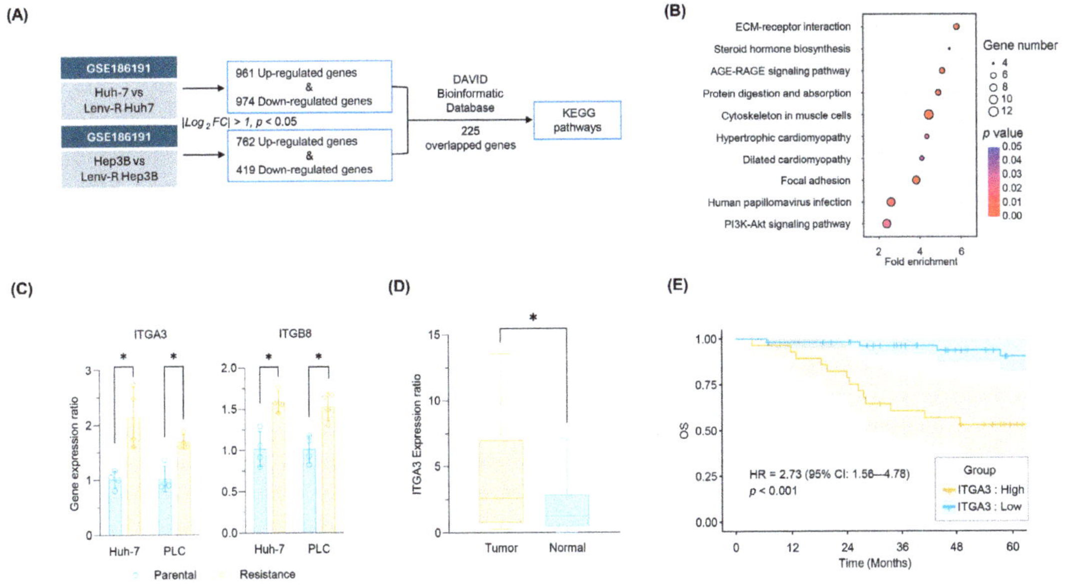

Figure 4. Gene Profiling Analysis Reveals Genes Involved in Lenvatinib Resistance. (**A**) Workflow showing the identification of differentially expressed genes from the GSE186191 dataset comparing parental and Lenvatinib-resistant Huh-7 and Hep3B cells. A total of 225 commonly altered genes were identified and analyzed using the DAVID Bioinformatics Database. (**B**) Pathway enrichment analysis of the 225 shared genes identified the top 10 KEGG pathways, with the ECM-receptor interaction pathway being the most enriched, including ITGA3 and ITGB8, which were also commonly found in the Focal Adhesion and PI3K/AKT signaling pathways. (**C**) qRT-PCR analysis of ITGA3 and ITGB8 expression in parental and rHuh-7 and rPLC cells. Both resistant cell lines exhibited significantly higher expression of these genes than their parental cell lines. (**D**) ITGA3 expression in 83 paired clinical samples (tumor tissue vs. adjacent non-tumor tissue). (**E**) Kaplan–Meier survival curve showing worse prognosis for patients with high ITGA3 expression ($p < 0.001$; HR = 2.73, 95% CI: 1.56–4.78). Data represent mean ± SD (* $p < 0.05$ vs. control).

2.5. siRNA-Mediated Knockdown of ITGA3 Suppresses Tumorigenic Features and Induces Anoikis Sensitivity in HCC Cells

To elucidate the role of ITGA3 in Lenvatinib resistance in HCC, we performed siRNA-mediated knockdown of ITGA3 in Lenvatinib-resistant HCC cell lines (rHuh-7 and rPLC). Combined ITGA3 knockdown and Lenvatinib treatment significantly inhibited cell proliferation in rHuh-7 ($p < 0.001$ for siRNA #1 and siRNA #2) and rPLC ($p = 0.002$ for siRNA #1 and $p < 0.001$ for siRNA #2 in both cell lines; Figure 5A). In addition to proliferation, we examined whether ITGA3 knockdown affected other malignant phenotypes of resistant HCC cells. ITGA3 knockdown markedly suppressed colony formation (Figure S1A), migration in wound-healing assays (Figure S1B), and invasion (Figure S1C), and also reduced the expression of stemness-related genes, including CD44, CD133, and OCT4 (Figure S1D). These findings indicate that ITGA3 regulates multiple aggressive characteristics of HCC cells.

To further evaluate the impact of ITGA3 knockdown on cell viability, apoptosis was quantified using Annexin V binding assays. Compared with cells transfected with negative control siRNA, ITGA3 knockdown significantly increased apoptosis in both rHuh-7 (FC = 2.58, $p < 0.01$ for siRNA #1; FC = 2.67, $p < 0.01$ for siRNA #2; Figure 5B) and rPLC (FC = 2.17, $p < 0.01$ for siRNA #1; FC = 2.93, $p < 0.01$ for siRNA #2; Figure 5B). Western blot analysis confirmed that ITGA3 knockdown markedly reduced ITGA3 protein expression and inhibited activation of the EGFR–AKT signaling pathway (Figure 5C). These findings suggest that ITGA3 is closely involved in the EGFR–AKT pathway, a crucial mediator of Lenvatinib resistance.

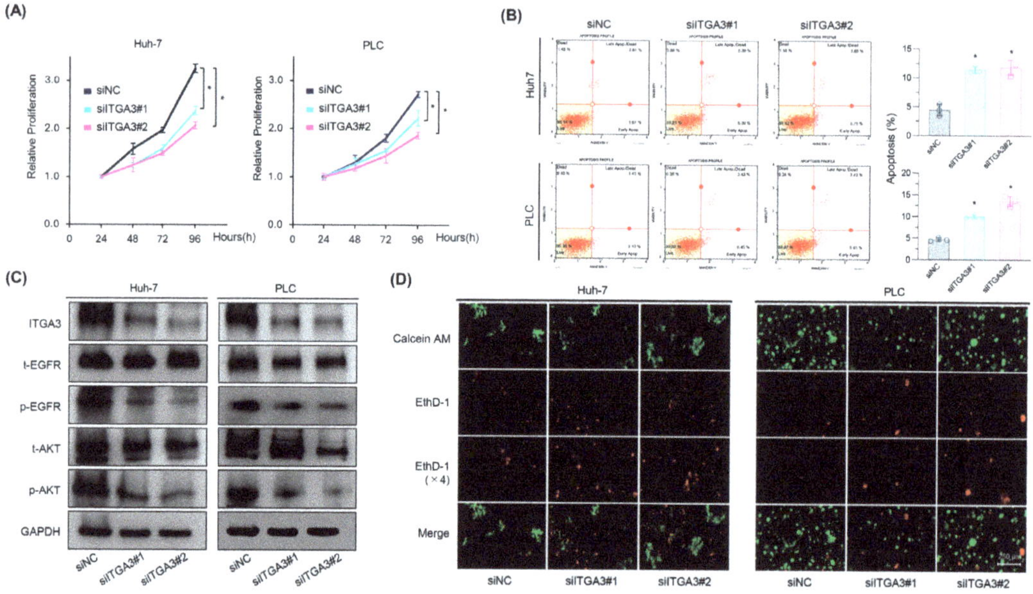

Figure 5. siRNA-mediated knockdown of ITGA3 suppresses tumorigenic phenotypes and induces apoptosis in HCC cell lines. (**A**) Proliferation assay after ITGA3 siRNA transfection. (**B**) Annexin V apoptosis assay in rHuh-7 and rPLC after ITGA3 knockdown. ITGA3 knockdown significantly increased apoptosis rates compared to control siRNA (siNC). (**C**) Western blot analysis showing decreased ITGA3 expression and inhibition of the EGFR–AKT signaling pathway following ITGA3 knockdown in rHuh-7 and rPLC. GAPDH was used as an internal control. (**D**) Representative images of anoikis assays in rHuh-7 and rPLC after ITGA3 knockdown. Calcein AM was used to stain viable cells (green), and EthD-1 was used to stain dead cells (red). Data represent mean ± SD (* $p < 0.05$ vs. control). (See also Figure S1 for functional assays demonstrating suppression of colony formation, migration, invasion, and stemness-related gene expression following ITGA3 knockdown).

Anoikis, a form of programmed cell death triggered by detachment from the ECM, is frequently circumvented in cancer cells via dysregulation of signaling pathways such as Ras/ERK and PI3K/AKT, as well as through remodeling of the ECM [27–29]. Anoikis resistance is strongly associated with chemotherapy resistance and represents a critical therapeutic target. Integrins, including ITGA3, have been implicated in promoting anoikis resistance and metastatic potential by interacting with receptor tyrosine kinases and activating survival signaling pathways that drive malignant transformation [30–34]. We hypothesized that ITGA3-mediated anoikis resistance contributes to Lenvatinib resistance in HCC. To test this, we performed anoikis assays following ITGA3 knockdown in Lenvatinib-resistant cells. As expected, ITGA3 knockdown significantly reduced anoikis resistance (Figure 5D). Collectively, these findings demonstrate that ITGA3 plays a critical role in multiple malignant phenotypes of HCC cells, including proliferation, colony formation, migration, invasion, stemness, apoptosis, and anoikis resistance, primarily through the activation of the EGFR–AKT pathway. Thus, ITGA3 represents a promising therapeutic target for overcoming Lenvatinib resistance in HCC.

2.6. Combined OPCs and Lenvatinib Therapy Restores Anoikis Sensitivity Through ITGA3–EGFR–AKT Pathway Inhibition

OPCs, widely studied for their anti-tumor properties, are known to inhibit multiple signaling pathways, thereby suppressing tumor growth, migration, and invasion [35–38]. Based on these characteristics, we hypothesized that OPCs may overcome Lenvatinib resistance by targeting the ITGA3–EGFR–AKT signaling axis and promoting anoikis. To test this hypothesis, we evaluated mRNA and protein expression levels of the ITGA3-EGFR–AKT signaling axis following OPCs treatment. In Lenvatinib-resistant rHuh-7 and rPLC, Lenvatinib monotherapy had a minimal effect on ITGA3 mRNA and protein levels (Figure 6A,B). In contrast, OPC treatment significantly downregulated ITGA3 expression. Notably, the combination of OPCs and Lenvatinib further suppressed ITGA3 expression compared to either treatment alone, accompanied by a marked reduction in EGFR and AKT phosphorylation (Figure 6A,B). Additionally, anoikis assays demonstrated that the combination therapy significantly restored anoikis sensitivity (Figure 6C), further supporting the role of ITGA3 in mediating anoikis resistance and its contribution to Lenvatinib resistance. These findings indicate that OPCs-mediated suppression of ITGA3 plays a central role in restoring Lenvatinib sensitivity in resistant HCC cells. Collectively, these results suggest that targeting ITGA3 through the combined use of OPCs and Lenvatinib represents a promising therapeutic strategy for overcoming Lenvatinib resistance in HCC.

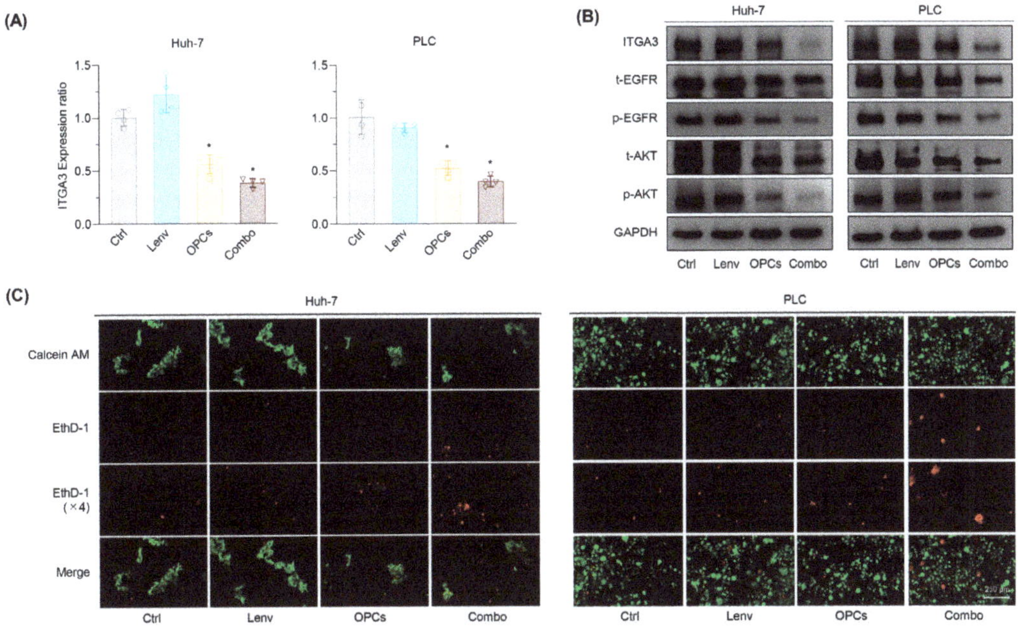

Figure 6. OPCs restore anoikis sensitivity and overcome Lenvatinib resistance by targeting ITGA3 and inhibiting EGFR–AKT signaling. (**A**) qRT-PCR analysis of ITGA3 expression in rHuh-7 and rPLC cell lines treated with Lenv, OPCs, or the combination of both. OPCs treatment significantly downregulated ITGA3 expression at the mRNA level. (**B**) Western blot analysis showing the effect of treatments on ITGA3 expression and EGFR–AKT signaling pathway activation in rHuh-7 and rPLC. OPCs and the combination treatment suppressed ITGA3 and the phosphorylation of EGFR, AKT. (**C**) Representative images from anoikis assays in rHuh-7 and rPLC treated with control, Lenvatinib, OPCs, or the combination. Calcein AM was used to stain viable cells (green), and EthD-1 was used to stain dead cells (red). Combination therapy restored anoikis sensitivity in both cell lines. Data represent mean ± SD (* $p < 0.05$ vs. control).

3. Discussion

HCC remains a major global health concern, representing the most common primary liver malignancy and the sixth most frequently diagnosed cancer worldwide [1]. While curative options such as surgical resection and liver transplantation are available for early-stage HCC, advanced cases typically require systemic therapies. Currently, Lenvatinib and the combination of Atezolizumab plus Bevacizumab are approved as first-line treatments [5,39]. Lenvatinib, a multi-tyrosine kinase inhibitor, is particularly effective in blocking several key growth factor receptors, including vascular endothelial growth factors and fibroblast growth factor receptors [40]. However, despite its clinical efficacy, the objective response rate of Lenvatinib is limited to approximately 24%, and the development of drug resistance is a significant clinical challenge [4]. The mechanisms underlying Lenvatinib resistance are complex and multifactorial. Our transcriptome analysis revealed that ECM-related signaling pathways, including the expression of ITGA3, were upregulated in Lenvatinib-resistant cells. In particular, integrins are known to mediate cell-ECM interactions and have been shown to play important roles in tumor progression, metastasis, anoikis resistance, and chemotherapy resistance through activation of downstream pathways such as the EGFR–AKT pathway [24–28,30,32].

Natural compounds with broad-spectrum anti-cancer activities, such as OPCs, offer a promising adjunctive approach. OPCs, naturally occurring polyphenols found in various fruits, vegetables, and plants, have demonstrated potent anti-tumor effects in a variety of cancers [21]. These effects are mediated through the modulation of several oncogenic signaling pathways, including growth signaling pathways, drug transporter systems, and metabolic pathways such as protein export, glutathione metabolism, and porphyrin metabolism [19,41,42]. The unique properties of OPCs, including their favorable safety profile and ability to target multiple pathways simultaneously, make them attractive candidates for combination therapy in cancer treatment.

In this study, we hypothesized that overexpression of ITGA3 activates the EGFR–AKT pathway through enhanced ECM pathways, contributing to Lenvatinib resistance in HCC. We further proposed that OPCs could overcome this resistance by targeting the ITGA3–EGFR–AKT signaling axis. Our results demonstrated that OPC treatment, particularly in combination with Lenvatinib, effectively inhibited proliferation and invasion in Lenvatinib-resistant HCC cells. Mechanistically, OPCs significantly downregulated the ITGA3–EGFR–AKT axis. We also observed that OPCs treatment reduced the spheroid-forming capacity of resistant cells, suggesting that it may suppress cancer stem cell-like properties. Moreover, ITGA3 overexpression was found to contribute to anoikis resistance, a known mechanism of chemoresistance. Importantly, co-administration of OPCs and Lenvatinib enhanced anoikis sensitivity and restored drug responsiveness in resistant cells. Apoptosis assays further confirmed that the combination therapy induced cell death, supporting its therapeutic potential.

We would like to acknowledge some of the limitations of this study. First, the current study employed only two Lenvatinib-resistant cell lines, which may limit the generalizability of the findings. Validation in a broader panel of HCC models is necessary. Second, although our results provide strong in vitro evidence, preclinical studies in animal models are essential to assess the in vivo efficacy and safety of the OPCs and Lenvatinib combination therapy. Nevertheless, this study is the first to demonstrate that ITGA3 plays a critical role in Lenvatinib resistance in HCC and that OPCs can potentially overcome this resistance by targeting the ITGA3–EGFR–AKT pathway. Moreover, our clinical sample analysis revealed a significant association between high ITGA3 expression and poor prognosis in HCC patients, further supporting ITGA3 as a promising and clinically relevant therapeutic target. Future studies should focus on validating these findings in vivo and exploring the therapeutic potential of OPCs in preclinical animal models.

4. Materials and Methods

4.1. Patient Cohort

This study included frozen tumor and normal tissue specimens from 83 HCC patients enrolled at Tokushima University, Japan. Patient characteristics are detailed in Table S1. All patients underwent surgical resection, and tumors were histologically confirmed as HCC. Tumors were classified according to the Union for International Cancer Control (UICC) TNM Classification of Malignant Tumors, version 7. The study was conducted in accordance with the ethical principles outlined in the Declaration of Helsinki, as revised in 2024, and was approved by the ethics committees of the participating institutions. Written informed consent was obtained from all patients prior to inclusion in the study.

4.2. Cell Culture and Materials

Two human HCC cell lines, Huh-7 and PLC-PRF-5 (PLC), were examined in this study and obtained from the RIKEN BioResource Center Cell Bank (Tsukuba, Japan). Both cell lines were cultured in Dulbecco's Modified Eagle's Medium (DMEM; Gibco, Carlsbad, CA, USA) containing 10% fetal bovine serum, and 1% penicillin and streptomycin, maintained in a humidified incubator at 37 °C in 5% CO_2.

4.3. Herbal Preparations and Drug Preparation

The OPCs used in this study were obtained from VX1®, a French grape seed extract (EuroPharma USA, Green Bay, WI, USA), standardized by the manufacturer to contain ≥99% total polyphenols and ≥80% low-molecular-weight OPCs (monomers, dimers, and trimers). The powder was dissolved in dimethyl sulfoxide (DMSO; Sigma-Aldrich, St. Louis, MO, USA) and further diluted in complete culture medium to obtain working concentrations for in vitro experiments.

Lenvatinib (Sigma-Aldrich) was dissolved in DMSO (Sigma-Aldrich). The stock solution of Lenvatinib was carefully stored at −20 °C in the dark, ensuring its stability and reliability. This stock solution was diluted with a complete culture medium to the necessary experimental concentrations before each application.

4.4. Cell Viability Assays

For these assays, 5×10^3 cells per well were seeded into 96-well plates under each culture condition. After overnight incubation for cell adherence to the plates, all cell lines were treated for 48h with Lenvatinib, OPCs, or their combination. Following completion of the treatments, Cell Counting Kit-8 (CCK-8) assays (Dojindo Molecular Technologies, Inc., Kumamoto, Japan; Cat# CK04) were performed according to the manufacturer's instructions. Synergy scores were calculated using SynergyFinder 3.0 (https://synergyfinder.fimm.fi), a freely available tool for interactive analysis and visualization of combination response outcomes [43].

4.5. Establishment of Lenvatinib-Resistant HCC Cell Lines

Lenvatinib-resistant cells were induced from continuous culture of Huh-7 and PLC cell lines in Lenvatinib-enriched medium. The parental cell lines were treated with increasing doses of Lenvatinib, with concentrations of 0.5 μM administered weekly over 10 months. Finally, resistant cells that could grow stably in medium containing 20 μM Lenvatinib were selected for further experiments.

4.6. Invasion Assay

For the invasion assay, cells (2.5×10^4 cells) treated with Lenvatinib, OPCs, and their combination for 48 h were grown in 24-well transwell chambers (8-μm pore size) coated with Matrigel (BD Biosciences, Franklin Lakes, NJ, USA). After 48 h, the invaded cells were fixed and stained with Diff-Quick (Thermo Fisher Scientific, Waltham, MA, USA) and then counted.

4.7. The Wound Healing Assay

For the wound healing assay, cells treated with Lenvatinib, OPCs, and their combination were seeded into 6-well plates and grown to 80% confluency. Wounds were made by scraping 200 μL of monolayer cells with a pipette tip (RAININ, LLC, Oakland, CA, USA). 24 h after wounding, treated and control cells were examined under a microscope (Zeiss, Oberkochen, Germany).

4.8. The Colony Formation Assay

For the colony formation assay, 5×10^2 cells treated with Lenvatinib, OPCs, and their combinations for 48 h were seeded into 6-well plates (Corning, Tehama County, CA, USA). Seven to ten days later, the number of colonies with 50 or more cells was counted, and relative changes were measured.

4.9. Apoptosis Assay

For the Annexin V binding apoptosis assay, cells were seeded in 6-well plates and then treated with Lenvatinib, OPCs, and their combinations for 48 h. Apoptotic cell fractions were then measured using the Muse Cell Analyzer (Millipore Corp, Billerica, MA, USA) and Annexin V and Dead Cell Kit (Luminex Corp, Austin, TX, USA) according to the manufacturer's instructions.

4.10. Spheroid Formation Assays

Methods for these assays have been described previously [44]. Briefly, Lenvatinib-resistant cell lines were seeded in serum-free DMEM-F12 medium (STEMCELL Technologies, Vancouver, BC, Canada) in ultra-low adherent plates (Corning); spheroids were formed over 5–10 days, and spheroid size and number were counted using ImageJ software (version 1.53; National Institutes of Health, Bethesda, MD, USA).

4.11. Identification of Differentially Expressed Genes and Functional Pathway Enrichment in Lenvatinib-Resistant HCC Cells

To identify genes that are differentially regulated in Lenvatinib-resistant HCC cells, we analyzed gene expression data obtained from the Gene Expression Omnibus (GEO) database (https://www.ncbi.nlm.nih.gov/geo/, accessed on 22 October 2024; GSE186191). Gene expression profiles of Lenv-R HCC cell lines were compared with those of parental HCC cell lines. Differentially regulated genes were defined by an FC > 1.0 or <−1.0 and a p-value < 0.05. Pathway enrichment analysis was conducted using the KEGG pathway analysis tool (https://david.ncifcrf.gov/, accessed on 22 October 2024). Enriched pathways were identified using the DAVID Bioinformatics Resources 2021 (https://david.ncifcrf.gov/, accessed on 22 October 2024) [23], with enrichment criteria of fold enrichment > 2.0 and $p < 0.05$. Scatter plots and heatmaps of the differentially regulated genes were generated based on the results of the enrichment analysis.

4.12. RNA Extraction and qRT-PCR

Total RNA was isolated from cancer cells treated with Lenvatinib, OPCs, or their combination for 24 h using the Qiagen miRNeasy Kit (Qiagen, Hilden, Germany). Complementary DNA (cDNA) was synthesized from the extracted RNA using a high-capacity cDNA reverse transcription kit (Thermo Fisher Scientific), QuantStudio 6/7 Flex RT-PCR System (Applied Biosystems, Foster City, CA, USA), and qRT-PCR was performed using SensiFAST SYBR Lo-ROX Kit (Bioline, London, UK). The housekeeping gene GAPDH was used as an internal control. Gene expression levels were quantified using the ΔCt method, which calculates the difference in Ct values between the target and control genes. The primer sequences used in this study are described in Table S2.

4.13. *Protein Isolation and Western Blotting*

Western blotting was performed according to previous studies [44,45]. Total protein was extracted from HCC cell lines treated with Lenvatinib, OPCs, or a combination of the two for 48 h. Cells were collected using a plastic scraper and washed three times with cold Phosphate-buffered saline (PBS). Cells were then lysed in ice-cold RIPA protein extract containing a protease inhibitor cocktail (Thermo Fisher Scientific). Extracted proteins were denatured in 4× Laemmli sample buffer (BIO-RAD, Hercules, CA, USA), which contains 5% 2-mercaptoethanol. Protein concentrations were determined using the BCA method (Thermo Fisher Scientific). Equal amounts of protein samples (60 μg) were separated by SDS-PAGE using 7.5% or 10% Mini-PROTEAN TGXTM Precast Gels (BIO-RAD), transferred to nitrocellulose membranes, and then transferred to 0.45 μm. The membranes were blocked with 5% bovine serum albumin (Sigma-Aldrich) in Tris-buffered saline (BIO-RAD) supplemented with 0.1% Tween-20 (Sigma-Aldrich) for 1 h at room temperature. Membranes were incubated overnight at 4 °C with the following primary antibodies: GAPDH (1:5000, Proteintech, Cat# 10494-1-AP), PARP (1:1000, CST, Cat# 9532S), Cleaved-PARP (1:1000, CST, Cat# 5625S), Caspase-3 (1:1000, CST, Cat# 9662S), Cleaved-Caspase-3 (1:1000, CST, Cat# 9661S), Bax (1:1000, CST, Cat# 41162), CD44 (1:1000, CST, Cat# 3570S), CD133 (1:1000, Merck Millipore, Cat# MAB4399), OCT4 (1:1000, CST, Cat# 75463S), ITGA3 (1:1000, Proteintech, Cat# 66070-1-Ig), EGFR (1:1000, CST, Cat# 4267T), Phospho-EGFR (Ser473, 1:1000, CST, Cat# 3777S), AKT (1:1000, CST, Cat# 9272), and Phospho-AKT (Ser473, 1:1000, CST, Cat# 4060S). After washing, membranes were incubated with HRP-conjugated secondary antibodies (CST) for 1 h at room temperature. Protein bands were visualized using an HRP-based chemiluminescence kit (Thermo Fisher Scientific) and imaged with Gel Imaging Systems (BIO-RAD). GAPDH was used as a loading control.

4.14. *Transfection of Small Interfering RNA*

In this study, 1×10^6 cells were reverse-transfected using Lipofectamine RNAiMAX (Thermo Fisher Scientific) with either ITGA3-specific siRNA (Cat. No. 2012881; Assay IDs: 107727 and 16478) or a negative control siRNA and subsequently plated in 6–cm dishes. After 48 h of transfection, the cells were utilized for RNA and protein extraction as well as additional assays.

4.15. *Anoikis Assay*

Anoikis resistance was assessed using the CytoSelect™ 96-Well Anoikis Assay (Cell Biolabs, San Diego, CA, USA; Cat# CBA-081). Huh-7 and PLC HCC cells were seeded at a density of 2×10^4 cells per well and cultured for 24 h at 37 °C in a 5% CO_2 atmosphere. For fluorometric detection, cells were stained with Calcein-AM (Invitrogen, Part No. 108002, 500X) and Ethidium Homodimer-1 (EthD-1; Invitrogen, Part No. 108003, 500X) diluted to 100X in culture medium. Live and dead cells were detected by fluorescence microscopy (Calcein-AM: Ex 485 nm/Em 515 nm; EthD-1: Ex 525 nm/Em 590 nm) and quantified using a fluorescence microplate reader (Tecan Trading AG, Männedorf, Switzerland).

4.16. Statistical Analysis

All experiments were conducted in triplicate, and the results were presented as mean ± standard deviation (SD). For statistical comparisons between two groups, the Wilcoxon rank-sum test (Mann–Whitney U test) was applied. A *p*-value of less than 0.05 was considered statistically significant. Kaplan–Meier survival curves were generated to evaluate OS, and differences between groups were assessed using the log-rank test. In addition, univariate Cox proportional hazards regression analysis was performed to calculate hazard ratios (HR) and 95% confidence intervals (CI) for each group. All statistical analyses, including survival analysis and HR calculation, were performed using R software (version 4.3.1), utilizing the survival and survminer packages.

5. Conclusions

In conclusion, our findings suggest that ITGA3-mediated activation of the EGFR–AKT pathway and associated anoikis resistance play critical roles in Lenvatinib resistance. Targeting this axis with OPCs restores anoikis sensitivity and resensitizes resistant HCC cells to Lenvatinib. These results highlight a novel therapeutic avenue for overcoming Lenvatinib resistance and provide a promising rationale for future clinical translation of OPCs-based combination strategies in HCC treatment.

Supplementary Materials: The following supporting information can be downloaded at: https://www.mdpi.com/article/10.3390/ph18091361/s1, Figure S1: Functional assays showing suppression of colony formation, migration, invasion, and stemness-related gene expression following ITGA3 knockdown; Figures S2–S5: Raw data of Western Blot; Table S1: Clinicopathological variables of HCC patients; Table S2: List of primers for RT-qPCR used in this study; Table S3: List of primary antibodies for Western blotting.

Author Contributions: Conceptualization, T.N., Y.L. and A.G.; formal analysis, T.N., Y.L.; resources, Y.W., Y.M., T.I., Y.S., S.Y., H.T., M.S.; clinical samples, Y.W., Y.M., T.I., Y.S., S.Y., H.T., M.S.; Lenvatinib-resistant cell lines, Y.W., Y.M., T.I., Y.S., S.Y., H.T., M.S., data curation, T.N., Y.L. and A.G.; writing—original draft preparation, T.N.; writing—review and editing, Y.L. and A.G.; visualization, T.N. and A.G.; supervision, A.G.; project administration, A.G.; funding acquisition, A.G. All authors have read and agreed to the published version of the manuscript.

Funding: This work was supported by the following grants from the National Cancer Institute, National Institutes of Health: CA72851, CA181572, CA184792, CA187956, CA202797, CA214254, and CA271443.

Institutional Review Board Statement: The study was conducted in accordance with the guidelines of the Declaration of Helsinki and was approved by the Institutional Review Board of City of Hope (protocol code 187811, dated 20 April 2020).

Informed Consent Statement: In accordance with the Declaration of Helsinki, all patients have provided written informed consent.

Data Availability Statement: The datasets generated and/or analyzed during the current study are available from the corresponding author on reasonable request.

Acknowledgments: The authors thank Caiming Xu, Silei Sui, Alessandro Mannucci, and Koichi Takiguchi for their thoughtful discussions and advice during this project.

Conflicts of Interest: The authors declare no conflicts of interest.

Abbreviations

The following abbreviations are used in this manuscript:

HCC	Hepatocellular carcinoma
ICIs	Immune checkpoint inhibitors
TKIs	Multi-tyrosine kinase inhibitors
OS	Overall survival
IC_{50}	Half-maximal inhibitory concentration
OPCs	Oligomeric proanthocyanidins
PLC	PLC-PRF-5
FC	Fold change
ECM	Extracellular matrix
EGFR	Epidermal growth factor receptor
DMEM	Dulbecco's Modified Eagle's medium
DMSO	Dimethyl sulfoxide
FBS	Fetal bovine serum
DAVID	Database for Annotation, Visualization, and Integrated Discovery
KEGG	Kyoto Encyclopedia of Genes and Genomes
CCK-8	Cell Counting Kit-8
PBS	Phosphate-buffered saline
SD	Standard deviation
HR	Hazard ratios
CI	Confidence intervals
cDNA	Complementary DNA
qRT-PCR	Quantitative reverse transcription polymerase chain reaction

References

1. Llovet, J.M.; Kelley, R.K.; Villanueva, A.; Singal, A.G.; Pikarsky, E.; Roayaie, S.; Lencioni, R.; Koike, K.; Zucman-Rossi, J.; Finn, R.S. Hepatocellular carcinoma. *Nat. Rev. Dis. Primers* **2021**, *7*, 6. [CrossRef]
2. Llovet, J.M.; Ricci, S.; Mazzaferro, V.; Hilgard, P.; Gane, E.; Blanc, J.F.; de Oliveira, A.C.; Santoro, A.; Raoul, J.L.; Forner, A.; et al. Sorafenib in advanced hepatocellular carcinoma. *N. Engl. J. Med.* **2008**, *359*, 378–390. [CrossRef]
3. Johnson, P.J.; Qin, S.; Park, J.W.; Poon, R.T.; Raoul, J.L.; Philip, P.A.; Hsu, C.H.; Hu, T.H.; Heo, J.; Xu, J.; et al. Brivanib versus sorafenib as first-line therapy in patients with unresectable, advanced hepatocellular carcinoma: Results from the randomized phase III BRISK-FL study. *J. Clin. Oncol.* **2013**, *31*, 3517–3524. [CrossRef]
4. Kudo, M.; Finn, R.S.; Qin, S.; Han, K.H.; Ikeda, K.; Piscaglia, F.; Baron, A.; Park, J.W.; Han, G.; Jassem, J.; et al. Lenvatinib versus sorafenib in first-line treatment of patients with unresectable hepatocellular carcinoma: A randomised phase 3 non-inferiority trial. *Lancet* **2018**, *391*, 1163–1173. [CrossRef] [PubMed]
5. Finn, R.S.; Qin, S.; Ikeda, M.; Galle, P.R.; Ducreux, M.; Kim, T.Y.; Kudo, M.; Breder, V.; Merle, P.; Kaseb, A.O.; et al. Atezolizumab plus Bevacizumab in Unresectable Hepatocellular Carcinoma. *N. Engl. J. Med.* **2020**, *382*, 1894–1905. [CrossRef]
6. Cheng, A.L.; Qin, S.; Ikeda, M.; Galle, P.R.; Ducreux, M.; Kim, T.Y.; Lim, H.Y.; Kudo, M.; Breder, V.; Merle, P.; et al. Updated efficacy and safety data from IMbrave150: Atezolizumab plus bevacizumab vs. sorafenib for unresectable hepatocellular carcinoma. *J. Hepatol.* **2022**, *76*, 862–873. [CrossRef] [PubMed]
7. Casadei-Gardini, A.; Rimini, M.; Tada, T.; Suda, G.; Shimose, S.; Kudo, M.; Cheon, J.; Finkelmeier, F.; Lim, H.Y.; Rimassa, L.; et al. Atezolizumab plus bevacizumab versus lenvatinib for unresectable hepatocellular carcinoma: A large real-life worldwide population. *Eur. J. Cancer* **2023**, *180*, 9–20. [CrossRef] [PubMed]
8. Estes, C.; Razavi, H.; Loomba, R.; Younossi, Z.; Sanyal, A.J. Modeling the epidemic of nonalcoholic fatty liver disease demonstrates an exponential increase in burden of disease. *Hepatology* **2018**, *67*, 123–133. [CrossRef]
9. Rimini, M.; Rimassa, L.; Ueshima, K.; Burgio, V.; Shigeo, S.; Tada, T.; Suda, G.; Yoo, C.; Cheon, J.; Pinato, D.J.; et al. Atezolizumab plus bevacizumab versus lenvatinib or sorafenib in non-viral unresectable hepatocellular carcinoma: An international propensity score matching analysis. *ESMO Open* **2022**, *7*, 100591. [CrossRef]
10. He, X.; Hikiba, Y.; Suzuki, Y.; Nakamori, Y.; Kanemaru, Y.; Sugimori, M.; Sato, T.; Nozaki, A.; Chuma, M.; Maeda, S. EGFR inhibition reverses resistance to lenvatinib in hepatocellular carcinoma cells. *Sci. Rep.* **2022**, *12*, 8007. [CrossRef]
11. Jin, H.; Shi, Y.; Lv, Y.; Yuan, S.; Ramirez, C.F.A.; Lieftink, C.; Wang, L.; Wang, S.; Wang, C.; Dias, M.H.; et al. EGFR activation limits the response of liver cancer to lenvatinib. *Nature* **2021**, *595*, 730–734. [CrossRef]

12. Wang, J.; Yu, H.; Dong, W.; Zhang, C.; Hu, M.; Ma, W.; Jiang, X.; Li, H.; Yang, P.; Xiang, D. N6-Methyladenosine-Mediated Up-Regulation of FZD10 Regulates Liver Cancer Stem Cells' Properties and Lenvatinib Resistance Through WNT/beta-Catenin and Hippo Signaling Pathways. *Gastroenterology* **2023**, *164*, 990–1005. [CrossRef]
13. Yu, T.; Yu, J.; Lu, L.; Zhang, Y.; Zhou, Y.; Zhou, Y.; Huang, F.; Sun, L.; Guo, Z.; Hou, G.; et al. MT1JP-mediated miR-24-3p/BCL2L2 axis promotes Lenvatinib resistance in hepatocellular carcinoma cells by inhibiting apoptosis. *Cell Oncol.* **2021**, *44*, 821–834. [CrossRef]
14. Bayat Mokhtari, R.; Homayouni, T.S.; Baluch, N.; Morgatskaya, E.; Kumar, S.; Das, B.; Yeger, H. Combination therapy in combating cancer. *Oncotarget* **2017**, *8*, 38022–38043. [CrossRef] [PubMed]
15. Chen, J.; Xiong, P.; Nie, M.; Pan, Y.; Wang, J.; Hu, D.; Zhou, Z.; Zhang, Y.; Chen, M.; Xu, L. The combination treatment strategy of lenvatinib for hepatocellular carcinoma: A real-world study. *J. Cancer Res. Clin. Oncol.* **2023**, *149*, 2491–2500. [CrossRef]
16. Bermudez-Soto, M.J.; Larrosa, M.; Garcia-Cantalejo, J.M.; Espin, J.C.; Tomas-Barberan, F.A.; Garcia-Conesa, M.T. Up-regulation of tumor suppressor carcinoembryonic antigen-related cell adhesion molecule 1 in human colon cancer Caco-2 cells following repetitive exposure to dietary levels of a polyphenol-rich chokeberry juice. *J. Nutr. Biochem.* **2007**, *18*, 259–271. [CrossRef]
17. Huai, Z.; Li, Z.; Xue, W.; Li, S.; Huang, Y.; Cao, X.; Wei, Q.; Wang, Y. Novel curcumin derivatives N17 exert anti-cancer effects through the CSNK1G3/AKT axis in triple-negative breast cancer. *Biochem. Pharmacol.* **2024**, *229*, 116472. [CrossRef]
18. Zhang, A.; Sun, H.; Wang, X. Potentiating therapeutic effects by enhancing synergism based on active constituents from traditional medicine. *Phytother. Res.* **2014**, *28*, 526–533. [CrossRef] [PubMed]
19. Shimura, T.; Sharma, P.; Sharma, G.G.; Banwait, J.K.; Goel, A. Enhanced anti-cancer activity of andrographis with oligomeric proanthocyanidins through activation of metabolic and ferroptosis pathways in colorectal cancer. *Sci. Rep.* **2021**, *11*, 7548. [CrossRef]
20. Ravindranathan, P.; Pasham, D.; Balaji, U.; Cardenas, J.; Gu, J.; Toden, S.; Goel, A. Mechanistic insights into anticancer properties of oligomeric proanthocyanidins from grape seeds in colorectal cancer. *Carcinogenesis* **2018**, *39*, 767–777. [CrossRef]
21. Ravindranathan, P.; Pasham, D.; Goel, A. Oligomeric proanthocyanidins (OPCs) from grape seed extract suppress the activity of ABC transporters in overcoming chemoresistance in colorectal cancer cells. *Carcinogenesis* **2019**, *40*, 412–421. [CrossRef] [PubMed]
22. Toden, S.; Ravindranathan, P.; Gu, J.; Cardenas, J.; Yuchang, M.; Goel, A. Oligomeric proanthocyanidins (OPCs) target cancer stem-like cells and suppress tumor organoid formation in colorectal cancer. *Sci. Rep.* **2018**, *8*, 3335. [CrossRef]
23. Sherman, B.T.; Hao, M.; Qiu, J.; Jiao, X.; Baseler, M.W.; Lane, H.C.; Imamichi, T.; Chang, W. DAVID: A web server for functional enrichment analysis and functional annotation of gene lists (2021 update). *Nucleic Acids Res.* **2022**, *50*, W216–W221. [CrossRef]
24. Cooper, J.; Giancotti, F.G. Integrin Signaling in Cancer: Mechanotransduction, Stemness, Epithelial Plasticity, and Therapeutic Resistance. *Cancer Cell* **2019**, *35*, 347–367. [CrossRef]
25. Kariya, Y.; Nishita, M. Integrins in Cancer Drug Resistance: Molecular Mechanisms and Clinical Implications. *Int. J. Mol. Sci.* **2025**, *26*, 3143. [CrossRef]
26. Nasimi Shad, A.; Moghbeli, M. Integrins as the pivotal regulators of cisplatin response in tumor cells. *Cell Commun. Signal* **2024**, *22*, 265. [CrossRef]
27. Paoli, P.; Giannoni, E.; Chiarugi, P. Anoikis molecular pathways and its role in cancer progression. *Biochim. Biophys. Acta* **2013**, *1833*, 3481–3498. [CrossRef]
28. Song, W.; Hu, H.; Yuan, Z.; Yao, H. A prognostic model for anoikis-related genes in pancreatic cancer. *Sci. Rep.* **2024**, *14*, 15200. [CrossRef] [PubMed]
29. Sa, K.D.; Zhang, X.; Li, X.F.; Gu, Z.P.; Yang, A.G.; Zhang, R.; Li, J.P.; Sun, J.Y. A miR-124/ITGA3 axis contributes to colorectal cancer metastasis by regulating anoikis susceptibility. *Biochem. Biophys. Res. Commun.* **2018**, *501*, 758–764. [CrossRef]
30. Guo, W.; Giancotti, F.G. Integrin signalling during tumour progression. *Nat. Rev. Mol. Cell Biol.* **2004**, *5*, 816–826. [CrossRef]
31. Hamidi, H.; Ivaska, J. Every step of the way: Integrins in cancer progression and metastasis. *Nat. Rev. Cancer* **2018**, *18*, 533–548. [CrossRef]
32. Dai, Y.; Zhang, X.; Ou, Y.; Zou, L.; Zhang, D.; Yang, Q.; Qin, Y.; Du, X.; Li, W.; Yuan, Z.; et al. Anoikis resistance--protagonists of breast cancer cells survive and metastasize after ECM detachment. *Cell Commun. Signal* **2023**, *21*, 190. [CrossRef]
33. Gonzalez-Llorente, L.; Santacatterina, F.; Garcia-Aguilar, A.; Nuevo-Tapioles, C.; Gonzalez-Garcia, S.; Tirpakova, Z.; Toribio, M.L.; Cuezva, J.M. Overexpression of Mitochondrial IF1 Prevents Metastatic Disease of Colorectal Cancer by Enhancing Anoikis and Tumor Infiltration of NK Cells. *Cancers* **2019**, *12*, 22. [CrossRef]
34. Wade, C.A.; Kyprianou, N. Profiling Prostate Cancer Therapeutic Resistance. *Int. J. Mol. Sci.* **2018**, *19*, 904. [CrossRef]
35. Nie, F.; Liu, L.; Cui, J.; Zhao, Y.; Zhang, D.; Zhou, D.; Wu, J.; Li, B.; Wang, T.; Li, M.; et al. Oligomeric Proanthocyanidins: An Updated Review of Their Natural Sources, Synthesis, and Potentials. *Antioxidants* **2023**, *12*, 1004. [CrossRef]
36. Liu, G.; Shi, A.; Wang, N.; Li, M.; He, X.; Yin, C.; Tu, Q.; Shen, X.; Tao, Y.; Wang, Q.; et al. Polyphenolic Proanthocyanidin-B2 suppresses proliferation of liver cancer cells and hepatocellular carcinogenesis through directly binding and inhibiting AKT activity. *Redox Biol.* **2020**, *37*, 101701. [CrossRef]

37. Al-Ishaq, R.K.; Overy, A.J.; Busselberg, D. Phytochemicals and Gastrointestinal Cancer: Cellular Mechanisms and Effects to Change Cancer Progression. *Biomolecules* **2020**, *10*, 105. [CrossRef]
38. Zhang, Y.P.; Liu, S.Y.; Sun, Q.Y.; Ren, J.; Liu, H.X.; Li, H. Proanthocyanidin B2 attenuates high-glucose-induced neurotoxicity of dorsal root ganglion neurons through the PI3K/Akt signaling pathway. *Neural Regen. Res.* **2018**, *13*, 1628–1636.
39. Vogel, A.; Qin, S.; Kudo, M.; Su, Y.; Hudgens, S.; Yamashita, T.; Yoon, J.H.; Fartoux, L.; Simon, K.; Lopez, C.; et al. Lenvatinib versus sorafenib for first-line treatment of unresectable hepatocellular carcinoma: Patient-reported outcomes from a randomised, open-label, non-inferiority, phase 3 trial. *Lancet Gastroenterol. Hepatol.* **2021**, *6*, 649–658. [CrossRef]
40. Capozzi, M.; De Divitiis, C.; Ottaiano, A.; von Arx, C.; Scala, S.; Tatangelo, F.; Delrio, P.; Tafuto, S. Lenvatinib, a molecule with versatile application: From preclinical evidence to future development in anti-cancer treatment. *Cancer Manag. Res.* **2019**, *11*, 3847–3860. [CrossRef] [PubMed]
41. Chen, S.; Hu, H.; Miao, S.; Zheng, J.; Xie, Z.; Zhao, H. Anti-tumor effect of cisplatin in human oral squamous cell carcinoma was enhanced by andrographolide via upregulation of phospho-p53 in vitro and in vivo. *Tumour. Biol.* **2017**, *39*, 1010428317705330. [CrossRef]
42. Sun, C.; Jin, W.; Shi, H. Oligomeric proanthocyanidins protects A549 cells against H_2O_2-induced oxidative stress via the Nrf2-ARE pathway. *Int. J. Mol. Med.* **2017**, *39*, 1548–1554. [CrossRef]
43. Ianevski, A.; Giri, A.K.; Aittokallio, T. SynergyFinder 3.0: An interactive analysis and consensus interpretation of multi-drug synergies across multiple samples. *Nucleic Acids Res.* **2022**, *50*, W739–W743. [CrossRef]
44. Roy, S.; Zhao, Y.; Yuan, Y.C.; Goel, A. Metformin and ICG-001 Act Synergistically to Abrogate Cancer Stem Cells-Mediated Chemoresistance in Colorectal Cancer by Promoting Apoptosis and Autophagy. *Cancers* **2022**, *14*, 1281. [CrossRef] [PubMed]
45. Zhao, Y.; Wang, C.; Goel, A. Andrographis overcomes 5-fluorouracil-associated chemoresistance through inhibition of DKK1 in colorectal cancer. *Carcinogenesis* **2021**, *42*, 814–825. [CrossRef]

pharmaceuticals

Article

Systems Network Integration of Transcriptomic, Proteomic, and Bioinformatic Analyses Reveals the Mechanism of XuanYunNing Tablets in Meniere's Disease via JAK-STAT Pathway Modulation

Zhengsen Jin [1], Chunguo Wang [2], Yifei Gao [1], Xiaoyu Tao [1], Chao Wu [1], Siyu Guo [1], Jiaqi Huang [1], Jiying Zhou [1], Chuanqi Qiao [1], Keyan Chai [1], Hua Chang [3], Chun Li [3], Xun Zou [3,*] and Jiarui Wu [1,*]

1 Department of Clinical Pharmacology of Traditional Chinese Medicine, School of Chinese Materia Medica, Beijing University of Chinese Medicine, Beijing 100029, China
2 Beijing Institute of Traditional Chinese Medicine, Beijing University of Chinese Medicine, Beijing 100029, China
3 Guilin Sanjin Pharmaceutical Co., Ltd., Guilin 541004, China
* Correspondence: xunzou@hotmail.com (X.Z.); exogamy@163.com (J.W.)

Abstract: Background: Meniere's disease (MD) is a rare inner ear disorder characterized by endolymphatic hydrops and symptoms such as vertigo and hearing loss, with no curative treatment currently available. XuanYunNing tablets (XYN) have been clinically used to treat MD, but their molecular mechanisms remain unclear. **Objective:** This study aimed to systematically evaluate the pharmacological effects of XYN in a guinea pig model of MD and to elucidate the underlying molecular mechanisms of both MD pathogenesis and XYN intervention through integrated multi-omics analyses, including transcriptomics, proteomics, and bioinformatics. **Methods:** A guinea pig model of endolymphatic hydrops was induced by intraperitoneal injection of desmopressin acetate (dDAVP). Pharmacodynamic efficacy was evaluated via behavioral scoring and histopathological analysis. The differentially expressed genes (DEGs) and differentially expressed proteins (DEPs) modulated by XYN treatment were identified using high-throughput transcriptomic and proteomic sequencing. These data were integrated through multi-omics bioinformatic analysis. Key molecular targets and signaling pathways were further validated using RT-qPCR and Western blotting. **Results:** Pharmacological evaluations showed that guinea pigs in the model group exhibited a 26% increase in endolymphatic hydrops area, while high-dose XYN treatment reduced this area by 19% and significantly improved functional parameters, including overall physiological condition (e.g., weight and general appearance), auricular reflexes to low-, medium-, and high-frequency sound stimuli, nystagmus, and the righting reflex. High-throughput sequencing combined with integrative omics analysis identified 513 potential molecular targets of XYN. Subsequent network and module analyses pinpointed the JAK-STAT signaling pathway as the central axis. Mendelian randomization (MR) analysis further supported a causal relationship between MD and metabolic, immune, and inflammatory traits, reinforcing the central role of JAK-STAT signaling in both MD progression and XYN-mediated intervention. Mechanistic studies confirmed that XYN downregulated IFNG, IFNGR1, JAK1, p-STAT3/STAT3, and AOX at both mRNA and protein levels, thereby inhibiting aberrant JAK-STAT pathway activation in MD model animals. In addition, a total of 125 chemical constituents were identified in XYN by UHPLC-MS analysis. ZBTB20 and other molecules were identified as potential blood-based biomarkers for MD. **Conclusions:** This study reveals that XYN alleviates MD symptoms by disrupting a pathological cycle driven by JAK-STAT signaling, inflammation, and metabolic dysfunction. These findings support the clinical potential of XYN in the treatment of Meniere's disease and may inform the development of novel therapeutic strategies.

 https://doi.org/10.3390/ph18091266

Keywords: Meniere's disease; endolymphatic hydrops; XuanYunNing tablets; transcriptomics; proteomics

1. Introduction

Ménière's disease (MD) is an inner ear disorder pathologically characterized by endolymphatic hydrops. Clinically, MD exhibits considerable heterogeneity, with a classic triad comprising episodic vestibular dysfunction and progressive auditory impairment. Its hallmark symptoms include recurrent episodes of rotational vertigo lasting from 20 min to 12 h, fluctuating sensorineural hearing loss predominantly affecting low-to-mid frequencies, and cochlear symptoms such as tinnitus or aural fullness. The disease typically follows a chronic and progressive course [1,2].

Although MD was first systematically described by Prosper Ménière in 1861, its precise pathogenesis remains incompletely understood [3]. Current evidence implicates a combination of factors, including structural and functional disturbances of the inner ear, ionic imbalance, as well as inflammatory and immune-related mechanisms [4,5]. The pathological hallmark and diagnostic gold standard of MD is endolymphatic hydrops [6].

MD predominantly affects middle-aged and older adults and exerts a profound impact on their quality of life [7,8]. Available treatment modalities include pharmacological and surgical approaches. However, current interventions are largely symptomatic and do not offer a definitive cure. Thus, the development of effective therapeutic strategies remains a key focus of ongoing MD research [9–11].

In recent years, traditional Chinese medicine (TCM) has demonstrated unique advantages in the prevention and treatment of inner ear disorders such as vertigo, tinnitus, and hearing loss. By adhering to the principle of syndrome differentiation and treatment, TCM aligns closely with the modern medical paradigms of "precision medicine" and "personalized therapy." It emphasizes a holistic approach, conceptually resonating with the principles of modern systems biology and aligning closely with the core tenets of network pharmacology, which integrates multi-target, multi-pathway, and multi-level analyses to elucidate the complex interactions between drugs and biological systems [12,13].

XYN is a proprietary Chinese medicine formulation composed of extracts from ten distinct medicinal herbs, selected according to traditional pharmacopeia principles. It is commonly prescribed in clinical settings to alleviate symptoms such as dizziness and tinnitus and has been applied in the treatment of MD [14,15]. However, existing clinical data are predominantly derived from studies with small sample sizes or combination therapies, and high-quality experimental evidence from basic research remains insufficient.

In light of the above, as shown in Figure 1, this study aims to undertake a comprehensive and systematic investigation of XYN and its potential therapeutic effects on MD. The therapeutic efficacy of XYN will first be evaluated using a guinea pig model of endolymphatic hydrops. Subsequently, transcriptomic and proteomic analyses will be employed to construct molecular regulatory networks and to identify key molecules and associated signaling pathways. Particular attention will be given to the JAK-STAT signaling pathway, which has been increasingly recognized for its pivotal role in mediating inflammation, immune responses, and cellular homeostasis—processes that are closely implicated in MD pathogenesis. This pathway also emerged as a high-confidence candidate in our integrative omics screening, supporting its selection as a focus for further mechanistic investigation. In addition, public databases and bioinformatics tools will be leveraged to preliminarily identify potential diagnostic biomarkers and risk factors for MD from an interaction network perspective.

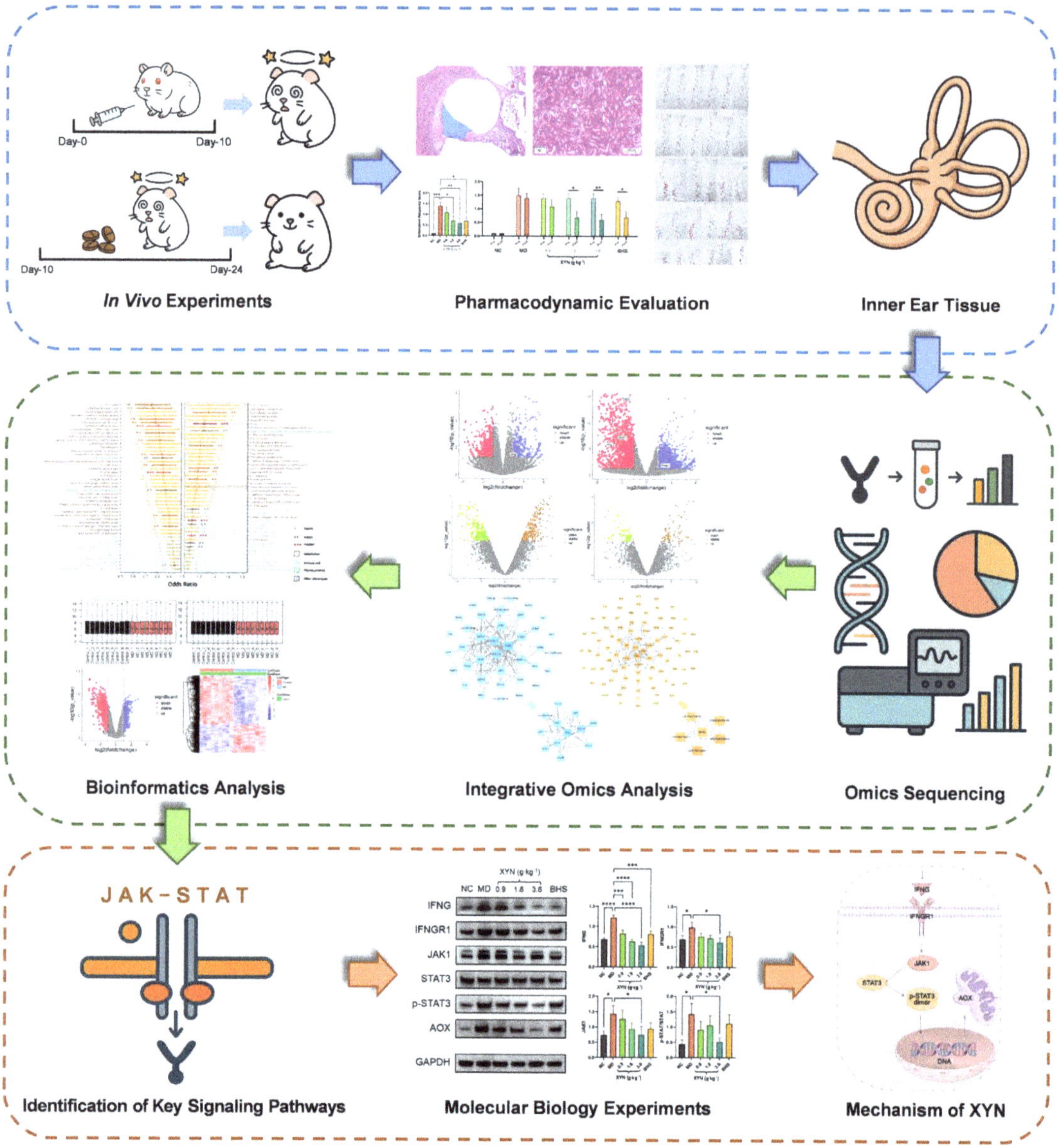

Figure 1. Overview of the proposed framework. Note: NC, normal control group; MD, model group; 0.9, low-dose XYN group; 1.8, medium-dose XYN group; 3.6, high-dose XYN group; BHS, positive control group treated with betahistine. * $p < 0.05$, ** $p < 0.01$, *** $p < 0.001$, **** $p < 0.0001$.

By integrating multi-level and multi-dimensional network-based approaches, this study endeavors to provide robust experimental and theoretical evidence supporting the clinical application of XYN in MD treatment, thereby establishing a solid foundation for the development of novel, safe, and effective therapeutic strategies.

2. Results

2.1. UHPLC-MS-Based Chemical Profiling of XYN

The extract of XYN was analyzed under positive ion mode. Major chromatographic peaks in the total ion chromatogram were systematically identified based on retention time, accurate mass measurements from high-resolution mass spectrometry, and MS/MS fragmentation patterns. The identification results are presented in Figure 2A. Similarly, the extract was analyzed under negative ion mode. The identification results are shown in Figure 2B.

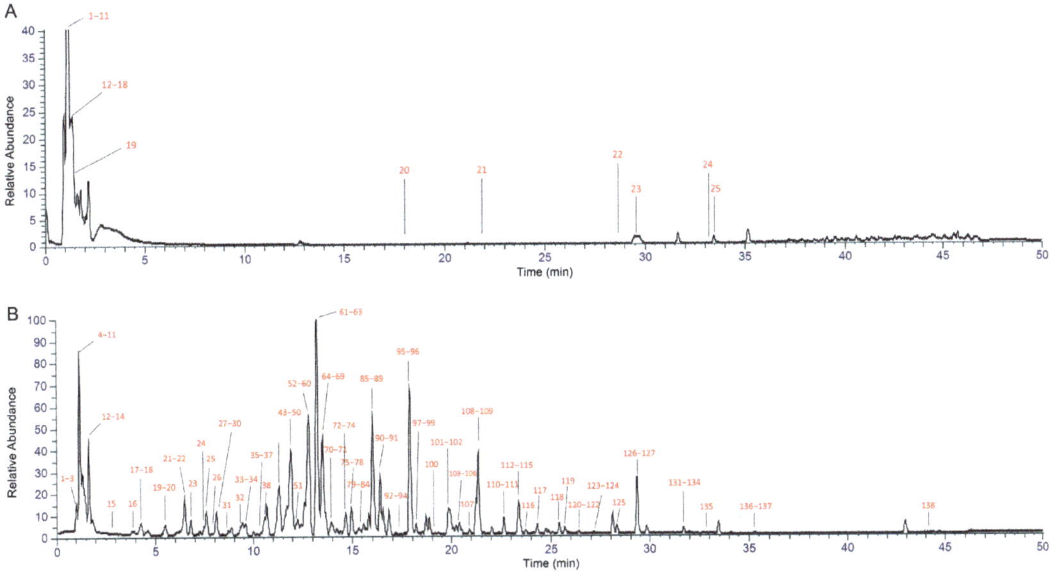

Figure 2. Total ion chromograms of XYN extract: (**A**) positive ion mode; (**B**) negative ion mode.

In total, 125 compounds were identified, comprising 45 flavonoids, 29 terpenoids, 17 phenylpropanoids, 14 alkaloids, 13 organic acids, 3 coumarins, 1 lignan, 1 quinone, and 2 others. The above results were obtained through manual interpretation without the use of reference standards. Further confirmation requires the acquisition and comparison of authentic reference compounds. Detailed information is provided in the Table S1.

2.2. XYN Administration Alleviates Endolymphatic Hydrops and Improves Associated Symptoms

2.2.1. Validation of the Endolymphatic Hydrops Model and Post-Modeling Re-Grouping

Baseline balance across groups following re-grouping is presented in the Figure S1. With the exception of the blank control group, guinea pigs in the remaining experimental groups exhibited relatively uniform distributions in terms of weight and behavioral indices, with no significant deviations observed. This indicates that re-grouping effectively eliminated individual and modeling-related differences and ensured consistent baseline conditions prior to drug administration.

In addition, guinea pigs in the model group demonstrated reduced weight and impaired behavioral performance, confirming the successful establishment of the endolymphatic hydrops model.

2.2.2. XYN Attenuates Endolymphatic Hydrops in the Cochlea

Figure 3 illustrates the degree of endolymphatic hydrops in the first turn of the cochlear scala media cross-sections across different groups. In the blank control group, the endolymphatic space accounted for approximately 21% of the cross-sectional area of the scala media. In contrast, this proportion increased to 47% in the model group. The proportions were 30%, 31%, and 28% in the low-, medium-, and high-dose XYN groups, respectively, and 26% in the betahistine (BHS)-treated group.

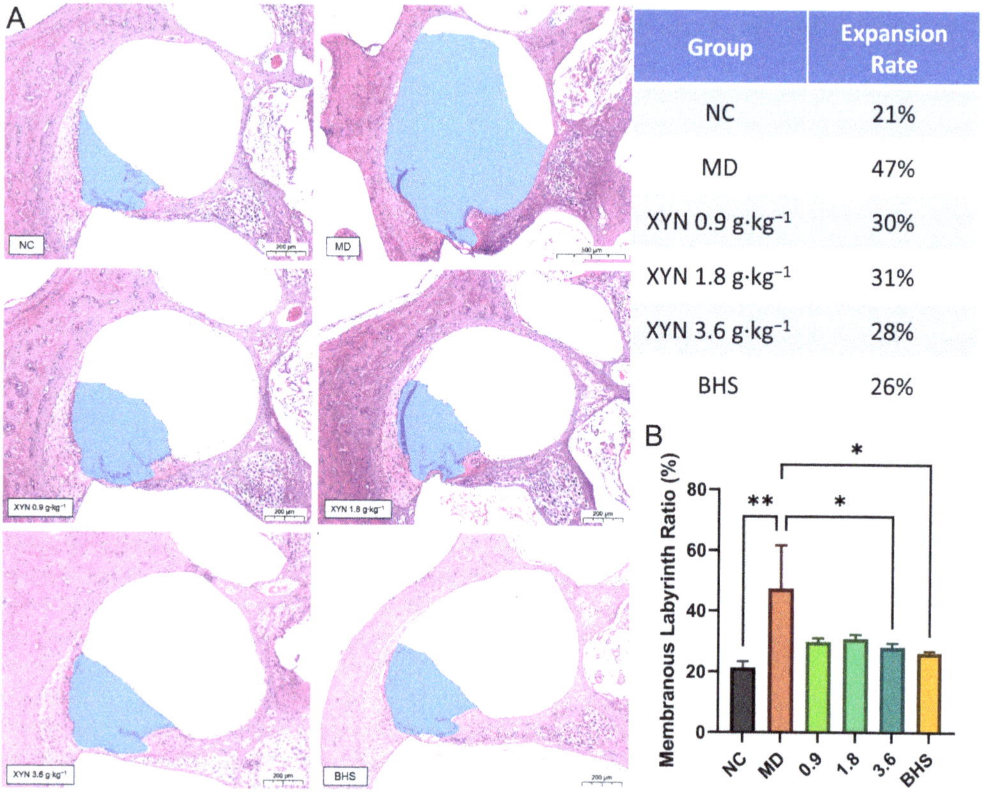

Figure 3. XYN alleviates endolymphatic hydrops in the first turn of the cochlear scala media. (**A**) Cross-sectional view of the endolymphatic labyrinth. The blue-shaded area indicates the endolymphatic labyrinth. (**B**) Quantitative analysis of cochlear cross-sections. The expansion rate refers to the ratio of the endolymphatic labyrinth area to the total cochlear area. Note: NC, normal control group; MD, model group; 0.9, low-dose XYN group; 1.8, medium-dose XYN group; 3.6, high-dose XYN group; BHS, positive control group treated with betahistine. * $p < 0.05$, ** $p < 0.01$; $n = 3$.

These findings indicate that, compared to the blank control group, guinea pigs in the model group exhibited clear enlargement of the endolymphatic space, confirming the presence of endolymphatic hydrops consistent with the pathological features of Meniere's disease. Relative to the model group, animals in all treatment groups showed a reduction in hydrops severity, suggesting that both XYN and BHS effectively alleviated endolymphatic hydrops in guinea pigs.

2.2.3. XYN Improves Gait Trajectories in Guinea Pigs

As shown in Figure 4A–C, gait anomaly detection was conducted using a convolutional neural network (CNN) for feature extraction combined with a one-class support vector machine (OCSVM) classifier. The results showed that in the model group, 18 out of 20 gait footprints were identified as abnormal. In contrast, the high-dose XYN group showed only 10 abnormal footprints, and all other treatment groups had fewer gait anomalies compared to the model group. These findings suggest that XYN can improve gait abnormalities to some extent in guinea pigs with endolymphatic hydrops.

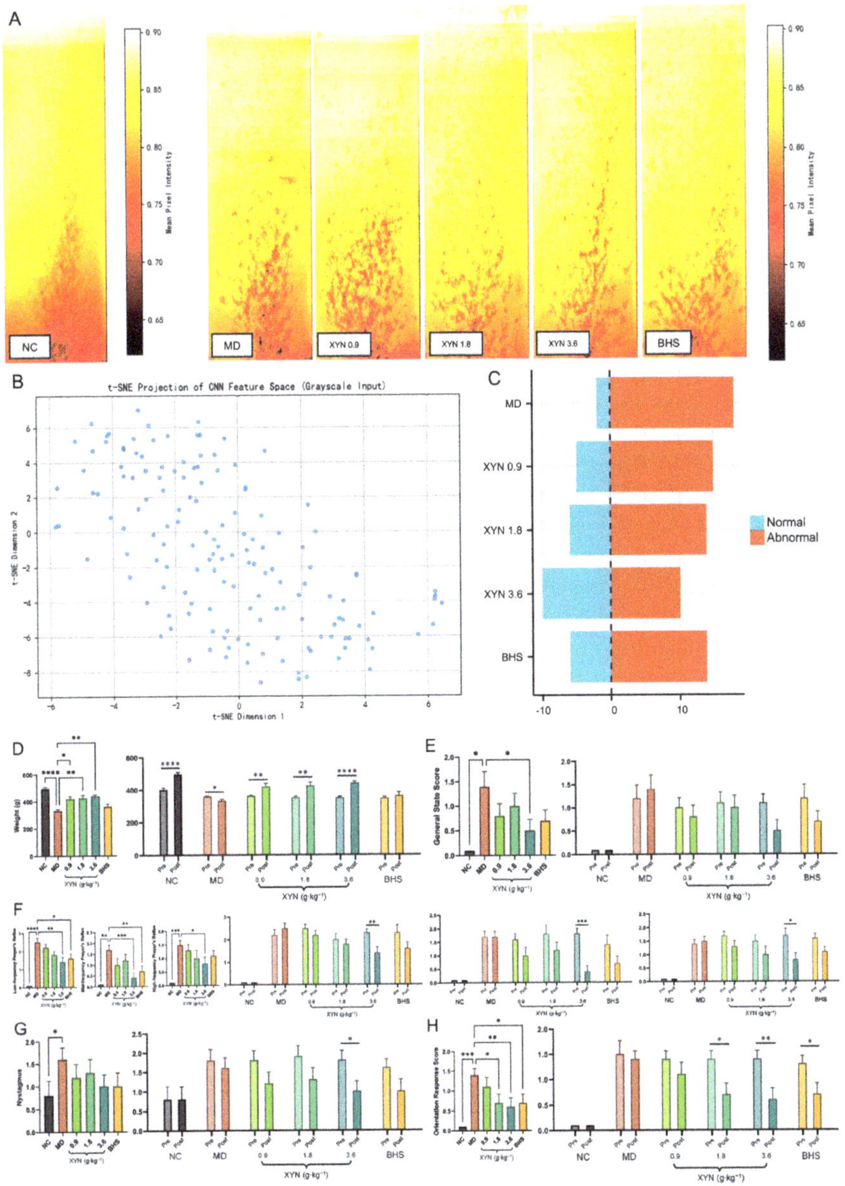

Figure 4. XYN improves behavioral performance in guinea pig. (**A**) Grayscale heatmaps of footprint distribution for the blank group (training set) and other groups. (**B**) t-SNE scatter plot showing dimensionality reduction and clustering. (**C**) Gait anomaly detection results based on the classification model. (**D**) Weight. (**E**) General condition. (**F**) Auricular reflex at low, medium, and high frequencies. (**G**) Nystagmus. (**H**) Righting reflex test. Note: NC, normal control group; MD, model group; 0.9, low-dose XYN group; 1.8, medium-dose XYN group; 3.6, high-dose XYN group; BHS, positive control group treated with betahistine. * $p < 0.05$, ** $p < 0.01$, *** $p < 0.001$, **** $p < 0.0001$; $n = 10$.

2.2.4. XYN Improves Behavioral Indices in Guinea Pigs Across Groups

Behavioral assessments in this study included general condition (weight and overall appearance), auricular reflexes (low-, medium-, and high-frequency stimulation), nystagmus, and righting reflex.

As shown on the left side of Figure 4D–F, the results showed that guinea pigs in the model group had significantly lower weight compared to the blank control group, while all other behavioral indices were significantly elevated, indicating more severe dysfunction. In contrast, guinea pigs in the high-dose XYN group exhibited significantly greater weight than those in the model group, along with marked improvements in all behavioral parameters.

2.2.5. XYN Improves Behavioral Indicators Before and After Treatment Within the Same Guinea Pigs

Considering that individual differences among guinea pigs may influence the precision of behavioral assessments, we further analyzed changes in behavioral indices before and after treatment within the same animals.

As shown on the right side of Figure 4D–F, in the blank control group, no significant differences were observed in any behavioral indicators before and after treatment, nor were there changes in general condition scores across all groups. In the model group, no statistically significant differences were detected before and after treatment; however, there was a trend toward worsening behavioral performance. In the high-dose XYN group, post-treatment assessments showed improvement in all behavioral indicators except general condition. Other treatment groups also demonstrated varying degrees of behavioral improvement, although none matched the efficacy observed in the high-dose group.

2.3. The JAK-STAT Signaling Pathway as a Core Axis in the Pathogenesis of Endolymphatic Hydrops and the Therapeutic Action of XYN

2.3.1. Differentially Expressed mRNAs and Proteins Associated with Endolymphatic Hydrops and XYN Intervention

According to Figure 5, transcriptomic analysis revealed that, compared to the blank control group, the model group exhibited 768 DEGs, with 296 upregulated and 472 downregulated. When comparing the high-dose XYN group to the model group, 2559 DEGs were identified, including 1191 upregulated and 1368 downregulated genes.

According to Figure 6, proteomic analysis showed 434 DEPs between the model and blank groups, with 348 upregulated and 86 downregulated. In comparison to the model group, the high-dose XYN group exhibited 150 DEPs, of which 48 were upregulated and 102 were downregulated.

GO and KEGG enrichment analyses were performed separately on DEGs and DEPs associated with disease onset and drug intervention, stratified by up- and downregulation. The enriched pathways were predominantly involved in immune response, inflammation, metabolism, and cytoskeletal regulation. Notably, both mRNA and protein datasets were significantly enriched in the cytokine–cytokine receptor interaction, JAK-STAT signaling pathway, and NF-κB signaling pathway, among others. Detailed enrichment analysis results are provided in the Figures S2–S5.

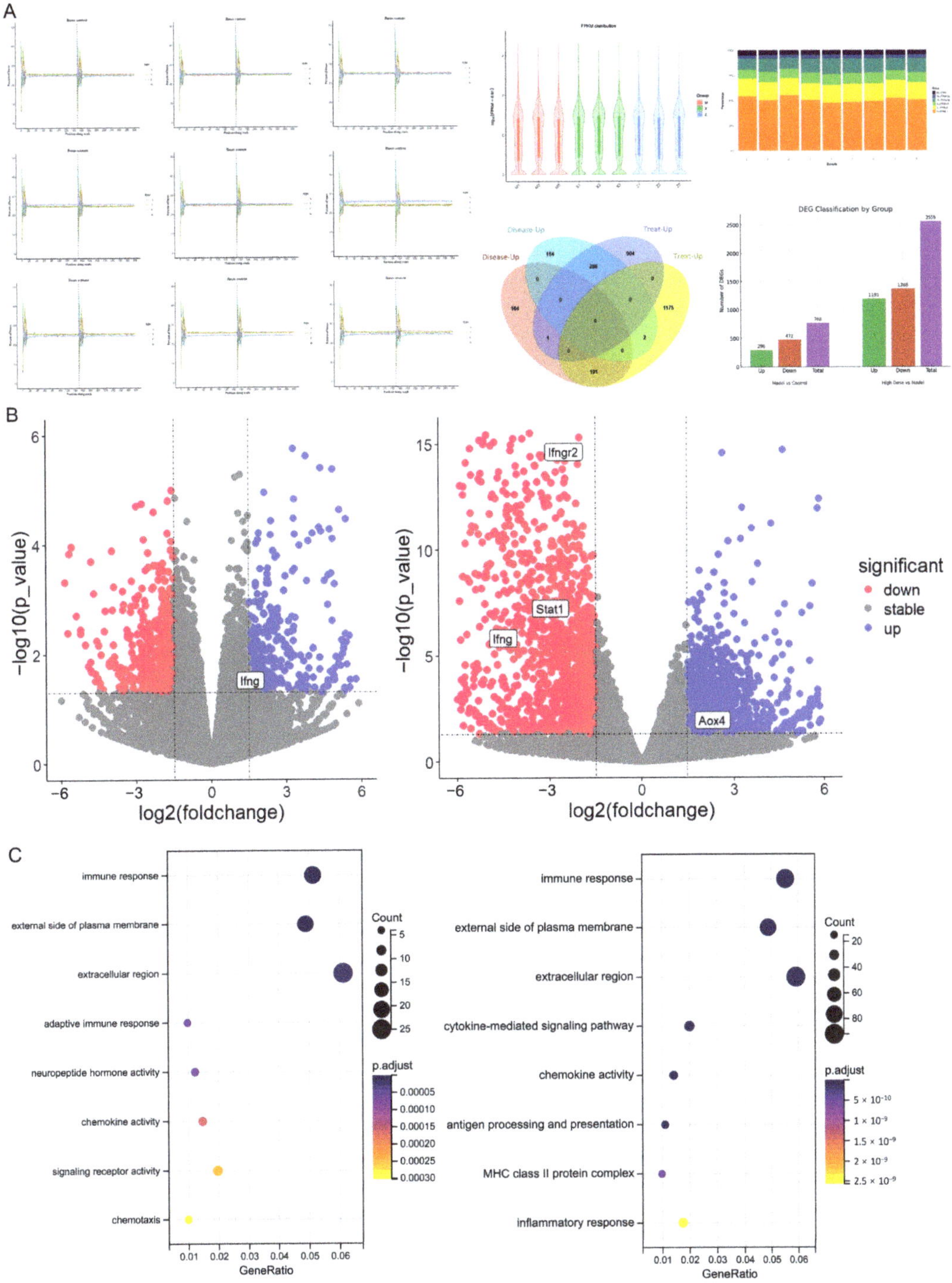

Figure 5. Transcriptomic analysis results. (**A**) Quality control of RNA sequencing data. (**B**) Volcano plot of DEGs. (**C**) Functional enrichment analysis of DEGs. Note: Inner ear tissues from guinea pigs were used for RNA sequencing (n = 3). No abnormalities were detected during quality control of the RNA sequencing data.

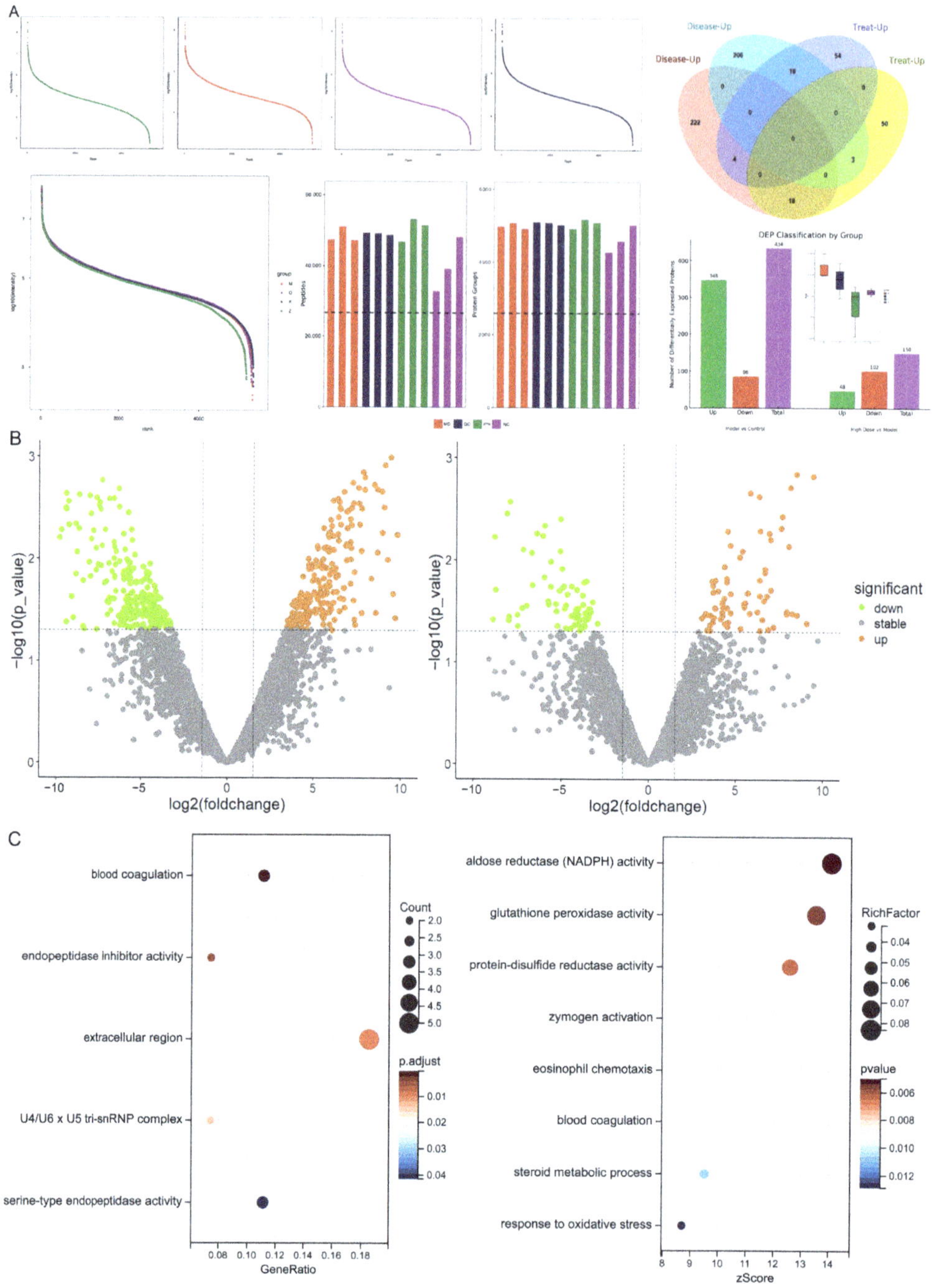

Figure 6. Proteomic analysis results. (**A**) Quality control of proteomic data. (**B**) Volcano plot of DEPs. (**C**) Functional enrichment analysis of DEPs. Note: Inner ear tissues from guinea pigs were used for proteomic analysis ($n = 3$). No abnormalities were detected during quality control of the proteomic data.

2.3.2. Metabolism, Inflammation, and Immunity-Related Phenotypes Are Associated with Meniere's Disease Onset

Given the lack of clearly defined research directions in MD, MR analysis was first performed to identify meaningful investigative targets, which subsequently guided the interpretation of high-throughput sequencing results in this study.

Based on previous research and the transcriptomic and proteomic findings outlined earlier, metabolic, immune, and inflammatory factors or pathways were prioritized for MR analysis. GWAS summary statistics for both exposures and outcomes were obtained from the Finnish biobank, with all relevant data accessed in September 2024. The Finnish data were derived from the most recent r-11 version of the database. Given the large size of the datasets, additional validation was conducted to ensure the robustness of the findings.

SNPs were selected based on a genome-wide significance threshold of $p < 5 \times 10^{-6}$ across all GWAS datasets, except for the immune cell phenotype dataset, where the threshold was relaxed to $p < 1 \times 10^{-5}$ to ensure adequate SNP inclusion for analysis. The dataset of potential related phenotypes of MD is provided in the Table S2.

A total of 2275 two-sample MR analyses were conducted, treating candidate phenotypes as exposure variables and MD as the outcome. All instrumental variables had F-statistics > 10, indicating sufficient strength. IVW analysis identified 112 exposure phenotypes with a causal relationship to MD, among which 57 phenotypes were positively associated (OR > 1, $p < 0.05$) and 55 were negatively associated (OR < 1, $p < 0.05$).

Specifically, out of 1400 metabolic traits, 75 were associated with MD. Among 731 immune cell phenotypes, 32 were associated. From 91 inflammatory circulating proteins, 3 were associated. Further analysis showed that 35 metabolic traits, 19 immune cell phenotypes, and 1 protein were positively associated with MD risk, while 40 metabolic traits, 13 immune phenotypes, and 2 proteins were negatively associated. In addition, both otitis media and anxiety disorders were found to have a significant positive correlation with MD risk.

To enhance reliability and confirm consistency, Bayesian-weighted MR analysis was conducted on 110 phenotypes from the three largest datasets. This analysis confirmed 90 significant exposure phenotypes with consistent effect directions in both standard and Bayesian MR approaches. As shown in Figure 7, including otitis media and anxiety, a total of 92 key exposure phenotypes were identified, forming a comprehensive risk factor profile for MD. Among them, 45 phenotypes were positively associated with MD risk, and 47 were negatively associated.

Overall, metabolism-related phenotypes exerted the strongest influence on MD risk, followed by inflammatory protein and immune cell–related phenotypes.

2.3.3. The JAK-STAT Signaling Pathway as a Core Axis in Endolymphatic Hydrops Pathogenesis and XYN Intervention

After stringent filtering, 191 genes were identified as pathologically upregulated in MD and downregulated following XYN treatment, whereas 286 genes exhibited the opposite trend—pathologically downregulated and pharmacologically upregulated. Similarly, 18 proteins were identified in each of the corresponding categories. Altogether, 209 molecules were classified as pathologically upregulated and pharmacologically downregulated, and 304 as pathologically downregulated and pharmacologically upregulated. These findings resulted in the identification of 513 potential molecular targets of XYN in the treatment of MD.

As shown in Figure 8, PPI network analysis was conducted after removing unconnected nodes. The resulting PPI network for these 513 candidate molecules consisted of 161 nodes and 368 edges. Using Molecular Complex Detection (MCODE), a Cytoscape plugin that identifies highly interconnected regions based on network topology, four subnetworks were identified according to node degree and clustering scores. Key nodes included IFNG, AOX2, STAT1, and IL22. These candidate molecules were primarily enriched in the JAK-STAT signaling pathway, cytokine–cytokine receptor interaction, and NF-κB signaling pathway, highlighting their relevance to inflammatory and immune responses.

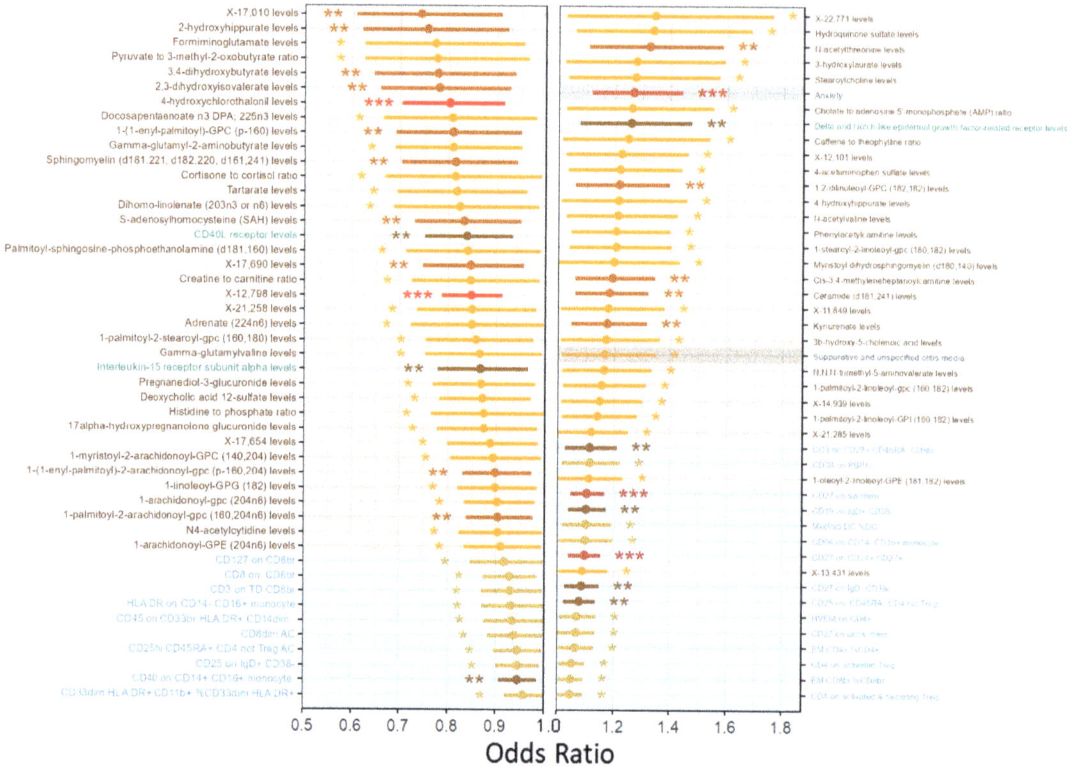

Figure 7. Risk factor landscape of MD. Note: 75 of 1400 metabolites, 32 of 731 immune cell phenotypes, and 3 of 91 inflammatory circulating proteins were linked to MD. Specifically, 35 metabolites, 19 immune cell phenotypes, and 1 protein showed a positive association, while 40 metabolites, 13 immune cell phenotypes, and 2 proteins were negatively associated with MD incidence. Additionally, otitis media and anxiety disorders both demonstrated a positive association with MD incidence. Sensitivity analyses revealed no heterogeneity (p-value of Q test > 0.05) or horizontal pleiotropy (p-value of MR-Egger intercept method > 0.05) among these exposure phenotypes. Bayesian-weighted MR was applied to 110 phenotypes from the top three largest datasets. This analysis identified 90 significant exposure phenotypes with consistent results across both primary MR and Bayesian-weighted MR analyses, all demonstrating the same effect direction. Including otitis media and anxiety disorders, this produced a total of 92 critical exposure phenotypes, forming the risk factor map for MD, * $p < 0.05$, ** $p < 0.01$, *** $p < 0.001$.

Further stratification of the PPI network into two subnetworks—based on pathological upregulation/pharmacological downregulation and vice versa—yielded the following: The 209 pathologically upregulated, pharmacologically downregulated molecules formed a subnetwork comprising 38 nodes and 136 edges. MCODE analysis identified IFNG and STAT1 as high-degree nodes, with IFNG emerging as a key molecule within the core subnetwork. The 304 pathologically downregulated, pharmacologically upregulated molecules formed a subnetwork of 86 nodes and 129 edges, where AOX2 was identified as a prominent node in the MCODE-defined core subnetwork.

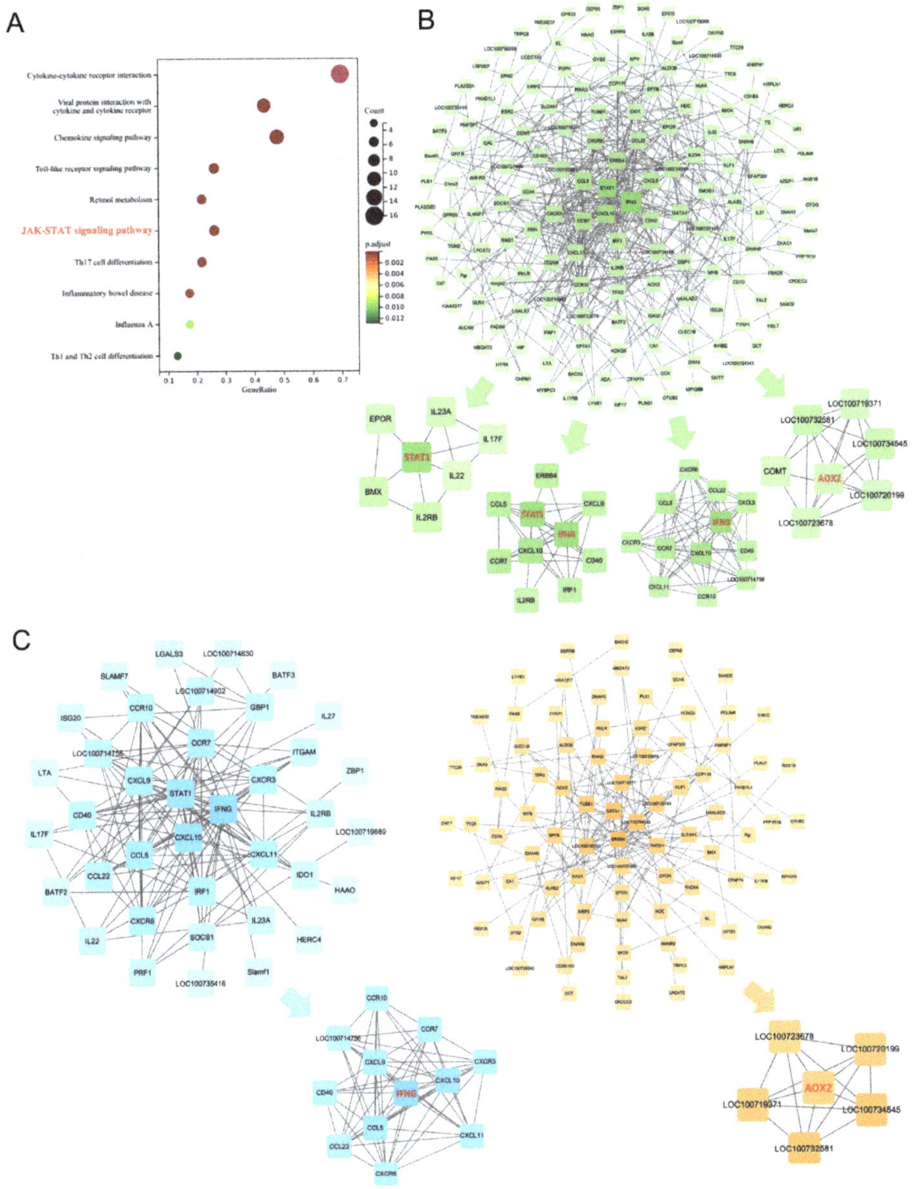

Figure 8. Integrated omics analysis. (**A**) KEGG enrichment analysis of potential molecular targets modulated by XYN Pian in MD. (**B**) PPI network and MCODE-derived subnetworks of potential targets. A total of 513 candidate targets were identified, including 209 molecules that were pathologically upregulated and pharmacologically downregulated, and 304 that were pathologically downregulated and pharmacologically upregulated. STAT1, IFNG, and AOX2 emerged as key nodes within the MCODE-defined subclusters. (**C**) Stratified PPI subnetworks based on differential regulation patterns. The left panel shows 209 molecules that were pathologically upregulated and pharmacologically downregulated, where MCODE analysis identified IFNG and STAT1 as core nodes. The right panel displays 304 molecules that were pathologically downregulated and pharmacologically upregulated, with AOX2 identified as a key node in the corresponding subnetwork.

Key nodes across these networks—including AOX2, IFNG, STAT1, and IL22—are well-recognized components of the JAK-STAT signaling pathway, and many (e.g., STAT and AOX family members) are closely associated with lipid metabolism. In conjunction with the MR analysis findings from Section 2.3.2, this strongly supports the JAK-STAT pathway as a central regulatory axis in both the pathogenesis of endolymphatic hydrops and the therapeutic mechanism of XYN.

2.3.4. The hsa-miR-3148/ZBTB20 Regulatory Axis as a Potential Blood Biomarker for Meniere's Disease

While findings from animal and basic research provide valuable mechanistic insights, a translational gap remains before clinical application can be achieved. Therefore, this section focuses on identifying potential blood biomarkers for MD using RNA sequencing data from clinical MD patients.

Two datasets—GSE202657 and GSE176560—were selected after initial screening for quality and relevance. In the GSE202657 dataset, 968 differentially expressed mRNAs were identified, comprising 355 upregulated and 613 downregulated transcripts. Functional enrichment analysis indicated that these dysregulated mRNAs were predominantly associated with immune system functions and fundamental cellular processes.

As shown in Figure 9, from the GSE176560 dataset, 34 differentially expressed miRNAs were identified, of which 21 were upregulated and 13 were downregulated. These miRNAs were analyzed using the miRDB and miRWALK databases, yielding 506 predicted target mRNAs. Functional enrichment analysis indicated that these targets were mainly associated with protein function, immune regulation, and developmental pathways.

The 34 differentially expressed miRNAs and their predicted target mRNAs were imported into Cytoscape to construct a miRNA–mRNA regulatory network, after removing isolated nodes and unconnected subnetworks. The resulting network consisted of 442 nodes and 457 edges, including 15 miRNAs and 427 mRNAs. Among these, hsa-miR-3148 had the highest node degree among miRNAs, and ZBTB20 had the highest node degree among mRNAs.

Intersecting the mRNA lists from both datasets led to the identification of 41 core mRNAs associated with MD pathogenesis. A refined miRNA–mRNA regulatory network was then constructed using these 41 mRNAs and the 34 differentially expressed miRNAs from GSE176560, excluding isolated nodes. The resulting network comprised 50 nodes and 41 edges, including 14 miRNAs and 36 mRNAs. Notably, hsa-miR-3148 and ZBTB20 remained the highest-degree nodes in the network, and a regulatory interaction between them was identified.

Importantly, ZBTB20 was also found to be significantly differentially expressed in both the transcriptomic and proteomic profiles of the guinea pig model in this study, further supporting its potential relevance as a clinical blood biomarker for MD.

2.4. Overactivation of the JAK-STAT Signaling Pathway in MD and Its Suppression by XYN Treatment

As shown in Figure 10, RT-qPCR results revealed that components of the JAK-STAT signaling pathway were significantly overactivated at the transcriptional level in the model group, with statistically significant differences observed. Treatment with XYN or BHS led to varying degrees of suppression of this pathway. IFNG and STAT3 expression levels were significantly downregulated in the medium- and high-dose XYN groups, as well as the BHS-treated group; IFNGR1 and AOX were significantly downregulated in the high-dose XYN group and the BHS group; JAK1 expression was significantly reduced only in the high-dose XYN group.

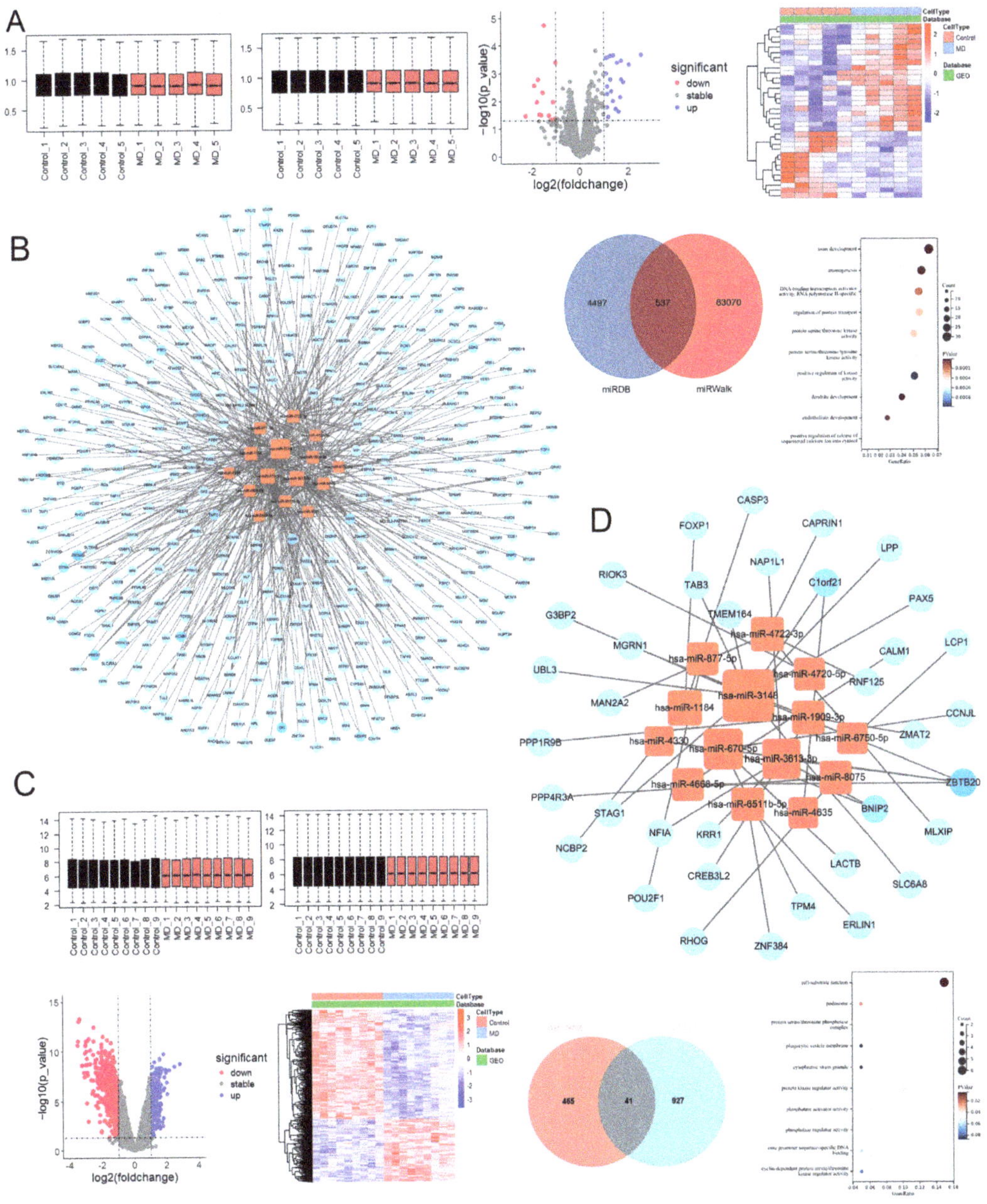

Figure 9. Analysis of blood biomarkers in MD patients. (**A**) Analysis and identification of differentially expressed molecules in the GSE176560 dataset; (**B**) miRNA–target interaction network based on the GSE176560 dataset; (**C**) analysis and identification of differentially expressed molecules in the GSE202657 dataset; (**D**) refined miRNA–mRNA regulatory network constructed from both datasets.

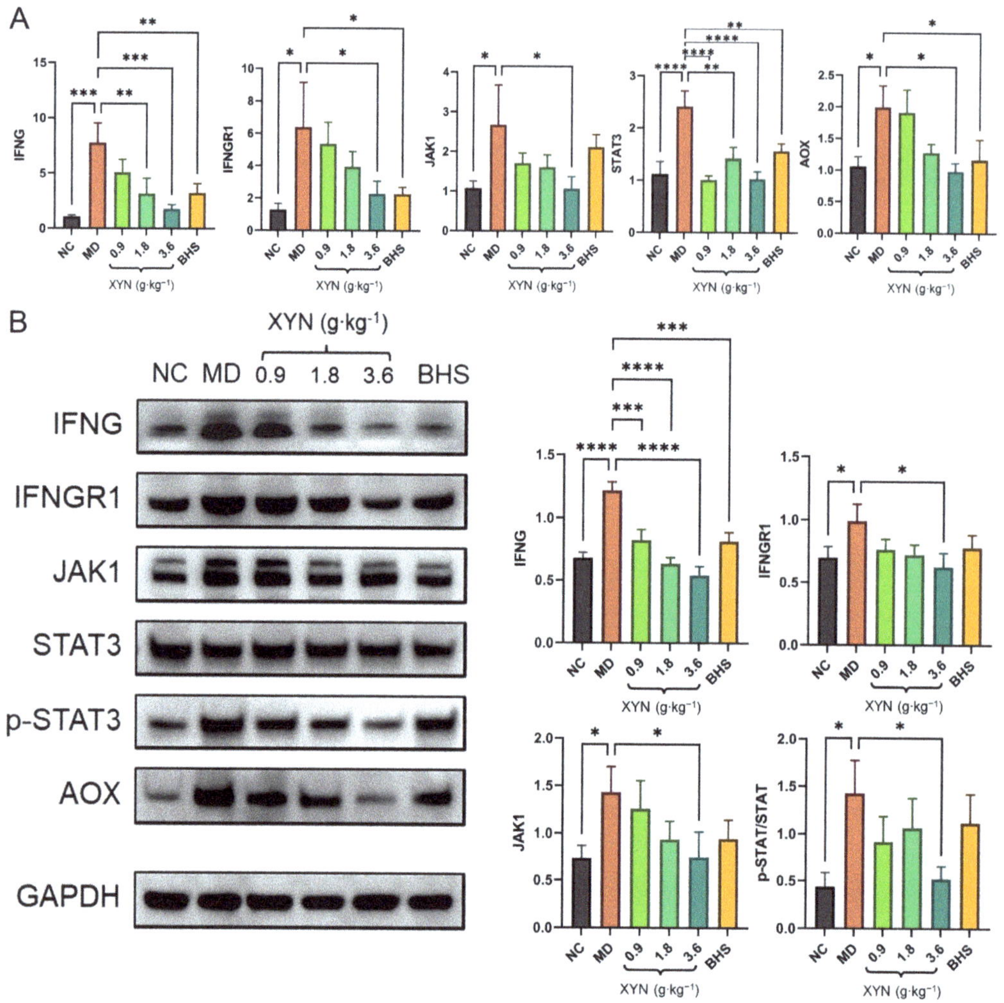

Figure 10. Molecular validation of the JAK-STAT signaling pathway. (**A**) Relative mRNA expression levels of key components in the JAK-STAT pathway; (**B**) Western blot bands and relative protein expression levels of corresponding molecules. Note: NC, normal control group; MD, model group; 0.9, low-dose XYN group; 1.8, medium-dose XYN group; 3.6, high-dose XYN group; BHS, positive control group treated with betahistine. * $p < 0.05$, ** $p < 0.01$, *** $p < 0.001$, **** $p < 0.0001$; $n = 6$.

Western blot results similarly demonstrated overactivation of JAK-STAT pathway proteins in the model group, with significant differences compared to controls. Treatment with XYN and BHS resulted in suppression of these protein expressions to varying extents. Expression levels of IFNG and AOX were significantly downregulated in all treatment groups; However, expression of IFNGR1, JAK1, and phosphorylated STAT/total STAT ratio (p-STAT/STAT) was significantly downregulated only in the high-dose XYN group. While other groups showed a downward trend, these changes were not statistically significant.

The sequences of primers and the details of antibodies used in the experiments are provided in Tables 1 and 2. Statistical summaries of significant differences in gene and protein expression levels across experimental groups are presented in Tables 3 and 4. For data that did not reach statistical significance, sensitivity analyses were not conducted.

Table 1. Primer information.

Gene	Primer Direction	Sequence (5′-3′)	Length
GAPDH	Forward	ATCAAGTGGGGTGATGCTGG	20
	Reverse	AAGATGCCTTTGAGGGAGCC	20
IFNG	Forward	AAGACAACAGCAGCAACAAGG	21
	Reverse	ACATGCTCGTCATTGACCGAAA	20
IFNGR1	Forward	GTGAACAGAAGTGAGACCCGA	21
	Reverse	AGAATACAGCAAGGGCACCG	20
JAK1	Forward	CCATGATGCGGAACATGCAG	20
	Reverse	GTTAATGCTGACCAGGGCCT	20
STAT3	Forward	CACCACAAAAGTCAGGCTGC	20
	Reverse	ACAGCCTGAGTAGTTCACGC	20
AOX	Forward	TCCCAGCTGGTGATCGAGTA	20
	Reverse	ACGGTGCTGGTTTCAGAGAG	20

Table 2. Antibody information.

Antibody	Catalog No.	Manufacturer	Dilution Ratio
HRP-conjugated Goat Anti-Rabbit IgG(H + L)	SA00001-2	Proteintech (Rosemont, IL, USA)	1:50,000
HRP-conjugated Goat Anti-Mouse IgG(H + L)	SA00001-1	Proteintech	1:10,000
STAT3 Rabbit Monoclonal antibody	A19566	ABclonal Technology (Wuhan, China)	1:10,000
Phospho-STAT3-Y705 Rabbit Monoclonal antibody	AP1468	ABclonal Technology	1:5000
IFN-gamma Rabbit Monoclonal antibody	A25684	ABclonal Technology	1:1000
JAK1 Monoclonal antibody	66466-1-Ig	Proteintech	1:3000
Aldehyde oxidase Polyclonal antibody	19495-1-AP	Proteintech	1:300
GAPDH Polyclonal antibody	10494-1-AP	Proteintech	1:20,000
IFN-gamma R1 Polyclonal antibody	10808-1-AP	Proteintech	1:600

Table 3. Significant mRNA-level differences.

Gene	Comparison	*p*-Value	Significance	Confidence Interval
IFNG	NC vs. MD	0.0002	***	−9.91 to −3.50
	MD vs. XYN-1.8	0.0064	**	1.39 to 7.81
	MD vs. XYN-3.6	0.0006	***	2.78 to 9.19
	MD vs. BHS	0.0072	**	1.32 to 7.73
IFNGR1	NC vs. MD	0.013	*	−9.08 to −1.16
	MD vs. XYN-3.6	0.0429	*	0.14 to 8.06
	MD vs. BHS	0.0421	*	0.16 to 8.08
JAK1	NC vs. MD	0.0252	*	−2.99 to −0.21
	MD vs. XYN-3.6	0.0254	*	0.21 to 2.99
STAT3	NC vs. MD	<0.0001	****	−1.88 to −0.71
	MD vs. XYN-0.9	<0.0001	****	0.82 to 1.99
	MD vs. XYN-1.8	0.0017	**	0.40 to 1.57
	MD vs. XYN-3.6	<0.0001	****	0.79 to 1.96
	MD vs. BHS	0.0061	**	0.26 to 1.43
AOX	NC vs. MD	0.0168	*	−1.69 to −0.18
	MD vs. XYN-3.6	0.0104	*	0.26 to 1.76
	MD vs. BHS	0.0324	*	0.07 to 1.58

* $p < 0.05$, ** $p < 0.01$, *** $p < 0.001$, **** $p < 0.0001$.

Table 4. Significant protein-level differences.

Protein	Comparison	*p*-Value	Significance	Confidence Interval
IFNG	NC vs. MD	<0.0001	****	−0.7333 to −0.3485
	MD vs. 0.9	0.0002	***	0.2048 to 0.5896
	MD vs. 1.8	<0.0001	****	0.3922 to 0.7771
	MD vs. 3.6	<0.0001	****	0.4851 to 0.8699
	MD vs. BHS	0.0002	***	0.2115 to 0.5963
IFNGR1	NC vs. MD	0.0482	*	−0.5889 to −0.002520
	MD vs. 3.6	0.0161	*	0.07293 to 0.6593
JAK1	NC vs. MD	0.0431	*	−1.372 to −0.02326
	MD vs. 3.6	0.0468	*	0.01032 to 1.359
p-STAT3/STAT3	NC vs. MD	0.013	*	−1.751 to −0.2238
	MD vs. 3.6	0.0222	*	0.1385 to 1.665
AOX	NC vs. MD	<0.0001	****	−1.857 to −0.9269
	NC vs. 0.9	0.0009	***	−1.302 to −0.3711
	MD vs. 0.9	0.0208	*	0.09051 to 1.021
	MD vs. 1.8	<0.0001	****	0.6883 to 1.619
	MD vs. 3.6	<0.0001	****	0.8443 to 1.775
	MD vs. BHS	0.0002	***	0.5183 to 1.449

* $p < 0.05$, *** $p < 0.001$, **** $p < 0.0001$.

3. Discussion

Traditional Chinese medicine (TCM) offers a distinctive perspective on the pathogenesis of vertigo. Classical TCM teachings suggest that "no vertigo occurs without phlegm" and "no vertigo occurs without deficiency," highlighting that impaired blood circulation, meridian obstruction, and failure of blood to nourish the brain are key mechanisms underlying the condition [16]. In the context of modern TCM theory, MD is classified under the syndromic categories of "Xuan Yun" (vertigo) and "Er Xuan Yun" (aural vertigo) [16–19]. Its core pathogenesis reflects a "root deficiency with branch excess" pattern [20–22].

Notably, the pathological hallmark of MD—endolymphatic hydrops—aligns closely with the TCM concept of "phlegm–fluid retention (tan yin)", which is believed to result from dysfunction in San Jiao (the Triple Energizer) and disrupted fluid metabolism [23].

XYN, composed of *Alisma plantago-aquatica* subsp. orientale Sam., *Atractylodes macrocephala* Koidz., *Wolfiporia cocos* (F.A. Wolf) Ryvarden & Gilb., *Pinellia ternate* (Thunb) Breit., *Ligustrum lucidum* Ait., *Eclipta prostrata* L., *Chrysanthemum morifolium* Ramat., *Achyranthes bidentata* Blume., *Citrus reticulata* Blanco., and *Glycyrrhiza uralensis* Fisch. (the plant name has been checked with http://www.worldfloraonline.org, accessed on 11 May 2025), was supplied by Guilin Sanjin Pharmaceutical Co., Ltd. (Guilin, China), batch number 230902. XYN exerts spleen-strengthening, dampness-draining, kidney-nourishing, and liver-pacifying effects. It is particularly effective for treating vertigo syndromes related to phlegm-dampness obstruction and deficiency of the liver and kidney [24,25], making it a promising candidate for the clinical management of MD. Clinical studies involving hundreds of patients have demonstrated that XYN provides a statistically significant higher total effective rate in treating MD compared to control treatments, suggesting its potential to effectively alleviate MD-related symptoms [14,15,25]. *Atractylodes macrocephala* has been reported to modulate the JAK-STAT signaling cascade as part of its synergistic mechanism in treating ulcerative colitis [26]. Network pharmacology studies have revealed that Citrus reticulata exerts therapeutic effects through targets significantly enriched in the JAK-STAT and related immune pathways [27]. Moreover, *Pinellia ternate* (Thunb) has been shown to activate the phosphorylation of JAK2, STAT1, STAT4, and STAT5 in a dose- and time-dependent manner, contributing to its immunomodulatory and antitumor activities [28]. These findings suggest that the JAK-STAT regulatory effects of XYN may be partly attributed to the concerted actions of its monomeric components.

Mechanistic studies on MD predominantly rely on the guinea pig model of endolymphatic hydrops, which can be reliably induced by arginine vasopressin (AVP) or its analog dDAVP [29]. Behavioral tests such as the rotating platform test and auricular reflex assessments are commonly used to evaluate vertigo and hearing impairment [9,10]. In this study, a guinea pig model of endolymphatic hydrops was successfully constructed and validated through cochlear pathology and multiple behavioral indicators. The therapeutic efficacy of XYN was comprehensively assessed in this model.

By integrating high-throughput sequencing with MR analysis, the JAK-STAT signaling pathway was identified as a central molecular axis involved both in the pathogenesis of endolymphatic hydrops and the therapeutic mechanism of XYN.

There is accumulating evidence supporting the immune-inflammatory mechanism underlying MD. In a subset of patients, anti-inner ear antibodies and circulating immune complexes have been detected in the serum [30]. Moreover, levels of inflammatory mediators such as interleukin-1β, IL-1 receptor antagonist, IL-6, heat shock protein 70, and tumor necrosis factor-α have been shown to correlate closely with hearing loss severity and disease progression [31,32]. In addition, total serum IgE is commonly elevated in MD patients and is positively associated with the grade of endolymphatic hydrops, the stage of hearing loss, and functional impairment scores [33–35].

At the molecular level, the JAK-STAT signaling pathway serves as a central node in cytokine-mediated inflammatory responses. It is composed of ligand–receptor pairs such as IFNG, members of the JAK family, and STATs [36,37]. Upon binding of pro-inflammatory cytokines like IFNG to their receptors, JAKs are activated and phosphorylate STATs, which in turn promote the polarization of M1-type macrophages and amplify the production of pro-inflammatory mediators [38,39]. Conversely, inhibition of this pathway has been shown to significantly reduce inflammation and tissue damage [40,41].

These findings suggest that humoral immune dysregulation and cytokine imbalance act synergistically, driving JAK-STAT-dependent inflammatory cascades, which represent a fundamental pathological basis for the progression and fluctuation of MD symptoms.

The JAK-STAT signaling pathway plays a pivotal role not only in immune and inflammatory regulation, but is also closely associated with a variety of metabolic disorders, including obesity, insulin resistance, non-alcoholic fatty liver disease, and atherosclerosis [42,43]. In the context of MD, metabolic disturbances may contribute to disease pathogenesis by disrupting the local inner ear environment. Specifically, lipid metabolism imbalance—such as cholesterol deposition or altered fatty acid composition—may impair the osmoregulatory function of the endolymphatic sac, potentially triggering or exacerbating endolymphatic hydrops [44,45].

The AOX family plays a key role in maintaining the homeostasis of omega-3 polyunsaturated fatty acids (e.g., DHA), thereby regulating membrane fluidity and signal transduction in inner ear cells, as well as alleviating local inflammation [46].

Notably, chronic activation of the JAK-STAT pathway in MD may exacerbate cochlear damage by amplifying oxidative stress. For example, STAT3 promotes the expression of NADPH oxidase complexes, leading to elevated reactive oxygen species levels. In parallel, peroxidation byproducts of lipid metabolism, such as 4-hydroxy-2-nonenal, require detoxification via the AOX system. However, this detoxification process itself generates additional oxidative species, such as superoxide and hydrogen peroxide, thereby further increasing oxidative burden [47,48]. Excessive ROS accumulation compromises the cochlea's antioxidant defense mechanisms, resulting in mitochondrial DNA damage and structural impairment of stereocilia proteins in sensory hair cells—lesions that are strongly associated with the sensorineural hearing loss observed in MD [49]. Additionally, ROS can oxidatively modify JAK kinases and their negative regulatory factors, disrupting feedback inhibition, sustaining JAK-STAT activation, and forming a positive feedback loop between oxidative stress and inflammation.

Although this study focused on the JAK-STAT signaling pathway as a central regulatory axis, other highly enriched pathways identified in our analysis may also hold significant relevance. Previous research has suggested that genetic alterations in Toll-like receptor pathways and cytokine-related signaling—particularly involving interleukin-1β and tumor necrosis factor-α—are closely associated with the inflammatory processes observed in Meniere's disease [50,51]. These findings highlight the potential importance of broader immune and inflammatory networks beyond JAK-STAT signaling. In addition, both the observed therapeutic effects in the guinea pig model and the proposed mechanisms of XYN action should be further corroborated using independent human datasets.

This study also explored potential biomarkers in the blood of MD patients. Notably, ZBTB20 deficiency has been shown to significantly reduce the endocochlear potential, disrupt the high-potassium/low-sodium environment of the endolymph, and induce hydrops by impairing fluid homeostasis [52,53]. ZBTB20 also suppresses the differentiation of root cells and the spiral prominence in the lateral wall, thereby reducing the expression of ion and water transport proteins such as Na^+/K^+-ATPase and AQP4, exacerbating fluid accumulation. Additionally, ZBTB20 is involved in the suprachiasmatic nucleus-driven circadian rhythm, and its deficiency has been linked to circadian disruption and hearing loss [54]. In immune cells, ZBTB20 also regulates the NF-κB pathway, and its deficiency can contribute to chronic low-grade inflammation [55]. These findings suggest that blood-based biomarkers such as ZBTB20 may hold promise for the clinical diagnosis or early screening of MD.

Despite the promising findings presented in this study, several limitations should be acknowledged. Currently, there is a significant lack of fundamental research on MD, and data concerning the effects of XYN on human tissues or patients remain extremely limited. As a result, no suitable external datasets are presently available for independent validation of our findings. Future studies will aim to investigate the mechanistic basis and therapeutic relevance of XYN using human-derived tissues and well-characterized clinical samples.

4. Materials and Methods

4.1. Component Identification Results of XYN

Ultra-high performance liquid chromatography coupled with high-resolution mass spectrometry was employed for the chemical analysis. Chromatographic separation was carried out on a Waters ACQUITY UPLC BEH C18 column (100 mm × 2.1 mm, 1.7 μm; Dublin, Ireland) using a Vanquish UHPLC system (Thermo Scientific, Waltham, MA, USA) equipped with a binary gradient pump, autosampler, column oven, and diode array detector. The mobile phase consisted of acetonitrile (A) and 0.1% formic acid in water (B), with the following gradient program: 0–2 min, 95% B; 2–42 min, 95% to 10% B; 42–44 min, 10% B; 44–45 min, 10% to 95% B; 45–50 min, 95% B. The flow rate was set at 0.3 mL/min, the injection volume was 3 μL, and the column temperature was maintained at 35 °C.

Mass spectrometric detection was performed on a Q-Exactive Orbitrap quadrupole-Orbitrap mass spectrometer (Thermo Scientific, USA) equipped with a heated electrospray ionization source and controlled by Xcalibur 4.1 software. In positive ion mode, the spray voltage was 3.5 kV, with the ion source temperature set at 350 °C, capillary temperature at 300 °C, and the S-Lens RF level at 60 V. Sheath and auxiliary gas (nitrogen, >99.99%) were supplied at 40 and 20 arbitrary units, respectively. In negative ion mode, the spray voltage was 3.2 kV, with sheath and auxiliary gas flow rates adjusted to 35 and 10 units, respectively. Data were acquired in both full-scan (m/z 200–2000) and data-dependent MS/MS modes, with resolving powers of 70,000 for full scan and 17,500 for MS/MS. Fragmentation was achieved using higher-energy collisional dissociation with a normalized collision energy of 30 and stepped NCE of 50%.

For sample preparation, XYN were finely pulverized, and 1.0 g of powder was accurately weighed into a stoppered conical flask. Methanol (50 mL) was added, and the mixture was subjected to ultrasonic extraction for 40 min. After cooling, the extract was weighed again and adjusted with methanol to compensate for solvent loss. The solution was thoroughly mixed, filtered, and passed through a 0.22 μm microporous membrane prior to UHPLC-HRMS analysis.

4.2. *Experimental Animals*

Male albino Hartley guinea pigs, weighing 250 ± 10 g, were obtained from Beijing Fangyuan Yuan Breeding Facility (License No. SCXK [Beijing] 2020-0001; Animal Quality Certificate No. 110334241100018953). All experiments were conducted at the Laboratory Animal Center of Beijing University of Chinese Medicine (Facility License No. SCXK [Beijing] 2023-0011), with ethical approval granted by the Institutional Animal Care and Use Committee of the university (Approval No. BUCM-2024022707-1091).

Animals were housed under controlled environmental conditions: temperature 18–22 °C, relative humidity 40–60%, and a 12 h light/dark cycle. All procedures involving animal care and use were conducted in strict accordance with the Regulations for the Administration of Laboratory Animals (China), as well as the guidelines and requirements of the Animal Ethics Committee of Beijing University of Chinese Medicine.

4.3. *Pharmacodynamic Evaluation Based on Endolymphatic Hydrops Model*

4.3.1. Establishment of the Guinea Pig Endolymphatic Hydrops Model

Intraperitoneal injection of dDAVP induces endolymphatic hydrops, leading to clinical manifestations such as vertigo and hearing loss, with minimal invasiveness and high safety [56,57]. Systemic administration of dDAVP has been successfully employed to model endolymphatic hydrops in experimental animals including rats, mice, and guinea pigs [58].

The modeling agent dDAVP was prepared at doses of 4 μg/kg and 8 μg/kg to generate low- and high-concentration solutions at 0.04 μg/μL and 0.08 μg/μL, respectively. Solutions were stored at −20 °C until use.

After a 7-day acclimation period, guinea pigs were intraperitoneally injected with the low-concentration dDAVP solution at a dose of 1 mL/kg daily for 7 consecutive days, followed by the high-concentration dDAVP solution at the same dose for 3 consecutive days. This protocol was used to induce endolymphatic hydrops in the guinea pigs.

4.3.2. Behavioral Assessments

Behavioral performance of the guinea pigs was evaluated using several criteria, including general condition, auricular reflex, presence of nystagmus, and righting reflex. Scoring was performed according to the standards outlined in Table 5. Detailed scoring criteria are provided in the Table S3.

Table 5. Behavioral assessment criteria.

Score	0	1	2	3
General condition	Normal	Mild gait instability	Gait instability with weight loss	Severe gait instability, inability to move normally, weight loss
Auricular reflex	Strong	Marked	Mild	Absent
Nystagmus	Absent	Mild	Moderate-frequency, moderate-amplitude	High-frequency, large-amplitude
Righting reflex	Rapid	Impaired righting response	Difficulty righting	No righting response

4.3.3. Re-Grouping and Drug Administration

To account for individual variability among guinea pigs and subtle differences introduced during the modeling process, animals with successfully induced endolymphatic hydrops were re-grouped to balance baseline characteristics and ensure the scientific rigor and reliability of experimental outcomes. Each group (excluding the blank control group) was balanced in terms of weight, auricular reflex, nystagmus, and righting response to minimize bias caused by group-level deviations.

Animals were randomly assigned into six groups (n = 10 per group): model group, low-dose XYN group (0.9 g/kg), medium-dose XYN group (1.8 g/kg), high-dose XYN group (3.6 g/kg), positive control group treated with BHS (22.5 mg/kg), and blank control group. These dosing levels were preliminarily assessed in our pilot study, which indicated that they were well tolerated in guinea pigs without signs of distress or adverse effects. Drug or placebo treatments were administered once daily by oral gavage for 14 consecutive days. The blank and model groups received an equivalent volume of normal saline.

Following the treatment period, behavioral assessments were conducted as described in Section 4.3.2. Afterward, guinea pigs were anesthetized, and cochlear and renal tissues were harvested for subsequent analyses.

4.4. High-Throughput Sequencing and Bioinformatics Analysis

4.4.1. Transcriptomic and Proteomic Analysis

Total RNA was extracted from guinea pig cochlear tissue and used for transcriptome library preparation. The libraries were sequenced on the Illumina NovaSeq 6000 platform, generating 150 bp paired-end reads. Data obtained from the Illumina (or BGI) platform were subsequently used for bioinformatics analysis.

For proteomic analysis, total protein was extracted from cochlear tissues. Peptides from each sample were analyzed using an Orbitrap™ Astral™ mass spectrometer (Thermo Scientific) coupled with a Vanquish Neo liquid chromatography system (Thermo Scientific) in data-independent acquisition (DIA) mode. DIA data were processed using DIA-NN version 1.8.1.

Both transcriptomic and proteomic data were aligned to the reference genome Cavia porcellus (NCBI Genome Assembly mCavPor4.1, https://www.ncbi.nlm.nih.gov/datasets/genome/-GCF_034190915.1/, accessed on 5 November 2023).

For downstream proteomic analysis, raw expression values were log2-transformed with a + 1 offset and linearly scaled to the range of 1–100. Differential expression analysis for both mRNA and proteins was performed using the limma package in R. Differentially expressed genes and proteins were defined based on a threshold of $|\log_2$ fold change $(\log_2 FC)| > 1.5$ and $p < 0.05$, with multiple testing correction performed using the Benjamini–Hochberg method.

Gene Ontology (http://geneontology.org/, accessed on 5 March 2024) and Kyoto Encyclopedia of Genes and Genomes (https://www.kegg.jp/, accessed on 5 March 2024) enrichment analyses were carried out using the clusterProfiler package in R. Enrichment was performed against the background gene set from NCBI (GCF_034190915.1-RS_2024_02, https://www.ncbi.nlm.nih.gov/datasets/gene/GCF_034190915.1/, accessed on 5 November 2023). Biological categories with $p < 0.05$ were considered significantly enriched.

4.4.2. Integrated Omics Analysis

To comprehensively identify key molecular targets, DEGs and DEPs were merged and categorized into two molecular subsets: (1) molecules upregulated under pathological conditions and downregulated after pharmacological treatment, (2) molecules downregulated under pathological conditions and upregulated following treatment. These subsets were considered potential molecular targets of XYN in the intervention of MD.

Each of the two molecular subsets, as well as their combined set, was imported into the STRING database (https://cn.string-db.org/, accessed on 5 March 2024) for protein–protein interaction (PPI) analysis. A high-confidence interaction score threshold ($\geq$0.7) was applied, and isolated nodes were hidden to enhance interpretability. The resulting PPI networks were visualized using Cytoscape (version 3.9.1). To identify densely connected regions potentially representing functional protein complexes or signaling modules, the Molecular Complex Detection (MCODE) plugin was employed. MCODE clustering was performed across the entire network using the following parameters: Degree Cutoff = 2, Node Score Cutoff = 0.2, K-Core = 2, and Max Depth = 100. The Haircut option was enabled to eliminate singly connected peripheral nodes from clusters, while the Fluff option was disabled to maintain strict cluster boundaries. Loops were included in the analysis. Core candidate molecules were subsequently screened based on node degree and their presence within MCODE-defined subnetworks.

4.4.3. Analysis of Risk Factors for Meniere's Disease

This study conducted an analysis based on publicly available genome-wide association study (GWAS) datasets, strictly adhering to the STROBE-MR (Strengthening the Reporting of Observational Studies in Epidemiology Using MR) guidelines to ensure methodological rigor and reliability of results [54]. All data used were ethically approved and obtained with informed consent; no personal or identifiable information was involved.

A comprehensive search was conducted in the PubMed database for factors associated with the onset of MD, using keywords such as "Meniere's disease etiology" and "risk factors for Meniere's disease."

Inclusion criteria required articles to directly address the etiology, pathophysiology, or risk factors of MD. Eligible literature types included scientific papers that contribute to understanding MD's etiology, specifically original research articles, review articles, and pertinent case reports.

Exclusion criteria eliminated articles unrelated to MD etiology, including those focused exclusively on treatment, prognosis, or other otologic disorders, as well as case reports lacking substantial etiological insights. Additionally, low-quality studies—such as non-peer-reviewed articles, conference abstracts, studies with insufficient methodological rigor, and duplicate publications—were excluded.

To retrieve relevant GWAS data, we searched databases such as the Finnish Database, GWAS Catalog, and PubMed for studies on associated risk factors and collected data on potential exposure phenotypes and outcomes related to MD.

To comprehensively examine the relationship between exposure phenotypes and MD across all GWAS datasets, we applied a genome-wide significance threshold of 5×10^{-6}. The F-statistic for each SNP was calculated to assess instrument strength, excluding any SNPs with an F-statistic below 10 to mitigate weak instrument bias.

To address linkage disequilibrium (LD) among SNPs and enhance the robustness of the analysis, we utilized reference data from the 1000 Genomes Project (https://github.com/mrcieu/gwasvcf/, accessed on 10 August 2024) as the reference panel for PLINK, the selected tool for LD calculation. Parameters were set to a 10,000 kb distance between SNPs, an r threshold of 0.001, and p1 and p2 thresholds set to 1. After merging exposure and outcome data, palindromic SNPs were excluded, leaving the remaining SNPs as the final IVs.

All statistical analyses were conducted in R (version 4.4.1). The primary MR analysis method was inverse variance weighted (IVW), implemented using the TwoSampleMR package in R. IVW is a meta-analysis-based approach that combines the Wald ratios of individual SNPs by weighting them inversely to their variance, assuming all instruments are valid and there is no horizontal pleiotropy. Post-analysis, heterogeneity was assessed via Cochran's Q test, where a p-value above 0.05 suggests no heterogeneity among the IVs. Horizontal pleiotropy was evaluated with the MR-Egger method, and a leave-one-out approach was employed to assess whether causal effects were impacted by any individual SNP.

Results are reported as odds ratios (ORs) with 95% confidence intervals (CIs). In this study, p-values were interpreted as indicators of evidence strength, with statistical significance set at $p < 0.05$. Visualizations were created using the R packages ggplot2 and ComplexUpset.

4.4.4. Analysis of Blood Biomarkers in Meniere's Disease Patients

The Gene Expression Omnibus (GEO) database (https://www.ncbi.nlm.nih.gov/geo/, accessed on 10 August 2024) was queried using the keyword "Ménière disease," and studies involving human blood samples were selected and screened for relevance. Both miRNA and mRNA datasets underwent preprocessing to ensure data quality and suitability for analysis.

Initial preprocessing steps included the removal of entries with missing values or duplicate data points. Subsequently, the data were normalized to bring all variables within a comparable range, facilitating reliable downstream analyses. Genes with missing expression values or duplicates were removed from the expression matrix, and those with expression levels below 5 were filtered out.

Differential expression analysis of miRNAs and mRNAs was performed using the limma package in R. Significant differentially expressed molecules were identified based on the criteria $|\log_2$ fold change $(\log_2 FC)| > 1.0$ and adjusted $p < 0.05$, with p-values corrected using the Benjamini–Hochberg method.

Target mRNAs regulated by differentially expressed miRNAs were predicted using the miRDB (https://mirdb.org/, accessed on 15 August 2024) and miRWALK (http://mirwalk.umm.uni-heidelberg.de/, accessed on 15 August 2024) databases. The intersection of predicted targets was defined as core mRNAs implicated in MD pathogenesis. These core mRNAs were then used to construct a miRNA–mRNA regulatory network associated with MD, visualized using Cytoscape.

4.5. Molecular Biology Experiments

To validate the expression of the key pathways and core molecules identified in the preceding analyses, RT-qPCR and Western blot assays were performed.

For RT-qPCR, total RNA was reverse transcribed using the ReverTra Ace qPCR RT Kit. The resulting cDNA was mixed with DEPC-treated water, target gene primers, and SYBR Green reagent to prepare a 10 μL reaction system. Amplification was carried out using a three-step PCR protocol, followed by analysis of melting and amplification curves. Relative expression levels of target genes were calculated using the $2^{-\Delta\Delta Ct}$ method.

For Western blotting, total protein concentrations in each group were quantified using the BCA assay and adjusted to uniform levels with PBS. Protein samples were separated on 10% SDS-PAGE gels, loaded by group, and transferred to NC membranes using a wet-transfer sandwich method. Membranes were blocked with BSA at room temperature for 1.5 h, then incubated with primary antibodies overnight at 4 °C. After washing with TBST five times, membranes were incubated with secondary antibodies at room temperature for

1.5 h, followed by another five washes with TBST. Protein bands were visualized using ECL detection reagents on a chemiluminescent imaging system.

Band intensities were quantified using ImageJ software 1.50i. The relative expression of target proteins was calculated as the ratio of the target protein band intensity to that of the internal reference protein.

4.6. Statistical Analysis

All statistical analyses were conducted using R software (version 4.4.1). For MR, the primary analytical method employed was IVW analysis, implemented via the TwoSampleMR package. To assess the reliability of the causal estimates, Cochran's Q test was used to evaluate heterogeneity among IVs, with $p > 0.05$ indicating no significant heterogeneity.

MR-Egger regression was applied to detect horizontal pleiotropy, and leave-one-out sensitivity analysis was used to determine whether the causal effect estimates were unduly influenced by any single SNP. Results were presented as odds ratios with 95% confidence intervals, and statistical significance was set at $p < 0.05$.

Data visualization was performed using the ggplot2 package in R to intuitively display the analytical outcomes. Quantitative results were expressed as the mean ± standard error of the mean. One-way ANOVA followed by Tukey's multiple comparison test was used to analyze differences among multiple groups.

5. Conclusions

This study, for the first time, systematically integrates transcriptomics, proteomics, animal experiments, and bioinformatics approaches to investigate the pathogenesis of MD and elucidate the therapeutic mechanisms of XYN from the perspective of molecular interaction networks. As shown in Figure 11, XYN administration alleviated endolymphatic hydrops in guinea pig models, accompanied by improvements in behavioral abnormalities such as vertigo and hearing loss, as confirmed by functional assessments and cochlear histopathology. Multi-omics and mechanistic analyses revealed dysregulation of several signaling pathways in MD, among which aberrant activation of the JAK-STAT pathway plays a central role by promoting a vicious cycle of inflammation, metabolic dysfunction, and oxidative stress. XYN intervention was shown to disrupt this pathological loop, thereby mitigating MD symptoms. ZBTB20 and other identified molecules emerged as potential blood-based biomarkers for the diagnosis and monitoring of MD.

In summary, these findings provide both experimental and theoretical support for the clinical application of XYN in MD treatment and contribute to the development of novel therapeutic strategies. Moreover, this integrative research framework offers valuable insights for exploring the role of traditional Chinese medicine in managing refractory and multifactorial diseases.

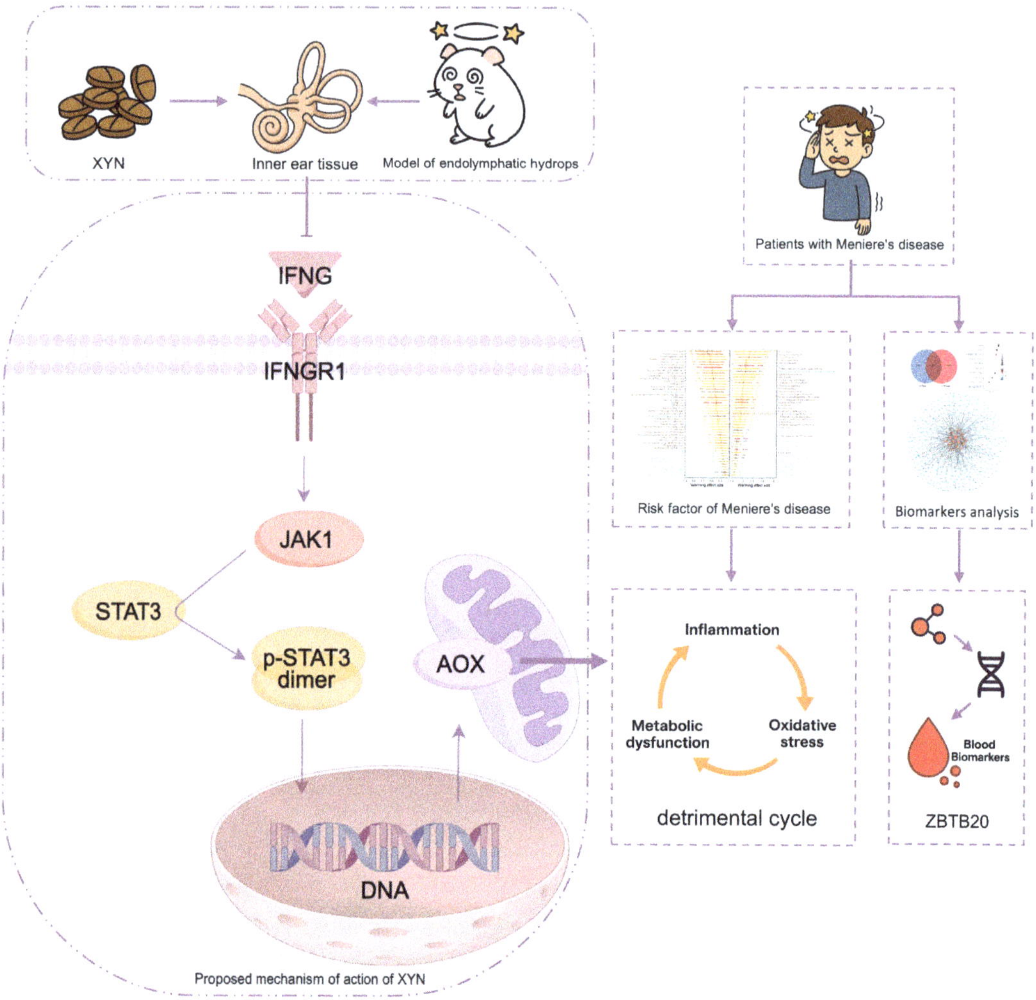

Figure 11. Schematic overview of the therapeutic mechanism of XYN and omics-based insights in MD. * $p < 0.05$, ** $p < 0.01$, *** $p < 0.001$.

Supplementary Materials: The following supporting information can be downloaded at https://www.mdpi.com/article/10.3390/ph18091266/s1, Table S1: Component Identification Results of XYN in Positive Ion Mode; Table S2: Potential Related Phenotypes of MD; Table S3: Scoring Criteria of Behavioral Assessments; Figure S1: Body weight and behavioral scores of guinea pigs in each group after regrouping; Figure S2: GO Enrichment Analysis of Differentially Expressed Genes; Figure S3: KEGG Enrichment Analysis of Differentially Expressed Genes; Figure S4: GO Enrichment Analysis of Differentially Expressed Proteins; Figure S5: KEGG Enrichment Analysis of Differentially Expressed Proteins.

Author Contributions: Data curation, Z.J.; funding acquisition, H.C., C.L., and X.Z.; methodology, Z.J., C.W. (Chao Wu), K.C., and C.W. (Chunguo Wang); project administration, J.W.; supervision, X.Z.; validation, Z.J., Y.G., X.T., S.G., J.H., J.Z., C.Q., and C.W. (Chunguo Wang); visualization, Z.J.; writing—original draft, Z.J., X.Z., and C.W. (Chunguo Wang); writing—review and editing, Z.J., Y.G., X.T., C.W. (Chao Wu), S.G., J.H., J.Z., C.Q., K.C., H.C., C.L., X.Z., and J.W. All authors have read and agreed to the published version of the manuscript.

Funding: This research was supported by Guilin Sanjin Pharmaceutical Co., Ltd. (Project No. BUCM-2023-JS-FW-060).

Institutional Review Board Statement: The animal study protocol was approved by the Institutional Animal Care and Use Committee of Beijing University of Chinese Medicine (Approval No. BUCM-2024022707-1091, approved on 27 February 2024). All experiments were conducted at the Laboratory Animal Center of Beijing University of Chinese Medicine (Facility License No. SCXK [Beijing] 2023-0011).

Informed Consent Statement: Not applicable.

Data Availability Statement: The data in this study were obtained from open public databases, and all relevant data are freely accessible on the respective websites.

Acknowledgments: The authors would like to thank the researchers who provided open access to the raw data.

Conflicts of Interest: The authors whose names are listed immediately below certify that they have NO conflicts of interest to declare: Zhengsen Jin, Chunguo Wang, Yifei Gao, Xiaoyu Tao, Chao Wu, Siyu Guo, Jiaqi Huang, Jiying Zhou, Chuanqi Qiao, Keyan Chai, and Jiarui Wu. Hua Chang, Chun Li, and Xun Zou are full-time employees of Guilin Sanjin Pharmaceutical Co., Ltd., which manufactures XuanYunNing tablets. The company contributed to the study by supplying the investigational drug, providing financial support, and sharing relevant proprietary information about the product. These authors were not involved in data analysis or interpretation to avoid potential bias.

Abbreviations

AQP	Aquaporin
AVP	Arginine vasopressin
BHS	Betahistine
CNN	Convolutional neural network
dDAVP	Diamino-Cys1, D-Arg8-vasopressin
DEGs	Differentially expressed genes
DEPs	Differentially expressed proteins
GWAS	Genome-wide association studies
IV	Instrumental variable
IVW	Inverse-variance weighted
LD	Linkage disequilibrium
MD	Ménière disease
MCODE	Molecular complex detection
MR	Mendelian randomization
OCSVM	One-class support vector machine
PBS	Phosphate-buffered saline
RT-qPCR	Real-time quantitative PCR
SNP	Single nucleotide polymorphism
TCM	Traditional Chinese medicine
WB	Western blot

References

1. "Meniere's Disease—Symptoms and Causes." Mayo Clinic. Available online: https://www.mayoclinic.org/diseases-conditions/menieres-disease/symptoms-causes/syc-20374910 (accessed on 22 November 2023).
2. "Meniere's Disease." American Hearing Research Foundation. Available online: https://www.american-hearing.org/disease/menieres-disease/ (accessed on 22 November 2023).
3. Ma, H.; Zhong, S.; Wen, Y. Regulatory Effect of Acetic Desmopressin on the Expression of Aquaporin-2 in the Cochlea of Guinea Pigs. *J. Audiol. Speech Pathol.* **2014**, *22*, 286–289.
4. Perez-Carpena, P.; Lopez-Escamez, J.A. Current Understanding and Clinical Management of Meniere's Disease: A Systematic Review. *Semin. Neurol.* **2019**, *40*, 138–150. [CrossRef]

5. Kwon, M.J.; Kang, H.S.; Kim, J.; Kim, J.H.; Bang, W.J.; Yoo, D.M.; Lee, N.-E.; Han, K.M.; Kim, N.Y.; Choi, H.G.; et al. Epidemiological Evidence for Upper Respiratory Infections as a Potential Risk Factor for Meniere's Disease: A Korean National Health Sample Cohort Study. *Microorganisms* **2024**, *12*, 2047. [CrossRef]
6. Alexander, T.H.; Harris, J.P. Current Epidemiology of Meniere's Syndrome. *Otolaryngol. Clin. N. Am.* **2010**, *43*, 965–970. [CrossRef]
7. Koenen, L.; Andaloro, C. Meniere Disease. In *StatPearls*; StatPearls Publishing: Treasure Island, FL, USA, 2023.
8. Basura, G.J.; Adams, M.E.; Monfared, A.; Schwartz, S.R.; Antonelli, P.J.; Burkard, R.; Bush, M.L.; Bykowski, J.; Colandrea, M.; Derebery, J.; et al. Clinical Practice Guideline: Ménière's Disease. *Otolaryngol. —Head Neck Surg.* **2020**, *162* (Suppl. S2), S1–S55. [CrossRef]
9. Adrion, C.; Fischer, C.S.; Wagner, J.; Gürkov, R.; Mansmann, U.; Strupp, M.; BEMED Study Group. Efficacy and Safety of Betahistine Treatment in Patients with Meniere's Disease: Primary Results of a Long-Term, Multicentre, Double-Blind, Randomised, Placebo-Controlled, Dose-Defining Trial (BEMED Trial). *Br. Med. Assoc.* **2016**, *352*, h6816. [CrossRef]
10. Esch, B.V.; Zaag-Loonen, H.V.D.; Bruintjes, T.; van Benthem, P.P. Betahistine in Ménière's Disease or Syndrome: A Systematic Review. *Audiol. Neurotol.* **2022**, *27*, 1–33. [CrossRef]
11. Rosenbaum, A.; Winter, M. Is Betahistine Effective for Ménière's Disease? *Medwave* **2017**, *17*, e7068. [CrossRef] [PubMed]
12. Zhang, P.; Zhang, D.; Zhou, W.; Wang, L.; Wang, B.; Zhang, T.; Li, S. Network pharmacology: Towards the artificial intelligence-based precision traditional Chinese medicine. *Brief. Bioinform.* **2023**, *25*, bbad518. [CrossRef] [PubMed]
13. Liu, Y.; Ren, Y.; Song, P. Traditional Chinese medicine for intractable and rare diseases: Research progress and future strategies. *Intractable Rare Dis. Res.* **2025**, *14*, 109–121. [CrossRef] [PubMed]
14. Zhao, S.; Ning, J.; Liu, D.; Yang, M. Clinical Study on Treating 120 Cases of Meniere's Disease with XYN. *China Med. Her.* **2012**, *10*, 611–613.
15. Wang, Z. Efficacy Analysis of XYN Decoction in Treating 200 Cases of Meniere's Disease. *Hebei J. Tradit. Chin. Med.* **1996**, 7–8. Available online: https://kns.cnki.net/kcms2/article/abstract?v=QUtgg5W7F1-o_g7KacxiiNnCXc20HBS_LCLGP4hYvJnmpdqV0UlYmLh-5qgZpMxOheNkzmC0Zn6FipoyiJfU68dZChYEz4pFsV8v124MbjKd6SGYn9V8DzM7QyGihFesk0iU_5EuVv44bRCwXgiROHVIhRPf1nVpfwYfbl2h2iM=&uniplatform=NZKPT&language=CHS (accessed on 1 May 2025).
16. Shi, Y. Observation of the Efficacy of XYN in Treating Vertigo Caused by Meniere's Disease. *Chin. Community Dr. Med.* **2010**, *12*, 124.
17. Wu, Z.; Wang, X.; Zhang, Y.; Yuan, J.J.; Wu, W.; Dong, Z.J.; Hong, Q.Y.; Su, Y.T.; Xin, Z.H.; Yan, Z.F.; et al. Research Review on the Advantages of Traditional Chinese Medicine in Treating Aural Vertigo and Meniere's Disease. *Chin. J. Exp. Tradit. Med. Formulae* **2023**, *29*, 196–203.
18. Zhai, Y. Treatment of 36 Cases of Meniere's Disease with XYN Tablets. *Guangming J. Chin. Med.* **2009**, *24*, 862–863.
19. Gu, H. Treatment of 72 Cases of Meniere's Syndrome with XYN Tablets. *Clin. Res. Tradit. Chin. Med.* **2011**, *3*, 97–99.
20. Luo, Y.; Tang, X.; Zhou, H.; Liu, T.; Zhong, S.J. Analysis of TCM Syndrome Patterns in 632 Emergency Patients with Vertigo. *New Chin. Med.* **2002**, 29–30.
21. Fu, M.; He, W. Exploring the Treatment of Meniere's Disease from the Perspective of Spleen and Stomach Theory. *China Med. Her.* **2020**, *17*, 149–152, 172.
22. Zhang, W.; Zhang, Y.; Huo, D. TCM Differentiation and Treatment During the Attack Phase of Meniere's Disease. *Jilin J. Tradit. Chin. Med.* **2009**, *29*, 571–572.
23. Li, T.; Leng, H. Exploring the Etiology and Treatment of Meniere's Disease Based on the "Phlegm-Retention Causing Dizziness" Theory. *Pract. J. Tradit. Chin. Intern. Med.* **2022**, *36*, 88–91.
24. Wang, Y.; Zhao, Y. Overview of Commonly Used Oral Chinese Patent Medicines for Treating Vertigo. *Mod. Distance Educ. Chin. Tradit. Med.* **2016**, *14*, 143–145.
25. Ding, Y. Clinical Study on XYN in Treating Meniere's Disease. *China Mod. Dr.* **2010**, *48*, 149–150.
26. Li, Y.; Li, Q.; Zhu, Y.; Huang, C.; Li, H.; Deng, Z.; Xu, C.; Wang, W.; Chen, L.; Zhang, S.; et al. Medicinal Plant-Derived Carbon Dots Nanozymes Ameliorate Ulcerative Colitis via Anti-inflammatory, Antioxidant, and Gut Barrier-Protective Effects. *ACS Appl. Mater. Interfaces* **2025**, *17*, 42751–42766. [CrossRef]
27. Ullah, A.; Sun, Q.; Li, J.; Li, J.; Khatun, P.; Kou, G.; Lyu, Q. Bioactive Compounds in Citrus reticulata Peel Are Potential Candidates for Alleviating Physical Fatigue through a Triad Approach of Network Pharmacology, Molecular Docking, and Molecular Dynamics Modeling. *Nutrients* **2024**, *16*, 1934. [CrossRef]
28. Wang, Y.; Lu, C.; Huang, H.; Yao, S.; Xu, C.; Ye, Y.; Gui, S.; Li, G. A lipid-soluble extract of Pinellia pedatisecta Schott orchestrates intratumoral dendritic cell-driven immune activation through SOCS1 signaling in cervical cancer. *J. Ethnopharmacol.* **2021**, *267*, 112837. [CrossRef]
29. Huang, Q.; Yin, S. Research Progress on the Relationship Between Sodium Channels, Aquaporins in Inner Ear Epithelium and Endolymph Metabolism. *J. Otolaryngol. Ophthalmol. Shandong Univ.* **2019**, *33*, 145–148.

30. Tan, C.; Cao, Y.; Liu, H.; Zhu, J.; He, X.; Du, C.; Zhou, M. Study on Immune-Related Factors in Meniere's Disease. *J. Clin. Otorhinolaryngol.* **1998**, 208–210. Available online: https://kns.cnki.net/kcms2/article/abstract?v=QUtgg5W7F18cQxpAgp1u6W3b1cob5s2YJC8bkhFPYQ9sNNnsSBjfQiOd6jNKHCoGksBX33yUl-qawNWB3AAu06uFhX2sXvFbYNcixIVIrx-VnMBdg7r8BlHbDn-TIgh1vumY6dXNeFa79xTgzdjVuavRxP1dfCOG_Z-41nbcNbTz2K1Et3AN85lNDCNj5ySxHJFrZmcHMMhad7rusOwf62ePm-ndVK5S-wk7q0599b4=&uniplatform=NZKPT (accessed on 1 May 2025).
31. Lee, A.; Webster, K.E.; George, B.; Harrington-Benton, N.A.; Judd, O.; Kaski, D.; Maarsingh, O.R.; MacKeith, S.; Ray, J.; Van Vugt, V.A. Surgical Interventions for Ménière's Disease. *Cochrane Database Syst. Rev.* **2023**, *2*, CD015249. [CrossRef]
32. Mohseni-Dargah, M.; Falahati, Z.; Pastras, C.; Khajeh, K.; Mukherjee, P.; Razmjou, A.; Stefani, S.; Asadnia, M. Meniere's Disease: Pathogenesis, Treatments, and Emerging Approaches for an Idiopathic Bioenvironmental Disorder. *Environ. Res.* **2023**, *238 Pt 1*, 116972. [CrossRef] [PubMed]
33. Sajjadi, H.; Paparella, M.M. Meniere's Disease. *Lancet* **2008**, *372*, 406–414. [CrossRef]
34. Burgess, S.; Butterworth, A.; Malarstig, A.; Thompson, S.G. Use of Mendelian Randomisation to Assess Potential Benefit of Clinical Intervention. *BMJ Clin. Res. Ed.* **2012**, *345*, e7325.
35. Skrivankova, V.W.; Richmond, R.C.; Woolf, B.A.R.; Davies, N.M.; Swanson, S.A.; VanderWeele, T.J.; Timpson, N.J.; Higgins, J.P.T.; Dimou, N.; Langenberg, C.; et al. Strengthening the Reporting of Observational Studies in Epidemiology Using Mendelian Randomisation (STROBE-MR): Explanation and Elaboration. *BMJ Clin. Res. Ed.* **2021**, *375*, n2233. [CrossRef]
36. Darnell, J.E.; Kerr, I.M.; Stark, G.R. Jak-STAT Pathways and Transcriptional Activation in Response to IFNs and Other Extracellular Signaling Proteins. *Science* **1994**, *264*, 1415–1421. [CrossRef]
37. Xue, C.; Yao, Q.; Gu, X.; Shi, Q.; Yuan, X.; Chu, Q.; Bao, Z.; Lu, J.; Li, L. Evolving Cognition of the JAK-STAT Signaling Pathway: Autoimmune Disorders and Cancer. *Signal Transduct. Target. Ther.* **2023**, *8*, 204. [CrossRef]
38. Mahjoor, M.; Mahmoudvand, G.; Farokhi, S.; Shadab, A.; Kashfi, M.; Afkhami, H. Double-Edged Sword of JAK/STAT Signaling Pathway in Viral Infections: Novel Insights into Virotherapy. *Cell Commun. Signal.* **2023**, *21*, 272. [CrossRef]
39. Xia, T.; Fu, S.; Yang, R.; Yang, K.; Lei, W.; Yang, Y.; Zhang, Q.; Zhao, Y.; Yu, J.; Yu, L.; et al. Advances in the Study of Macrophage Polarization in Inflammatory Immune Skin Diseases. *J. Inflamm.* **2023**, *20*, 33. [CrossRef]
40. Sarapultsev, A.; Gusev, E.; Komelkova, M.; Utepova, I.; Luo, S.; Hu, D. JAK-STAT Signaling in Inflammation and Stress-Related Diseases: Implications for Therapeutic Interventions. *Mol. Biomed.* **2023**, *4*, 40. [CrossRef] [PubMed]
41. Ding, Q.; Hu, W.; Wang, R.; Yang, Q.; Zhu, M.; Li, M.; Cai, J.; Rose, P.; Mao, J.; Zhu, Y.Z. Signaling Pathways in Rheumatoid Arthritis: Implications for Targeted Therapy. *Signal Transduct. Target. Ther.* **2023**, *8*, 68. [CrossRef] [PubMed]
42. He, W.; Mu, X.; Wu, X.; Liu, Y.; Deng, J.; Liu, Y.; Han, F.; Nie, X. The cGAS-STING Pathway: A Therapeutic Target in Diabetes and Its Complications. *Burn. Trauma* **2024**, *12*, tkad050. [CrossRef] [PubMed]
43. Decout, A.; Katz, J.D.; Venkatraman, S.; Ablasser, A. The cGAS–STING Pathway as a Therapeutic Target in Inflammatory Diseases. *Nat. Rev. Immunol.* **2021**, *21*, 548–569. [CrossRef] [PubMed]
44. Zatterale, F.; Longo, M.; Naderi, J.; Raciti, G.A.; Desiderio, A.; Miele, C.; Beguinot, F. Chronic Adipose Tissue Inflammation Linking Obesity to Insulin Resistance and Type 2 Diabetes. *Front. Physiol.* **2019**, *10*, 1607. [CrossRef]
45. Lu, D.; He, A.; Tan, M.; Mrad, M.; El Daibani, A.; Hu, D.; Liu, X.; Kleiboeker, B.; Che, T.; Hsu, F.F.; et al. Liver ACOX1 Regulates Levels of Circulating Lipids That Promote Metabolic Health Through Adipose Remodeling. *Nat. Commun.* **2024**, *15*, 4214. [CrossRef]
46. Albernaz, P.L.M. Menière's Disease and Disorders of the Carbohydrate Metabolism Involving the Inner Ear. *Int. Arch. Otorhinolaryngol.* **2019**, *23*, 218–220. [CrossRef]
47. Rossmeisl, M.; Jilkova, Z.M.; Kuda, O.; Jelenik, T.; Medrikova, D.; Stankova, B.; Kristinsson, B.; Haraldsson, G.G.; Svensen, H.; Stoknes, I.; et al. Metabolic Effects of n-3 PUFA as Phospholipids Are Superior to Triglycerides in Mice Fed a High-Fat Diet: Possible Role of Endocannabinoids. *PLoS ONE* **2012**, *7*, e38834. [CrossRef]
48. Marchitti, S.A.; Brocker, C.; Stagos, D.; Vasiliou, V. Non-P450 Aldehyde Oxidizing Enzymes: The Aldehyde Dehydrogenase Superfamily. *Expert Opin. Drug Metab. Toxicol.* **2008**, *4*, 697–720. [CrossRef]
49. Terao, M.; Garattini, E.; Romão, M.J.; Leimkühler, S. Evolution, Expression, and Substrate Specificities of Aldehyde Oxidase Enzymes in Eukaryotes. *J. Biol. Chem.* **2020**, *295*, 5377–5389. [CrossRef]
50. Yang, M.; Wu, C.; Lin, Y.; Tsai, M.; Hwang, C.; Yang, C. Dissecting the Circadian Clock and Toll-like Receptor Gene Alterations in Meniere's Disease and Vestibular Migraine. *Otolaryngol.—Head Neck Surg.* **2025**, *172*, 999–1005. [CrossRef] [PubMed]
51. Frejo, L.; Lopez-Escamez, J.A. Cytokines and Inflammation in Meniere Disease. *Clin. Exp. Otorhinolaryngol.* **2022**, *15*, 49–59. [CrossRef] [PubMed]
52. Teraoka, M.; Hato, N.; Inufusa, H.; You, F. Role of Oxidative Stress in Sensorineural Hearing Loss. *Int. J. Mol. Sci.* **2024**, *25*, 4146. [CrossRef] [PubMed]
53. Xie, Z.; Ma, X.H.; Bai, Q.F.; Tang, J.; Sun, J.H.; Jiang, F.; Guo, W.; Wang, C.M.; Yang, R.; Wen, Y.C.; et al. ZBTB20 is Essential for Cochlear Maturation and Hearing in Mice. *Proc. Natl. Acad. Sci. USA* **2023**, *120*, e2220867120. [CrossRef]

54. Salt, A.N.; Plontke, S.K. Endolymphatic Hydrops: Pathophysiology and Experimental Models. *Otolaryngol. Clin. N. Am.* **2010**, *43*, 971–983. [CrossRef]
55. Liu, X.; Zhang, P.; Bao, Y.; Han, Y.; Wang, Y.; Zhang, Q.; Zhan, Z.; Meng, J.; Li, Y.; Li, N. Zinc Finger Protein ZBTB20 Promotes Toll-like Receptor-Triggered Innate Immune Responses by Repressing IκBα Gene Transcription. *Proc. Natl. Acad. Sci. USA* **2013**, *110*, 11097–11102. [CrossRef]
56. Seo, Y.J.; Brown, D. Experimental Animal Models for Meniere's Disease: A Mini-Review. *J. Audiol. Otol.* **2020**, *24*, 53–60. [CrossRef] [PubMed]
57. Kakigi, A.; Egami, N.; Uehara, N.; Fujita, T.; Nibu, K.I.; Yamashita, S.; Yamasoba, T. Live imaging and functional changes of the inner ear in an animal model of Meniere's disease. *Sci. Rep.* **2020**, *10*, 12271. [CrossRef] [PubMed]
58. Meddens, S.F.W.; de Vlaming, R.; Bowers, P.; Burik, C.A.P.; Linnér, R.K.; Lee, C.; Okbay, A.; Turley, P.; Rietveld, C.A.; Fontana, M.A.; et al. Genomic Analysis of Diet Composition Finds Novel Loci and Associations with Health and Lifestyle. *Mol. Psychiatry* **2021**, *26*, 2056–2069. [CrossRef] [PubMed]

pharmaceuticals

MDPI

Article

Network Pharmacology and Machine Learning Identify Flavonoids as Potential Senotherapeutics

Jose Alberto Santiago-de-la-Cruz [1,2], Nadia Alejandra Rivero-Segura [1], María Elizbeth Alvarez-Sánchez [2] and Juan Carlos Gomez-Verjan [1,*]

1 Dirección de Investigación, Instituto Nacional Geriatría (INGER), Mexico City 10200, Mexico; alberto.santiago@alumnos.uacm.edu.mx (J.A.S.-d.-l.-C.); nrivero@inger.gob.mx (N.A.R.-S.)

2 Posgrado en Ciencias Genómicas, Universidad Autónoma de la Ciudad de México, San Lorenzo 290, Col. Del Valle, Mexico City 03100, Mexico; maria.alvarez@uacm.edu.mx

* Correspondence: jverjan@inger.gob.mx; Tel.: +52-55738601 (ext. 54521)

Abstract: Background/Objectives: Cellular senescence is characterised by irreversible cell cycle arrest and the secretion of a proinflammatory phenotype. In recent years, senescent cell accumulation and senescence-associated secretory phenotype (SASP) secretion have been linked to the onset of chronic degenerative diseases associated with ageing. In this context, the senotherapeutic compounds have emerged as promising drugs that specifically eliminate senescent cells (senolytics) or diminish the damage caused by SASP (senomorphics). On the other hand, computational approaches, such as network pharmacology and machine learning, have revolutionised the identification of novel drugs. These tools enable the analysis of large volumes of compounds and the optimisation of the search for the most promising ones as potential drugs. Therefore, we employed such approaches in the present study to identify potential senotherapeutic compounds. **Methods:** First, we constructed drug-protein interaction networks related to cellular senescence. Then, using three machine learning models (Random Forest, Support Vector Machine, and K-Nearest Neighbours), we classified these compounds based on their therapeutic potential against senescence. **Results:** Our results enabled us to identify 714 compounds with potential senescent therapeutic activity, of which 270 exhibited desirable medicinal chemistry properties, and we developed an interactive web tool freely accessible to the scientific community. **Conclusions:** we found that flavonoids were the most abundant compound class from which 18 have never been reported as senotherapeutics.

Keywords: senescence; flavonoids; network pharmacology; machine learning; ageing

1. Introduction

Cellular senescence is an irreversible state of proliferative arrest characterised by various morphological, biochemical, and genetic changes [1]. In this sense, although senescence initially contributes to developmental processes of tissue repair, regeneration, and immune surveillance, it also induces detrimental effects in the organism, contributing to the development of the most common age-related diseases. Moreover, senescent cells secrete numerous factors, collectively referred to as the senescence-associated secretory phenotype (SASP), which includes proinflammatory cytokines, chemokines, proteases, and inhibitory molecules [2]. The molecular mechanisms leading to cellular senescence are diverse and complex, encompassing DNA damage, telomeric shortening, oncogene activation, mutation accumulation, increased reactive oxygen species (ROS), and mitochondrial dysfunction [3].

The dysfunction in senescent cells (SCs) elimination intensifies with age, leading to their tissue accumulation and increased senescence-associated secretory phenotype (SASP), which perpetuates molecular damage in a feedback loop that accelerates ageing [4,5]. Concomitantly, immunosenescence, the decline of the immune system in number and function, reduces the number and activity of immune cells, weakening the recognition and elimination of SCs through NK cells, macrophages, and cytotoxic T lymphocytes [6]. Simultaneously, accumulated SCs secrete pro-inflammatory cytokines, chemokines, and growth factors that contribute to the chronic low-grade inflammatory state (inflammaging), further deteriorating immune function and creating a vicious cycle between cellular senescence and immunosenescence [7]. They are also linked to neurodegenerative and cardiovascular diseases, as well as some types of cancer [8]. This bidirectional interaction not only accelerates the ageing process but also increases susceptibility to age-related diseases, underscoring the critical importance of developing geroprotective therapies that can disrupt these interconnected pathological mechanisms [9].

In recent years, senotherapy has emerged as a promising pharmacological strategy for healthy ageing [9,10], focusing on two main strategies: senolytics, which eliminate senescent cells, and senomorphics, which inhibit the adverse effects of SASP [11,12]. Among the most studied senotherapeutics are metformin [13], navitoclax [14], quercetin, and dasatinib [15]. However, only a combination of dasatinib and quercetin has reached clinical trials [16,17].

The development of senotherapeutic drugs faces significant challenges due to the specificity and potential toxicity in non-senescent cells [18]. To address these limitations, current research is focusing on two innovative approaches: network pharmacology [19] and machine learning (ML) [20]. Network pharmacology is an approach that uses systems biology to identify and predict multiple drug targets in complex treatments, focusing on interactions within signalling networks [20]. In contrast, machine learning is a fundamental branch of artificial intelligence, which seeks to develop algorithms and models that enable computer systems to learn from data, optimising their performance, such as category classification or regression [21]. Interestingly, in recent years, both network pharmacology and machine learning have been applied for target identification, drug discovery and optimisation, predicting drug-target interactions, and virtual screening of vast libraries of chemical compounds to identify promising candidates before they are synthesised and tested [22–25]. In this context, previous studies reported the use of chemoinformatics analysis based on chemical descriptors and pharmacokinetic properties to identify a set of natural compounds as candidates against cellular senescence [9]; nevertheless, many of the targets of these identified drugs have not yet been fully explored, meaning that other putative senolytics identified through fingerprint analysis, but not selected in this study, might also exhibit senolytic activity due to their structural similarity. Besides, they only restrict the use of network pharmacology for the identification of potential senolytic candidates, increasing the bias in the results. Conversely, Smer-Barreto et al. employed machine learning techniques to identify three senolytics—ginkgetin, oleandrin, and periplocin—which were validated in vitro [20]. However, the study notes that oleandrin is cardiotoxic and that further studies are required to ensure the safety of such compounds. This limitation arises from the fact that the authors focused solely on using machine learning algorithms to identify potential senolytic compounds, disregarding relevant pharmacological properties. Another limitation of the study is the class imbalance in the training data, with non-senolytics (negative) overrepresented relative to senolytics (positive), which leads to inflated performance metrics. Overall, this evidence suggests that using both tools together could be a novel strategy for accelerating drug discovery and developing new therapies that could improve quality of life during ageing by reducing the number of experiments required and enhancing the types of molecules screened. Therefore, the present study aims to identify chemical compounds with potential senotherapeutic activity by combining network pharmacology and supervised machine learning approaches.

2. Results

We mapped 249 proteins involved in cellular senescence that were imported into CTD to obtain gene-compound interactions. Once we eliminated redundancy and non-human species, we found that 65,339 compounds interact with proteins related to cellular senescence (Figure 1). The interactome represents proteins or chemical compounds as nodes, while the edges represent the interactions between these nodes, with all edges having the same weight. The largest nodes are key proteins or compounds that act as hubs within the interaction network, including p53, ERK2, ERK1, TGF-β1, IL-6, AKT1, mTOR, cyclin D1, and p21; additionally, Resveratrol, Quercetin, Curcumin, Doxorubicin, Cisplatin, and Azoles were also detected.

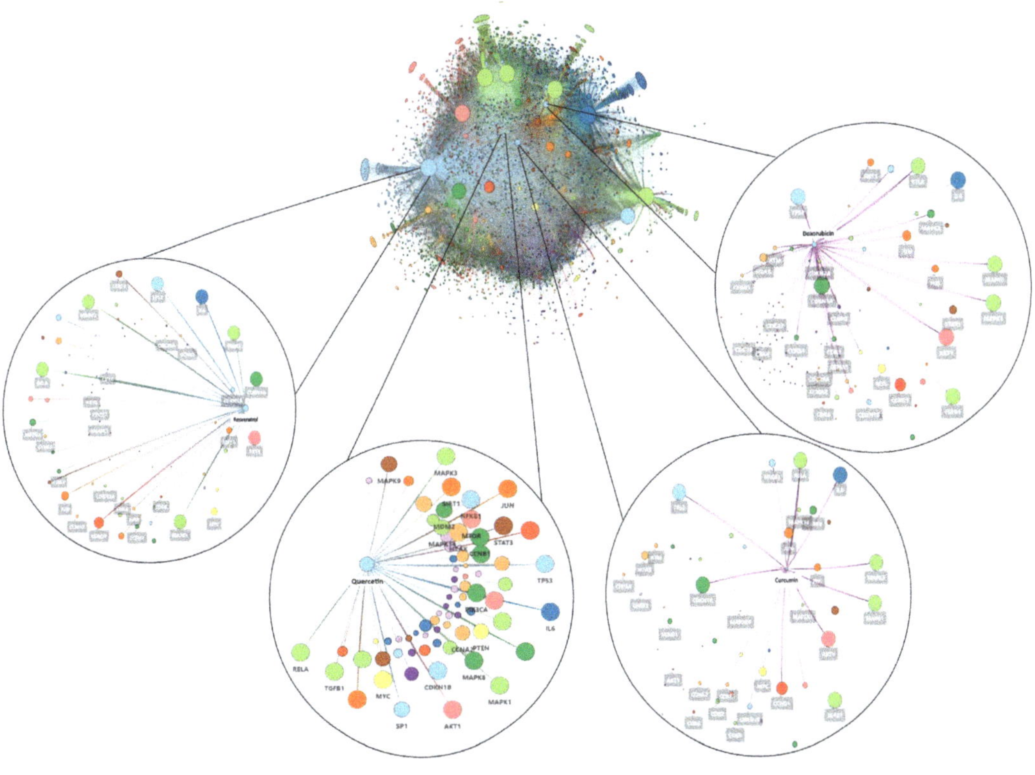

Figure 1. Drug-protein senescence interactome. The interactome shows the connections between the chemical compounds (65,339) and the 249 proteins associated with senescence. Nodes represent proteins and chemicals. The colour of the nodes is random. The edges indicate the different interactions between chemicals and proteins as reported by CTD without any size. The size of the nodes is approximately proportional to their degree value.

Subsequently, we identify the SMILES of 54,401 compounds out of 65,339 total compounds, for which 39 molecular descriptors were calculated, as described in the methods section. The RF, SVM, and KNN models were evaluated using the metrics accuracy, specificity, precision, Recall, F1-score, and Kappa value (Table 1).

Table 1. Results from three ML classifier models. Accuracy (performance), specificity (actual negative cases), recall (sensitivity), F1 (precision), and Kappa (agreement) proportions from 0 to 1.

	RF	SVM	KNN
Accuracy	0.88 *	0.76	0.76
Specificity	0.92	0.71	0.88
Precision	0.90	0.71	0.88
Recall	0.92	0.83	0.67
F1-Score	0.89	0.76	0.76
Kappa	0.76 *	0.54	0.53

* Best performance.

Our results indicate that the RF model obtained the best overall performance among the three algorithms evaluated. It received an accuracy of 0.88, suggesting that it correctly classified 88% of the cases. It achieved a specificity of 0.92, indicating a high ability to identify negatives correctly. Additionally, the Kappa coefficient for this model was 0.76, confirming substantial agreement and suggesting that the model performs significantly better than chance.

On the other hand, SVM and KNN demonstrated similar overall performance, with identical F1 scores (0.76), but distinct strengths. The SVM showed good sensitivity (0.83) but inferior accuracy and specificity, with a Kappa of 0.54 indicating moderate agreement. KNN was notable for its accuracy (0.88) and specificity (0.88), but had a low sensitivity (0.67), making it more suitable for minimising false positives. Therefore, to enhance the robustness and accuracy of our classification, we selected only compounds classified as senotherapeutics by all three models (Figure 2).

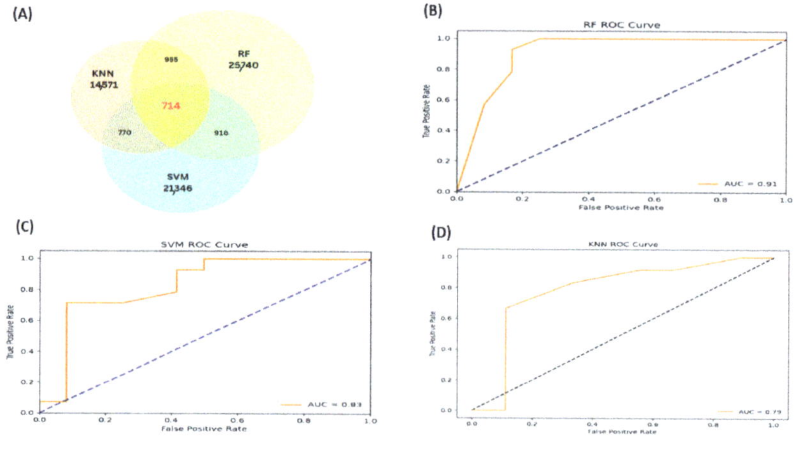

Figure 2. Venn diagram and ROC curves of the ML models. (**A**) Venn diagram of the compounds classified across the three models as possible senotherapeutic molecules. (**B**) ROC curve of the RF model. (**C**) ROC curve of the SVM model. (**D**) ROC curve of the KNN model.

Our results suggest that only 714 compounds were positively scored by the three ML models (Figure 2A). ROC curves illustrate the relationship between the actual and false favourable rates as the decision threshold of the model varies. The area under the curve (AUC) was evaluated, which indicates the probability that the ML model correctly classifies a randomly selected compound as positive; the closer this value is to 1, the better the model's performance. Our AUC values are 0.91 for RF (Figure 2B), 0.83 for

SVM (Figure 2C), and 0.79 for KNN (Figure 2D), indicating that our models effectively distinguish between categorical classes or classifications.

Once we filtered the compounds according to Lipinski's rules, 270 compounds met the desired physicochemical characteristics. These compounds were stored in a freely accessible database published online on March 2025 (https://gcoixc-laboratorio0de0bioinform0tic-inger.shinyapps.io/Senotherapeutics_Shiny/).

Finally, we analysed the chemical family of these 270 compounds (Figure 3). Interestingly, 9.3% of the entire database consisted of flavonoids, from which only 18 flavonoids have not been previously reported as senotherapeutics (3′,4′,7-trihydroxyisoflavone, daidzin, catechin, eriodictyol, auriculasin, pomiferin, 4′-O-methylalpinumisoflavone, tephrosin, 5,7-dihydroxy-3-(3-hydroxy-4-methoxybenzyl)-6-methoxychroman-4-one, calycosin-7-O-beta-D-glucoside, (R)-hesperetin, glycitein, glycitin, jaceosidin, silybin, isosilybin A, eupafolin, and skullcapflavone II).

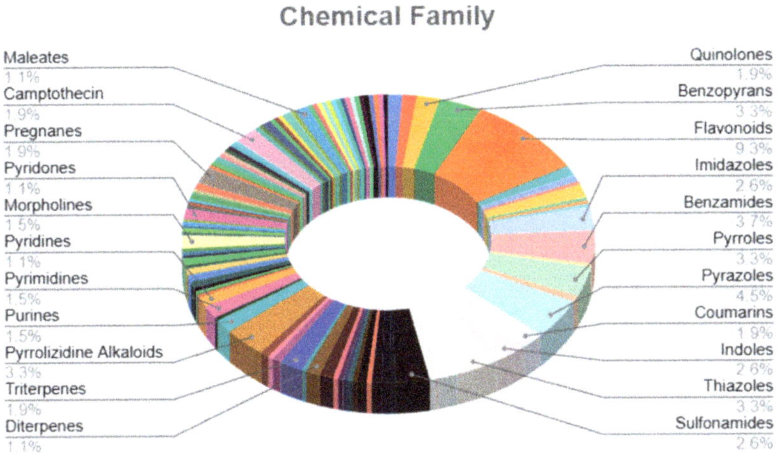

Figure 3. Compound family analysis of senotherapeutic compounds identified by ML. The pie chart shows the chemical families to which our senotherapeutics belong, highlighting flavonoids with the highest percentage.

Finally, to validate the potential senolytic effect of flavonoids, the most abundant chemical family, as indicated by our results above, we performed a docking analysis. All proteins were selected since they have already been reported to interact with flavonoids. In this context, according to the results (Table 2 and Supplementary Materials) we obtain 18 blind couplings between the selected proteins (p53, c-Fos, Cyclin D1, Trx, p21, AKT1, CDK1, NORE1, p65, c-Jun, and p38α) and compounds (3′,4′,7-trihydroxyisoflavone, daidzin, catechin, eriodictyol, auriculasin, pomiferin, 4′-O-methylalpinumisoflavone, tephrosin, 5,7,3′-trihydroxy-3,4′-dimethoxyflavone, calycosin-7-O-beta-D-glucoside, 5,7-dihydroxy-3-(3-hydroxy-4-methoxybenzyl)-6-methoxychroman-4-one, glycitein, glycitin, jaceosidin, silybin, isosilybin A, eupafolin, and skullcapflavone II). Interestingly, their interactions exhibit a moderate affinity (values between −6 and −9 kcal/mol) [26], and only a few compounds show high affinity (tephrosin, 5,7-dihydroxy-3-(3-hydroxy-4-methoxybenzyl)-6-methoxychroman-4-one, and isosilybin A, as they exhibit values between −9 and −12 kcal/mol) or weak affinity (jaceosidin and eupafolin, which show values between −4 and −6 kcal/mol), suggesting that such compounds with high or moderate affinity may be considered for further experimental validation.

Table 2. Docking results for tested flavonoids (Table 2 and Supplementary Materials) and their protein targets according to network pharmacology (Figure 1).

Protein Target	Flavonoid	ΔG (kcal/mol)
p53	3′,4′,7-trihydroxyisoflavone	−6.3
	Catechin	−6.8
	Auriculasin	−7.4
	Glycitein	−6.1
	Silybin	−7.3
AKT1	Tephrosin	−11.2
	5,7-dihydroxy-3-(3-hydroxy-4-methoxybenzyl)-6-methoxychroman-4-one	−9.2
Trx	Pomiferin	−6.9
	Calycosin-7-O-beta-D-glucoside	−6.1
Cyclin D1	Eriodictyol	−7.2
p21	4′-O-methylalpinumisoflavone	−6.4
c-Fos	Daidzin	−6.0
CDK1	5,7,3′-trihydroxy-3,4′-dimethoxyflavone	−8.9
NORE1	Glycitin	−7.0
p65	Jaceosidin	−4.4
CDK1	Isosilybin A	−9.7
c-Jun	Eupafolin	−5.9
p38α	Skullcapflavone II	−8.5

3. Discussion

Computational assays have revolutionised the pharmaceutical industry by offering innovative tools to speed up and optimise traditionally slow and costly processes. They do not replace traditional methods, but they are critical accelerators in the era of precision medicine. Their ability to analyse big data makes them pillars of modern pharmaceutical discovery.

In this sense, our research group employed a chemoinformatics analysis based on chemical descriptors and filtered by medicinal chemistry properties, such as Lipinski's rules, to identify terpenoids and naphthalenes as natural compounds that could be candidates for combating cellular senescence [6]. On the other hand, using a machine learning approach based on a structure-activity relationship network, Smer-Barreto et al., 2023, identified three compounds with potential as senolytics (ginkgetin, oleandrin, and periplocin); interestingly, ginkgetin is a biflavonoid [20]. Such a study demonstrates the potential for integrating network pharmacology and machine learning (ML) to accelerate the discovery of senotherapeutics, a critical challenge in ageing medicine.

In this sense, our results demonstrate that the construction of the drug-protein interactome enabled the mapping of key molecular dynamics associated with senescence, highlighting central nodes such as p53, ERK2, TGF-β1, IL-6, and AKT1, which are essential in cell cycle regulation and the DNA damage response [3]. These findings align with previous studies that have linked these proteins to SASP and their role in chronic diseases [1,2]. Moreover, it is essential to highlight that the compounds mentioned above are currently being investigated as potential senotherapeutics [27,28] or geroprotectors [29].

Our study identifies 270 compounds as candidates for use as senotherapeutic agents through the use of three machine learning models (RFC, SVM, and KNN), significantly reducing the number of molecules (65,339 compounds) to be experimentally analysed. Interestingly, 49 of these compounds are already FDA-approved drugs, opening up the possibility of their pharmacological repositioning. This strategy can effectively accelerate their validation as senotherapeutic agents. Moreover, the presence of antioxidants (e.g., resveratrol) and chemotherapeutics (e.g., fluorouracil) in the results reinforces the hypothesis that molecules with dual mechanisms of action (proapoptotic and antioxidant) could selectively modulate senescence, as already reported in preclinical studies by Hickson et al., who treated 15 patients with diabetic kidney disease with a combination of Dasatinib + Quercetine, most of whom had reduced numbers of senescent cells in blood and adipose tissue after treatment [16]. We developed a free web tool to disseminate the database of the 270 compounds that may be potential senolytic compounds. This database serves as a valuable resource for the scientific community, facilitating open access to data and fostering interdisciplinary collaborations.

Additionally, our study reveals that 9.3% of the compounds identified by ML models are flavonoids from which only 18 have not been previously reported as senotherapeutics (3′,4′,7-trihydroxyisoflavone, daidzin, catechin, eriodictyol, auriculasin, pomiferin, 4′-O-methylalpinumisoflavone, tephrosin, 5,7-dihydroxy-3-(3-hydroxy-4-methoxybenzyl)-6-methoxychroman-4-one, calycosin-7-O-beta-D-glucoside, (R)-hesperetin, glycitein, glycitin, jaceosidin, silybin, isosilybin A, eupafolin and skullcapflavone II). Such results are quite relevant since flavonoids exhibit a wide range of biological activities, including anti-cancer, anti-inflammatory, antidiabetic, and neuroprotective effects [30], suggesting that combining these compounds with other therapies may yield more effective senotherapies. Nevertheless, it is essential to mention that many flavonoids exhibit poor bioavailability due to their low aqueous solubility, poor absorption, metabolic transformation, and limited distribution in organs and tissues [31]. This suggests that if flavonoids are to be used as senotherapeutic agents, they need to be improved by structural transformations, absorption enhancers, or using pharmacological technologies as mentioned in [32] to improve pharmacokinetic properties. For instance, synthetic flavonoids have been recently developed to enhance the stability and modulation of platelet function [33].

Interestingly, upon performing the docking validation, we found that only tephrosin, 5,7-dihydroxy-3-(3-hydroxy-4-methoxybenzyl)-6-methoxychroman-4-one, and isosilybin A exhibit higher energetic values (−9 and −12 kcal/mol) between their receptors and the molecules. This suggests that these compounds may be suitable for further experimental analysis.

Finally, our results from the docking assay reveals that the identified flavonoid showed moderate to high binding affinity to senescence-related target proteins, many of which have been classified as PAINS (pan-assay interference compounds) or IMPS (invalid metabolic panaceas) [34,35], suggesting possible nonspecific effects in biological assays; flavonoids represent a remarkable template for the development of numerous compounds with diverse biological properties [36].

Limitations of the Study

This study is based exclusively on computational analysis and therefore lacks experimental validation. Furthermore, some of the selected compounds, such as several flavonoids, have been reported in the literature as frequent interferents in biological assays (PAINS), with low bioavailability and unfavourable metabolism. Therefore, the findings presented should be considered exploratory and require additional experimental validation to confirm their senotherapeutic relevance.

4. Materials and Methods

4.1. Network Pharmacology

A drug-protein interactome was constructed to investigate the interactions between compounds and proteins involved in cellular senescence. To build this interactome, we identified 249 proteins relevant to cellular senescence using the freely accessed databases KEGG (https://www.genome.jp/kegg/pathway.html) (accessed on 11 November 2024) and Reactome (https://reactome.org/content/detail/R-HSA-2559583) (accessed on 11 November 2024), and duplicates were manually removed. We prioritise the use of KEGG and Reactome databases since both are constantly curated and updated, making them quite suitable for different research needs. To gain insight into the compounds interacting with these proteins, data on these interactions were extracted from the freely accessed database Comparative Toxicogenomics Database (CTD) (https://ctdbase.org) [37] (accessed on 11 November 2024), with a focus on interactions in humans. The network was constructed and analysed using Graphistry v1.0 (https://www.graphistry.com/) via the Application Programming Interface (API) in Python v3.0.

4.2. Molecular Descriptors

Molecular descriptors (1–3D) were calculated for each dataset using the freely available DataWarrior v5.5.0 software (https://openmolecules.org/datawarrior). We calculated the following physicochemical, medicinal chemistry, and toxicoinformatic properties [38]: Total Molweight, Monoisotopic Mass, cLogP, cLogS, H-Acceptors, H-Donors, Total Surface Area, Relative PSA, Polar Surface Area, Druglikeness, Shape Index, Molecular Flexibility, Molecular Complexity, Fragments, Non-H Atoms, Non-C/H Atoms, Metal-Atoms, Electronegative Atoms, Stereo Centers, Rotatable Bonds, Rings Closures, Aromatic Atoms, sp3-Atoms, Symmetric atoms, Small Rings, Carbo-Rings, Hetero-Rings, Saturated Rings, Non-Aromatic Rings, Aromatic Rings, Saturated Carbo-Rings, Non-Aromatic Carbo-Rings, Carbo-Aromatic Rings, Saturated Hetero-Rings, Non-Aromatic Hetero-Rings, Hetero-Aromatic Rings, Amides, Amines, Alkyl-Amines, Aromatic Amines, Aromatic Nitrogens, Basic Nitrogens, and Acidic Oxygens.

4.3. Supervised ML Analysis (SVM, KNN, and RFC)

Among ML algorithms, we found Random Forest (RF), which builds multiple decision trees during the training process and determines the most frequent class for classification [39]; Support Vector Machine (SVM), which searches for the optimal hyperplane to separate different classes of data in a high-dimensional space [40]; and K-Nearest Neighbors (KNN), which classifies data according to the predominant class of its nearest neighbours in the feature space [41].

We utilised the Scikit-learn package v1.7.1 (https://scikit-learn.org/stable/index.html) in Python 3.0 to generate the models, which implement various statistical and machine learning algorithms. We constructed a classifier using the training set data of already reported senotherapeutic compounds by Lei Zhang [42]. Additionally, to increase the specificity of our model, we used a set of non-related senotherapeutic compounds randomly extracted from the ChEMBL database (https://www.ebi.ac.uk/chembl/) accessed on 25 November 2024.

Subsequently, the data were divided into training (75%) and test (25%) subsets by stratified random sampling, with the subsets further divided into positive and negative senotherapeutics. We used three machine learning models (RF, SVM, and KNN) to generate three classifiers.

The receiver operating characteristic area under the curve (ROC-AUC) was used to evaluate the predictive accuracy of our models. We used a metric indicating the performance of the models, with values ranging from 0 to 1, where 1 represents perfect prediction. For each model's accuracy, we calculated and assessed the overall effectiveness and specificity to determine whether true negatives were correctly classified. Similarly, we evaluated the balance between accuracy and sensitivity using the F1-score [43]. Additionally, to provide a more robust and nuanced evaluation of classification model performance, we calculated the Kappa statistics for each model.

Once we had the classifier for each algorithm, we used it to select the potential senotherapeutic compounds from the interactome obtained by network pharmacology, extracted from the CTD. We selected only those compounds that were shared across all three classifiers to enhance the robustness and accuracy of our calculations.

4.4. Druglikeness by Lipinski Rules

The compounds positively predicted by the three models were integrated and filtered using druglikeness analysis based on Lipinski's rules [44] to preliminarily filter only those compounds with suitable physicochemical properties, suggesting good absorption. Additionally, using DataWarrior v.5.5.0 [38], we determined the toxicoinformatic properties of the compounds and eliminated those that could be tumorigenic, mutagenic, carcinogenic, or irritating: toxicoinformatic analysis to assign mutagenicity, based on the ability of a compound to cause changes in DNA through a structure comparison with molecules reported as hazardous; tumorigenicity, based on the potential of a compound to cause tumours or cancer through a structure comparison with molecules reported as hazardous; irritant based on the likelihood of a compound irritating skin, through a structure comparison with molecules reported as dangerous; and reproductive effective based on the potential for a compound to harm reproductive organs or cause developmental defects [38].

4.5. Development of a Web Tool and Chemical Classification

The dataset of new senotherapeutic compounds obtained from the consensus of the three algorithms was organised using a web tool based on the freely available R language package ShinyApp v1.11.1. Finally, we analysed the chemical classification to which each compound belonged to identify the chemical families.

4.6. Docking Analysis

We explore the potential senolytic effect of flavonoids through docking analysis between these compounds and their reported targets, as described below. It is essential to mention that proteins were selected since they have been previously reported to interact with flavonoids.

4.6.1. Protein Structures Acquisition

We retrieve protein structures from the Protein Databank in the PDB format (.pdb) (https://www.rcsb.org/, accessed on 30 June 2025). The proteins retrieved are as follows: p53 (ID: 2OCJ), c-Fos (ID: 1FOS), Cyclin D1 (ID: 2W9Z), Trx (ID: 1ERT), p21 (ID: 6P8H), AKT1 (ID: 3O96), CDK1 (ID: 5HQ0), NORE1 (ID: 3DDC), p65 (ID: 6QHL), c-Jun (ID: 5T01), and p38α (ID: 3HVC).

Subsequently, protein pre-processing was generated with USCF Chimera v1.15 software [45] according to the following parameters: water residues were removed, solvent residues were removed, ions that are free or not part of the proteins were removed, coupled nucleic acids and associated ligands were removed. All protein complexes were removed, and only monomers were used for further processes.

Additionally, a protein optimisation process was generated using the USCF Chimera v1.15 interface, according to the following parameters: (1) Correction of chains and addition of hydrogens, to reflect a realistic structure and to establish the correct interactions with the ligand; (2) Partial charges, AMBER ff14SB partial charges improve the accuracy of docking, ensuring that the protein has a proper electrostatic representation, as they describe the geometry, bonds, and partial charges of the amino acids to model their interactions correctly; and (3) Energy minimisation, to reduce possible distortions, thereby improving the accuracy of the docking.

4.6.2. Compounds Structure Obtention for Docking Analysis

We retrieved the 2D compound structure in .sdf format from the PubChem database (https://pubchem.ncbi.nlm.nih.gov/, accessed on 7 July 2025): 3′,4′,7-trihydroxyisoflavone (ID: 5284648), daidzin (ID: 107971), catechin (ID: 9064), eriodictyol (ID: 440735), auriculasin (ID: 5358846), pomiferin (ID: 4871), 4′-O-methylalpinumisoflavone (ID: 15596285), tephrosin (ID: 114909), 5,7,3′-trihydroxy-3,4′-dimethoxyflavone (ID: 5380905), calycosin-7-O-beta-D-glucoside (ID: 5318267), 5,7-dihydroxy-3-(3-hydroxy-4-methoxybenzyl)-6-methoxychroman-4-one (ID: 21676260), glycitein (ID: 5317750), glycitin (ID: 187808), jaceosidin (ID: 5379096), silybin (ID: 31553), isosilybin A (ID: 11059920), eupafolin (ID: 5317284), and skullcapflavone II (ID: 124211).

The 2D structures of the compounds were downloaded in .sdf format from the PubChem database and converted to three-dimensional structures using geometric optimisation performed in Avogadro v1.2.0 (https://avogadro.cc/releases/avogadro_120/) accessed on 9 December 2024, using the MMFF94 molecular mechanics algorithm. They were then prepared in UCSF Chimera v1.15 by adding hydrogens, assigning partial charges AMBER ff14SB, and minimising energy (1000 steepest descent steps and 100 conjugate gradient steps, 0.02 Å step size). The AM1-BCC force fields were applied for proteins and Gasteiger for compounds, under vacuum conditions and with the removal of non-biological residues, generating stable structures for docking analysis.

4.6.3. Molecular Docking

Once the above compounds were chosen, we used the USCF Chimera version 1.15 interface to run Autodock Vina version 1.1.2 [46], a software that predicts binding modes between different target proteins and ligands.

Each compound was loaded with each protein in the USCF Chimera software, the total protein area was set, and blind docking was performed for each ligand-protein.

5. Conclusions

The present study identified 270 compounds with senotherapeutic potential, with flavonoids being the most abundant compound class. Notably, 18 of these compounds represent novel senolytics that warrant experimental validation due to their interesting pharmacological properties. Among these, tephrosin, 5,7-dihydroxy-3-(3-hydroxy-4-methoxybenzyl)-6-methoxychroman-4-one, and isosilybin are particularly deserving of experimental verification for further development. Nevertheless, these results are exploratory and based solely on computational models; further experimental studies and chemical modifications are necessary to improve their specificity, safety, and efficacy as senotherapeutics.

Supplementary Materials: The following supporting information can be downloaded at: https://www.mdpi.com/article/10.3390/ph18081176/s1, Table S1: Docking test for compounds.

Author Contributions: J.C.G.-V.: Conceptualisation, investigation, writing—original draft and editing. J.A.S.-d.-l.-C.: Supervision and project administration, investigation, data curation, web application development, writing—original draft, editing, and visualisation. N.A.R.-S.: Validation, formal analysis, writing—review, editing, and visualisation. M.E.A.-S.: Supervision and project, editing, and visualisation. All authors have read and agreed to the published version of the manuscript.

Funding: This study was part of a registered project at the Instituto Nacional de Geriatría DI-PI-008-2021 (JCGV). We thank the Consejo Nacional de Humanidades, Ciencias y Tecnologías (CONAHCYT), which has become Secretaría de Ciencia, Humanidades, Tecnología e Innovación (SECIHTI), for funding and the support of this research through the project 319706 ¿Se puede revertir el envejecimiento con fármacos?

Data Availability Statement: The code and models developed in this study are available at https://github.com/BioAgeLab/Senotherapeutics_Project_INGER-UACM. The database is freely available at: https://gcoixc-laboratorio0de0bioinform0tic-inger.shinyapps.io/Senotherapeutics_Shiny/.

Acknowledgments: This article aims to enable José Alberto Santiago de la Cruz to obtain his doctoral degree. We would like to thank the Graduate Program in Genomic Sciences at the Autonomous University of Mexico City. The publication of this paper was conducted by the Instituto Nacional de Geriatría, México, and was financially supported by the Consejo Nacional de Humanidades, Ciencias y Tecnologías, México; Project 319706 "¿Se puede revertir el envejecimiento con fármacos?".

Conflicts of Interest: The authors declare no conflicts of interest.

Abbreviations

The following abbreviations are used in this manuscript:

SASP	Senescence-associated secretory phenotype
AI	Artificial intelligence
ML	Machine learning
RFC	Random Forest Classifier
SVM	Supand Vector Machine
KNN	K-Nearest Neighbors
CTD	Comparative Toxicogenomics Database
PPI	Protein-Protein Interactions
ROC	Receiver Operating Characteristic
AUC	Area under the curve
FDA	Food and Drug Administration

References

1. Huang, W.; Hickson, L.J.; Eirin, A.; Kirkland, J.L.; Lerman, L.O. Cellular Senescence: The Good, the Bad and the Unknown. *Nat. Rev. Nephrol.* **2022**, *18*, 611–627. [CrossRef]
2. Childs, B.G.; Durik, M.; Baker, D.J.; van Deursen, J.M. Cellular Senescence in Aging and Age-Related Disease: From Mechanisms to Therapy. *Nat. Med.* **2015**, *21*, 1424–1435. [CrossRef]
3. Mylonas, A.; O'Loghlen, A. Cellular Senescence and Ageing: Mechanisms and Interventions. *Front. Aging* **2022**, *3*, 866718. [CrossRef]
4. Zarneshan, S.N.; Fakhri, S.; Bachtel, G.; Bishayee, A. Exploiting Pivotal Mechanisms behind the Senescence-like Cell Cycle Arrest in Cancer. *Adv. Protein Chem. Struct. Biol.* **2023**, *135*, 1–19.
5. Borghesan, M.; Hoogaars, W.M.H.; Varela-Eirin, M.; Talma, N.; Demaria, M. A Senescence-Centric View of Aging: Implications for Longevity and Disease. *Trends Cell Biol.* **2020**, *30*, 777–791. [CrossRef]
6. Lewis, E.D.; Wu, D.; Meydani, S.N. Age-Associated Alterations in Immune Function and Inflammation. *Prog. Neuropsychopharmacol. Biol. Psychiatry* **2022**, *118*, 110576. [CrossRef]
7. Hazeldine, J.; Lord, J.M. Immunesenescence and Compromised Removal of Senescent Cells: Implications for Health in Old Age. In *Healthy Ageing and Longevity*; Springer International Publishing: Cham, Switzerland, 2022; pp. 23–52. ISBN 9783030875312.
8. McHugh, D.; Gil, J. Senescence and Aging: Causes, Consequences, and Therapeutic Avenues. *J. Cell Biol.* **2018**, *217*, 65–77. [CrossRef]
9. Barrera-Vázquez, O.S.; Magos-Guerrero, G.A.; Escobar-Ramírez, J.L.; Gomez-Verjan, J.C. Natural Products as a Major Source of Candidates for Potential Senolytic Compounds Obtained by Screening. *Med. Chem.* **2023**, *19*, 653–668. [CrossRef] [PubMed]
10. Niedernhofer, L.J.; Robbins, P.D. Senotherapeutics for Healthy Ageing. *Nat. Rev. Drug Discov.* **2018**, *17*, 377. [CrossRef]
11. Zhang, L.J.; Salekeen, R.; Soto-Palma, C.; He, Y.; Elsallabi, O.; Hughes, B.; Nunes, A.; Xu, W.; Zhang, B.; Mohamed, A.; et al. Development of Novel Flavonoid Senolytics through Phenotypic Drug Screening and Drug Design. *bioRxiv* **2024**, *10*, 620529. [CrossRef]
12. Pacifico, F.; Magni, F.; Leonardi, A.; Crescenzi, E. Therapy-Induced Senescence: Novel Approaches for Markers Identification. *Int. J. Mol. Sci.* **2024**, *25*, 8448. [CrossRef] [PubMed]
13. Chen, M.; Fu, Y.; Wang, X.; Wu, R.; Su, D.; Zhou, N.; Qi, Y. Metformin Protects Lens Epithelial Cells against Senescence in a Naturally Aged Mouse Model. *Cell Death Discov.* **2022**, *8*, 8. [CrossRef]

14. Walaszczyk, A.; Dookun, E.; Redgrave, R.; Tual-Chalot, S.; Victorelli, S.; Spyridopoulos, I.; Owens, A.; Arthur, H.M.; Passos, J.F.; Richardson, G.D. Pharmacological Clearance of Senescent Cells Improves Survival and Recovery in Aged Mice Following Acute Myocardial Infarction. *Aging Cell* **2019**, *18*, e12945. [CrossRef]
15. Islam, M.T.; Tuday, E.; Allen, S.; Kim, J.; Trott, D.W.; Holland, W.L.; Donato, A.J.; Lesniewski, L.A. Senolytic Drugs, Dasatinib and Quercetin, Attenuate Adipose Tissue Inflammation, and Ameliorate Metabolic Function in Old Age. *Aging Cell* **2023**, *22*, e13767. [CrossRef]
16. Hickson, L.J.; Langhi Prata, L.G.P.; Bobart, S.A.; Evans, T.K.; Giorgadze, N.; Hashmi, S.K.; Herrmann, S.M.; Jensen, M.D.; Jia, Q.; Jordan, K.L.; et al. Senolytics Decrease Senescent Cells in Humans: Preliminary Report from a Clinical Trial of Dasatinib plus Quercetin in Individuals with Diabetic Kidney Disease. *EBioMedicine* **2019**, *47*, 446–456. [CrossRef] [PubMed]
17. Alzforum Dasatinib + Quercetin. Available online: https://www.alzforum.org/therapeutics/dasatinib-quercetin (accessed on 22 April 2025).
18. He, Y.; Zheng, G.; Zhou, D. Senolytic Drug Development. In *Healthy Ageing and Longevity*; Springer International Publishing: Cham, Switzerland, 2020; pp. 3–20. ISBN 9783030449025.
19. Muthuramalingam, P.; Jeyasri, R.; Varadharajan, V.; Priya, A.; Dhanapal, A.R.; Shin, H.; Thiruvengadam, M.; Ramesh, M.; Krishnan, M.; Omosimua, R.O.; et al. Network Pharmacology: An Efficient but Underutilized Approach in Oral, Head and Neck Cancer Therapy-a Review. *Front. Pharmacol.* **2024**, *15*, 1410942. [CrossRef]
20. Smer-Barreto, V.; Quintanilla, A.; Elliott, R.J.R.; Dawson, J.C.; Sun, J.; Campa, V.M.; Lorente-Macías, Á.; Unciti-Broceta, A.; Carragher, N.O.; Acosta, J.C.; et al. Discovery of Senolytics Using Machine Learning. *Nat. Commun.* **2023**, *14*, 3445. [CrossRef]
21. Meenakshi, M.; Ruban, S.; Nandhini, T.J.; Loganayagi, S.; Sayed, R.M.; Hassan, E.; Al-Saidi, I.A.-D.H. A Framework Design of ML Classifier Algorithm for Retrieve the Information about the Drugs and Its Quality. In Proceedings of the 2024 4th International Conference on Advance Computing and Innovative Technologies in Engineering (ICACITE), Greater Noida, India, 14 May 2024; pp. 409–412.
22. Priya, S.; Tripathi, G.; Singh, D.B.; Jain, P.; Kumar, A. Machine Learning Approaches and Their Applications in Drug Discovery and Design. *Chem. Biol. Drug Des.* **2022**, *100*, 136–153. [CrossRef] [PubMed]
23. Ferreira, F.J.N.; Carneiro, A.S. AI-Driven Drug Discovery: A Comprehensive Review. *ACS Omega* **2025**, *10*, 23889–23903. [CrossRef]
24. Shah, A.; Patel, V.; Jain, M.; Parmar, G. Network Pharmacology and Systems Biology in Drug Discovery. In *Interdisciplinary Biotechnological Advances*; Springer Nature: Singapore, 2023; pp. 231–252. ISBN 9789819913152.
25. Arrell, D.K.; Terzic, A. Network Systems Biology for Drug Discovery. *Clin. Pharmacol. Ther.* **2010**, *88*, 120–125. [CrossRef]
26. Knegtel, R.M.A.; Grootenhuis, P.D.J. Binding Affinities and Non-Bonded Interaction Energies. In *3D QSAR in Drug Design*; Kluwer Academic Publishers: Dordrecht, The Netherlands, 2005; pp. 99–114. ISBN 9780792347903.
27. Kong, X.; Xu, J.; Hussain, S.A.; Alrubie, T.M.; Maddu, N.; Wei, H. Combination of Quercetin and Curcumin modulates NF-κB inflammatory signaling pathway in murine model of esophageal erosive reflux disease erosive reflux disease. *Folia Morphol. (Warsz), Online ahead of print*. 2025. [CrossRef] [PubMed]
28. Ahmadinejad, F.; Bos, T.; Hu, B.; Britt, E.; Koblinski, J.; Souers, A.J.; Leverson, J.D.; Faber, A.C.; Gewirtz, D.A.; Harada, H. Senolytic-Mediated Elimination of Head and Neck Tumor Cells Induced Into Senescence by Cisplatin. *Mol. Pharmacol.* **2022**, *101*, 168–180. [CrossRef]
29. Proshkina, E.; Koval, L.; Platonova, E.; Golubev, D.; Ulyasheva, N.; Babak, T.; Shaposhnikov, M.; Moskalev, A. Polyphenols as Potential Geroprotectors. *Antioxid. Redox Signal.* **2024**, *40*, 564–593. [CrossRef]
30. Tiwari, A.K.; Singh, M.V. Insights into the Origin and Therapeutic Implications of Benzopyran and Its Derivatives. *ChemistrySelect* **2023**, *8*, e202300220. [CrossRef]
31. Yuan, D.; Guo, Y.; Pu, F.; Yang, C.; Xiao, X.; Du, H.; He, J.; Lu, S. Opportunities and Challenges in Enhancing the Bioavailability and Bioactivity of Dietary Flavonoids: A Novel Delivery System Perspective. *Food Chem.* **2024**, *430*, 137115. [CrossRef]
32. Zhao, J.; Yang, J.; Xie, Y. Improvement Strategies for the Oral Bioavailability of Poorly Water-Soluble Flavonoids: An Overview. *Int. J. Pharm.* **2019**, *570*, 118642. [CrossRef]
33. Vallance, T.M.; Ravishankar, D.; Albadawi, D.A.I.; Osborn, H.M.I.; Vaiyapuri, S. Synthetic Flavonoids as Novel Modulators of Platelet Function and Thrombosis. *Int. J. Mol. Sci.* **2019**, *20*, 3106. [CrossRef] [PubMed]
34. Bisson, J.; McAlpine, J.B.; Friesen, J.B.; Chen, S.-N.; Graham, J.; Pauli, G.F. Can Invalid Bioactives Undermine Natural Product-Based Drug Discovery? *J. Med. Chem.* **2016**, *59*, 1671–1690. [CrossRef]
35. Baell, J.; Walters, M.A. Chemistry: Chemical Con Artists Foil Drug Discovery. *Nature* **2014**, *513*, 481–483. [CrossRef] [PubMed]
36. Uivarosi, V.; Munteanu, A.-C.; Nițulescu, G.M. An Overview of Synthetic and Semisynthetic Flavonoid Derivatives and Analogues: Perspectives in Drug Discovery. In *Studies in Natural Products Chemistry*; Studies in natural products chemistry; Elsevier: Amsterdam, The Netherlands, 2019; pp. 29–84. ISBN 9780444641816.
37. Mattingly, C.J.; Rosenstein, M.C.; Davis, A.P.; Colby, G.T.; Forrest, J.N., Jr.; Boyer, J.L. The Comparative Toxicogenomics Database: A Cross-Species Resource for Building Chemical-Gene Interaction Networks. *Toxicol. Sci.* **2006**, *92*, 587–595. [CrossRef] [PubMed]

38. Sander, T.; Freyss, J.; von Korff, M.; Rufener, C. DataWarrior: An Open-Source Program for Chemistry Aware Data Visualization and Analysis. *J. Chem. Inf. Model.* **2015**, *55*, 460–473. [CrossRef]
39. Salman, H.A.; Kalakech, A.; Steiti, A. Random Forest Algorithm Overview. *Babylon. J. Mach. Learn.* **2024**, *2024*, 69–79. [CrossRef] [PubMed]
40. Schonlau, M. Support Vector Machines. In *Statistics and Computing*; Springer International Publishing: Cham, The Netherlands, 2023; pp. 237–266. ISBN 9783031333897.
41. Mladenova, T.; Valova, I. Classification with K-Nearest Neighbors Algorithm: Comparative Analysis between the Manual and Automatic Methods for K-Selection. *Int. J. Adv. Comput. Sci. Appl.* **2023**, *14*, 396–404. [CrossRef]
42. Zhang, L.; Pitcher, L.E.; Prahalad, V.; Niedernhofer, L.J.; Robbins, P.D. Targeting Cellular Senescence with Senotherapeutics: Senolytics and Senomorphics. *FEBS J.* **2023**, *290*, 1362–1383. [CrossRef]
43. Naidu, G.; Zuva, T.; Sibanda, E.M. A Review of Evaluation Metrics in Machine Learning Algorithms. In *Lecture Notes in Networks and Systems*; Springer International Publishing: Cham, The Netherlands, 2023; pp. 15–25. ISBN 9783031353130.
44. Pillai, O.; Dhanikula, A.B.; Panchagnula, R. Drug Delivery: An Odyssey of 100 Years. *Curr. Opin. Chem. Biol.* **2001**, *5*, 439–446. [CrossRef]
45. Pettersen, E.F.; Goddard, T.D.; Huang, C.C.; Couch, G.S.; Greenblatt, D.M.; Meng, E.C.; Ferrin, T.E. UCSF Chimera--a Visualization System for Exploratory Research and Analysis. *J. Comput. Chem.* **2004**, *25*, 1605–1612. [CrossRef] [PubMed]
46. Trott, O.; Olson, A.J. AutoDock Vina: Improving the Speed and Accuracy of Docking with a New Scoring Function, Efficient Optimization, and Multithreading. *J. Comput. Chem.* **2010**, *31*, 455–461. [CrossRef] [PubMed]

pharmaceuticals

MDPI

Article

Integrative In Silico and In Vivo Analysis of Banhasasim-Tang for Irritable Bowel Syndrome: Mechanistic Insights into Inflammation-Related Pathways

Woo-Gyun Choi [1,†], Seok-Jae Ko [2,3,†], Jung-Ha Shim [1], Chang-Hwan Bae [4], Seungtae Kim [4], Jae-Woo Park [2,3,*] and Byung-Joo Kim [1,*]

1 Department of Longevity and Biofunctional Medicine, School of Korean Medicine, Pusan National University, Yangsan 50612, Republic of Korea; ak0510@hanmail.net (W.-G.C.); luckydunk@naver.com (J.-H.S.)
2 Department of Clinical Korean Medicine, Graduate School, Kyung Hee University, Seoul 02447, Republic of Korea; kokokoko119@daum.net
3 Department of Gastroenterology, College of Korean Medicine, Kyung Hee University, Seoul 02447, Republic of Korea
4 Department of Korean Medical Science, School of Korean Medicine, Pusan National University, Yangsan 50612, Republic of Korea; kimst@pusan.ac.kr (S.K.)
* Correspondence: pjw2907@khu.ac.kr (J.-W.P.); vision@pusan.ac.kr (B.-J.K.)
† These authors contributed equally to this work.

Abstract: Background/Objectives: Banhasasim-tang (BHSST) is a traditional herbal formula commonly used to treat gastrointestinal (GI) disorders and has been considered a potential therapeutic option for irritable bowel syndrome (IBS). This study aimed to explore the molecular targets and underlying mechanisms of BHSST in IBS using a combination of network pharmacology, molecular docking, molecular dynamics simulations, and in vivo validation. **Methods:** Active compounds in BHSST were screened based on drug-likeness and oral bioavailability. Potential targets were predicted using ChEMBL, and IBS-related targets were obtained from GeneCards and DisGeNET. A compound–target–disease network was constructed and analyzed via Gene Ontology and KEGG pathway enrichment. Compound–target interactions were further assessed using molecular docking and molecular dynamics simulations. The in vivo effects of eudesm-4(14)-en-11-ol, elemol, and BHSST were evaluated in a zymosan-induced IBS mouse model. **Results:** Twelve BHSST-related targets were associated with IBS, with enrichment analysis identifying TNF signaling and apoptosis as key pathways. In silico simulations suggested stable binding of eudesm-4(14)-en-11-ol to TNF-α and kanzonol T to PIK3CD, whereas elemol showed weak interaction with PRKCD. In vivo, eudesm-4(14)-en-11-ol improved colon length, weight, stool consistency, TNF-α levels, and pain-related behaviors—effects comparable to those of BHSST. Elemol, however, showed no therapeutic benefit. **Conclusions:** These findings provide preliminary mechanistic insight into the anti-inflammatory potential of BHSST in IBS. The integrated in silico and in vivo approaches support the contribution of specific components, such as eudesm-4(14)-en-11-ol, to its observed effects, warranting further investigation.

Keywords: Banhasasim-tang; irritable bowel syndrome; network pharmacology; molecular docking; molecular dynamics

1. Introduction

Irritable bowel syndrome (IBS) is a common functional gastrointestinal (GI) disorder characterized by recurrent abdominal pain and altered bowel habits. It affects approximately 11% of the global population [1] and significantly impairs patients' quality of life [2]. The pathogenesis of IBS is multifactorial, involving psychological stress, gut microbiota imbalance, intestinal dysmotility, visceral hypersensitivity, and prior infections [3]. Although IBS does not cause structural damage to the GI tract, it leads to persistent discomfort, reduced quality of life, and a substantial healthcare burden [4–6].

Since its emergence in 2007, network pharmacology has become a valuable approach in drug discovery, offering insights into polypharmacology and the complexity of biological systems [7]. By integrating computational tools, network pharmacology enables the analysis of protein–protein interactions, compound–target–disease (CTD) networks, and the identification of key therapeutic pathways, particularly in traditional medicine. Given that herbal formulas typically contain multiple bioactive compounds, this systems-level approach is especially useful for elucidating their mechanisms of action from a holistic perspective. For example, Zhou and Wu demonstrated that the mitogen-activated protein kinase (MAPK) pathway is a potential target of *Eucommia ulmoides* cortex in the treatment of osteoporosis [8]. Similarly, Dou et al. reported that tanshinone II, a compound from *Salvia miltiorrhiza* Bunge, exerted protective effects in an acute kidney injury model by activating the pregnane X receptor [9].

Banhasasim-Tang (BHSST), known as Hange-shashin-to in Japan, and an-xia-xiexin-tang in China, is a traditional herbal medicine formula composed of Coptidis Rhizoma (CR), Ginseng Radix (GR), Glycyrrhizae Radix et Rhizoma (GRR), Pinelliae Tuber (PT), Scutellariae Radix (SR), Zizyphi Fructus (ZF), Zingiberis Rhizoma (ZR), and Zingiberis Rhizoma Recens (ZRR). BHSST is primarily used for treating GI disorders such as dyspepsia, gastric ulcers, pharyngitis, colitis, diarrhea, gastroesophageal reflux disease, and esophageal ulcers caused by chronic reflux [10–17]. Additionally, BHSST is an effective mouthwash for treating oral mucosal inflammation and reducing PGE2 concentration in oral keratinocytes [18,19]. Moreover, it functions as an anti-inflammatory, antioxidant, and antimicrobial agent by inhibiting the COX-2 activity related to inflammation [19–23].

Although IBS has traditionally been considered a functional disorder, recent studies suggest that mucosal inflammation and immune activation may contribute to its pathogenesis [24]. Increased numbers of mast cells and other immune cells in the gut mucosa can release pro-inflammatory cytokines such as TNF-α and IL-6, leading to visceral hypersensitivity and altered motility [25]. Post-infectious IBS further supports the role of persistent inflammation in symptom development, possibly mediated through gut microbiota changes and gut–brain axis dysregulation [26].

Although traditional use and various studies—including our previous experimental research demonstrating the efficacy of BHSST in IBS models [27]—suggest a potential benefit of herbal medicines in IBS management [15,28,29], mechanistic evidence remains limited. Given the complexity of BHSST, which contains numerous phytochemicals, fully elucidating its mechanism of action is not feasible. Therefore, we adopted a representative compound-based approach to explore potential molecular interactions.

In this study, we employed network pharmacology and in silico simulations to predict interactions between selected active compounds in BHSST and IBS-related targets. Among them, eudesm-4(14)-en-11-ol and kanzonol T were identified as potential modulators of inflammatory pathways associated with IBS pathophysiology. To support these computational predictions, we conducted in vivo experiments using a zymosan-induced IBS mouse model. Eudesm-4(14)-en-11-ol significantly alleviated colon shortening, abnormal colon weight gain, altered stool consistency, elevated TNF-α levels, and pain-related behaviors. In contrast, elemol did not exhibit therapeutic efficacy.

While we acknowledge the limitations of extrapolating these findings to the full BHSST formulation or to human IBS, our results offer preliminary mechanistic insights into how individual components—particularly eudesm-4(14)-en-11-ol—may contribute to the observed effects of BHSST in IBS.

2. Results

2.1. Screening of Active Compounds in BHSST

The objective of this study was to investigate the human intestinal absorption of the individual compounds in BHSST using the log P method (WLogP), based on the BOILED-Egg model developed by Wildman and Crippen (Figure 1). This approach assesses two physicochemical properties: the topological polar surface area (TPSA) and lipophilicity [30]. The list of filtered compounds was refined to ensure suitability for further pharmacological analyses. After excluding compounds with predicted human oral bioavailability below 20%, and those that violated Lipinski's "Rule of Five" or were P-glycoprotein substrates, we identified 23 out of 128 compounds from CR, 131 out of 716 compounds from GR, 285 out of 599 compounds from GRR, 78 out of 169 compounds from PT, 70 out of 232 compounds from SR, 181 out of 380 compounds from ZF, 281 out of 566 compounds from ZR, and 176 out of 442 compounds from ZRR. After removing duplicates, 982 compounds were identified as active compounds. The light histogram represents the entire set of compounds present in the formulation. In contrast, the dark histogram illustrates the distribution of the physicochemical properties of the 982 compounds that met the established criteria of high drug similarity and oral bioavailability (Figure 2). A comprehensive list of the active compounds is provided in Supplementary Material Table S1.

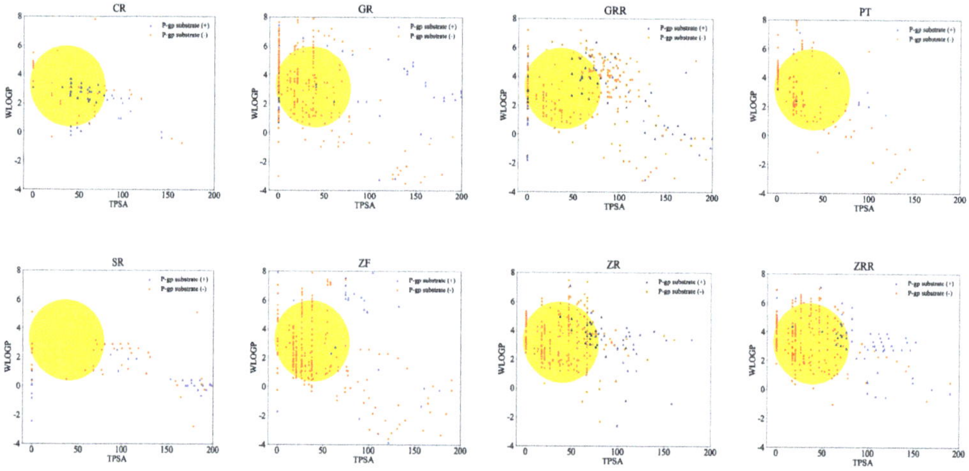

Figure 1. Predicted plots of the intestinal absorption and P-glycoprotein substrate potential of individual herbs in Banhasasim-tang. Compounds within the white ellipses indicate the human intestinal absorption potential. In particular, compounds within the yellow ellipse are predicted to cross the blood–brain barrier. Orange dots represent negative substrates for P-glycoprotein, whereas blue triangles denote positive substrates that are expected to be effluxed by P-glycoprotein. TPSA, topological polar surface area; CR, Coptidis Rhizoma; GR, Ginseng Radix; GRR, Glycyrrhizae Radix et Rhizoma; PT, Pinelliae Tuber; SR, Scutellariae Radix; ZF, Zizyphi Fructus; ZR, Zingiberis Rhizoma; ZRR, Zingiberis Rhizoma Recens.

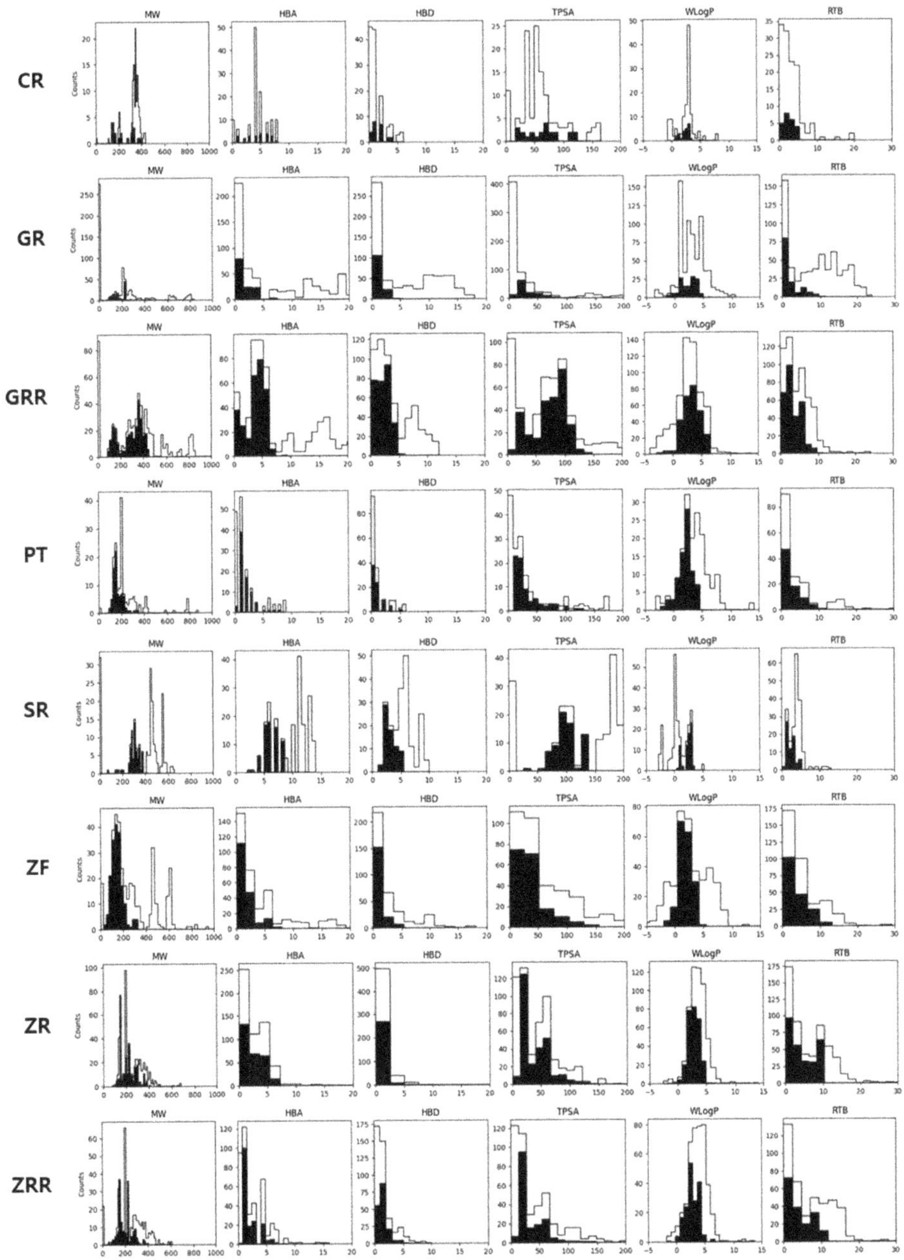

Figure 2. Histograms of the physicochemical properties of the active compounds in each BHSST formulation. The white histograms depict the distribution of all compounds within the formulation, whereas the black histograms illustrate the distribution of active compounds that meet the drug-likeness and oral bioavailability criteria. MW, Molecular Weight; HBA, Hydrogen Bond Acceptors; HBD, Hydrogen Bond Donors; TPSA, Topological Polar Surface Area; WLogP, Water Partition Coefficient; RTB, Rotatable Bonds; CR, Coptidis Rhizoma; GR, Ginseng Radix; GRR, Glycyrrhizae Radix et Rhizoma; PT, Pinelliae Tuber; SR, Scutellariae Radix; ZF, Zizyphi Fructus; ZR, Zingiberis Rhizoma; ZRR, Zingiberis Rhizoma Recens.

2.2. Candidate Target Proteins

Version 33 of the ChEMBL database was used to predict candidate target proteins for each compound. The SMILES of the compounds were queried, and targets with a probability of 0.7 or higher were classified. After removing duplicates and retaining those relevant to Homo sapiens, 328 candidate targets for BHSST were identified (Figure 3; Supplementary Material Table S1). Supplementary Material Table S1 also shows the composition of the compound–target protein pairs.

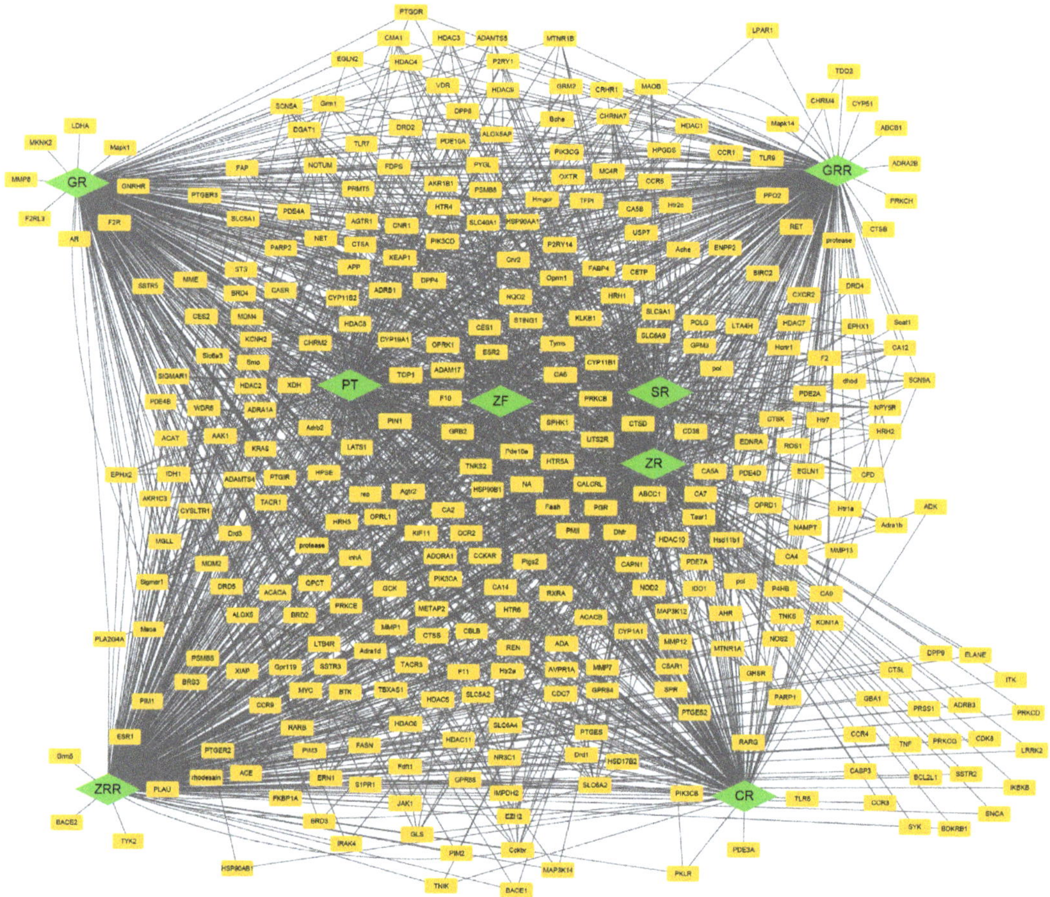

Figure 3. Network of components and target proteins. Green diamonds represent the components, while orange rectangles denote the target proteins. CR, Coptidis Rhizoma; GR, Ginseng Radix; GRR, Glycyrrhizae Radix et Rhizoma; PT, Pinelliae Tuber; SR, Scutellariae Radix; ZF, Zizyphi Fructus; ZR, Zingiberis Rhizoma; ZRR, Zingiberis Rhizoma Recens.

2.3. Disease Gene Association

To identify disease-related genes, we searched for the term "Irritable Bowel Syndrome" in the DisGeNET and GeneCards databases. This process yielded 414 IBS-related genes from DisGeNET, filtered for an evidence index of 0.7 or higher. Additionally, we identified 343 IBS-related protein-coding genes from the top 10% of the scores in the GeneCards database. Consequently, 43 overlapping targets were selected for further analysis (Figure 4).

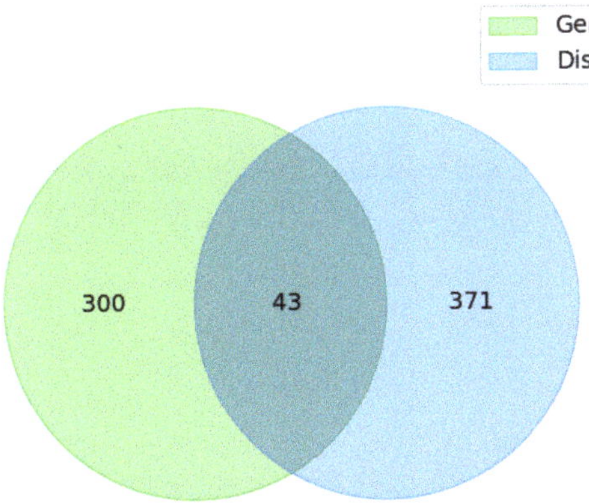

Figure 4. Venn diagram illustrating the overlap of IBS-related targets. Targets were selected on the basis of the top 10% of protein-coding genes from GeneCards and on the basis of targets with an evidence score of 0.7 or higher from DisGeNET.

2.4. Network Analysis

The CTD network connecting BHSST with IBS was constructed using Cytoscape software and data from the STRING database (Figure 5A). Network centrality was assessed using the CytoNCA plug-in of Cytoscape (Table 1) [31]. The overlapping protein–protein interaction network between BHSST and IBS comprised 12 nodes and 16 edges (Figure 5B). In terms of degree centrality, TNF-α exhibited the highest centrality with a score of six, followed by PRKCD and PIK3CD. Regarding the eigenvector centrality, which reflects the centrality weights of neighboring nodes, TNF-α, PIK3CD, and PRKCD displayed relatively high eigenvector centrality, followed by XIAP and ABCB1. Specifically, we filtered key target proteins based on the 75th percentile of degree and eigenvector centrality. The third-quartile values were 4 for degree centrality and approximately 0.378 for eigenvector centrality. Accordingly, TNF-α (degree centrality: 6, eigenvector centrality: 0.526), PIK3CD (degree centrality: 4, eigenvector centrality: 0.394), and PRKCD (degree centrality: 4, eigenvector centrality: 0.371) were recognized as key targets (Table 1).

Table 1. Centrality analysis of 12 candidate target proteins related to irritable bowel syndrome in Banhasasim-tang.

Protein Name	Gene Symbol	Degree	Eigenvector	Betweenness	Closeness
Tumor necrosis factor, membrane form	*TNF-α*	6	0.526	52	0.407
Phosphatidylinositol 4,5-bisphosphate 3-kinase catalytic subunit delta isoform	*PIK3CD*	4	0.394	29	0.393
Protein kinase C delta-type regulatory subunit	*PRKCD*	4	0.371	23	0.379
ATP-dependent translocase ABCB1	*ABCB1*	3	0.304	1	0.324
E3 ubiquitin-protein ligase XIAP	*XIAP*	3	0.304	1	0.324
Phosphatidylinositol 4,5-bisphosphate 3-kinase catalytic subunit alpha isoform	*PIK3CA*	3	0.277	4	0.333
Sodium-dependent serotonin transporter	*SLC6A4*	2	0.236	0	0.314
Nucleotide-binding oligomerization domain-containing protein 2	*NOD2*	2	0.236	0	0.314
Extracellular cell-membrane anchored RET cadherin 120 kDa fragment	*RET*	3	0.208	18	0.324
Nuclear protein 1	*NUPR1*	1	0.106	0	0.289
Extracellular calcium-sensing receptor	*CASR*	1	0.059	0	0.256
Sodium channel protein type 5 subunit alpha	*SCN5A*	0	0.000	0	0.083

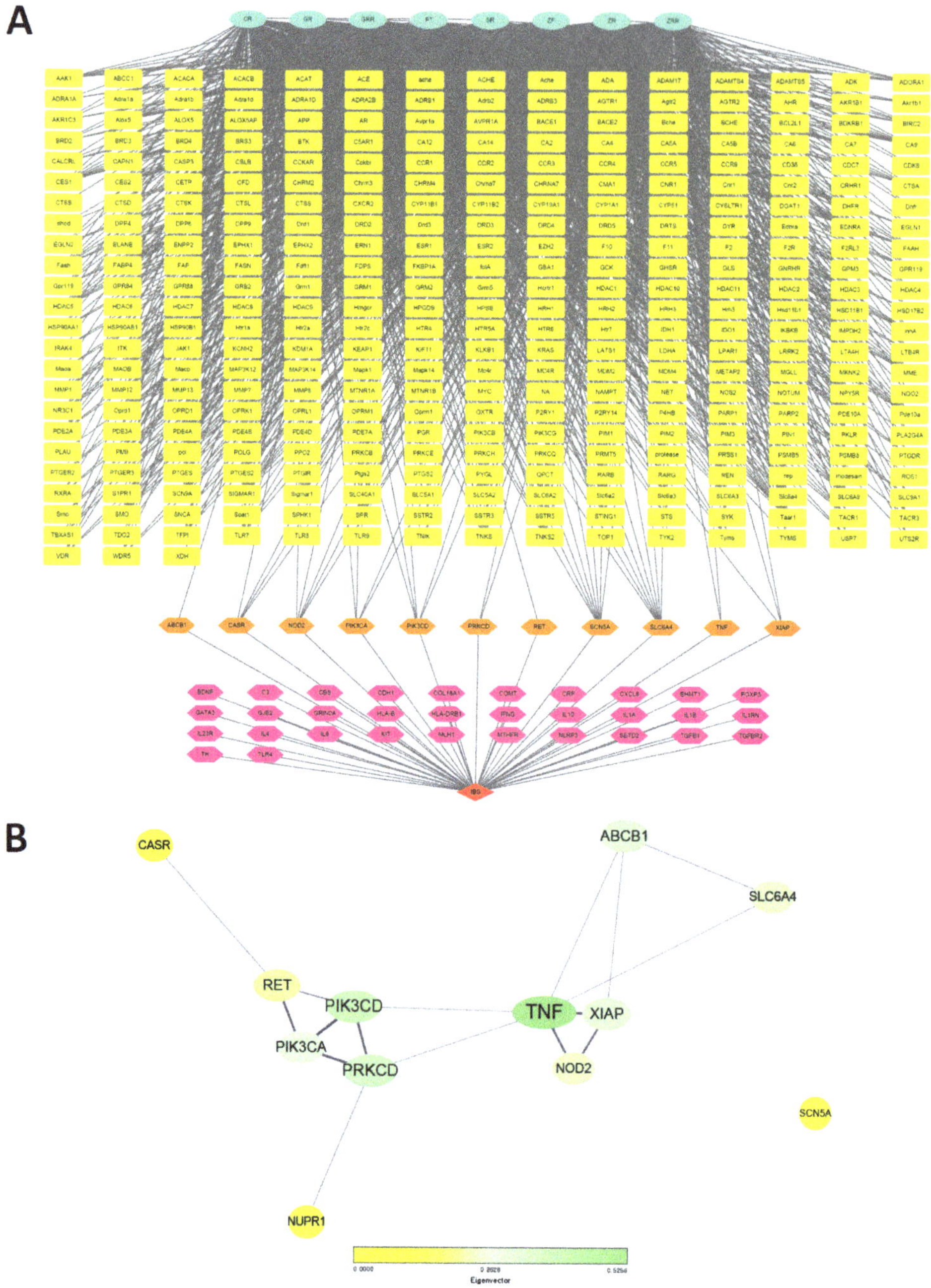

Figure 5. (**A**) Component–target–disease network for BHSST and IBS. Mint circles, yellow squares, pink hexagons, and red diamonds represent the components of BHSST, targets of BHSST, IBS-related targets, and IBS, respectively. Orange hexagons indicate potential BHSST targets involved in IBS pathogenesis. (**B**) Protein–protein interactions of 12 candidate target proteins from BHSST involved in IBS, as shown in panel (**A**). Node size and color represent degree and eigenvector centrality. CR: Coptidis Rhizoma, GR: Ginseng Radix, GRR: Glycyrrhizae Radix et Rhizoma, PT: Pinelliae Tuber, SR: Scutellariae Radix, ZF: Zizyphi Fructus, ZR: Zingiberis Rhizoma, ZRR: Zingiberis Rhizoma Recens.

2.5. Enrichment Analysis of GO and KEGG Pathways

GO enrichment analysis was conducted to explore the biological processes related to the 12 overlapping target candidates of BHSST implicated in IBS. The GO analysis results were categorized according to high-fold enrichment and low false discovery rates. The results indicated enrichment in the following biological processes: regulation of anatomical structure size, immune response-regulating signaling pathways, circulatory system processes, positive regulation of transport, and positive regulation of intracellular signal transduction. The predicted candidate locations for cellular components included the phosphatidylinositol 3-kinase complex class IA, phosphatidylinositol 3-kinase complex class IB, phosphatidylinositol 3-kinase complex class I, the external side of the apical plasma membrane, and the phosphatidylinositol 3-kinase complex. The following activities were enriched: phosphatidylinositol-4,5-bisphosphate 3-kinase activity; phosphatidylinositol-3,4-bisphosphate 5-kinase activity; 1-phosphatidylinositol-4-phosphate 3-kinase; 1-phosphatidylinositol-3-kinase; and insulin receptor substrate binding (Figure 6). To further elucidate the potential mechanisms, we investigated enriched biological pathways using the KEGG database. The results showed significant enrichment of pathways related to type II diabetes mellitus, central carbon metabolism in cancer, aldosterone-regulated sodium reabsorption, carbohydrate digestion and absorption, non-small-cell lung cancer, and platinum drug resistance (Figure 7). Excluding diseases unrelated to IBS, the TNF-α signaling pathway was notably enriched. Overall, TNF-α signaling-related proteins are potential candidates for the regulatory effects of BHSST on IBS.

2.6. Molecular Docking Simulation

Based on the network and enrichment analyses that identified TNF-α, PIK3CD, and PRKCD as key targets, molecular docking simulations were performed to determine whether the active compounds of BHSST could stably bind to these core proteins. Ligand-binding pockets of each protein were identified using the Protein Data Bank and literature sources. Ten independent molecular docking simulations were conducted for active compounds targeting TNF-α, PIK3CD, and PRKCD. Most of the simulation results showed stable binding positions consistent with those of known inhibitors. Binding poses with binding affinities lower than −5 kcal/mol are generally considered stable. Molecular docking simulations showed binding poses with affinities primarily below −5 kcal/mol (Supplementary Material Table S2). Specifically, the lowest binding affinity for TNF-α (PDB ID: 5MU8) with eudesm-4(14)-en-11-ol from ZR was −6.8212 kcal/mol, that for PIK3CD (PDB ID: 6PYR) with kanzonol T from GRR was −8.6546 kcal/mol, and that for PRKCD (PDB ID: 1YRK) with elemol from ZR and ZRR was −5.8467 kcal/mol (Figure 8, Table 2). A list of other candidate binding positions is provided in Supplementary Material Table S2.

Table 2. Representative molecular docking simulation results for active compounds in BHSST with their target proteins.

Medicine	Compound Name	PubChem ID	Target Protein (PDB ID)	Binding Affinity (kcal/mol)
ZR	eudesm-4(14)-en-11-ol	10557	TNF-α (5MU8)	−6.8212
GRR	kanzonol T	999902	PIK3CD (6PYR)	−8.6546
ZR, ZRR	elemol	92138	PRKCD (1YRK)	−5.8467

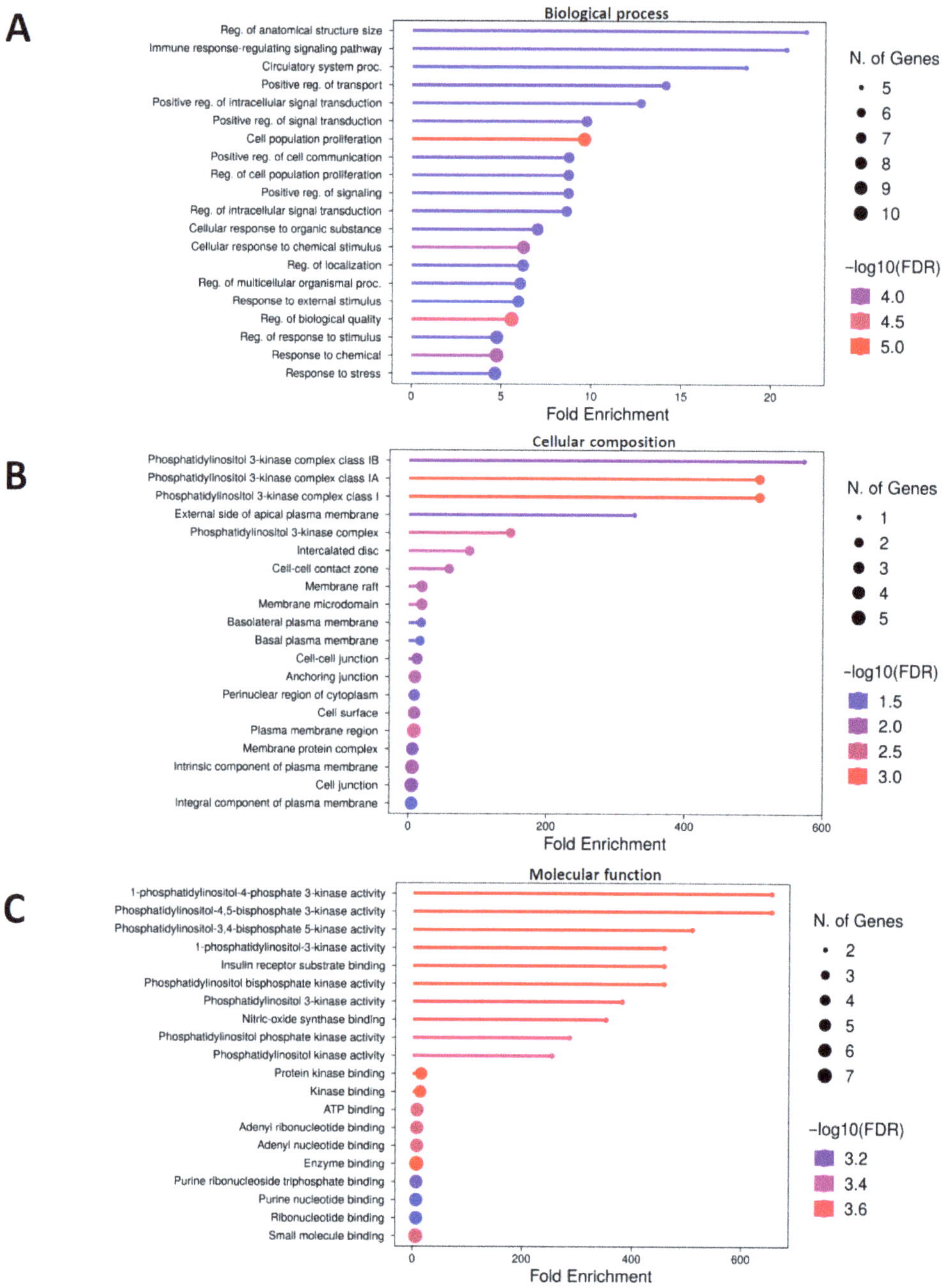

Figure 6. Gene ontology enrichment analysis. (**A**) Biological process, (**B**) cellular composition, and (**C**) molecular function. Based on the fold enrichment, the data are sorted in descending order. Bubble size represents the number of genes associated with each term (FDR cutoff < 0.05).

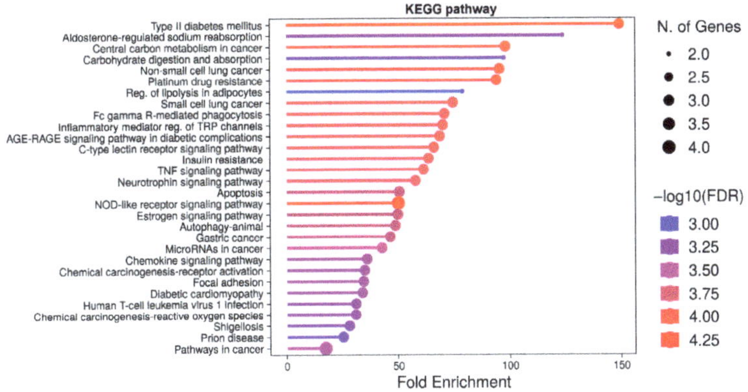

Figure 7. Enrichment analysis of the top 30 pathways from the Kyoto Encyclopedia of Genes and Genomes (KEGG). Based on fold enrichment, data are sorted in descending order. Bubble size represents the number of genes associated with each term (FDR cutoff < 0.05).

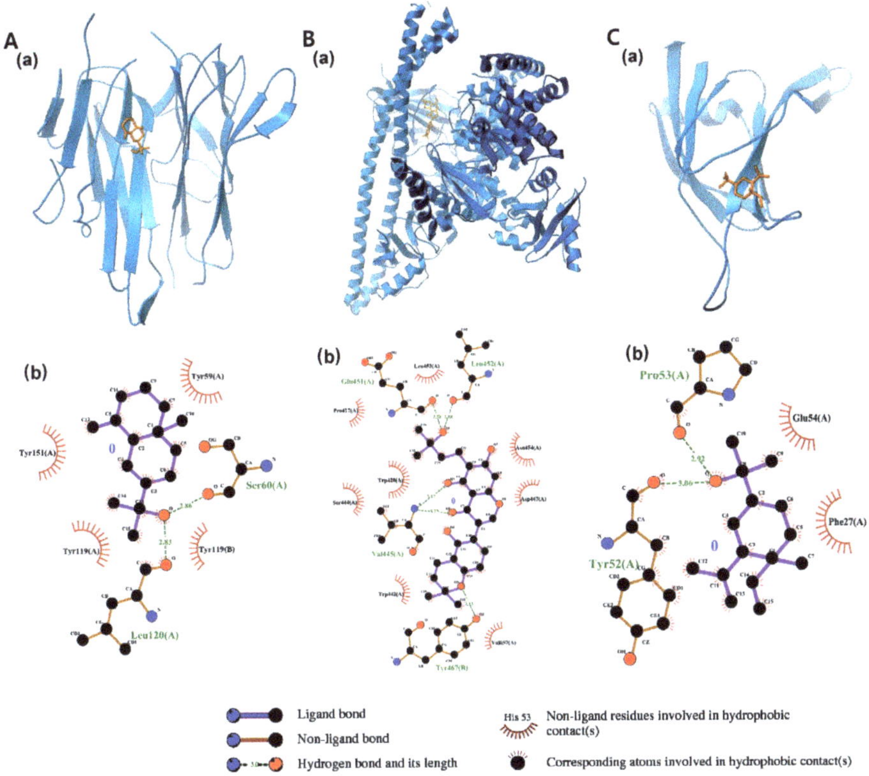

Figure 8. Representative stable binding poses from molecular docking simulations. The top panel shows the docking poses of the ligand (orange) with the protein (blue cartoon). The bottom panel illustrates the molecular interactions between the ligand and the protein, indicating the residues and chains involved in the interactions. Hydrogen bonds are depicted as green dashed lines with distances (in Ångströms). (**A**) Eudem-4(14)-en-11-ol with TNF-α. (**B**) Kanzonol T with PIK3CD. (**C**) Elemol with PRKCD. Black beads represent carbon, red beads represent oxygen, and blue beads represent nitrogen.

2.7. Molecular Dynamics Results

To corroborate the results obtained from the molecular docking analysis, a series of molecular dynamics (MD) simulations were conducted using GROMACS software in conjunction with the Charmm36 force field. The simulation results for TNF-α indicated that eudem-4(14)-en-11-ol stably bound to the protein over 50 ns. The RMSD of the distance between eu-dem-4(14)-en-11-ol and TNF-α was 0.16 nm, with a standard deviation of 0.02 nm. To gain insight into the trajectory of the ligand and protein, three data points were obtained at 25 ns intervals. Eudem-4(14)-en-11-ol remained stable within the cavity between the TNF-α dimers throughout the simulation. It was further demonstrated that the consistently maintained hydrogen bond interactions provided additional support for the binding of eu-dem-4(14)-en-11-ol to TNF-α (Figure 9).

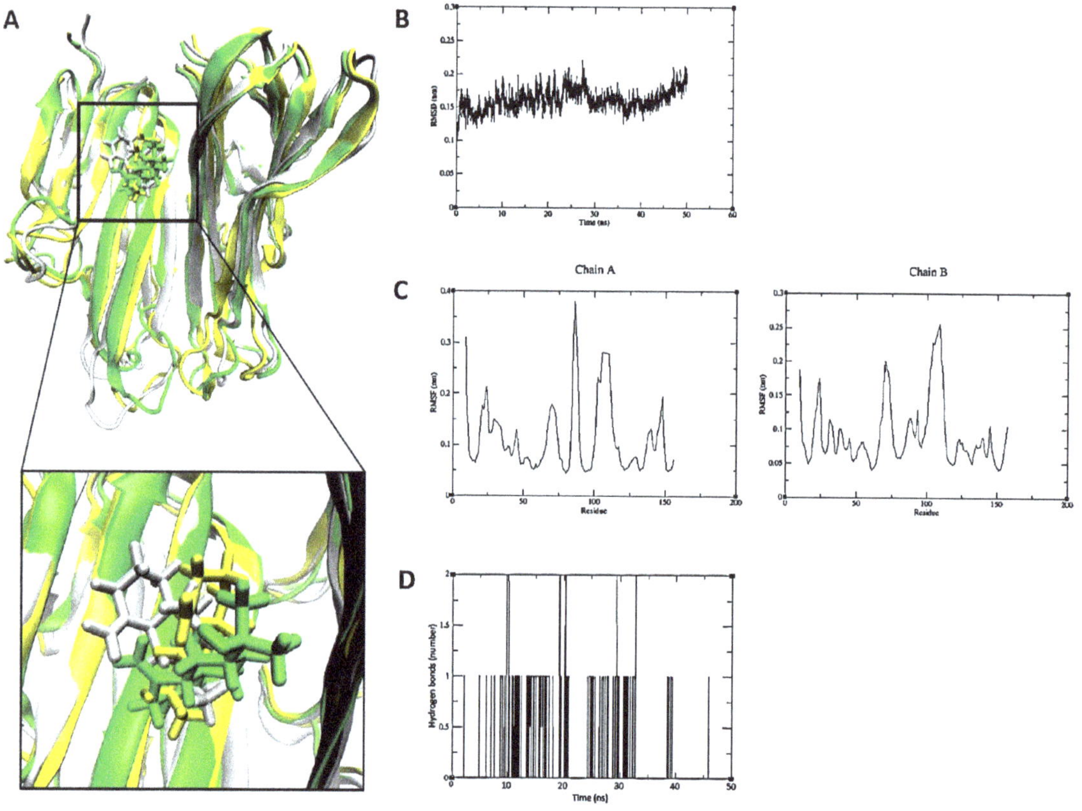

Figure 9. Molecular dynamics simulation analysis of eudem-4(14)-en-11-ol binding to the TNF-α dimer. (**A**) Three conformational snapshots merged at 25 ns intervals during the simulation (white: 0 ns; yellow: 25 ns; green: 50 ns). (**B**) RMSD between eudem-4(14)-en-11-ol and TNF-α. (**C**) RMSF of TNF-α. (**D**) Hydrogen bond interactions between eudem-4(14)-en-11-ol and TNF-α.

The binding of kanzonol T to PIK3CD was maintained at the active site. Although the planar conformation folded quickly, the portion of the structure bound near the active site pocket remained stable throughout the simulation. The RMSD of the distance was calculated to be 0.6 nm, with a standard deviation of 0.14 nm. Hydrogen bonding interactions remained consistently stable (Figure 10).

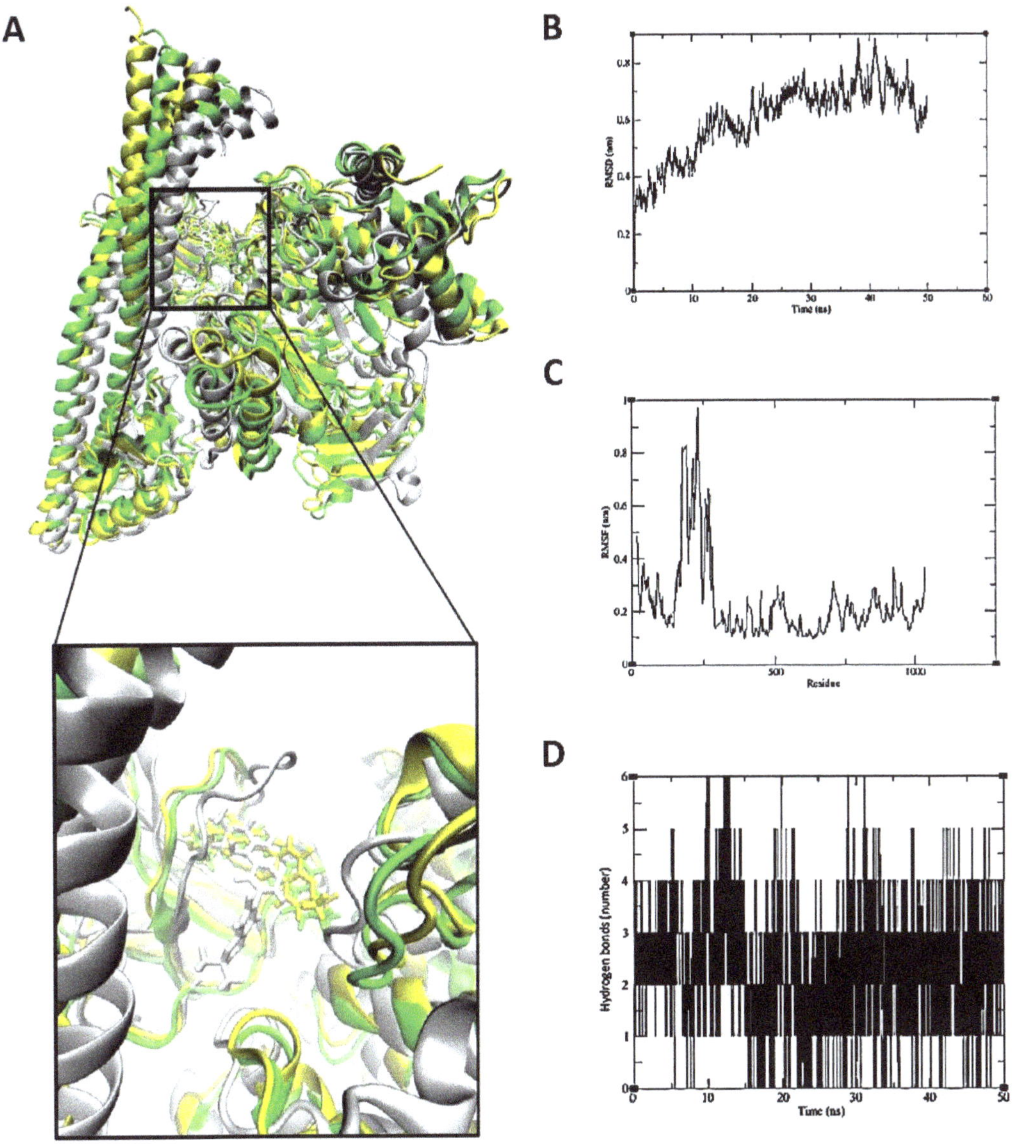

Figure 10. Analysis of the binding of Kanzonol T to PIK3CD by molecular dynamics simulation. (**A**) Three conformational snapshots taken at 25 ns intervals during the simulation (white: 0 ns; yellow: 25 ns; green: 50 ns). The molecular surface of PIK3CD is shown in white at 50 ns. (**B**) RMSD between Kanzonol T and PIK3CD. (**C**) RMSF of PIK3CD. (**D**) Interactions of the hydrogen bonds between Kanzonol T and PIK3CD.

However, MD simulation of elemol with PRKCD yielded results that differed from those obtained by molecular docking. The average RMSD was 0.28 nm, with a standard deviation of 0.11 nm. Elemol maintained its binding position from the start of the simulation until approximately 25 ns; however, at 50 ns it deviated slightly from the catalytic region (Figure 11).

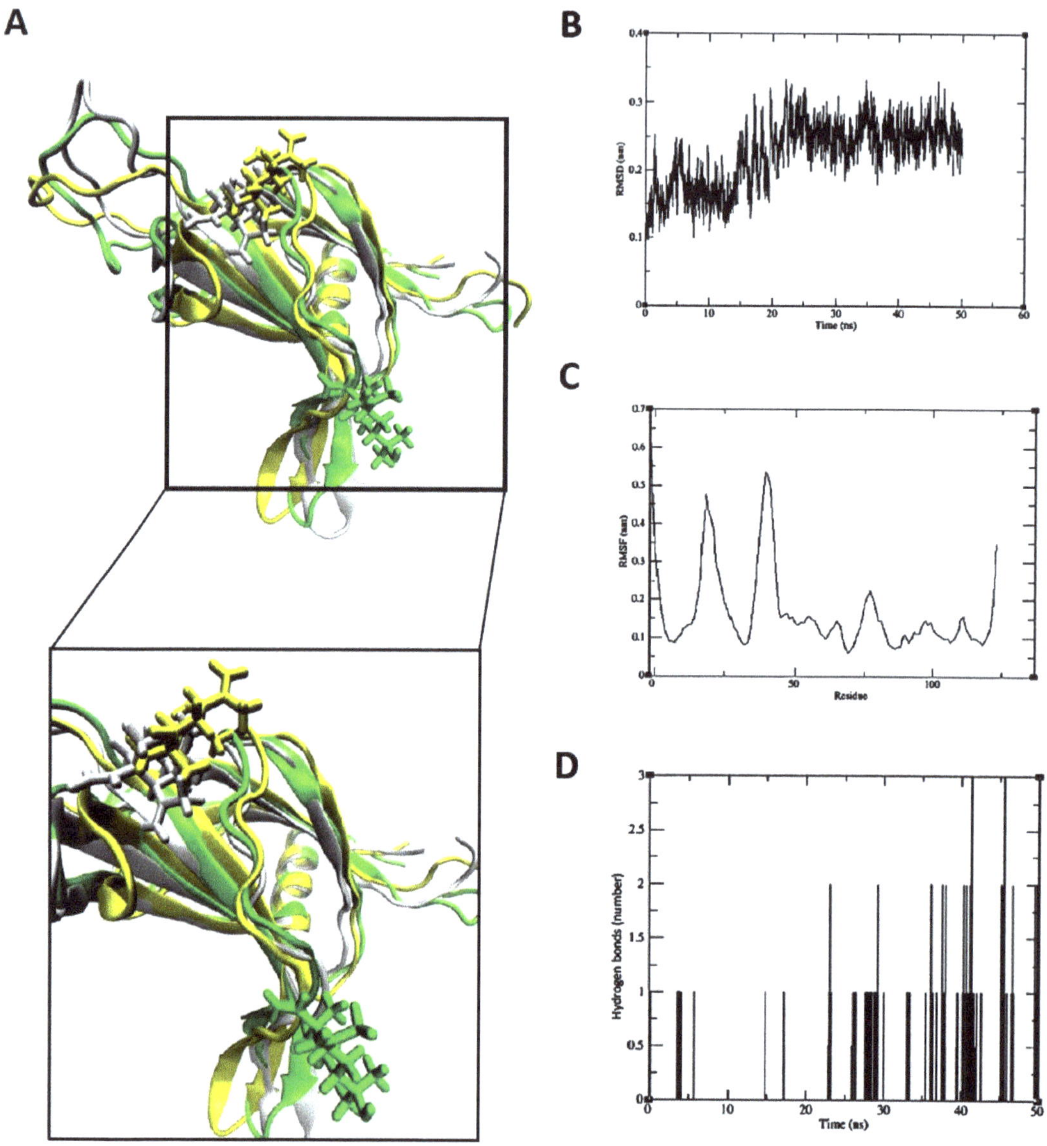

Figure 11. Analysis of the binding of elemol binding to PRKCD by molecular dynamics simulation. (**A**) Four conformational snapshots taken during the simulation and merged (white: 0 ns; yellow: 25 ns; green: 50 ns). Elemol moved away from the initial binding site on the catalytic domain over the course of the simulation. The molecular surface of PRKCD is shown in white at 50 ns. (**B**) RMSD between elemol and PRKCD. (**C**) RMSF of PRKCD. (**D**) Interactions of the hydrogen bonds between elemol and PRKCD.

2.8. Effects of Eudesm-4(14)-en-11-ol, Elemol, and BHSST on Zymosan-Induced Colon Alterations in IBS Mouse Models

To evaluate the therapeutic potential of eudesm-4(14)-en-11-ol, elemol, and BHSST, we assessed colon length and weight, stool characteristics, TNF-α levels, and pain-related behaviors in a zymosan-induced IBS colitis mouse model. Zymosan administration significantly shortened colon length and increased colon weight compared to healthy controls, confirming the successful induction of colitis. Treatment with eudesm-4(14)-en-11-ol (100 mg/kg) significantly restored colon length and reduced colon weight, while elemol (100 mg/kg) showed no measurable effect. BHSST (500 mg/kg) produced outcomes comparable to those of eudesm-4(14)-en-11-ol (Figure 12A,B). Zymosan also induced stool abnormalities, including watery, discolored feces and increased stool consistency scores. These alterations were significantly ameliorated by both eudesm-4(14)-en-11-ol and BHSST but remained unchanged with elemol treatment (Figure 12C). Furthermore, eudesm-4(14)-en-11-ol and BHSST both significantly reduced TNF-α expression and attenuated pain-related behaviors, while elemol did not demonstrate any beneficial effects (Figure 12D,E). Collectively, these findings suggest that eudesm-4(14)-en-11-ol, a bioactive component of BHSST, contributes substantially to the alleviation of zymosan-induced colitis and its associated symptoms.

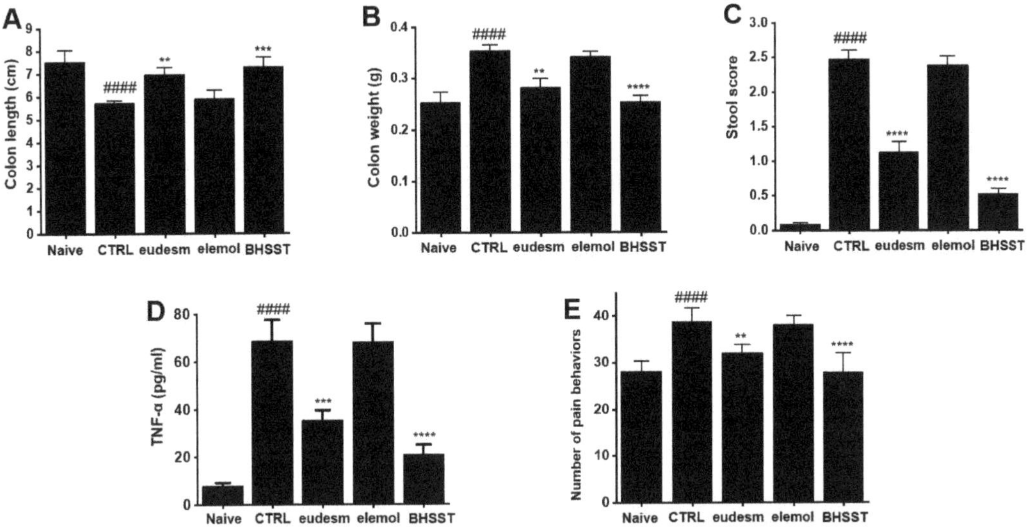

Figure 12. Effects of eudesm-4(14)-en-11-ol, elemol, and BHSST on colonic characteristics, stool consistency, TNF-α mRNA expression, and nociceptive behaviors in a zymosan-induced IBS animal model. (**A**) Colonic length and (**B**) weight were measured. (**C**) Stool consistency was assessed using a scoring system. (**D**) TNF-α mRNA levels were quantified by RT-qPCR. (E) Visceral pain-related behaviors were examined. Data are presented as mean ± SE. #### $p < 0.0001$ compared to the naïve group; ** $p < 0.01$, *** $p < 0.001$ and **** $p < 0.0001$ compared to the control group. CTRL: Control group; Eudesm: eudesm-4(14)-en-11-ol; BHSST: Banhasasim-tang.

3. Discussion

This study employed network pharmacology to explore the potential therapeutic targets and pathways of BHSST in the context of IBS. Prior to conducting the analysis, it was necessary to identify the physicochemical properties of the individual compounds present in each herbal component of BHSST, which required access to comprehensive metadata. Several specialized databases provide systematically curated information on traditional medicines, including the TM-MC, Zhongyaocai Integrated Database, TCM Database@Taiwan, and the Traditional Chinese Medicine Systems Pharmacology Database and Analysis Platform [32–35]. Among these, TM-MC was selected as the primary resource for the following three main reasons: (1) it focuses on traditional medicines commonly used in Northeast Asia; (2) the database is curated by subject-matter experts, including biologists and traditional medicine practitioners, based on up-to-date literature; (3) it offers clearly referenced and well-structured data sources.

To screen candidate therapeutic compounds, two criteria were applied: drug-likeness and oral bioavailability. While the definition of drug-likeness may vary across studies, compounds with higher drug-likeness scores are generally considered more likely to exhibit therapeutic effects. Oral bioavailability refers to the proportion of an orally administered compound that reaches systemic circulation and is thus available for pharmacological action [36].

Lipinski reported that compounds with poor absorption and permeability are more likely to fail in early-phase clinical trials and, thus, are considered to have low drug-likeness [37]. To address this, he proposed the well-known "Rule of 5", which outlines four criteria for optimal drug-likeness: a molecular weight under 500 Da, no more than five hydrogen bond donors, no more than ten hydrogen bond acceptors, and a calculated LogP below 5 [38]. Although several approved drugs, including antibiotics and antifungals, violate this rule, it remains a widely used guideline for predicting oral bioavailability. Similarly, Veber suggested that favorable oral bioavailability is associated with specific molecular properties, such as fewer than 10 rotatable bonds and a topological polar surface area (TPSA) below 140 $Å^2$ [39]. Based on these principles, the BOILED-Egg model was applied in our study to predict human intestinal absorption and blood–brain barrier (BBB) permeability. This model, developed from experimental datasets [40], utilizes two key physicochemical parameters—TPSA and WLogP—to classify compounds. The supervised learning algorithm used in the BOILED-Egg model demonstrated reliable predictive power, with a Matthews correlation coefficient of 0.6531 and an accuracy of 0.9156 for intestinal absorption [30]. Compounds predicted to be poorly absorbed were excluded from further analysis. Additionally, compounds identified as P-glycoprotein substrates were removed as P-glycoprotein plays a critical role in effluxing xenobiotics and their metabolites, thereby limiting therapeutic efficacy [41]. Oral bioavailability was further evaluated using Wei's model, applying a 20% cutoff threshold [37]. This model, trained on 1142 molecules and validated with 287 test molecules, showed robust predictive performance. Interestingly, among over 1000 molecular descriptors, topological indices exhibited a negative correlation with oral bioavailability [37,42].

After removing duplicates, 328 compounds were identified as active constituents of BHSST. Given the limitations of rule-based drug screening approaches, we combined both rule-based criteria and machine learning models to select candidate compounds predicted to have favorable drug-likeness and oral bioavailability in silico. Figure 2 illustrates the histograms of the physicochemical properties of BHSST compounds: active compounds (black) versus all compounds (white). The observed distributional differences underscore the insufficiency of rule-based methods alone in accurately identifying bioactive compounds. Subsequently, IBS-related genes were retrieved from the GeneCards and DisGeNET databases. From GeneCards the top 10% of genes ranked by relevance score were selected, while from DisGeNET genes with an evidence index ≥ 0.7 were included. The overlapping genes were subjected to further analysis.

To examine the potential interaction between BHSST and IBS-related targets, a compound–target–disease (CTD) network was constructed. The intersection of compound-derived and disease-related targets suggested mechanistic links through which BHSST might exert therapeutic effects in IBS. From this network, 12 hub targets (pivot candidates) were identified, and their protein–protein interaction (PPI) networks were analyzed. Such topological network analysis is known to provide novel insights into biological complexity and supports drug repurposing efforts [43].

Centrality measures, commonly applied in topological analyses, help to assess the importance of individual nodes within a biological network. Degree centrality quantifies the number of direct interactions, while eigenvector centrality reflects node influence based on the connectivity of neighboring nodes [44]. Although betweenness and closeness centralities are also standard metrics, they require biological interpretation and were not the primary focus of this study. Instead, we emphasized degree and eigenvector centralities to assess node importance. Nonetheless, for reference, data on betweenness and closeness centrality are also provided (Table 1).

Degree and eigenvector centrality analyses identified TNF-α, PIK3CD, and PRKCD as key regulatory nodes in IBS pathophysiology. TNF-α is a pivotal mediator of inflammation, and the monoclonal antibody infliximab, which targets TNF-α, is widely used to treat inflammatory diseases such as Crohn's disease and ulcerative colitis [45]. Anti-TNF-α therapies not only reduce inflammation but also help restore gut microbiota composition toward a healthier state in patients with Crohn's disease [46]. Given increasing evidence that low-grade inflammation and dysbiosis contribute to IBS symptoms, modulation of TNF-α may offer therapeutic benefits in specific IBS subtypes, especially those characterized by immune activation or post-infectious features. PIK3CD plays a critical role in immune cell signaling [47]. Gain-of-function mutations in PIK3CD have been linked to immunodeficiency syndromes presenting with gastrointestinal symptoms, including chronic diarrhea, intestinal lymphoid hyperplasia, and mucosal inflammation [48]. These manifestations overlap with clinical features observed in inflammatory IBS subtypes. Therefore, targeting PIK3CD signaling may represent a promising approach to modulate aberrant immune responses and restore gut homeostasis in IBS patients with underlying immune dysregulation. PRKCD, a member of the protein kinase C family, regulates diverse cellular functions such as apoptosis, proliferation, and immune cell activity [49]. Within the gut, PRKCD may influence epithelial barrier integrity and immune tolerance through its context-dependent pro- or anti-apoptotic effects [50]. Dysregulation of PRKCD signaling could contribute to mucosal immune imbalance, visceral hypersensitivity, or impaired epithelial repair in IBS. Thus, modulating PRKCD activity may have therapeutic relevance, although further studies are necessary to elucidate its precise role in IBS pathogenesis.

Molecular docking is a computational technique used to predict the preferred binding positions of ligands to target proteins. In this study, docking simulations revealed stable binding affinities between active compounds from BHSST and the key target proteins TNF-α, PIK3CD, and PRKCD. Previous research suggests that binding affinities around −5 kcal/mol indicate stable ligand–protein interactions [51,52]. Consistently, several active compounds in our study exhibited binding affinities of −5 kcal/mol or lower, implying potential effective interactions with these targets (see Supplementary Material Table S2). MD simulations, based on molecular mechanics, provide a dynamic view by tracking the trajectories of molecules over time [53]. While molecular docking offers a high-throughput assessment of ligand–receptor interactions, it represents a static snapshot and cannot capture the full dynamic behavior of molecular complexes. Therefore, we complemented docking results with MD simulations to further validate and characterize the stability and dynamics of the ligand–target interactions.

However, this study has several limitations. First, although Lipinski's rule of five was used to screen drug-like compounds, it may not be fully applicable to complex herbal formulations like BHSST, which contain a broad range of phytochemicals that do not conform to typical synthetic drug properties. Second, the oral bioavailability and systemic exposure of the predicted active compounds, including eudesm-4(14)-en-11-ol, have not been evaluated in humans. Therefore, their actual therapeutic potential in clinical settings remains to be validated. Also, while molecular docking and dynamics analyses suggest plausible target interactions, these findings should be supported by further pharmacokinetic and pharmacodynamic studies. In addition, although in silico approaches such as molecular docking and dynamics simulations provided valuable insights into potential compound–target interactions, these computational findings ideally require further validation through in vitro assays, including enzymatic inhibition tests or biophysical binding analyses such as surface plasmon resonance, isothermal titration calorimetry, or microscale thermophoresis. Due to current laboratory limitations, we were unable to perform such in vitro validation in this study. Instead, we focused on in vivo experiments to partially support the predicted mechanisms. Nevertheless, future studies incorporating these functional assays will be essential to confirm the direct molecular interactions and further substantiate the pharmacological relevance of the identified compounds. Furthermore, the extract used in this study was provided as a finished product by a pharmaceutical company, and critical manufacturing details such as the drug extract ratio (DER) and precise phytochemical composition were not disclosed. This lack of quantitative characterization may affect the consistency and reproducibility of pharmacological effects across different batches. Future studies should aim to include comprehensive phytochemical profiling and batch standardization to ensure product quality and replicable biological activity. Moreover, while selected compounds such as eudesm-4(14)-en-11-ol and elemol were administered in animal experiments based on available literature, their actual content within the BHSST extract was not quantified. This limits our ability to directly correlate their concentrations with observed pharmacological outcomes. Inclusion of validated analytical methods to determine the levels of such constituents would enhance the reliability and reproducibility of future research.

Consequently, eudesm-4(14)-en-11-ol was found to bind stably within the central cavity of the TNF-α dimer (Figure 9). The stable root mean square deviation (RMSD) and trajectory analysis indicate a tight and sustained interaction between eudesm-4(14)-en-11-ol and TNF-α. The substrate-binding pocket of PIK3CD, comprising residues Trp442, Leu452, and Tyr467, mediates interactions with various substrates and inhibitors primarily through hydrogen bonding. Molecular dynamics simulations demonstrated that kanzonol T maintained a stable binding conformation within this pocket (Figure 10). Interestingly, the MD analysis of elemol binding to PRKCD revealed results that differed from the initial molecular docking predictions. Although docking simulations suggested a stable binding pose with an affinity of −5.8467 kcal/mol, MD simulations showed that elemol deviated from its initial binding position after approximately 50 ns (Figure 11), indicating reduced stability in a dynamic environment.

Among the molecular candidates identified, eudesm-4(14)-en-11-ol and kanzonol T were prioritized for further evaluation due to their predicted biological activity. However, owing to the unavailability of commercially sourced kanzonol T, we were unable to include it in the in vivo experiments and thus could only confirm the therapeutic efficacy of eudesm-4(14)-en-11-ol in the IBS model. As a complementary control, elemol was also evaluated and showed no therapeutic effect. Notably, BHSST treatment produced beneficial effects comparable to those of eudesm-4(14)-en-11-ol (Figure 12). Future studies will focus on the isolation or synthesis of kanzonol T to enable its biological evaluation in similar in vivo models.

4. Materials and Methods

4.1. Screening Active Compounds

The list of compounds in BHSST was retrieved from the Traditional Medicine Materials and Chemical Compounds Database of Northeast Asia (https://informatics.kiom.re.kr/compound/, accessed on 2 May 2024) [32]. The Simplified Molecular Input Line

Entry System (SMILES) for each compound was retrieved and validated using the PubChem database (https://pubchem.ncbi.nlm.nih.gov/, accessed on 2 May 2024). If the isomeric SMILES of a compound was not available in the PubChem database, the standard SMILES was selected for analysis. Compounds predicted to be negative for P-glycoprotein substrates and to exhibit human intestinal absorption were classified using SwissADME (http://www.swissadme.ch/index.php/, accessed on 7 May 2024) based on SMILES representations of up to 200 characters. The remaining compounds, which did not violate Lipinski's "Rule of Five" and were predicted to have an oral bioavailability exceeding 20%, were identified as active compounds [37,38].

4.2. Selection of Disease-Related Genes

IBS-related genes were retrieved from GeneCards (https://www.genecards.org/, accessed on 7 May 2024) and DisGeNET (https://www.disgenet.org/, accessed on 7 May 2024) databases [54,55]. To maintain a high level of relevance between diseases and genes, the top 10% protein-coding genes from GeneCards and those with an evidence index of 0.7 or above from DisGeNET were selected.

4.3. Target Prediction

The target proteins of the active compounds in BHSST were predicted using models from version 33 of the ChEMBL database (https://www.ebi.ac.uk/chembl/, accessed on 13 May 2024) [56,57]. The SMILES of each compound were queried using the ChEMBL multitask neural network model (https://github.com/chembl/chembl_multitask_model accessed on 13 May 2024), and the target proteins were filtered for those with a probability of 0.7 or higher for human targets.

4.4. Network Construction

To elucidate the associations among active compounds, target candidates, and diseases, a CTD network was constructed. Key protein–protein interactions were obtained using Cytoscape 3.9.1 software (Boston, MA, USA) [56]. Critical nodes in the protein–protein interactions were identified using the third quartile of eigenvector centrality and degree centrality.

4.5. Gene Ontology (GO) and Kyoto Encyclopedia of Genes and Genomes (KEGG) Pathway Analysis

To elucidate the contributions of BHSST to the functional and underlying pathways, GO and KEGG pathways were analyzed [57,58]. GO and KEGG pathway analyses were conducted using ShinyGO version 0.80 (http://bioinformatics.sdstate.edu/go/, accessed on 29 May 2024) [59]. A statistical cutoff threshold of 0.05 was established. The top 20 GO results and the top 30 KEGG pathway results were reported based on fold enrichment, which reflected the false discovery rate and gene count.

4.6. Molecular Docking

The crystal structures of the target proteins were sourced from the RCSB Protein Data Bank (https://www.rcsb.org/, accessed on 11 June 2024), and the three-dimensional structures of each ligand were prepared using the PubChem database. Prior to the docking simulations, heteroatoms, including ions and water molecules, were removed. The ligand files were converted into AutoDock-compatible formats (.sdf to .pdb) using PyMOL software (V3.0.5; Schrödinger LLC., New York, NY, USA). Ligands were prepared to identify rotatable bonds, charges, and unnecessary hydrogen atoms. Proteins were processed to adjust charges, add hydrogen atoms, and merge non-polar hydrogen atoms for docking. A binding site search grid was configured to cover the entire surface of the protein. To ensure accuracy, ten independent docking simulations were conducted for each ligand, with the simulation completeness set to 32. The docking simulations were performed using AutoDock Tools version 1.5.7 and AutoDock Vina version 1.2.3 [60–62]. The pose exhibiting the lowest binding affinity (kcal/mol) between the active compounds and proteins was considered the most stable protein–ligand binding pose. Data visualization was performed using PyMOL version 2.6 and LigPlot+ version 2.2 software [63].

4.7. Molecular Dynamics Simulation

GROMACS software version 2024.2 was used for the molecular dynamics (MD) simulations [64]. Prior to initiating the simulations, each protein structure was subjected to a preparation process wherein water molecules and heteroatoms were removed from the coordinate files in accordance with established protocols. The coordinates of the active compounds were selected based on the results of molecular docking simulations, which identified the most stable binding poses. The coordinates and parameters of each active compound were configured according to the CHARMM36 force field in the context of MD [65]. In order to model the solvation under periodic boundary conditions, the TIP3P explicit water model was employed. The objective of this study was to introduce sodium and chloride ions at a concentration of 0.154 M to achieve physiological conditions. Additional sodium ions were added to neutralize the system. The system was subsequently subjected to energy minimization. For NVT and NPT equilibrations, the Berendsen thermostat and Parrinello–Rahman barostat, respectively, were utilized. In this study, long-range electrostatics were investigated using the Particle Mesh Ewald method [66]. A neighbor-searching operation was conducted using the Verlet algorithm. Following a 50 ns simulation, the root mean square deviation (RMSD) and root mean square fluctuation (RMSF) were analyzed. The hydrogen bonding interactions during the simulation were evaluated using the VMD software (V1.9.4.) [67], employing distance and angle cutoffs of 3.5 nm and 30°, respectively. The results were rendered in a three-dimensional visual form using PyMOL software.

4.8. Instrument and Reagents

BHSST was donated by HANKOOKSHINYAK Pharmaceutical Co., Ltd. (Nonsan, Republic of Korea). The dried extract powder of BHSST, which was prepared using a water extraction method, was used in the present study. The analysis was conducted using an ACQUITY™ UPLC system (Waters, Milford, MA, USA), equipped with a photodiode array (PDA) detector and an ACQUITY™ BEH C18 column (1.7 μm, 2.1 × 100 mm). Data acquisition and processing were carried out using Empower software (V3.8.0). For sample extraction, a microwave extractor (Power Sonic 405, HWA-SHIN TECH, Seoul, Republic of Korea) was employed. The solvents used included methanol (Junsei, Tokyo, Japan), acetonitrile (JT BAKER, Phillipsburg, NJ, USA), and triple-distilled water. The individual initial components of BHSST are presented in Table 3. Reference standards—6-gingerol, glycyrrhizinic acid, liquiritin, isoliquiritigenin, berberine, baicalin, and ginsenoside Rb1—were obtained from Sigma-Aldrich (St. Louis, MO, USA) [27,68].

4.9. Preparation of Standard Solutions

For quantitative analysis, precise amounts of each reference compound—6-gingerol, glycyrrhizinic acid, liquiritin, isoliquiritigenin, berberine, baicalin, and ginsenoside Rb1—were accurately weighed and dissolved in methanol to prepare stock solutions at a concentration of 1 μg/mL. These stock solutions were subsequently diluted with methanol to obtain working standard solutions at concentrations of 1, 5, and 10 ng/mL [27,68].

Table 3. Initial composition of BHSST used in this study.

Latin Name	Scientific Name	Amount (g)
Pinelliae rhizoma	*Pinellia ternata* Breitenbach	0.63
Scutellariae radix	*Scutellaria baicalensis* Georgi	0.85
Zingiberis rhizoma siccus	*Zingiber officinale*	0.03
Ginseng radix	*Panax ginseng* C. A. Meyer	0.45
Glycyrrhizae Radix	*Glycyrrhiza uralensis* Fischer	0.51
Jujubae fructus	*Zizyphus jujuba Mill*	0.34
Coptidis rhizoma	*Coptis chinensis* Franch	0.11
Zingiberis Rhizoma	*Zingiber officinale* Roscoe	0.28
	Total	3.20

4.10. *Preparation of Test Solution for Quantitative Analysis*

For the quantitative analysis, each test solution was prepared by accurately weighing 0.1 g of the BHSST sample, which had been uniformly mixed with the respective test liquid. The weighed sample was then extracted with 10 mL of 50% methanol using microwave-assisted extraction for 1 h. After extraction, the mixture was filtered through a membrane filter with a pore size of less than 0.45 μm, and the resulting filtrate was collected for analysis [27,68].

4.11. *Quantification of BHSST*

Quantitative analysis of BHSST was performed using a Waters ACQUITY™ UPLC system equipped with a photodiode array (PDA) detector and an ACQUITY™ BEH C18 column (1.7 μm, 2.1 × 100 mm, Waters, Milford, MA, USA). Data acquisition was managed using Empower software. The column was maintained at ambient temperature. The PDA detection wavelengths for the analytes were as follows: 6-gingerol at 280 nm; glycyrrhizinic acid, liquiritin, and isoliquiritigenin at 254 nm; berberine at 345 nm; and baicalin at 277 nm. The mobile phase consisted of acetonitrile and water containing 0.1% formic acid. Detailed chromatographic conditions are provided in Table 4. Each sample (10 μL) was injected with a flow rate of 1.0 mL/min. Identification was based on retention times, and quantification was carried out using the peak area method.

Table 4. BHSST used in this study. The analysis condition of 6-Gingerol, Glycyrrhizinic acid, Liquiritin, Isoliquiritigenin, Berberine, and Baicalin. FA: Formic Acid.

Time (min)	0.1% FA/Water (%)	0.1% FA/Acetonitrile (%)	Flow Rate (mL/min)
0	98	2	0.40
1.0	98	2	0.40
3.0	90	10	0.40
7.0	40	60	0.40
10.0	20	80	0.40
12.0	0	100	0.40
14.0	98	2	0.40
16.0	98	2	0.40

For the analysis of ginsenoside Rg1, PDA detection was performed at 203 nm. The mobile phase consisted of a binary mixture of acetonitrile and water. Analytical parameters specific to Rg1 are summarized in Table 5. In this case, a 2 μL sample was injected with a flow rate of 0.4 mL/min. As with the other analytes, identification was determined by retention time, and quantification was based on peak area [27,68].

Table 5. The analysis condition of Ginsenoside Rg1.

Time (min)	Water (%)	Acetonitrile (%)	Flow Rate (mL/min)
0	85	15	0.40
1.0	85	15	0.40
14.0	70	30	0.40
15.0	68	32	0.40
16.0	60	40	0.40
17.0	45	55	0.40
19.0	45	55	0.40
21.0	10	90	0.40
22.0	10	90	0.40
23.0	85	15	0.40

4.12. *Quantitative Analysis of Marker Compounds in BHSST*

The concentrations of 6-gingerol, glycyrrhizinic acid, liquiritin, isoliquiritigenin, berberine, baicalin, and ginsenoside Rb1 in BHSST were determined by UPLC. Quantification was performed based on calibration curves generated from each corresponding reference standard, as shown in Table 6. Method validation confirmed the analytical procedure to be stable and reliable, enabling consistent and effective separation of the seven major constituents in BHSST [27,68].

Table 6. Contents of the seven marker compounds in the dried, powdered BHSST extract, measured by UPLC.

Compound (Marker)	Content in Extract (mg/g)	Calculated Marker Dose (mg/kg)
6-Gingerol	0.00106 ± 0.00020	0.00053 ± 0.00010
Glycyrrhizinic acid	0.01057 ± 0.00130	0.00529 ± 0.00065
Liquiritin	0.00353 ± 0.00015	0.00177 ± 0.00008
Isoliquiritigenin	0.00073 ± 0.00003	0.00037 ± 0.00002
Berberine	0.03300 ± 0.00075	0.01650 ± 0.00038
Baicalin	0.00111 ± 0.00027	0.00056 ± 0.00014
Ginsenoside Rb1	0.00153 ± 0.00013	0.00077 ± 0.00007

4.13. *IBS Animal Model and Treatment*

Colitis was induced in 6-week-old C57BL/6 mice via transanal administration of 0.1 mL of a zymosan suspension (30 mg/mL) using a feeding needle. Mice were then orally administered one of the following treatments once daily for three consecutive days: PBS, eudesm-4(14)-en-11-ol (100 mg/kg; Sigma-Aldrich, St. Louis, MO, USA) [69], elemol (100 mg/kg; Angene Chemical, London, UK), or BHSST (500 mg/kg) [27,68]. On day four all experimental assessments were conducted. The zymosan-treated mice were divided into the following five groups (n = 8 per group): PBS naïve, zymosan control, eudesm-4(14)-en-11-ol-treated, elemol-treated, and BHSST-treated.

4.14. *Macroscopic Evaluation*

After fecal matter was removed, colon length (from cecum to anus) and weight were measured. Stool consistency was scored independently by three blinded observers using a four-point scale: 0 = normal, 1 = loose, 2 = soft/sticky, and 3 = diarrhea.

4.15. *Quantification of TNF-α Expression by RT-qPCR*

Total RNA was extracted from colonic tissue using TRIzol reagent (Invitrogen, Waltham, MA, USA). Complementary DNA (cDNA) was synthesized from the isolated

RNA using an M-MLV reverse transcriptase kit (Promega, Madison, WI, USA). TNF-α mRNA expression levels were quantified using real-time quantitative PCR (RT-qPCR).

4.16. Assessment of Pain-Related Behaviors

Pain-related behaviors were evaluated by observing specific actions such as abdominal licking, full-body stretching, pressing the abdomen against the floor, and arching of the back caused by visceral contractions. Two independent observers recorded these behaviors during a 10 min observation period.

4.17. Statistical Analysis

Data are presented as mean ± standard error (SE). Statistical comparisons among groups were performed using a one-way analysis of variance (ANOVA), followed by Dunnett's post hoc test. Analyses were conducted using GraphPad Prism 8 software, with statistical significance set at $p < 0.05$.

5. Conclusions

This study employed network pharmacology, molecular docking, and molecular dynamics simulations to explore the potential mechanisms of BHSST in IBS. In silico analyses identified 12 candidate targets, highlighting the TNF-α signaling and apoptosis pathways. Among the compounds analyzed, eudesm-4(14)-en-11-ol and kanzonol T showed potential interactions with TNF-α and PIK3CD, respectively. In vivo validation using a zymosan-induced IBS mouse model confirmed the therapeutic potential of eudesm-4(14)-en-11-ol, while elemol, predicted to be inactive, showed no effect. BHSST itself produced similar improvements to eudesm-4(14)-en-11-ol across key parameters. These findings offer preliminary mechanistic insights into the anti-inflammatory actions of BHSST and support its potential relevance in IBS management, warranting further investigation.

Supplementary Materials: The following supporting information can be downloaded at: https://www.mdpi.com/article/10.3390/ph18081123/s1. Table S1: List of all active compound–target pairs and candidate target proteins for BHSST; Table S2: Additional molecular docking simulation results for active compounds of BHSST against TNF-α, PIK3CD, and PRKCD.

Author Contributions: Conceptualization, W.-G.C., S.-J.K., J.-W.P., and B.-J.K.; methodology, W.-G.C., S.-J.K., J.-H.S., C.-H.B., and S.K.; software, W.-G.C.; validation, W.-G.C., S.-J.K., J.-H.S., C.-H.B., and S.K.; formal analysis, W.-G.C., S.-J.K., and J.-H.S.; investigation, W.-G.C., S.-J.K., and J.-H.S.; resources, W.-G.C., S.-J.K., C.-H.B., and S.K.; data curation, W.-G.C., J.-H.S., C.-H.B., and S.K.; writing—original draft preparation, W.-G.C., J.-W.P., and B.-J.K.; writing—review and editing, W.-G.C., S.-J.K., J.-W.P., and B.-J.K.; visualization, W.-G.C., S.-J.K., J.-H.S., C.-H.B., and S.K.; supervision, J.-W.P. and B.-J.K.; project administration, J.-W.P. and B.-J.K.; funding acquisition, J.-W.P. and B.-J.K. All authors have read and agreed to the published version of the manuscript.

Funding: This study was supported by the Basic Science Research Program through the National Research Foundation of Korea (NRF) funded by the Ministry of Education (RS-2021-NR065896) and by the Bio & Medical Technology Development Program of the National Research Foundation (NRF) funded by the Korean government (MSIT) (No. RS-2022-NR067333).

Institutional Review Board Statement: The animal experiments were conducted in accordance with the guidelines of the Institutional Animal Care and Use Committee (IACUC) of Pusan National University (Busan, Republic of Korea; PNU-2025-0577, Approval day: 1 March 2025).

Informed Consent Statement: Not applicable.

Data Availability Statement: The original data are available upon reasonable request to the corresponding author. The data are not publicly available due to privacy and ethical restrictions.

Conflicts of Interest: The authors declare no conflicts of interest.

References

1. Canavan, C.; West, J.; Card, T. The Epidemiology of Irritable Bowel Syndrome. *Clin. Epidemiol.* **2014**, *6*, 71–80.
2. Chen, M.; Ruan, G.; Chen, L.; Ying, S.; Li, G.; Xu, F.; Xiao, Z.; Tian, Y.; Lv, L.; Ping, Y.; et al. Neurotransmitter and Intestinal Interactions: Focus on the Microbiota-Gut-Brain Axis in Irritable Bowel Syndrome. *Front. Endocrinol.* **2022**, *13*, 817100. [CrossRef]
3. Hellström, P.M. Pathophysiology of the Irritable Bowel Syndrome—Reflections of Today. *Best Pract. Res. Clin. Gastroenterol.* **2019**, *40–41*, 101620. [CrossRef]
4. Jang, D.E.; Bae, J.H.; Chang, Y.J.; Lee, Y.H.; Nam, K.T.; Kim, I.Y.; Seong, J.K.; Lee, Y.C.; Yeom, S.C. Neuronal Nitric Oxide Synthase Is a Novel Biomarker for the Interstitial Cells of Cajal in Stress-Induced Diarrhea-Dominant Irritable Bowel Syndrome. *Dig. Dis. Sci.* **2018**, *63*, 619–627. [CrossRef]
5. Shih, Y.C.T.; Barghout, V.E.; Sandler, R.S.; Jhingran, P.; Sasane, M.; Cook, S.; Gibbons, D.C.; Halpern, M. Resource Utilization Associated with Irritable Bowel Syndrome in the United States 1987–1997. *Dig. Dis. Sci.* **2002**, *47*, 1705–1715. [CrossRef]
6. Fuentes, I.M.; Christianson, J.A. Ion Channels, Ion Channel Receptors, and Visceral Hypersensitivity in Irritable Bowel Syndrome. *Neurogastroenterol. Motil.* **2016**, *28*, 1613–1618. [CrossRef]
7. Hopkins, A.L. Network Pharmacology. *Nat. Biotechnol.* **2007**, *25*, 1110–1111. [CrossRef]
8. Zhou, L.; Wu, T. A Network Pharmacology-Based Study on Vital Pharmacological Pathways and Targets of Eucommiae Cortex Acting on Osteoporosis. *BioMed Res. Int.* **2022**, *2022*, 8510842. [CrossRef]
9. Dou, J.Y.; Zhang, M.; Cen, H.; Chen, Y.Q.; Wu, Y.F.; Lu, F.; Zhou, J.; Liu, X.S.; Gu, Y.Y. *Salvia miltiorrhiza* Bunge (Danshen) and Bioactive Compound Tanshinone IIA Alleviates Cisplatin-Induced Acute Kidney Injury Through Regulating PXR/NF-κB Signaling. *Front. Pharmacol.* **2022**, *13*, 860383. [CrossRef]
10. Lee, S.K.; Zetterling, C.M.; Östling, M.; Moon, B.M. Electrical Characterization of Titanium-Based Ohmic Contacts to 4H-Silicon Carbide for High-Power and High-Temperature Operation. *J. Korean Phys. Soc.* **2002**, *40*, 572.
11. Kawashima, K.; Nomura, A.; Makino, T.; Saito, K.; Kano, Y. Pharmacological Properties of Traditional Medicine (XXIX): Effect of Hange-Shashin-to and the Combinations of Its Herbal Constituents on Rat Experimental Colitis. *Biol. Pharm. Bull.* **2004**, *27*, 1599–1603. [CrossRef]
12. Xu, G. Treatment of Reflux Laryngopharyngitis with Modified Banxia Xiexin Tang (*Pinellia* Decoction for Draining the Heart)—A Report of 40 Cases. *J. Tradit. Chin. Med.* **2006**, *26*, 127–131.
13. Chen, F.; Chen, F.; Jong, M.; Tsai, H.; Wang, J.; Hwang, S. Modern Use of Chinese Herbal Formulae from Shang-Han Lun. *Chin. Med. J.* **2009**, *122*, 1889–1894.
14. Shin, M.R.; Seo, B.I.; Son, C.G.; Roh, S.S.; An, H.J. Banhasasim-Tang Treatment Reduces the Severity of Esophageal Mucosal Ulcer on Chronic Acid Reflux Esophagitis in Rats. *BioMed Res. Int.* **2017**, *2017*, 7157212. [CrossRef]
15. Kil, B.H.; Park, J.S.; Jo, H.M.; Jung, D.H.; Jeong, Y.K.; Won, J.Y.; Kim, D.W. A Case Report of Irritable Bowel Syndrome in a Patient that Improved with Banhasasim-tang and Yukgunja-tang-gami. *J. Int. Korean Med.* **2020**, *41*, 877–884. [CrossRef]
16. Park, J.W.; Ko, S.J.; Han, G.; Yeo, I.; Ryu, B.; Kim, J. The Effects of Banhasasim-tang on Dyspeptic Symptoms and Gastric Motility in Cases of Functional Dyspepsia: A Randomized, Double-Blind, Placebo-Controlled, and Two-Center Trial. *Evid. Based Complement. Alternat. Med.* **2013**, *2013*, 265035. [CrossRef] [PubMed]
17. Jeon, Y.J.; Lee, J.S.; Cho, Y.R.; Lee, S.B.; Kim, W.Y.; Roh, S.S.; Joung, J.Y.; Lee, H.D.; Moon, S.O.; Cho, J.H.; et al. Banhasasim-tang improves gastrointestinal function in loperamide-induced functional dyspepsia mouse model. *J. Ethnopharmacol.* **2019**, *238*, 111834. [CrossRef] [PubMed]
18. Aoyama, T.; Nishikawa, K.; Takiguchi, N.; Tanabe, K.; Imano, M.; Fukushima, R.; Sakamoto, J.; Oba, M.S.; Morita, S.; Kono, T.; et al. Double-Blind, Placebo-Controlled, Randomized Phase II Study of TJ-14 (Hangeshashinto) for Gastric Cancer Chemotherapy-Induced Oral Mucositis. *Cancer Chemother. Pharmacol.* **2014**, *73*, 1047–1054. [CrossRef]
19. Kono, T.; Kaneko, A.; Matsumoto, C.; Miyagi, C.; Ohbuchi, K.; Mizuhara, Y.; Miyano, K.; Uezono, Y. Multitargeted Effects of Hangeshashinto for Treatment of Chemotherapy-Induced Oral Mucositis on Inducible Prostaglandin E2 Production in Human Oral Keratinocytes. *Integr. Cancer Ther.* **2014**, *13*, 435–445. [CrossRef]
20. Kase, Y.; Saitoh, K.; Ishige, A.; Komatsu, Y. Mechanisms by Which Hange-Shashin-to Reduces Prostaglandin E2 Levels. *Biol. Pharma. Bull.* **1998**, *21*, 1277–1281. [CrossRef]
21. Kamide, D.; Yamashita, T.; Araki, K.; Tomifuji, M.; Shiotani, A. Hangeshashinto (TJ-14) Prevents Radiation-Induced Mucositis by Suppressing Cyclooxygenase-2 Expression and Chemotaxis of Inflammatory Cells. *Clin. Transl. Oncol.* **2017**, *19*, 1329–1336. [CrossRef]
22. Fukamachi, H.; Matsumoto, C.; Omiya, Y.; Arimoto, T.; Morisaki, H.; Kataoka, H.; Kadena, M.; Funatsu, T.; Fukutake, M.; Kase, Y.; et al. Effects of Hangeshashinto on Growth of Oral Microorganisms. *Evid.-Based Complement. Alternat. Med.* **2015**, *2015*, 1–6. [CrossRef]

23. Hitomi, S.; Ono, K.; Yamaguchi, K.; Terawaki, K.; Imai, R.; Kubota, K.; Omiya, Y.; Hattori, T.; Kase, Y.; Inenaga, K. The Traditional Japanese Medicine Hangeshashinto Alleviates Oral Ulcer-Induced Pain in a Rat Model. *Arch. Oral. Biol.* **2016**, *66*, 30–37. [CrossRef]
24. Ohman, L.; Simrén, M. Pathogenesis of IBS: Role of inflammation, immunity and neuroimmune interactions. *Nat. Rev. Gastroenterol. Hepatol.* **2010**, *7*, 163–173. [CrossRef] [PubMed]
25. Ng, Q.X.; Soh, A.Y.S.; Loke, W.; Lim, D.Y.; Yeo, W.S. The role of inflammation in irritable bowel syndrome (IBS). *J. Inflamm. Res.* **2018**, *11*, 345–349. [CrossRef]
26. Sinagra, E.; Pompei, G.; Tomasello, G.; Cappello, F.; Morreale, G.C.; Amvrosiadis, G.; Rossi, F.; Lo Monte, A.I.; Rizzo, A.G.; Raimondo, D. Inflammation in irritable bowel syndrome: Myth or new treatment target? *World J. Gastroenterol.* **2016**, *22*, 2242–2255. [CrossRef]
27. Choi, N.R.; Kwon, M.J.; Choi, W.G.; Kim, S.C.; Park, J.W.; Nam, J.H.; Kim, B.J. The traditional herbal medicines mixture, Banhasasim-tang, relieves the symptoms of irritable bowel syndrome via modulation of TRPA1, NaV1.5 and NaV1.7 channels. *J. Ethnopharmacol.* **2023**, *312*, 116499. [CrossRef] [PubMed]
28. Tang, Z. Traditional Chinese Medicine Clinical Experience of the Treatment for Irritable Bowel Syndrome. *Chin. J. Integr. Med.* **2009**, *15*, 93–94. [CrossRef]
29. Li, H.; Xia, J.; Zhang, W.; Gu, L.; Pan, C.; Tian, Y. Xifeng Huashi Formula Presents Therapeutic Effect on Diarrhea Predominant Irritable Bowel Syndrome through Regulating Brain-Gut Axis and SCF/C-KIT Signaling Pathway. *Int. J. Clin. Exp. Med.* **2017**, *10*, 15789–15797.
30. Daina, A.; Zoete, V. A BOILED-Egg to Predict Gastrointestinal Absorption and Brain Penetration of Small Molecules. *Chem. Med. Chem.* **2016**, *11*, 1117–1121. [CrossRef]
31. Tang, Y.; Li, M.; Wang, J.; Pan, Y.; Wu, F.-X. CytoNCA: A Cytoscape Plugin for Centrality Analysis and Evaluation of Protein Interaction Networks. *Biosystems* **2015**, *127*, 67–72. [CrossRef]
32. Kim, S.K.; Nam, S.; Jang, H.; Kim, A.; Lee, J.J. TM-MC: A Database of Medicinal Materials and Chemical Compounds in Northeast Asian Traditional Medicine. *BMC Complement. Altern. Med.* **2015**, *15*, 218. [CrossRef]
33. Xue, R.; Fang, Z.; Zhang, M.; Yi, Z.; Wen, C.; Shi, T. TCMID: Traditional Chinese Medicine Integrative Database for Herb Molecular Mechanism Analysis. *N. Acids Res.* **2012**, *41*, D1089–D1095. [CrossRef]
34. Chen, C.Y.-C. TCM Database@Taiwan: The World's Largest Traditional Chinese Medicine Database for Drug Screening In Silico. *PLoS ONE* **2011**, *6*, e15939. [CrossRef]
35. Ru, J.; Li, P.; Wang, J.; Zhou, W.; Li, B.; Huang, C.; Li, P.; Guo, Z.; Tao, W.; Yang, Y.; et al. TCMSP: A Database of Systems Pharmacology for Drug Discovery from Herbal Medicines. *J. Cheminform.* **2014**, *6*, 13. [CrossRef]
36. Kim, M.T.; Sedykh, A.; Chakravarti, S.K.; Saiakhov, R.D.; Zhu, H. Critical Evaluation of Human Oral Bioavailability for Pharmaceutical Drugs by Using Various Cheminformatics Approaches. *Pharm. Res.* **2014**, *31*, 1002–1014. [CrossRef]
37. Wei, M.; Zhang, X.; Pan, X.; Wang, B.; Ji, C.; Qi, Y.; Zhang, J.Z.H. HobPre: Accurate Prediction of Human Oral Bioavailability for Small Molecules. *J. Cheminform.* **2022**, *14*, 1. [CrossRef]
38. Lipinski, C.A.; Lombardo, F.; Dominy, B.W.; Feeney, P.J. Experimental and Computational Approaches to Estimate Solubility and Permeability in Drug Discovery and Development Settings. *Adv. Drug Deliv. Rev.* **2001**, *46*, 3–26. [CrossRef]
39. Veber, D.F.; Johnson, S.R.; Cheng, H.-Y.; Smith, B.R.; Ward, K.W.; Kopple, K.D. Molecular Properties That Influence the Oral Bioavailability of Drug Candidates. *J. Med. Chem.* **2002**, *45*, 2615–2623. [CrossRef]
40. Falcón-Cano, G.; Molina, C.; Cabrera-Pérez, M.Á. ADME Prediction with KNIME: Development and Validation of a Publicly Available Workflow for the Prediction of Human Oral Bioavailability. *J. Chem. Inf. Model.* **2020**, *60*, 2660–2667. [CrossRef]
41. Lin, J.H.; Yamazaki, M. Role of P-Glycoprotein in Pharmacokinetics: Clinical Implications. *Clin. Pharmacokinet.* **2003**, *42*, 59–98. [CrossRef]
42. Moriwaki, H.; Tian, Y.S.; Kawashita, N.; Takagi, T. Mordred: A Molecular Descriptor Calculator. *J. Cheminform.* **2018**, *10*, 4. [CrossRef]
43. Badkas, A.; De Landtsheer, S.; Sauter, T. Topological Network Measures for Drug Repositioning. *Brief. Bioinform.* **2021**, *22*, bbaa357. [CrossRef]
44. Lohmann, G.; Margulies, D.S.; Horstmann, A.; Pleger, B.; Lepsien, J.; Goldhahn, D.; Schloegl, H.; Stumvoll, M.; Villringer, A.; Turner, R. Eigenvector Centrality Mapping for Analyzing Connectivity Patterns in fMRI Data of the Human Brain. *PLoS ONE* **2010**, *5*, e10232. [CrossRef]
45. Nikkonen, A.; Kolho, K. Infliximab and Its Biosimilar Produced Similar First-year Therapy Outcomes in Patients with Inflammatory Bowel Disease. *Acta Paediatr.* **2020**, *109*, 836–841. [CrossRef]
46. Busquets, D.; Mas-de-Xaxars, T.; López-Siles, M.; Martínez-Medina, M.; Bahí, A.; Sàbat, M.; Louvriex, R.; Miquel-Cusachs, J.O.; Garcia-Gil, J.L.; Aldeguer, X. Anti-Tumour Necrosis Factor Treatment with Adalimumab Induces Changes in the Microbiota of Crohn's Disease. *J. Crohns Colitis* **2015**, *9*, 899–906. [CrossRef]

47. Okkenhaug, K.; Vanhaesebroeck, B. PI3K in lymphocyte development, differentiation and activation. *Nat. Rev. Immunol.* **2003**, *3*, 317–330. [CrossRef]
48. Farachi, S.; Werner, L.; Konnikova, L.; Rea, F.; Vardi, I.; Romeo, E.; Barel, O.; De Angelis, P.; Dall'Oglio, L.; Rechavi, G.; et al. DOP010 Activating PIK3CD Mutations Cause Severe Intestinal Lymphonodular Hyperplasia and an IBD-like Phenotype. *J. Crohns Colitis* **2018**, *12*, S036–S037. [CrossRef]
49. Huppi, K.; Siwarski, D.; Goodnight, J.; Mischak, H. Assignment of the Protein Kinase C Delta Polypeptide Gene (PRKCD) to Human Chromosome 3 and Mouse Chromosome 14. *Genomics* **1994**, *19*, 161–162. [CrossRef]
50. Kikkawa, U.; Matsuzaki, H.; Yamamoto, T. Protein Kinase C Delta (PKC Delta): Activation Mechanisms and Functions. *J. Biochem.* **2002**, *132*, 831–839. [CrossRef]
51. Wu, C.; Cao, L.; Liu, M.; Zhang, W.; Chen, H.; Wang, R.; Liu, C.; He, Z. Exploring the Mechanisms Underlying the Therapeutic Effect of the Drug Pair Rhubarb-Coptis in Diabetic Nephropathy Using Network Pharmacology and Molecular Docking Analysis. *Ann. Transl. Med.* **2022**, *10*, 1343. [CrossRef]
52. Zhao, J.; Zhao, F.C.; Li, G. A Network Pharmacology-Based Study of Potential Targets of Angelicae Pubescentis-Herba Taxilli Compound for the Treatment of Osteoarthritis. *Comput. Math. Methods Med.* **2022**, *2022*, 1–10. [CrossRef]
53. Salmaso, V.; Moro, S. Bridging Molecular Docking to Molecular Dynamics in Exploring Ligand-Protein Recognition Process: An Overview. *Front. Pharmacol.* **2018**, *9*, 923. [CrossRef]
54. Piñero, J.; Bravo, À.; Queralt-Rosinach, N.; Gutiérrez-Sacristán, A.; Deu-Pons, J.; Centeno, E.; García-García, J.; Sanz, F.; Furlong, L.I. DisGeNET: A Comprehensive Platform Integrating Information on Human Disease-Associated Genes and Variants. *N. Acids Res.* **2017**, *45*, D833–D839. [CrossRef]
55. Safran, M.; Rosen, N.; Twik, M.; BarShir, R.; Stein, T.I.; Dahary, D.; Fishilevich, S.; Lancet, D. The GeneCards Suite. In *Practical Guide to Life Science Databases*; Abugessaisa, I., Kasukawa, T., Eds.; Springer Nature: Singapore, 2021; pp. 27–56.
56. Shannon, P.; Markiel, A.; Ozier, O.; Baliga, N.S.; Wang, J.T.; Ramage, D.; Amin, N.; Schwikowski, B.; Ideker, T. Cytoscape: A Software Environment for Integrated Models of Biomolecular Interaction Networks. *Genome Res.* **2003**, *13*, 2498–2504. [CrossRef]
57. Gene Ontology Consortium. The Gene Ontology Resource: Enriching a GOld Mine. *N. Acids Res.* **2021**, *49*, D325–D334. [CrossRef]
58. Kanehisa, M. KEGG: Kyoto Encyclopedia of Genes and Genomes. *Nucleic Acids Res.* **2000**, *28*, 27–30. [CrossRef]
59. Ge, S.X.; Jung, D.; Yao, R. ShinyGO: A Graphical Gene-Set Enrichment Tool for Animals and Plants. *Bioinformatics* **2020**, *36*, 2628–2629. [CrossRef]
60. Trott, O.; Olson, A.J. AutoDock Vina: Improving the Speed and Accuracy of Docking with a New Scoring Function, Efficient Optimization, and Multithreading. *J. Comput. Chem.* **2010**, *31*, 455–461. [CrossRef]
61. Eberhardt, J.; Santos-Martins, D.; Tillack, A.F.; Forli, S. AutoDock Vina 1.2.0: New Docking Methods, Expanded Force Field, and Python Bindings. *J. Chem. Inf. Model.* **2021**, *61*, 3891–3898. [CrossRef]
62. Sanner, M.F. Python: A Programming Language for Software Integration and Development. *J. Mol. Graph. Model.* **1999**, *17*, 57–61.
63. Laskowski, R.A.; Swindells, M.B. LigPlot+: Multiple Ligand-Protein Interaction Diagrams for Drug Discovery. *J. Chem. Inf. Model.* **2011**, *51*, 2778–2786. [CrossRef]
64. Abraham, M.J.; Murtola, T.; Schulz, R.; Páll, S.; Smith, J.C.; Hess, B.; Lindahl, E. GROMACS: High Performance Molecular Simulations through Multi-Level Parallelism from Laptops to Supercomputers. *SoftwareX* **2015**, *1–2*, 19–25. [CrossRef]
65. Huang, J.; MacKerell, A.D. CHARMM36 All-Atom Additive Protein Force Field: Validation Based on Comparison to NMR Data. *J. Comput. Chem.* **2013**, *34*, 2135–2145. [CrossRef]
66. Petersen, H.G. Accuracy and Efficiency of the Particle Mesh Ewald Method. *J. Chem. Phys.* **1995**, *103*, 3668–3679. [CrossRef]
67. Humphrey, W.; Dalke, A.; Schulten, K. VMD: Visual Molecular Dynamics. *J. Mol. Graph.* **1996**, *14*, 33–38. [CrossRef]
68. Kim, J.N.; Nam, J.H.; Lee, J.R.; Kim, S.C.; Kim, B.J. The Traditional Medicine Banhasasim-Tang Depolarizes Pacemaker Potentials of Cultured Interstitial Cells of Cajal through M3 Muscarinic and 5-HT3 Receptors in Murine Small Intestine. *Digestion* **2020**, *101*, 536–551. [CrossRef] [PubMed]
69. Plengsuriyakarn, T.; Karbwang, J.; Na-Bangchang, K. Anticancer activity using positron emission tomography-computed tomography and pharmacokinetics of β-eudesmol in human cholangiocarcinoma xenografted nude mouse model. *Clin. Exp. Pharmacol. Physiol.* **2015**, *42*, 293–304. [CrossRef] [PubMed]

pharmaceuticals

Article

Natural Products for Drug Discovery in Cognitive Disabilities: Bibliometric Hotspots, Research Trends, Conceptual Framework, and Future Directions

Mohammed Albratty [1,2,*], Maryam Halawi [2,3] and Ali Mufraih Albarrati [4]

1 Department of Pharmaceutical Chemistry and Pharmacognosy, College of Pharmacy, Jazan University, Jazan 45142, Saudi Arabia
2 King Salman Centre for Disability Research, Riyadh 11614, Saudi Arabia; halawima@cardiff.ac.uk
3 Department of Haematology, College of Medicine, Cardiff University, Cardiff CF14 4XN, UK
4 Department of Rehabilitation Sciences, College of Applied Medical Sciences, King Saud University, Riyadh 11451, Saudi Arabia; albarrati@ksu.edu.sa
* Correspondence: malbratty@jazanu.edu.sa

Abstract: Background: The therapeutic potential of natural products in cognitive disabilities has drawn growing attention, yet a comprehensive analysis of trends and key contributors is lacking. This study provides a bibliometric overview highlighting growth patterns, themes, and future directions. **Methods**: A comprehensive Scopus search with multistep filtering was conducted by applying keywords related to natural products and cognitive disabilities to titles, abstracts, and keywords, initially retrieving 10,011 documents. Filters for original articles and English language reduced the results to 5688. Data extracted in October 2024 were analyzed using Excel and the R-package, yielding performance and citation indices. Differential proliferation was visualized using a Sankey diagram, while thematic maps highlighted key research themes, geographic trends, and subject clusters. **Results**: The field exhibited an annual growth rate of 12.36% from 1971 to 2024, with 2021 being the most productive year (497 articles). In recent decades, citation metrics have highlighted significant impacts. Thematic maps and Sankey diagrams revealed the research focus, geographic trends, and collaboration. Alzheimer's disease dominates the field, alongside topics such as oxidative stress, neuroprotection, and molecular docking. Emerging trends include ferroptosis, UPLC-Q-TOF-MS, and network pharmacology, which have marked advancements in therapeutic and computational approaches. **Conclusions**: This analysis underscores the dynamic and interdisciplinary nature of this field, highlighting areas for future exploration, particularly underrepresented cognitive disorders and novel therapeutic approaches.

Keywords: natural products; cognitive disabilities; bibliometric analysis; neuroprotection; emerging trends

1. Introduction

Cognitive disabilities refer to a broad range of conditions that affect an individual's ability to process information, learn, communicate, and perform everyday tasks [1]. These disabilities can arise from various causes including genetic disorders, developmental abnormalities, brain injuries, and neurodegenerative diseases [2]. Common examples of cognitive impairment include autism spectrum disorder (ASD), attention deficit hyperactivity disorder (ADHD), Down syndrome, Alzheimer's disease, dyslexia, cerebral palsy, and intellectual disabilities [3]. Cognitive disabilities can significantly affect an individual's quality of life, limiting independence and the ability to participate fully in educational, social, and occupational settings [4]. The severity of these impairments varies widely, ranging from mild difficulties in memory or attention to profound challenges in communication and decision making [5]. Advances in neuroscience and psychology have shed light on the mechanisms underlying these conditions, enabling the development of targeted therapies and interventions [6,7]. However, many individuals with cognitive disabilities continue to face social stigma and have limited access to resources, particularly in low-resource settings [8]. Increasing awareness, promoting inclusivity, and investing in evidence-based treatments remains critical for improving outcomes [9,10]. Recent research has also explored the role of natural products, including plant-derived compounds, in the management of cognitive disabilities, offering promising avenues for therapeutic innovation through their neuroprotective and anti-inflammatory properties [5,11–17].

Neuropharmacology examines the impact of medications on nervous system function and the neural mechanisms that mediate their effects on behavior [18]. Neuropharmacology comprises two primary branches: behavioral and molecular [16,19]. Behavioral neuropharmacology examines the impact of pharmaceuticals on human behavior, encompassing the effects of drug dependence and addiction on the brain [20]. Molecular neuropharmacology encompasses the examination of neurons and their neurochemical interactions, aiming to create pharmaceuticals that positively influence brain function. These topics are intricately linked, as they both focus on the interactions of neurotransmitters, neuropeptides, neurohormones, neuromodulators, enzymes, second messengers, co-transporters, ion channels, and receptor proteins within the central and peripheral nervous systems [21]. Researchers are developing pharmaceuticals to address various neurological problems, including pain, neurodegenerative diseases like Parkinson's and Alzheimer's, psychological disorders, addiction, and others, by examining these connections [22].

Cognitive disabilities are characterized by significant limitations in intellectual functioning and adaptive behavior. According to the American Association on Intellectual and Developmental Disabilities (AAIDD), this includes: (1) an IQ below 70, (2) limitations in adaptive behaviors such as communication and self-care, and (3) onset before the age of 18 for developmental forms [23,24]. Cognitive disabilities can be developmental or acquired, and their severity may range from mild to profound. Cognitive disabilities encompass a broad range of conditions that affect intellectual functioning and adaptive behavior. These include developmental and acquired disorders such as intellectual disability (ID), Down syndrome, autism spectrum disorder (ASD), and traumatic brain injury (TBI). Specific learning disabilities like dyslexia (reading), dyscalculia (math), and dysgraphia (writing) are also recognized as forms of cognitive impairment. Other conditions include attention-deficit/hyperactivity disorder (ADHD), fetal alcohol spectrum disorders (FASD), and neurodegenerative diseases such as Alzheimer's disease and mild cognitive impairment (MCI). Language-related disorders like aphasia, as well as genetic and developmental syndromes including fragile X syndrome, Rett syndrome, and Williams syndrome, are part of this spectrum. Additionally, developmental delay in early childhood and cerebral palsy—particularly when accompanied by cognitive deficits—are considered under the umbrella of cognitive disabilities [1,2,25–27].

Natural therapies are increasingly being recognized for their potential to safeguard brain structures, diminish inflammation, and enhance cognitive function in the treatment of cognitive disorders [7,14,28]. Despite increasing interest, no systematic bibliometric analysis has been performed on the advancement of research [29,30] in the intricate domain linking cognitive impairments and natural products [14,31]. In this respect, evidence highlights the relevance of focus for determining the scope and trends of studies and maps the scientific terrain. Bibliometric analysis enabled this study to quantify the number of publications, identify significant authors, assess journal influence and scope, and evaluate worldwide cooperation within the field [30,32]. Furthermore, it identifies areas of deficiency and novel elements, which will assist in the design and planning of subsequent initiatives to enhance treatment modalities [33]. The results are significant for researchers, international institutions, and grant agencies, facilitating informed decisions concerning the development of novel plant-based treatment approaches for Alzheimer's disease, ADHD, Down syndrome, and autism spectrum disorder. This study, lacking comparable bibliometric analyses, is uniquely positioned to evaluate global research activity patterns and their relationship with clinical factors, thereby aiding in the formulation of effective strategies to enhance the quality of life of individuals with cognitive impairments.

2. Results

2.1. Annual Growth and Citation Dynamics

The bibliometric analysis of natural products and cognitive disorders from 1971 to 2024 showed a fair increase in publication output and citing dynamics (Figure 1). An impressive annual growth rate of 12.36% indicates that 5688 documents were found from 1370 sources. The average age of documents stood at 7.21 years, which indicates an increase in research activity that has not been in this volume form recently. The greatest number of original articles (data-driven studies) were published annually between the 2020s, the peak year being 2021, with 497 articles marking this decade as the most productive. Citation dynamics (Figure 1) also showed notable growth. An average document was cited 31.08 times a year (mean TCperYear). In 2007, the highest mean number of citations, no less than five a year, was reported at 5.87, followed by the totals in 2008 (5.56) and 2000 (5.29). Such a pattern indicates that some very important studies conducted in these years have had major impacts on other future studies. The earlier years, in this case the 1970s and 1980s, were characterized by very low citations, with a mean below 0.1 per year, which signifies the emergence of research in that field during those times. At the general level, this review suggests that it is a lively and rapidly developing field of research, with the greatest progress and awareness in the field being achieved in the past few decades.

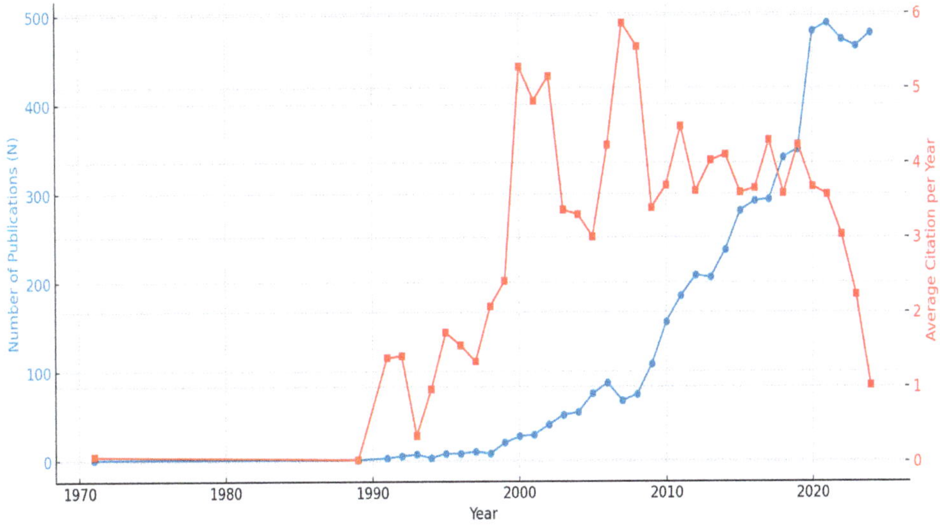

Figure 1. Annual growth and citation dynamics.

2.2. Key Contributors in the Field

Table 1 highlights the primary contributors to the research on natural products and cognitive disabilities. Among the authors, Zengin, G. stands out as the most productive with 42 publications, followed by Oh, M.S. (28), Choi, J.S. (27), and Shin, D.H. (26). The leading affiliations include the Ministry of Education of the People's Republic of China (166 publications), Kyung Hee University (133), Chinese Academy of Sciences (95), and Seoul National University (65). In terms of country contributions, China leads with 1270 publications, followed by India (777), the United States (700), and South Korea (627). The most productive sources were the Journal of Ethnopharmacology (187 publications), Molecules (131), Phytomedicine (91), and Frontiers in Pharmacology (75). Figure 2 provides additional insights through a Sankey diagram that visually represents the connections between authors, countries, and sources. In bibliometrics, a Sankey diagram visually represents the connections between authors, countries, and sources. Authors, countries, and sources are shown as nodes, with links indicating flows, such as publications or collaborations between them. This visualization helps analyze patterns of collaboration, publication distribution, and information flow in the research data. The key contributors shift when focusing on the most relevant sources. Wang, Y., Zhang, Y., Liu, J., and Zhang, J. emerged as the top authors, while China, Korea, Japan, the USA, India, and Italy remained the leading countries. The key journals in this refined analysis were consistent, including the Journal of Ethnopharmacology, Phytomedicine, Molecules, and Frontiers in Pharmacology. The discrepancies between Table 1 and Figure 2 are due to the narrowed focus in Figure 2 on the most relevant sources. For instance, while Zengin, G. was the most productive author overall (Table 1), Wang, Y. was identified as the most prolific author when limited to highly relevant publications (Figure 2). This difference highlights the variability in the productivity metrics based on source selection.

Table 1. Key contributors in the field.

Authors	N	Affiliation	N	Sources	N	Country	N
Zengin, G.	42	Ministry of Education of the People's Republic of China	166	Journal of Ethnopharmacology	187	China	1270
Oh, M.S.	28	Kyung Hee University	133	Molecules	131	India	777
Choi, J.S.	27	Chinese Academy of Sciences	95	Phytomedicine	91	United States	700
Shin, D.H.	26	Seoul National University	65	Frontiers in Pharmacology	75	South Korea	627
Ryu, J.H.	23	Shenyang Pharmaceutical University	62	International Journal of Molecular Sciences	75	Japan	389
Oboh, G.	22	King Saud University	58	Journal of Alzheimer's Disease	75	Italy	240
Hritcu, L.	21	Chinese Academy of Medical Sciences & Peking Union Medical College	55	Phytotherapy Research	74	Iran	235
Jung, H.A.	21	Selçuk Üniversitesi	52	Nutrients	71	Turkey	214
Bi, K.	20	National Research Centre	51	Evidence-Based Complementary and Alternative Medicine	69	Saudi Arabia	199
Choi, S.J.	20	King Abdulaziz University	50	PLOS One	68	Germany	197

N: number of documents.

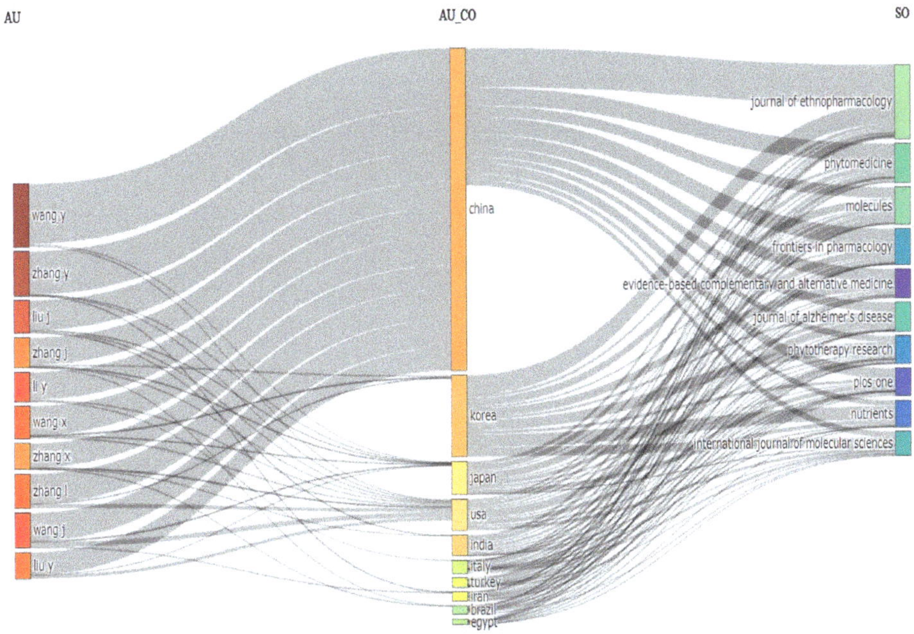

Figure 2. Sankey diagram. Visually representation of the connections between authors, countries, and sources. In bibliometrics, a Sankey diagram can visually represent the connections between authors, countries, and sources. Authors, countries, and sources are shown as nodes, with links indicating flows such as publications or collaborations between them.

2.3. Top-Cited and Collaborative Countries

Figure 3 provides insights into the top-cited (Figure 3A) and most collaborative (Figure 3B) countries in terms of research on natural products and cognitive disabilities. In terms of total citations (TC), the USA had 32,010 citations, followed by China (25,884), Korea (15,298), and India (10,730). Other notable contributors included Japan (7901), the United Kingdom (5659), Italy (5339), Iran (5274), Germany (3881), and Turkey (3873). These metrics highlight the significant influence of the research outputs from these countries in advancing the field. Collaboration metrics show that the percentage of international co-authorships is 25.91%, reflecting a strong global research network. Publications were categorized into single-country publications (SCP) and multiple-country publications (MCP), with the MCP ratio indicating the extent of international collaboration. Among the most collaborative countries, Turkey (MCP ratio: 0.387) and Italy (0.377) demonstrated the highest levels of international partnerships, followed by the USA (0.281). On the other hand, countries such as China and India, despite their large output (1129 and 593 articles, respectively), exhibited relatively lower MCP ratios (0.148 and 0.164), indicating a higher prevalence of domestic research activities. These findings reveal a dual landscape in which countries like the USA and China dominate in citations and output, while smaller players such as Turkey and Italy excel in fostering international collaboration. This balance underscores the importance of both citation impact and collaborative effort in shaping global research.

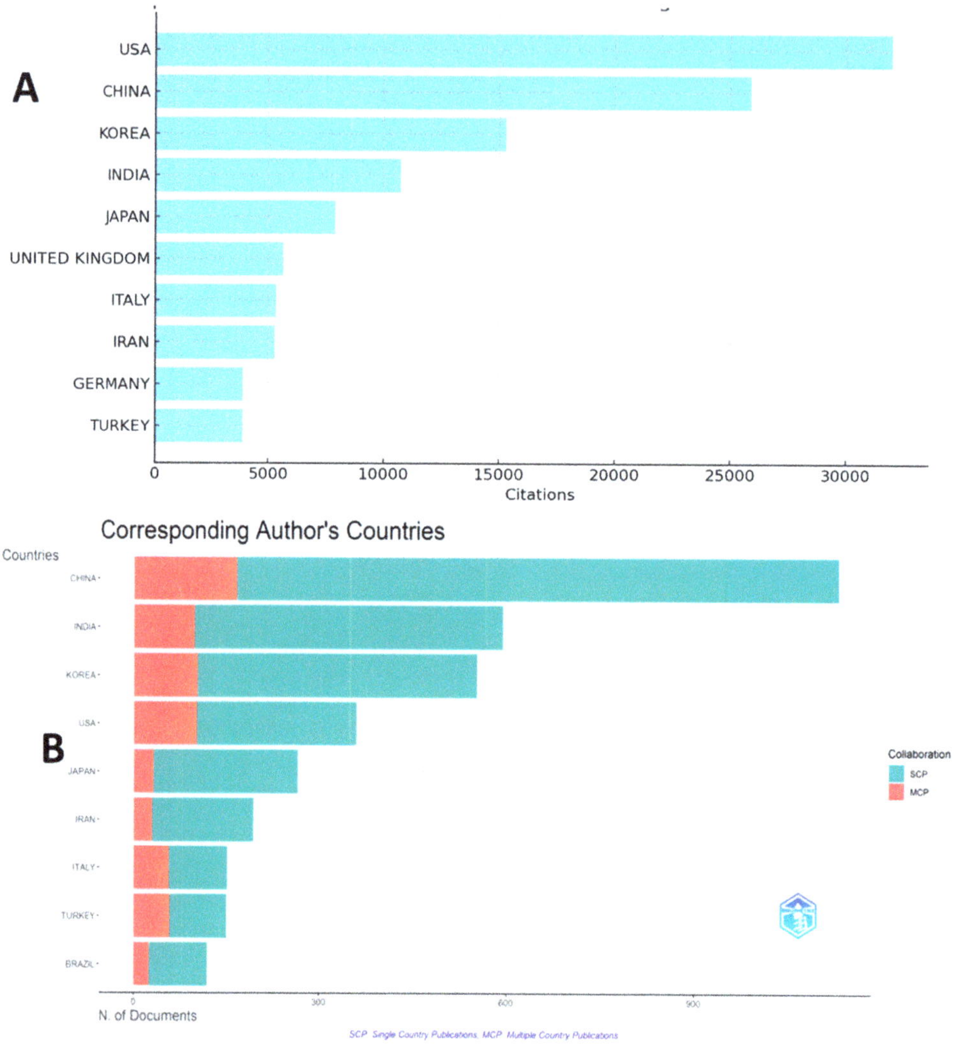

Figure 3. Top-cited (**A**) and collaborative (**B**) countries.

2.4. Authors' Keyword Co-Occurrence Analysis

Authors' keyword co-occurrence analysis (Figure 4) identifies major research themes, emerging trends, interdisciplinary links, and research gaps, offering insights into topic relationships and guiding future studies through visualized research networks. The most frequently occurring terms in research on natural products and cognitive disabilities are the key areas of focus. Alzheimer's disease dominates with 1935 mentions, reflecting its significance as the primary research topic in this field. Other prominent terms include oxidative stress (387), acetylcholinesterase (372), antioxidants (258), and neuroprotection (253), emphasizing the importance of understanding oxidative damage and neuroprotective mechanisms. Emerging methodologies such as molecular docking (236) underscore the integration of computational tools for drug discovery. Conditions such as dementia (215) and processes such as neuroinflammation (190) and apoptosis (130) further demonstrate the breadth of research topics exploring the underlying pathologies of cognitive impairment. Natural compounds and their bioactivities are represented by terms such as natural products (115), antioxidant activity (106), and flavonoids (94), highlighting the need for plant-based therapies. Additionally, specific enzymes, such as butyrylcholinesterase (100), and models, such as scopolamine (98), suggest targeted biochemical approaches in therapeutic development. This term analysis revealed a strong focus on neurodegenerative diseases, oxidative mechanisms, and natural product-based interventions, reflecting the interdisciplinary and translational nature of research in this field.

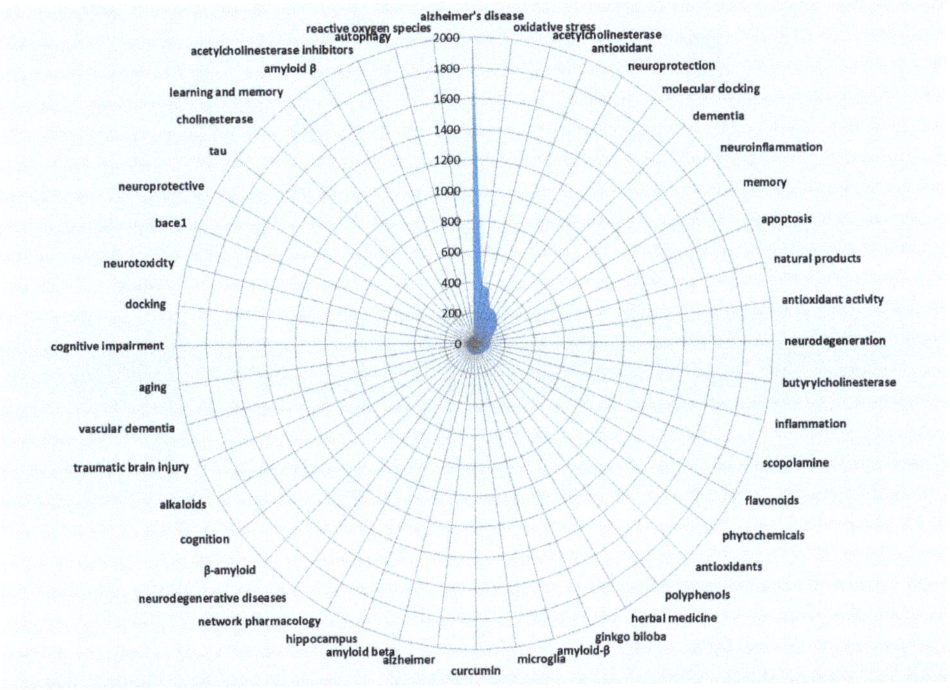

Figure 4. Authors' keyword co-occurrence analysis.

2.5. *Progression of Themes in Research*

Figure 5 illustrates the thematic evolution of research in the field of natural products and cognitive disabilities, from 1971 to 2024. During the early period (1971–2015), the focus was predominantly on acetylcholinesterase, acetylcholinesterase inhibitors, antioxidant activity, Alzheimer's disease, dementia, oxidative stress, and related mechanisms, indicating a foundational exploration of neurochemical pathways and degenerative brain conditions. In the subsequent phase (2016–2021), research themes transitioned towards integrating broader therapeutic approaches. Alzheimer's disease remains a dominant topic alongside emerging interests in antioxidant activity, oxidative stress, herbal medicine, and reactive oxygen species. This phase is characterized by the evolution of natural products to deal with cognitive impairments, for example, their antioxidative and neuroprotective roles. Over the past two years (2022–2024), there is evidence that further diversification has occurred within central themes. Other than Alzheimer's disease, which remained the predominant issue, more emphasis was placed on enzyme inhibition, alkaloids, and traumatic head injuries. Themes such as autism spectrum disorder and virtual screening seem to point to a widening focus on how natural products may be applied to other cognitive disabilities, as well as drug design through computational methods. This development suggests that this is a vibrant area of research in which research on neurochemistry has expanded to encompass many aspects in relation to other cognitive disorders with a strong focus on the use of natural products. The new direction in this area of research also shows that there could be brighter prospects for addressing intricate brain disorder problems.

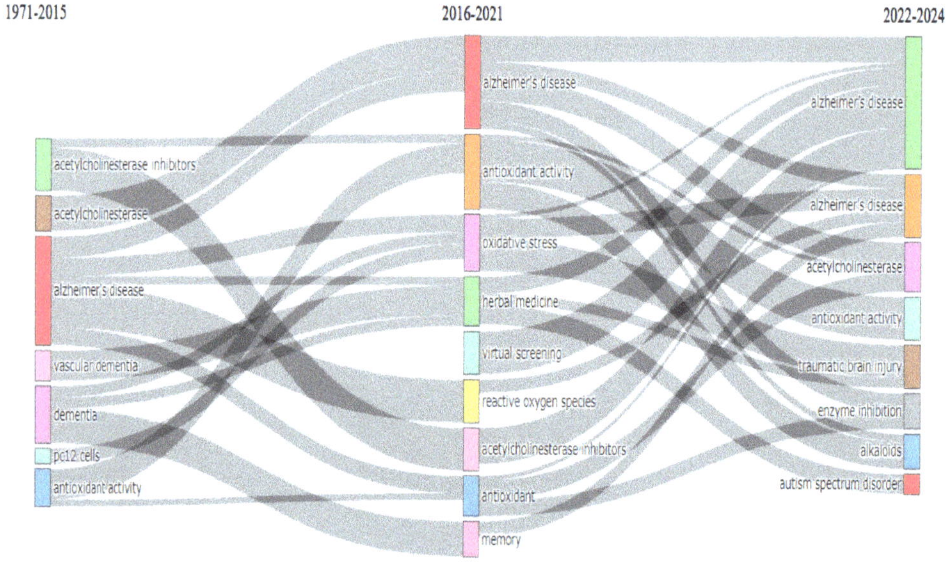

Figure 5. Thematic evolution of the research on natural products and cognitive disabilities.

2.6. Conceptual Structure

Authors' keywords were used because they directly reflect the researchers' intended focus and terminology. They are essential for identifying thematic trends, keyword co-occurrence, and emerging topics, making them well-suited for bibliometric mapping and conceptual analysis. Thematic map analysis, conducted using the R package, categorized research themes in natural products and cognitive disabilities based on their centrality (importance) and density (development). Basic themes, such as acetylcholinesterase, molecular docking, antioxidant activity, natural products, and virtual screening form the foundational knowledge essential for understanding therapeutic mechanisms and advancing drug discovery. Motor themes, which are well developed and central to the field, include Alzheimer's disease, oxidative stress, neuroprotection, neuroinflammation, apoptosis, and amyloid-β, focusing on neurodegenerative processes and therapeutic interventions. Additionally, memory and dementia-related topics, including scopolamine, acetylcholine, cognitive function, and traditional Chinese medicine, highlight experimental approaches and established therapies, such as donepezil. A niche theme, represented by Amaryllidaceae, explores specialized plant-based bioactive compounds, reflecting focused but isolated research. In contrast, declining or emerging themes such as herbal medicine, *Ginkgo biloba*, vascular dementia, and mild cognitive impairment represent areas transitioning in relevance or being integrated into broader topics. The analysis underscores the dominance of motor themes, such as neurodegeneration and Alzheimer's disease, foundational insights from basic themes, and the potential for exploring niche areas, offering a roadmap for future research directions and highlighting critical areas requiring further development.

2.7. Emerging Topics

Table 2 highlights emerging topics in research on natural products and cognitive disabilities, showing their frequency and temporal progression. Recent advancements have resulted in a growing interest in cutting-edge methodologies and evolving therapeutic approaches. Key emerging technologies include UPLC-Q-TOF-MS (first quartile [Q1] 2023, median 2024), ferroptosis (Q1 2022, median 2024), and network pharmacology (Q1 2021, median 2022), all of which emphasize the application of advanced analytical and computational tools to unravel complex biological mechanisms. Molecular dynamics simulation (Q1 2021, median 2023) and molecular docking (Q1 2020, median 2022) demonstrated an increasing reliance on computational modeling for understanding drug–target interactions. Topics such as absorption, distribution, metabolism, excretion, and toxicity (Q1 2021, median 2023) and MD simulations further underscore the emphasis on computational pharmacology in optimizing drug discovery. Emerging biological processes, including ferroptosis, autophagy (Q1 2019, median 2022), and neuroinflammation (Q1 2018, median 2021), indicate a focus on novel pathological pathways in cognitive disorders. Long-standing yet continually evolving topics, such as antioxidant activity, oxidative stress, and phytochemicals, have maintained their relevance, bridging traditional and modern therapeutic approaches. Among the diseases, Alzheimer's disease is the most frequently studied emerging topic, with consistent growth (Q1 2019, median 2021), reflecting its significance in neurodegenerative research. These trends highlight the interdisciplinary nature of this field, which combines natural products, computational approaches, and advanced methodologies to address cognitive disabilities.

Table 2. Emerging topics.

Item	Frequency	Year_q1	Year_med	Year_q3
UPLC-Q-TOF-MS	6	2023	2024	2024
Ferroptosis	9	2022	2024	2024
Network pharmacology	65	2021	2022	2024
Molecular dynamics simulation	28	2021	2023	2024
ADMET	18	2021	2023	2024
Molecular docking	236	2020	2022	2023
Alzheimer's disease	628	2019	2021	2023
Phytochemicals	85	2019	2021	2023
Autophagy	48	2019	2022	2023
Neuroinflammation	190	2018	2021	2023
Neurodegeneration	106	2016	2020	2022
Antioxidant	258	2015	2019	2022
Antioxidant activity	106	2015	2019	2022
Flavonoids	94	2015	2020	2022
Oxidative stress	387	2014	2019	2022

Abbreviations: med: median; UPLC-Q-TOF-MS: ultra-performance liquid chromatography quadrupole time-of-flight mass spectrometry; ADMET: absorption, distribution, metabolism, excretion, and toxicity.

3. Discussion

Research on natural products and cognitive illnesses from 1971 to 2024 demonstrates a dynamic and rapidly evolving field characterized by an impressive annual growth rate of 12.36%. The publication of 5688 papers from 1370 sources indicates a consistent increase in research output, underscoring the global recognition of natural products as a valuable area of study. The peak year of 2021, with 497 articles, indicates heightened interest, which may be driven by advancements in technology, such as molecular docking [16,17], and an increasing understanding of plant-based therapies for neurological disorders [9,34,35]. The escalation in citation dynamics underscores the significance of fundamental research as it has influenced subsequent studies and positioned natural products [9,34,35] as a cornerstone of innovation in therapeutic development. These results complement earlier research, stressing the need for natural products to treat several diseases, including cancer [27], cardiovascular diseases [36], diabetes [37], and neurological diseases such as Alzheimer's disease [2,10,34]. Although countries like China and India produce a high volume of research, they tend to have lower levels of international collaboration—possibly due to robust domestic research networks, language preferences, or national funding priorities—underscoring the importance of encouraging more global partnerships in future studies.

This work supports the importance of natural chemicals in medication development, especially their bioactive characteristics that support antioxidant, anti-inflammatory, and neuroprotective activities. Through trend mapping and research impact analysis, this study supports the increasing agreement that natural products are viable strategies for controlling complicated disorders and for developing therapeutic treatments worldwide.

This research indicates that China is the leading country in terms of output in the field of natural products and cognitive disabilities more probably under the influence that traditional Chinese medicine (TCM) plays in this area. TCM has been known for a long time to combine natural products and holistic approaches for the treatment of neurological and cognitive dysfunctions, which to some extent explains the high volume of research activities in China [15,31,38]. Newer research has drawn attention to the use of traditional medicine in modern paradigms for the treatment of cognitive disabilities, stressing its place in rehabilitation and treatment [15]. TCM has been shown to be effective in the management of cognitive deficits following stroke. Combining TCM with new practices such as virtual reality (VR) can help enhance memory and executive function recovery in stroke survivors [26]. Additionally, there have been developments in neuroprosthetics and brain–computer interfaces that reportedly show better results in cognitive rehabilitation and are said to be based on TCM [39]. Another traditional approach that has been applied in a number of post-stroke patients is music therapy, which has been used in the treatment of emotional and cognitive rehabilitation [40]. Newer techniques, such as dynamic brain network mapping and deep brain stimulation (DBS), also advocate the combination of traditional techniques with new methods for the treatment of neurological and cognitive disorders. The incorporation of traditional medicine into holistic approaches, such as the biopsychosocial model, has effective implications in steadying the complete recovery of older populations from both mental and physical aspects [16,27,36]. Understanding the role of TCM and other traditional medicines is essential in developing methods for cognitive rehabilitation and dealing with highly complex neurological disorders [15].

Zengin, G., a leading scholar in natural product research, has significantly advanced the understanding of plant-based therapies for managing chronic conditions such as diabetes, Alzheimer's disease, and oxidative stress. His work emphasizes phytochemical profiling, enzyme inhibition, and antioxidant activity using both in vitro and in silico methodologies. Notable studies include the evaluation of *Salvia syriaca* L. for its antidiabetic, anti-Alzheimer's, and antioxidant properties [28] and *Ajuga chamaecistus* for its neuroprotective and skin-care applications [41]. Zengin's research on mangiferin and essential oils from *Sideritis galatica* demonstrated their inhibitory effects on enzymes associated with Alzheimer's disease and diabetes, thus providing molecular insights into their therapeutic roles [16,37]. Using advanced techniques, such as HPLC-MS/MS, Zengin profiled phenolic compounds in species such as *Ferula halophila* and *Scrophularia lucida*, combining these analyses with antioxidant, anti-inflammatory, and docking studies to explore their multifunctional applications [42]. Comparative studies of Apiaceae species have highlighted their antioxidant, antimicrobial, and cytotoxic properties, emphasizing their potential against cancer [43]. By integrating cutting-edge analytical approaches with pharmacological evaluations, Zengin bridges phytochemistry and therapeutic innovation, offering diverse applications for natural products in combating chronic diseases and oxidative stress-related conditions [28,37,41–48].

This conceptual shift has focused research after 2022 on antioxidants and their use to regulate cholinesterase, which plays a role in the pathology of Alzheimer's, according to the analysis of the study's objectives. Alzheimer's disease, the most prevalent form of dementia, degrades brain functions over time. As the condition advances, acetylcholine levels in aged brains decrease, causing cognitive decline. Acetylcholinesterase inhibitors (AChEIs) increase synaptic acetylcholine levels and restore cholinergic neurotransmission [2,10,31,34]. Current drugs may not sufficiently modulate acetylcholine levels to provide a complete therapeutic response, and selective cholinesterase inhibitors without dose-limiting adverse effects are unavailable [49]. Synthetic drugs such as tacrine, donepezil, and rivastigmine can also induce gastrointestinal and bioavailability issues. Thus, the search for more effective AChEIs, especially from natural sources, is ongoing. Reactive oxygen species (ROS) generate oxidative stress, which oxidizes biomolecules and damages cells, thereby causing aging. Recently, plant antioxidants have garnered attention because they reduce oxidative damage and may prevent aging and neurological illnesses.

Neuroprotection has become one of the central motor themes in research concerning natural compounds with respect to the degenerative diseases such as Alzheimer's disease [50]. The natural compound extracts provided in these studies tend to have functional properties, including the ability to manage oxidative stress, inhibit β-amyloid (Aβ) aggregation, and modulate inflammatory pathways [2,6,10,34,51]. These compounds can reduce age-related neurodegeneration. Such work basically extends the findings of Bastianetto et al., who demonstrated that catechin gallates from extracts of green and black tea-infused cultures could protect cells from the Aβ-induced toxicity by inhibiting the apoptotic events and aggregation of Aβ [34]. Similarly, Chu et al. confirmed that treatment with Ginsenoside Rg5 isolated from Panax ginseng had remedial effects on cognitive deficits in rats by reducing neuroinflammation and Aβ deposition and increasing acetylcholine levels [2]. *Bacopa monnieri* has been extensively studied for its anti-nutritional properties. It was found to be protective against Aβ-induced neurotoxicity and to improve cognitive function due to its antioxidant and acetylcholinesterase inhibitory properties [52]. In addition, beta-asarone from *Acorus tatarinowii* was found to prevent cognitive impairment and neuronal apoptosis in Aβ-injected rats through the reversal of caspase activation and JNK phosphorylation processes [10]. These studies highlight that neuroprotection is an area worthy of focus in research by creating strategies that are based on both modern and traditional wisdom concerning natural products through the use of antioxidant activity, anti-inflammatory activity, and Aβ aggregation inhibition to solve cognitive decline.

A bibliometric analysis of trends in UPLC-Q-TOF-MS usage shows its growing relevance as a revolutionary technique for the study of the application of natural products in the treatment of cognitive dysfunction. In addition, this technique of analysis is the most useful in identifying and explaining the mechanism of action of bioactive compounds in the case of neurodegenerative diseases, which include but are not restricted to Alzheimer's disease. Recent studies have further bolstered their relevance. Qiu et al. performed UPLC-Q-TOF-MS on *Aurantii Fructus* and *Aurantii Fructus Immaturus* and reported the discovery of 50 compounds with neuroprotective effects categorized as Alzheimer's, NF-κB signaling, and apoptosis pathways [53]. Wang et al. investigated the anti-Alzheimer's properties of Mume Flos using UHPLC-Q-Orbitrap-MS/MS and noted that rutin and chlorogenic acid were inferior to others in terms of their efficacy in the inhibition of Aβ deposition in *Caenorhabditis elegans* models [54]. Similarly, Zhang et al. used high-resolution LC-Q-TOF-MS to demonstrate the significant microinhibitory activity of nitidine from *Zanthoxylum nitidum* as a strong candidate for acetylcholinesterase activity inhibition [55]. These findings illustrate the potential power of UPLC-Q-TOF-MS techniques for the development and application of natural product-derived medicine against cognitive disorders, and highlight the possible advancements that such techniques would herald for the integration of herbal research and contemporary pharmacology.

Bibliometric analysis showed that research on the processes of regulation of cell death, such as ferroptosis, has been a hot topic in the areas of cognitive disorders; however, recent studies have highlighted the importance of these processes in Alzheimer's disease and several other degenerative diseases. Gong et al. showed that curculigoside significantly restrained the progression of Alzheimer's disease and ameliorated cognitive dysfunction by upregulating GPX4 and inhibiting the SLC7A11 pathway [31]. A similar effort was made by Li et al., who investigated avicularin as a means to ameliorate cognitive defects associated with Alzheimer's disease by modifying the NOX4/Nrf2 axis in PC12 cell lines and transgenic models of AD [17]. Long et al. investigated the neuronal protection offered by the SuanZaoRen decoction and its ability to inhibit Alzheimer's disease-mediated neuronal loss and improve synaptic connectivity by targeting the DJ-1/Nrf2 signaling pathway [16]. Tao et al. evaluated the biochemical and physiological effects of oleanonic acid on ferroptosis and mitochondrial damage via Nrf2/HO-1 signaling [14]. More recently, Yong et al. characterized Thonningianin A, a new compound that inhibits ferroptosis and described its use in Alzheimer's disease therapy via GPX4 stimulation through the AMPK/Nrf2 pathway [12]. Moreover, *Penthorum chinense* Pursh (PEF) has been shown to inhibit ferroptosis in Alzheimer's disease cellular and C. elegans models by targeting oxidative stress and lipid peroxidation processes [11]. These studies confirm the bibliometric findings by showcasing ferroptosis as a key factor in neurodegenerative diseases, and natural products have been proposed as potential anti-ferroptotic agents to improve cognition. While emerging topics such as ferroptosis and UPLC-Q-TOF-MS signal promising directions, their clinical translation remains limited by challenges in validation, including biological complexity, lack of standardized protocols, and the need for robust in vivo and clinical evidence to support their therapeutic feasibility.

4. Limitations

Scopus- and English-exclusive databases have constraints. Examples of these problems include inadequate citation coverage, publishing bias, language and geographical discrepancies, subject limitations, and data-input inaccuracies. Researchers ought to employ several databases, examine scholarly papers in different languages, engage in interdisciplinary collaboration, and investigate supplementary publications to mitigate these limitations. This guarantees a comprehensive and reliable research environment.

5. Materials and Methods

5.1. Search Strategy and Data Extraction

A comprehensive and multistep search was conducted in the Scopus database to identify relevant literature on the use of natural products to address cognitive disabilities and related conditions. The search terms included keywords related to natural products, such as "phytotherapy", "herbal medicines", "plant extract", "natural product", "natural compound", "natural molecule", "phytochemical", "secondary metabolite", "bioactive compounds", "biologically active compounds", "phytonutrient", "plant-derived chemical", and "plant-derived compound," combined with terms associated with cognitive disabilities and related conditions, including "degenerative brain disease", "cognitive disability", "dementia", "autism spectrum disorder", "ADHD", "Down syndrome", "fragile X syndrome", "traumatic brain injury", "Alzheimer's disease", "cerebral palsy", "aphasia", "dyslexia", and "intellectual disabilities". These keywords were extracted from an extensive search in the related literature [1,7,17,19,27,54]. To ensure the quality and relevance of the data, specific filters were applied during the search process. Only original research articles were included, and the language was restricted to English. These filters were applied after the initial retrieval of 10,011 documents, resulting in a refined dataset of 5688 articles suitable for bibliometric analysis. This approach ensured the inclusion of peer-reviewed, research-focused studies relevant to natural products and cognitive disabilities. The search results were exported in the CSV and BibTeX formats, and the data were extracted in October 2024.

5.2. *Analysis and Visualizations*

Annual trends were examined using Microsoft Excel, while bibliometric statistics and visualizations were produced using the R-package software Version 5.0.1 [55], enabling comprehensive mapping of research focus points, geographical research regions, and subject clusters. The package measures the intensity of the linkages or connections among authors, institutions, and keywords inside a network map. The thematic map depicts the primary issues in the field according to the author keywords. The objective of constructing a thematic map was to understand the present conditions and assess the future direction of research progress on the subject. The map depicts the strength of internal density, highlighting inter-cluster development and external connections, and underscoring the significance of the study to a specific focal location. It is partitioned into four quadrants. The term thematic map classifies the principal study themes and subjects within a certain domain [55,56].

6. Conclusions

This study shows that research on natural products and cognitive disabilities is rapidly evolving, with a notable surge in global interest and collaboration. The field has been growing at an annual rate of 12.36%, with a sharp rise in citations since 2021, reflecting its increasing relevance. Major contributions from countries like China, the USA, and South Korea have helped shape this progress. The research landscape has expanded from early focus areas—such as oxidative stress and acetylcholinesterase inhibition—to newer themes like ferroptosis and advanced computational tools, underscoring the field's interdisciplinary growth.

Despite this progress, several gaps remain. Alzheimer's disease continues to dominate the research spotlight, often overshadowing other important cognitive conditions like autism spectrum disorders and traumatic brain injuries. Additionally, many potentially valuable bioactive compounds from less-studied plant species remain underexplored. Topics such as vascular dementia, which once received more attention, are now on the decline and require renewed scientific focus. Promising innovations, including UPLC-Q-TOF-MS and studies on ferroptosis, show potential but still need validation through clinical trials.

To move the field forward, researchers are encouraged to broaden their focus to include a wider range of cognitive disorders, enhance international collaboration to share resources and expertise, and utilize emerging technologies to uncover new therapeutic pathways. Emphasizing translational research and improving data sharing will also help bridge the gap between lab-based discoveries and real-world clinical impact. By addressing these challenges while continuing to build on core strengths, the field can make meaningful advances in the development of therapies for cognitive disabilities.

Author Contributions: Conceptualization, M.A. and A.M.A.; methodology, M.H.; formal analysis, M.H. and A.M.A.; writing—original draft preparation, M.A. and A.M.A.; writing—review and editing, M.A. and M.H.; funding acquisition, M.A. All authors have read and agreed to the published version of the manuscript.

Funding: The authors extend their appreciation to the King Salman Center for Disability Research for funding this work through Research Group no KSRG-2024-178.

Institutional Review Board Statement: Not applicable.

Informed Consent Statement: Not applicable.

Data Availability Statement: The original contributions presented in this study are included in the article. Further inquiries can be directed to the corresponding author.

Acknowledgments: The authors extend their appreciation to the King Salman Center for Disability Research for funding this work through Research Group no KSRG-2024-178.

Conflicts of Interest: The authors have no conflicts of interest.

References

1. Uabundit, N.; Wattanathorn, J.; Mucimapura, S.; Ingkaninan, K. Cognitive enhancement and neuroprotective effects of *Bacopa monnieri* in Alzheimer's disease model. *J. Ethnopharmacol.* **2010**, *127*, 26–31. [CrossRef]
2. Chu, S.; Gu, J.; Feng, L.; Liu, J.; Zhang, M.; Jia, X.; Liu, M.; Yao, D. Ginsenoside Rg5 improves cognitive dysfunction and beta-amyloid deposition in STZ-induced memory impaired rats via attenuating neuroinflammatory responses. *Int. Immunopharmacol.* **2014**, *19*, 317–326. [CrossRef] [PubMed]
3. Sigafoos, J.; Roche, L.; O'Reilly, M.F.; Lancioni, G.E. Persistence of primitive reflexes in developmental disorders. *Curr. Dev. Disord. Rep.* **2021**, *8*, 98–105. [CrossRef]
4. Yeung, P.; Breheny, M. Quality of life among older people with a disability: The role of purpose in life and capabilities. *Disabil. Rehabil.* **2021**, *43*, 181–191. [CrossRef]
5. Megari, K.; Thomaidou, E.; Chatzidimitriou, E. Highlighting the Neuropsychological Consequences of COVID-19: Evidence From a Narrative Review. *INQUIRY J. Health Care Organ. Provis. Financ.* **2024**, *61*, 00469580241262442. [CrossRef] [PubMed]
6. Lim, G.P.; Chu, T.; Yang, F.; Beech, W.; Frautschy, S.A.; Cole, G.M. The curry spice curcumin reduces oxidative damage and amyloid pathology in an Alzheimer transgenic mouse. *J. Neurosci.* **2001**, *21*, 8370–8377. [CrossRef]
7. Park, C.H.; Choi, S.H.; Koo, J.W.; Seo, J.H.; Kim, H.S.; Jeong, S.J.; Suh, Y.H. Novel cognitive improving and neuroprotective activities of *Polygala tenuifolia* willdenow extract, BT-11. *J. Neurosci. Res.* **2002**, *70*, 484–492. [CrossRef]
8. Hepperlen, R.A.; Biggs, J.; Mwandileya, W.; Rabaey, P.; Ngulube, E.; Hearst, M.O. Using community-based interventions to reduce public stigma of children with disabilities: A feasibility study. *J. Appl. Res. Intellect. Disabil.* **2021**, *34*, 1499–1510. [CrossRef]
9. Budzynska, B.; Boguszewska-Czubara, A.; Kruk-Slomka, M.; Skalicka-Wozniak, K.; Michalak, A.; Musik, I.; Biala, G. Effects of imperatorin on scopolamine-induced cognitive impairment and oxidative stress in mice. *Psychopharmacology* **2015**, *232*, 931–942. [CrossRef]
10. Geng, Y.; Li, C.; Liu, J.; Xing, G.; Zhou, L.; Dong, M.; Li, X.; Niu, Y. Beta-asarone improves cognitive function by suppressing neuronal apoptosis in the beta-amyloid hippocampus injection rats. *Biol. Pharm. Bull.* **2010**, *33*, 836–843. [CrossRef]
11. Yong, Y.Y.; Yan, L.; Wang, B.D.; Fan, D.S.; Guo, M.S.; Yu, L.; Wu, J.M.; Qin, D.L.; Law, B.Y.K.; Wong, V.K.W.; et al. *Penthorum chinense* Pursh inhibits ferroptosis in cellular and *Caenorhabditis elegans* models of Alzheimer's disease. *Phytomedicine* **2024**, *127*, 155463. [CrossRef]
12. Yong, Y.; Yan, L.; Wei, J.; Feng, C.; Yu, L.; Wu, J.; Guo, M.; Fan, D.; Yu, C.; Qin, D.; et al. A novel ferroptosis inhibitor, Thonningianin A, improves Alzheimer's disease by activating GPX4. *Theranostics* **2024**, *14*, 6161–6184. [CrossRef]
13. Tao, L.; Liu, Z.; Li, X.; Wang, H.; Wang, Y.; Zhou, D.; Zhang, H. Oleanonic acid ameliorates mutant Aβ precursor protein-induced oxidative stress, autophagy deficits, ferroptosis, mitochondrial damage, and ER stress in vitro. *Biochim. Biophys. Acta Mol. Basis Dis.* **2024**, *1870*, 167459. [CrossRef]
14. Tang, H.; He, K.; Zhao, K.; Zheng, C.; Wu, W.; Jin, W.; Yang, L.; Xie, B. Protective Effects of Hinokitiol on Neuronal Ferroptosis by Activating the Keap1/Nrf2/HO-1 Pathway in Traumatic Brain Injury. *J. Neurotrauma* **2024**, *41*, 734–750. [CrossRef]

15. Qiu, M.; Zhang, J.; Wei, W.; Zhang, Y.; Li, M.; Bai, Y.; Wang, H.; Meng, Q.; Guo, D.A. Integrated UPLC/Q-TOF-MS/MS Analysis and Network Pharmacology to Reveal the Neuroprotective Mechanisms and Potential Pharmacological Ingredients of Aurantii Fructus Immaturus and Aurantii Fructus. *Pharmaceuticals* **2024**, *17*, 239. [CrossRef]
16. Long, Q.; Li, T.; Zhu, Q.; He, L.; Zhao, B. SuanZaoRen decoction alleviates neuronal loss, synaptic damage and ferroptosis of AD via activating DJ-1/Nrf2 signaling pathway. *J. Ethnopharmacol.* **2024**, *323*, 117679. [CrossRef]
17. Li, Z.; Lu, Y.; Zhen, Y.; Jin, W.; Ma, X.; Yuan, Z.; Liu, B.; Zhou, X.L.; Zhang, L. Avicularin inhibits ferroptosis and improves cognitive impairments in Alzheimer's disease by modulating the NOX4/Nrf2 axis. *Phytomedicine* **2024**, *135*, 156209. [CrossRef]
18. Mishra, V.H.; Khade, A.; Noman, O. Drug effects on the nervous system: Mechanisms and future directions in neuropharmacological therapy. *Adv. Hum. Biol.* **2025**, *15*, 291–292. [CrossRef]
19. Um, M.Y.; Choi, W.H.; Aan, J.Y.; Kim, S.R.; Ha, T.Y. Protective effect of Polygonum multiflorum Thunb on amyloid β-peptide 25-35 induced cognitive deficits in mice. *J. Ethnopharmacol.* **2006**, *104*, 144–148. [CrossRef]
20. Ghallab, Y.K.; Elassal, O.S. Biochemical and Neuropharmacology of Psychiatric Disorders. In *Nutrition and Psychiatric Disorders: An Evidence-Based Approach to Understanding the Diet-Brain Connection*; Springer: Berlin/Heidelberg, Germany, 2024; pp. 25–47.
21. Orchard, I.; Leyria, J.; Al-Dailami, A.; Lange, A.B. Fluid secretion by Malpighian tubules of Rhodnius prolixus: Neuroendocrine control with new insights from a transcriptome analysis. *Front. Endocrinol.* **2021**, *12*, 722487. [CrossRef]
22. Oyebanjo, O.T.; Adetuyi, B.O.; Adeoye, A.D.; Adetuyi, O.A.; Oni, P.G.; Ogunlana, O.O. Neuropharmacology and neurotherapeutics: Advancing the understanding and treatment of neurological disorders. In *Biochemical and Molecular Pharmacology in Drug Discovery*; Elsevier: Amsterdam, The Netherlands, 2024; pp. 403–425.
23. Tassé, M.J.; Luckasson, R.; Schalock, R.L. The relation between intellectual functioning and adaptive behavior in the diagnosis of intellectual disability. *Intellect. Dev. Disabil.* **2016**, *54*, 381–390. [CrossRef]
24. Tassé, M.J.; Grover, M. American association on intellectual and developmental disabilities (aaidd). In *Encyclopedia of Autism Spectrum Disorders*; Springer: Berlin/Heidelberg, Germany, 2021; pp. 165–168.
25. Boat, T.F.; Wu, J.T.; Committee to Evaluate the Supplemental Security Income Disability Program for Children with Mental Disorders; Board on the Health of Select Populations; Board on Children, Youth, and Families; Institute of Medicine; The National Academies of Sciences, Engineering, and Medicine. Clinical characteristics of intellectual disabilities. In *Mental Disorders and Disabilities Among Low-Income Children*; National Academies Press (US): Washington, DC, USA, 2015.
26. Bao, X.; Song, X.; Deng, H.; Jiang, L. The Impact of Virtual Reality Training Combined with Traditional Chinese Medicine Health Preservation Therapy on Cognitive Function, Neurological Function, and Physical Function of Stroke Patients. *Int. J. Neurosci.* **2024**. [CrossRef]
27. Li, L.; Li, W.J.; Zheng, X.R.; Liu, Q.L.; Du, Q.; Lai, Y.J.; Liu, S.Q. Eriodictyol ameliorates cognitive dysfunction in APP/PS1 mice by inhibiting ferroptosis via vitamin D receptor-mediated Nrf2 activation. *Mol. Med.* **2022**, *28*, 11. [CrossRef]
28. Bahadori, M.B.; Dinparast, L.; Zengin, G.; Sarikurkcu, C.; Bahadori, S.; Asghari, B.; Movahhedin, N. Functional components, antidiabetic, anti-Alzheimer's disease, and antioxidant activities of *Salvia syriaca* L. *Int. J. Food Prop.* **2017**, *20*, 1761–1772. [CrossRef]
29. Abdelwahab, S.I.; Taha, M.M.E.; Mariod, A.A. Performance analysis, conceptual mapping, and emerging trends for Gum Arabic research: A comprehensive bibliometric analysis from 1916 to 2023. *Food Prod. Process. Nutr.* **2025**, *7*, 4. [CrossRef]
30. Abdelwahab, S.I.; Farasani, A.; Alfaifi, H.A.; Hassan, W. Trends and dynamics in facelift surgery research: A bibliometric analysis of the top 50 most cited papers. *Chin. J. Plast. Reconstr. Surg.* **2024**, *7*, 11–17. [CrossRef]
31. Gong, Y.; Wang, Y.; Li, Y.; Weng, F.; Chen, T.; He, L. Curculigoside, a traditional Chinese medicine monomer, ameliorates oxidative stress in Alzheimer's disease mouse model via suppressing ferroptosis. *Phytother. Res.* **2024**, *38*, 2462–2481. [CrossRef]
32. Van Eck, N.; Waltman, L. Software survey: VOSviewer, a computer program for bibliometric mapping. *Scientometrics* **2010**, *84*, 523–538. [CrossRef]
33. Bérdi, M. Bibliometric analysis of Hungarian-related publications in suicidal behavior research of the last three decades. *Psychiatr. Hung.* **2023**, *38*, 189–202.
34. Bastianetto, S.; Yao, Z.X.; Papadopoulos, V.; Quirion, R. Neuroprotective effects of green and black teas and their catechin gallate esters against β-amyloid-induced toxicity. *Eur. J. Neurosci.* **2006**, *23*, 55–64. [CrossRef]
35. Das, A.; Shanker, G.; Nath, C.; Pal, R.; Singh, S.; Singh, H.K. A comparative study in rodents of standardized extracts of *Bacopa monniera* and *Ginkgo biloba*—Anticholinesterase and cognitive enhancing activities. *Pharmacol. Biochem. Behav.* **2002**, *73*, 893–900. [CrossRef] [PubMed]
36. Hybertson, B.M.; Gao, B.; Bose, S.K.; McCord, J.M. Oxidative stress in health and disease: The therapeutic potential of Nrf2 activation. *Mol. Asp. Med.* **2011**, *32*, 234–246. [CrossRef] [PubMed]
37. Picot, M.C.N.; Zengin, G.; Mollica, A.; Stefanucci, A.; Carradori, S.; Mahomoodally, M.F. In vitro and in silico studies of mangiferin from aphloia theiformis on key enzymes linked to diabetes type 2 and associated complications. *Med. Chem.* **2017**, *13*, 633–640. [CrossRef] [PubMed]

38. Wang, X.; Zhao, H.; Wu, M.; Gan, Y.; Zhang, S.; Wu, D.; Ou, J.; Jin, C.; Zhang, W. Integrated UHPLC-Q-Orbitrap-MS/MS Method and Network Pharmacology for Exploring the Active Components and Potential Mechanisms of Neuroprotective Effect of the n-Butanol Part of Mume Flos. *Nat. Prod. Commun.* **2024**, *19*. [CrossRef]
39. Tao, Q.; Chao, H.; Fang, D.; Dou, D. Progress in neurorehabilitation research and the support by the National Natural Science Foundation of China from 2010 to 2022. *Neural Regen. Res.* **2024**, *19*, 226–232. [CrossRef]
40. Lin, F.; Huang, D.; He, N.; Gu, Y.; Wu, Y. Effect of music therapy derived from the five elements in Traditional Chinese Medicine on post-stroke depression. *J. Tradit. Chin. Med.* **2017**, *37*, 675–680. [PubMed]
41. Movahhedin, N.; Zengin, G.; Bahadori, M.B.; Sarikurkcu, C.; Bahadori, S.; Dinparast, L. *Ajuga chamaecistus* subsp. scoparia (Boiss.) Rech.f.: A new source of phytochemicals for antidiabetic, skin-care, and neuroprotective uses. *Ind. Crops Prod.* **2016**, *94*, 89–96. [CrossRef]
42. Zengin, G.; Uysal, A.; Diuzheva, A.; Gunes, E.; Jekő, J.; Cziáky, Z.; Picot-Allain, C.M.N.; Mahomoodally, M.F. Characterization of phytochemical components of *Ferula halophila* extracts using HPLC-MS/MS and their pharmacological potentials: A multi-functional insight. *J. Pharm. Biomed. Anal.* **2018**, *160*, 374–382. [CrossRef]
43. Zengin, G.; Sinan, K.I.; Ak, G.; Mahomoodally, M.F.; Paksoy, M.Y.; Picot-Allain, C.; Glamocilja, J.; Sokovic, M.; Jekő, J.; Cziáky, Z.; et al. Chemical profile, antioxidant, antimicrobial, enzyme inhibitory, and cytotoxicity of seven Apiaceae species from Turkey: A comparative study. *Ind. Crops Prod.* **2020**, *153*, 112572. [CrossRef]
44. Savran, A.; Zengin, G.; Aktumsek, A.; Mocan, A.; Glamoćlija, J.; Ćirić, A.; Soković, M. Phenolic compounds and biological effects of edible: *Rumex scutatus* and *Pseudosempervivum sempervivum*: Potential sources of natural agents with health benefits. *Food Funct.* **2016**, *7*, 3252–3262. [CrossRef]
45. Zengin, G.; Nithiyanantham, S.; Locatelli, M.; Ceylan, R.; Uysal, S.; Aktumsek, A.; Selvi, P.K.; Maskovic, P. Screening of in vitro antioxidant and enzyme inhibitory activities of different extracts from two uninvestigated wild plants: *Centranthus longiflorus* subsp. *longiflorus and Cerinthe minor subsp. auriculata. Eur. J. Integr. Med.* **2016**, *8*, 286–292. [CrossRef]
46. Zengin, G.; Sarıkürkçü, C.; Aktümsek, A.; Ceylan, R. Antioxidant potential and inhibition of key enzymes linked to Alzheimer's diseases and diabetes mellitus by monoterpene-rich essential oil from *Sideritis galatica* Bornm. Endemic to Turkey. *Rec. Nat. Prod.* **2015**, *10*, 195–206.
47. Zengin, G.; Sarikurkcu, C.; Gunes, E.; Uysal, A.; Ceylan, R.; Uysal, S.; Gungor, H.; Aktumsek, A. Two Ganoderma species: Profiling of phenolic compounds by HPLC-DAD, antioxidant, antimicrobial and inhibitory activities on key enzymes linked to diabetes mellitus, Alzheimer's disease and skin disorders. *Food Funct.* **2015**, *6*, 2794–2802. [CrossRef]
48. Zengin, G.; Stefanucci, A.; Rodrigues, M.J.; Mollica, A.; Custodio, L.; Aumeeruddy, M.Z.; Mahomoodally, M.F. *Scrophularia lucida* L. as a valuable source of bioactive compounds for pharmaceutical applications: In vitro antioxidant, anti-inflammatory, enzyme inhibitory properties, in silico studies, and HPLC profiles. *J. Pharm. Biomed. Anal.* **2019**, *162*, 225–233. [CrossRef] [PubMed]
49. Mukherjee, P.K.; Kumar, V.; Mal, M.; Houghton, P.J. Acetylcholinesterase inhibitors from plants. *Phytomedicine* **2007**, *14*, 289–300. [CrossRef]
50. Heo, H.J.; Kim, D.O.; Shin, S.C.; Kim, M.J.; Kim, B.G.; Shin, D.H. Effect of Antioxidant Flavanone, Naringenin, from *Citrus junos* on Neuroprotection. *J. Agric. Food Chem.* **2004**, *52*, 1520–1525. [CrossRef]
51. Yu, M.S.; Leung, S.K.Y.; Lai, S.W.; Che, C.M.; Zee, S.Y.; So, K.F.; Yuen, W.H.; Chang, R.C.C. Neuroprotective effects of anti-aging oriental medicine *Lycium barbarum* against β-amyloid peptide neurotoxicity. *Exp. Gerontol.* **2005**, *40*, 716–727. [CrossRef] [PubMed]
52. Limpeanchob, N.; Jaipan, S.; Rattanakaruna, S.; Phrompittayarat, W.; Ingkaninan, K. Neuroprotective effect of *Bacopa monnieri* on beta-amyloid-induced cell death in primary cortical culture. *J. Ethnopharmacol.* **2008**, *120*, 112–117. [CrossRef]
53. Zhang, J.-N.; Pei, Z.-D.; Wang, W.-Y.; Zhao, M.-Y.; Pei, W.-H.; Zhang, H.; Yin, H.-B.; Wang, T.-M.; Xin, G.-Z.; Xie, M. Integration of High-Resolution LC-Q-TOF Mass Spectrometry and Multidimensional Chemical-Biological Analysis to Detect Nanomolar-Level Acetylcholinesterase Inhibitors from Different Parts of *Zanthoxylum nitidum*. *J. Agric. Food Chem.* **2024**, *72*, 17328–17342. [CrossRef] [PubMed]
54. McCarney, R.; Warner, J.; Iliffe, S.; Van Haselen, R.; Griffin, M.; Fisher, P. The Hawthorne Effect: A randomised, controlled trial. *BMC Med. Res. Methodol.* **2007**, *7*, 30. [CrossRef] [PubMed]
55. Aria, M.; Cuccurullo, C. bibliometrix: An R-tool for comprehensive science mapping analysis. *J. Informetr.* **2017**, *11*, 959–975. [CrossRef]
56. Alkhammash, R. Bibliometric, network, and thematic mapping analyses of metaphor and discourse in COVID-19 publications from 2020 to 2022. *Front. Psychol.* **2023**, *13*, 1062943. [CrossRef]

pharmaceuticals

Review

Pleiotropic Bioactivity of Caterpillar Fungus, Orange Cordyceps, and Cordycepin: Insight from Integrated Network Pharmacology and Food and Drug Regulatory Framework

Alexander Panossian

Research & Development, Phytomed AB, 59344 Västervick, Sweden; ap@phytomed.se

Abstract

Background/Objectives: The medical mushroom *Ophiocordyceps sinensis* (Caterpillar Fungus), known for its ability to enhance "vitality," is one of the most popular medicines in Asian traditional medical systems. According to the Chinese *Pharmacopeia*, *O. sinensis* is standardized for its adenosine content, the precursor of ATP, which mediates numerous physiological and pathological processes in many diseases. The related fungus of order Hypocreales, *Cordyceps militaris*, and its major bioactive constituents, 3′-deoxyadenosine (cordycepin), also exhibit pleiotropic biological activities. This review aims to provide a rationale for the adaptogenic and resilience-supporting effects of these medicinal fungi and to align food and drug regulation in Western countries. **Methods:** In this narrative review, we integrated results from chemical, pharmacokinetic, network pharmacology, preclinical, and clinical studies of *O. sinensis*, *C. militaris*, and cordycepin using network pharmacology and bioinformatics tools. **Results:** Across studies, recurrent mechanistic hubs included PI3K–Akt, AMPK–mTOR, MAPK, NF-κB, apoptosis, and adaptive stress-response signaling pathways, linking immune regulation and metabolic homeostasis. Experimental studies confirmed modulation of cytokine production, kinase signaling, and mitochondrial regulators. Clinical meta-analyses demonstrate consistent adjunctive benefits in renal and pulmonary disorders, although heterogeneity in preparation and methodological limitations remains significant. The review reveals controversy regarding the bioavailability of cordycepin in vivo and its concentration in vitro studies, raising the hypothesis that cordycepin may act as a driver, triggering the organism's adaptive stress response in stress-induced and aging-related diseases. Pharmacokinetic data indicate that systemic cordycepin concentrations after oral administration remain in the nanomolar range, suggesting that some predicted molecular interactions may occur indirectly or through systems-level mechanisms. The review, for the first time, suggests establishing a regulatory category for resilience-supporting physiological modulators to align food and drug regulation in the EU with contemporary systems biology, thereby complementing the work of EFSA, EMA, FDA, and Asian authorities. **Conclusions:** *O. sinensis*, *C. militaris*, and 3-deoxyadenosine share a common adaptogenic mechanism for maintaining homeostasis of cellular and integrated biological system functions. The systems-level network analysis and reductionistic molecular ligand preceptor pharmacology provide complementary approaches for understanding the multi-target bioactivity of these fungi. This review clarifies conceptual and regulatory barriers to recognizing resilience-supporting interventions and informs future regulatory innovation.

Keywords: *Ophiocordyceps sinensis*; *Cordyceps militaris*; cordycepin; adaptogen; resilience; fungi; botanicals; network pharmacology

1. Introduction

Ophiocordyceps sinensis (Berk.) G.H. Sung, J.M. Sung, Hywel-Jones and Spatafora, 2007 (Caterpillar Fungus) [1] and *Cordyceps militaris* (L.) Fr., 1818 (Orange Cordyceps) [2] are botanicals [3] belonging to the fungi kingdom [4–6], traditionally valued across East Asia [7–12] for their tonic, energy-enhancing, aphrodisiac, and respiratory ailments, lung invigoration, and kidney-nourishing actions [13–19], Appendix A Tables A1 and A2. Their therapeutic applications span inflammatory, respiratory disorders, fatigue, metabolic diseases (atherosclerosis, hyperlipidemia, glucose metabolism), kidney diseases, fertility, sexual-restorative functions, which are associated with immune, nervous, endocrine, cardiovascular, respiratory, renal, hepatic systems [14,20–25]. These attributes align with the modern concept of adaptogens as a therapeutic category of herbal medicines and nutritional products, characterized by increased human adaptability, survival, and resilience in response to stress by triggering intracellular and extracellular adaptive signaling pathways within cellular and organismal defense systems, including the neuroendocrine-immune complex [26]. In 1968, the term adaptogen (phytoadaptogen) was applied to medicinal plants, herbal medicines, and phytomedicines, reflecting their origin in the plant kingdom [27]. Phytoadaptogens are plant secondary metabolites, particularly tetracyclic terpenoids, and phenethyl- or phenylpropanoid derivatives of the defense system, chemically similar to steroidal and phenolic hormones of the human stress system [28].

Several studies claim that *O. sinensis* is an adaptogen [29–32] that triggers various adaptive stress–response signaling pathways [33–38]. However, the rationale for polyvalent action and the molecular mechanisms of *O. sinensis* have not been sufficiently studied or understood. Furthermore, clinical efficacy was not unambiguously demonstrated, and potential new indications for *O. sinensis* should be evaluated.

Unlike phytoadaptogens derived from the green plant kingdom Viridiplantae, *O. sinensis* [1,2,5,39,40], commonly known as Caterpillar Fungus or Winter Worm-Summer Grass, is an entomopathogenic fungus of the phylum Ascomycota, with a quite different biological nature compared to typical edible mushrooms (Basidiomycota). Initially described as *Sphaeria sinensis* by Berkeley in 1843, it was later named *Cordyceps sinensis* by Saccardo in 1878, and in 2007 it was renamed *Ophiocordyceps sinensis*, a member of the genus *Ophiocordyceps* (family Ophiocordycipitaceae, order Hypocreales), based on phylogenetic studies [3,4,10,25].

Caterpillar Fungus symbiotically parasitizes the larvae of ghost moths (*Fam. Hepialidae, Hepialus* spp./*Thitarodes* spp.) to survive, producing a characteristic club-shaped stroma that emerges from the mummified caterpillar [13,14,16,21,29,30,41,42]. As the larva's self-defense mechanism weakens, the fungal cells spread throughout the body, forming the sexual stroma, which grows upward above the soil surface while remaining connected to the dead larva/host below, creating the unique insect/fungus combination [43–46].

This medicinal fungus is endemic to high-altitude regions of the Tibetan Plateau and the Himalayas [47,48] and has a long history in traditional medical systems of China, Nepal, India, Bhutan, Republic of Korea, Vietnam, Thailand, and Japan as a tonic to replenish bodily health [19,39]. Caterpillar Fungus is officially recognized as a medicinal fungus in the pharmacopeias of several countries, especially in East Asia, where it is highly valued for energy, immune, and respiratory support [49]. In *Pharmacopeia* of the People's Republic of China, Chinese Caterpillar Fungus, Cordyceps (Dongchongxiacao) is classified as a *Chinese Materia Medica* crude drug, indicated for deficiency of kidney essence, impotence and seminal emission, limp aching in the lower back and knees, chronic cough and dyspnea of deficiency type, cough caused by consumptive diseases, and hemoptysis in daily dosage 3–9 g corresponding to ~1 mg of adenosine [50], Figure 1.

https://doi.org/10.3390/ph19030519

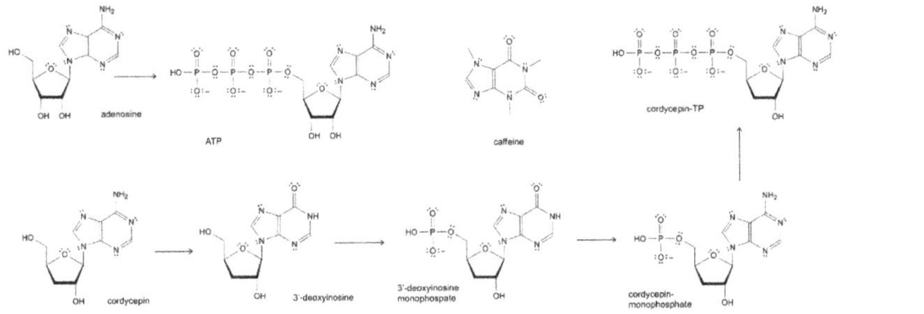

Figure 1. Chemical structure of purine alkaloids adenosine, cordycepin, 3′-deoxyinosine, and phosphorylated nucleoside ATP, cordycepin-TP, 3′-deoxyinosine-monophosphate. (primary metabolites of *O. sinensis* and *C. militaris*) and caffeine (a comparator-major active constituent of coffee and green tea).

Related species, *C. militaris* [2], also known as the Scarlet Caterpillar Club and in Chinese as Northern Cordyceps, is cultivated on silkworm pupae and used for medicinal purposes, as a health supplement, and as a pharmaceutical drug on a large scale, especially in China [25,51]. Numerous studies on the chemical constituents and pharmacological activities of *C. militaris* [20,22,52–54] and its bioactive marker, cordycepin [53,54], reveal multiple effects on the neuroendocrine-immune complex [36,37,42,55–62], which is typical of adaptogens [22]. In the course of the search for new fungal antibiotics in 1950, Cunningham et al. found that the mold *C. militaris* secretes a substance called cordycepin, which inhibits the growth of several bacteria [63], increases the survival time of mice with Ehrlich ascites tumors, and inhibits the growth of human tumor cells in culture. In 1980, the chemical structure of cordycepin was elucidated as the nucleoside 3′-deoxyadenosine [64], a copy of adenosine with one oxygen atom removed from its structure (Figure 1).

Both fungi contain diverse bioactive metabolites, including nucleosides, sterols, peptides, polysaccharides, and secondary metabolites (Appendix A Figure A1 and Tables A3–A6).

The pharmacological breadth of both species suggests multi-target effects rather than classical single-receptor drug actions (Appendix A Tables A4 and A5). Network pharmacology has become a significant framework for elucidating the complex, multi-target actions of such herbal and fungal preparations, providing a systematic approach to deciphering these interactions by integrating predicted targets, signaling pathways, molecular docking, and multi-omics data. However, most reports remain scattered, disease-specific, or lacking integration with wet-lab validation. A unified synthesis is needed to understand the core pharmacological principles of *O. sinensis* and *C. militaris*.

Despite numerous studies, no comprehensive synthesis has unified the mechanistic insights across species, compounds, and disease contexts. This narrative study integrates 37 network pharmacology investigations and 10 experimental validation studies to define the adaptogenic potential and systems-level pharmacology of these fungi and their active constituent, 3-deoxyadenosine (cordycepin).

Network pharmacology provides a valuable framework for understanding these multi- component, multi-target interactions. Nevertheless, existing studies are often disease-specific and fragmented, lacking an integrated mechanistic synthesis. This work consolidates findings from 37 network pharmacology studies, including 22 experimentally validated investigations, to establish a unified systems-level model for the adaptogenic activity of Caterpillar Fungus, Orange Cordyceps, and 3-deoxy-adenosine.

The adaptogenic concept represents a systems-level interpretation of complex physiological responses characteristic of holistic Traditional Chinese Medicine (TCM) and Ayurvedic concepts, whereas European Food Safety Authority (EFSA) regulatory frameworks lack concepts for resilience and adaptive capacity and operate at the level of single, well-defined functional outcomes, which raises regulatory issues for food and drugs in Western countries.

https://doi.org/10.3390/ph19030519

The implementation of European standards by EMA drug regulatory authorities for traditional herbal medicines and other botanicals developed under regulatory conditions in Asian countries creates problems for their regulation in Europe. This is mainly due to the core conceptual differences between reductionistic, mechanistic, and Systems-based, integrative, and holistic approaches to medicine in Western and Oriental countries, as well as to insufficient clinical evidence and limited well-established use. Another limitation in EU countries is that the EFSA does not accept the definitions of stress, fatigue, and adaptogens as dietary supplements or food additives, despite their worldwide scientific recognition. The reason is that EFSA considers these products for use only in healthy subjects, whereas medicines are used to treat or prevent defined diseases. However, the same products are used in China, India, Japan, and other Asian countries to restore balance and resilience. In this review, we sought to harmonize these complementary paradigms to address the gap and reach consensus.

Overall, this literature review primarily aims to justify a rationale for the pleiotropic adaptogenic potential of two traditionally used botanicals from the fungal species, Caterpillar Fungus and Orange Cordyceps, and its active constituent, 3-deoxyadenosine (cordycepin), using a network pharmacology approach The secondary aim was to establish a regulatory category for resilience-supporting physiological modulators that could align food and drug regulation in the EU with contemporary systems biology, and regulatory acceptance of adaptogenic botanicals across the European Union (EU), United States (US), and selected Asian jurisdictions.

2. Results

2.1. Bioactive Compounds of *O. sinensis* and *C. militaris* Fungi and Their Pharmacological Activity

Overall, 90 primary and secondary metabolites in *O. sinensis* and 26 constituents in *C. militaris* were identified in an extensive review, covering its traditional uses, chemistry, and pharmacology [19], as shown in Appendix A Tables A3 and A4 and Figure A1.

Studies of chemical compositions of *O. sinensis* [21,29,65] and *C. militaris* [23,29,66,67] show the presence of host–parasite symbiotic interactions, four types of primary metabolites: (i)—amino acids and peptides, (ii)—nucleotides/nucleosides, (iii)—lipids, including sterols and fatty acids, and (iv)—carbohydrates, including polysaccharides. All of them are essential for the parasite's growth and development, as well as for the host's adaptive stress response (Appendix A Tables A4–A6). Some secondary metabolites that function in defense responses include cytotoxic alkaloids and antioxidant phenolic compounds. These compounds were isolated and identified in *O. sinensis* growing under wild conditions, but not in cultivated *O. sinensis* and *C. militaris* (Appendix A Figure A1).

Many primary metabolites of mushrooms, including nucleosides, sterols, and polysaccharides, have been specified as physiologically active markers of *O. synensis* in both in vitro and in vivo studies [68]. Meanwhile, several novel compounds characteristic of *O. sinensis* have been identified, including epipolythiodioxopiperazines, gliocladicillins A, B, and 11,11′-dideoxyverticillin, which are capable of inhibiting the growth of tumor cells [16,69,70]. Exclusive to *O. sinensis*, five anti-inflammatory alkaloids, named cordysinin (A–E), have also been reported for the first time [16,19, 71].

At present, cordycepin, adenosine, total nucleosides, ergosterol, and polysaccharides are commonly used quality control markers for *O. sinensis* and *C. militaris* products (Tables 1 and A5) [18,71–97]. However, they are not regarded as efficacy markers for therapeutic or nutritional purposes for several reasons, including poor oral bioavailability, instability, nonspecific (cordycepin, adenosine) or inconsistent actions (polysaccharides, ergosterol), and a lack of direct correlation between marker levels and clinical effects in humans [84,85].

https://doi.org/10.3390/ph19030519

Table 1. Key analytical markers and typical ranges in *O. sinensis* and *C. militaris* products.

Markers	*O. sinensis*, mg/g	*C. militaris*, mg/g	References
Adenosine	≈0.2–10	0.3–2.5	[86–88]
Cordycepin	<0.2 (0.006–0.075)	~6.6 (3–26)	[53,87–90]
Polysaccharides	≥60 (≈50–100)	≥80 (~30–150)	[16,88,91]
Total nucleosides	~2.0–3.1		[92–94]
Total Ergosterol	~1.9–2.7	~2–3	[95,96]
Mattitol	25.6–115.7		[89,97]

O. sinensis exhibits broad biological and pharmacological actions in hepatic, renal, cardiovascular, and immunological systems, and has anticancer activity as well [15,97]. Over 30 different bioactivities have been reported for *O. sinensis*, including anti-inflammatory, immunomodulatory, antioxidant, antibacterial, hepatoprotective, antifatigue, antiaging, steroid hormones production, antidepressant, sedative, and the ability to promote endurance capacity, improve learning-memory in vitro, in vivo, or ex vivo studies, as shown in Appendix A Table A4 [97].

In the course of the search for new fungal antibiotics in 1950, Cunningham et al. found that the mold *C. militaris* secretes a substance called cordycepin, which inhibits the growth of several bacteria [63], increases the survival time of mice with Ehrlich ascites tumors, and inhibits the growth of human tumor cells in culture. In 1980, the chemical structure of cordycepin was elucidated as the nucleoside 3′-deoxyadenosine [64] (Figure 1). One of its modes of action is by inhibition of RNA synthesis. It is incorporated as 3′-deoxyadenosine triphosphate at the 3′ end of the RNA molecule, thereby preventing further elongation [98]. Phosphorylated adenosine, adenosinetriphosphate (ATP), is known as an "energy currency" in the metabolism of the organism. A cellular energy sensor, AMPK (AMP-activated protein kinase (PRKAA1/2/PRKAG1) is one of the key mediators of adaptive stress–response signaling pathways. Phosphorylated cordycepin (cordycepin triphosphate, COR-tp) competes with ATP, resulting in its incorporation into enzymatic processes where it acts as a substitute for ATP [99,100]. This molecular mimicry may underlie the diverse biological activities of cordycepin, leading to abnormal purine metabolism and inhibiting or aberrantly activating ATP-targeted protein kinases [35,62]. Consequently, it is not surprising that cordycepin may have beneficial health effects in stress-induced metabolic diseases and aging disorders, showing anticancer, antiviral, antioxidant, anti-aging, and anti-inflammatory activities [33–38,42,55,61,101–104].

Overall, the pharmacological activity of *O. sinensis* and *C. militaris* product preparations is unlikely to be attributable to a single active constituent, as compounds such as cordycepin and adenosine suffer from poor oral bioavailability and limited pharmacokinetic stability. Instead, it is reasonable to hypothesize that the overall therapeutic profile arises from the synergistic action of multiple metabolites—including nucleosides, polysaccharides, sterols, and peptides—that interact with diverse molecular targets. At present, the validity of this hypothesis rests primarily on the outcomes of randomized controlled clinical trials, rather than on any single chemical marker. In this context, network pharmacology approaches combined with gene expression analyses may be suitable tools for elucidating the complex, multi-target interactions underlying the putative synergistic effects of *O. sinensis* and *C. militaris* ingredients.

2.2. Nucleosides Adenosine and Cordycepin as Mediators of Adaptive Stress Response Andanti-Fatigue Activity of O. sinensis, and C. militaris

The choice of adenosine as an active marker for the standardization of Cordyceps (Dongchongxiacao), Chinese Caterpillar Fungus [50] and Patented Traditional Chinese Medicines (TCM) Bailing capsule [105], containing fermented *O. sinensis* powder standardized for 0.4 mg of adenosine, is presumably due to: (i) its high content in *O. sinensis* and (ii) its physiological functions.

https://doi.org/10.3390/ph19030519

Adenosine functions as an energy metabolite (part of the ATP/AMP balance) and as a signaling molecule via cell-surface receptors and intracellular actions in the nervous, cardiovascular, immune, respiratory, and renal systems [106–111]. Adenosine is a byproduct of the "energy fuel", adenosine triphosphate (ATP) breakdown during stress (hypoxia, ischemia, exercise), matching oxygen supply with demand as a local, short-lived homeostatic regulator, and coordinating energy balance, vascular tone, neuronal excitability, and immune activity [112–118]. During low-energy states, adenosine acts as a local signal to increase energy supply. Adenosine indirectly regulates AMP-activated protein kinase (AMPK) activity through AMP/adenosine balance. High AMP/ATP ratios activate AMP-activated protein kinase (AMPK), promoting energy-conserving processes. Adenosine can also directly activate receptors, and its balance with AMP is maintained by enzymes such as adenosine kinase (ADK), as shown in Figure 1. Its primary molecular targets are the four adenosine GPCRs (A1, A2A, A2B, A3), as well as metabolic enzymes and transporters that control its levels [117,119–122].

Adenosine is the endogenous agonist of GPCR adenosine receptors (A1, A2A, A2B, A3, high affinity; EC50 in the low-nanomolar range), producing inhibitory neuromodulation that promotes sleep, decreases neuronal firing, and increases the subjective sensation of fatigue [101,123], Table 2. In contrast, caffeine acts as a competitive antagonist at A1 and A2A receptors (non-selective; micromolar affinities, Ki ~2–50 μM), thereby blocking adenosine's inhibitory signaling and producing stimulatory effects on arousal, mood, reduced fatigue, and physical performance [124–126], Table 2. Cordycepin (3′-deoxyadenosine), despite structural similarity to adenosine, can act as an agonist in vitro (at A3 in many cell studies and A1/A2A in some reports), and has minimal functional interaction with adenosine receptors in vivo because it is rapidly deaminated to 3′-deoxyinosine, exhibits very low plasma nano-molar levels after oral ingestion [127,128], and demonstrates poor blood–brain barrier penetration, meanwhile in cell/animal models cordycepin's effects (anti-inflammatory, antiproliferative) are often attributed to A3 agonism or other intracellular actions (AMPK activation, PI3K/mTOR inhibition) [101,129,130]. Consequently, cordycepin does not meaningfully modulate adenosine receptor activity and cannot reproduce either the inhibitory effects of adenosine or the stimulatory effects of caffeine. The net result is that adenosine is fatigue-promoting, caffeine is fatigue-reducing, and cordycepin is functionally neutral in the context of central fatigue regulation (Table 2).

Table 2. Mental and physical fatigue effects.

Compound	Receptor Action	Net CNS Effect	Fatigue Impact	Mechanistic Reason
Adenosine	Agonist at A1, A2A	Sedative	Increases fatigue	Inhibits neuronal firing, promotes sleep pressure
Caffeine	Antagonist at A1, A2A	Stimulant	Reduces fatigue	Blocks adenosine, increases dopamine + cortical activity
Cordycepin	Minimal activity (in vivo)	Neutral	No proven effect	Rapid deamination, poor BBB penetration, weak receptor affinity

Cordycepin cannot meaningfully act as a CNS adenosine receptor ligand, yet *O. sinensis* and *C. militaris* extracts and purified cordycepin repeatedly show anti-fatigue effects in animals and humans. This appears contradictory only if one assumes that fatigue modulation must occur via central adenosinergic signaling. Apparently, the anti-fatigue effects of *O. sinensis* and *C. militaris* are mediated by non-adenosinergic, non-CNS mechanisms, though somewhat peripheral.

Cordycepin has poor intestinal permeability and low bioavailability due to rapid hepatic degradation by the enzyme adenosine deaminase, which converts it to the inactive 3′-deoxyinosine. However, 3′-deoxyinosine has significant bioavailability following oral administration of cordycepin, when absorbed into the systemic circulation, and can be phosphorylated to the active cordycepin 5′-triphosphate, an analog of ATP [131], Figure 1, and therefore could be responsible for the therapeutic effects of cordycepin when administered orally. These findings offer important insights into

https://doi.org/10.3390/ph19030519

the mechanisms underlying the therapeutic effects of cordycepin. Moreover, this metabolic pathway could play an important role in the activity of adenosine and other adenosine analog drugs. The metabolized products (i.e., the inactive metabolite of cordycepin, 3′-deoxyinosine) are available in the systemic circulation instead. They can return to the phosphorylation pathway of their parent form, as shown in this study [131].

The bioavailability of cordycepin is very low; a 10 mg/kg intravenous dose in rats yields a peak concentration of 2.1 ± 0.9 μg/mL (8366 nM). However, when cordycepin is administered orally to rats at a 10-fold higher dose of 100 mg/kg, it results in a relatively low peak plasma concentration, averaging approximately 0.004 ± 0.001 μg/mL (16 nM) [127]. The Cmax values of cordycepin in the rat blood and brain after exposure (10 mg/kg, i.p.) were 7.8 ng/mL (31 nM) and 5.4 ng/mL (21 nM), respectively [128]. Pharmacokinetic and brain research studies [127,128,131,132] reveal that the concentration of cordicepin in blood, kidney > liver > heart > lung > spleen > brain is dramatically lower than observed in vitro studies [127]. After systemic dosing with 10 mg cordycepin, its concentration in rat brain tissue is on the order of ~10–50 nM [127,128], while most published microglia/astrocyte studies use 10–50 μM cordycepin, which is 1000-fold higher than the presumed brain levels from a 9 g/day *O. sinensis* crude dose. These μM levels are clearly supra-physiological compared with the nM brain levels observed in PK studies; they are more like "pharmacological screening" than strict dose translation.

Obviously, the active concentrations of cordicepin, *O. sinensis*, and *C. militaris* preparations used in vitro studies are 1000-fold higher than those used in animal studies and do not match the effective therapeutic human daily dose of 9 g of *O. sinensis* and *C. militaris* crude drugs [50], which are traditionally used.

2.3. Efficacy and Safety of Ophiocordyceps sinensis and Cordyceps militaris in Human Subjects

2.3.1. Traditional Use

Oriental medical systems, TCM and Ayurveda, are based on a holistic approach, multi-target and polyvalent actions, but rely on archaic theories. In contrast, Western conventional medicine is based on a reductional approach, selective targeting, and specific action in the treatment of diseases, relying on another archaic theory of galenic preparations that ignores interactions and overlaps among regulatory systems and the effects of other constituents in multi-component plant extracts. In fact, both approaches are complementary, particularly in the treatment of diseases of complex pathology associated with the stress system interacting with other regulatory systems. The concomitant administration of several Western conventional medicines that selectively act on various receptors provides more effective treatment in hypertension, post-stroke rehabilitation, viral infections, etc. The "ready for use" of complex botanicals and botanical hybrid products used in the Eastern world acts similarly. The challenge is to understand the mechanisms of action and scientifically validate their efficacy, quality, and safety.

According to traditional Chinese medicine (TCM) theory, the organ functions concepts differ from Western physiology and pathology, suggesting that Caterpillar Fungus goes to the "Lung" and the "Kidney" meridians, supporting "lung protection," "kidney improvement," and so-called "YinYang double invigoration" [133]. Since the kidneys are considered "the root of life" in TCM, they store "Jing," a substance described as an undifferentiated, prime organic material that is "the source of reproduction, development, and maturation" [133]. Conception is made possible by the power of Jing; growth to maturity is the blossoming of Jing; and the decline into old age reflects the weakening of Jing. Over time, the Jing decreases in both vitality and quantity. Consequently, according to TCM, reproductive problems such as sterility or impotence and developmental disorders like retarded growth or lack of sexual maturation are seen as a dysfunction of the kidney's storing of Jing [133]. Moreover, according to TCM theory, the kidneys enable the fundamental "energy of life, so-called the Natural Air", Qi/chi, to penetrate deeply, completing the inhalation process by what is called "grasping the Qi." The kidneys are thus the root of Qi, while the lungs

https://doi.org/10.3390/ph19030519

are the "foundation of Qi." Proper breathing thus depends on the kidneys, and kidney disharmonies may result in respiratory problems, especially chronic asthma. In a "disharmony of the Lungs," a deficient Qi can result in any area of the body, and the power of resistance of the "protective Qi will be poor" [13,133]. Both TCM and Ayurveda have a notion of "life vital energy" and activating the body and mind: the qi in TCM and the prana in Ayurveda. Herbalists refer to adaptogens as restoratives, qi-tonics, rasayanas, or rejuvenating herbs [134].

According to TCM, Caterpillar Fungus goes to the "Lung" and the "Kidney" meridians, supporting "lung protection," "kidney improvement," and so-called "YinYang double invigoration" [133] and therefor was used to treat "lung" and "kidney" asthenia syndromes describing groups of symptoms associated with respiratory and renal diseases and other disease conditions such as fatigue, asthenia after severe illness, night sweating, male and female hyposexualities, including impotence, hyperglycemia, hyperlipidemia, respiratory diseases, renal dysfunction and renal failure, liver diseases, arrhythmias and other heart diseases [13]. They have been included as a dietary supplement to maintain health and prevent disease (Appendix A Table A7) [13,135].

It has been found that most local folk/traditional healers use Caterpillar Fungus to treat 21 ailments, including erectile dysfunction, female aphrodisia, malignant tumors, bronchial asthma, bronchitis, diabetes, cough and cold, jaundice, alcoholic hepatitis, and others [21,97].

2.3.2. Clinical Studies

2.3.2.1. Systematic Reviews and Meta-Analyses of Randomized Clinical Trials

Several systematic reviews and meta-analyses of randomized clinical trials of *O. sinensis* in dialysis patients [136,137] with renal dysfunction [137], acute kidney injury [138], chronic kidney disease [139], diabetic kidney disease [140], lung cancer [141], chronic obstructive pulmonary disease [142,143] and in healthy human subjects [144,145] were conducted, Table 3. These meta-analyses support the efficacy and safety of *O. sinensis* for immune and respiratory health, making it a promising adjunct in both healthy and clinical populations.

An umbrella-level synthesis of these systematic reviews and meta-analyses of randomized controlled trials (RCTs) evaluating *O. sinensis* was conducted by AI assistance. The objective was to assess the strength and consistency of the clinical evidence, stratified by species and preparation type, and to grade the overall level of evidence in accordance with the European Medicines Agency (EMA) criteria for well-established use (WEU) herbal medicinal products. Evidence was synthesized narratively and comparatively, without re-pooling individual trial data, in line with accepted methodology for overviews of systematic reviews [146].

Table 3 summarizes the totality of clinical evidence from nine systematic reviews, stratified by species and indication, and maps the findings against the key elements required for well-established use according to EMA/HMPC principles. Figure 2 illustrates the conceptual pathway from individual randomized trials to regulatory-relevant evidence grading, highlighting the points at which the current evidence base fails to meet WEU requirements despite consistent efficacy signals.

Table 3. Summary of clinical evidence from systematic reviews of *O. sinensis* and grading against EMA well-established use criteria.

References	Main Preparations Studied	Indications (Systematic Reviews)	No. of SRs/Meta-analyses	Approx. No. of RCTs (Patients)	Consistency of Clinical Effects	Methodological Quality Certainty of Evidence	Key Limitations	EMA WEU Relevance
Liu et al., 2024; Wu et al., 2025 Pu et al., 2024; Tao et al., 2024; Xue et al., 2024; [136–140]	Fermented mycelium (Bailing, Jinshuibao, Zhiling, others)	Dialysis (HD/PD), DKD, CKD, CA-AKI prevention, renal dysfunction	5	>210 RCTs (>16,000 pts, overlapping);	Consistent improvement in renal and inflammatory surrogate markers (Scr, BUN, CRP, proteinuria); reduced CA-AKI incidence when used preventively	Low to very low (GRADE); majority of SRs critically low (AMSTAR-2)	Open-label RCTs; short follow-up; surrogate endpoints; heterogeneous preparations	Does not meet WEU (efficacy signal present, but insufficient robustness and preparation definition)
Wang et al., 2024; Yu et al., 2019; Ma & Jin, 2024 [141–143]	Bailing capsule, cultivated mycelia, mixed CS preparations	COPD, lung cancer (adjunctive),	3	~80–100 RCTs (>5000 pts)	Consistent adjunctive benefits (lung function, QoL, immune markers, tumor response rate)	Low to moderate	Lack of blinding; all trials conducted in China; unclear allocation concealment; adjunctive designs only	Does not meet WEU (methodological and EU-use limitations)
Welch et al., 2023; Dewi & Khemtong, 2025 * [144,145]	Supplements (varied)	Healthy volunteers/exercise performance	2	7 RCTs (286 pts)	Inconsistent, small effects	Low	Small samples; heterogeneous outcomes; limited clinical relevance	Not relevant for WEU

Abbreviations: CA-AKI, contrast-associated acute kidney injury; CKD, chronic kidney disease; DKD—diabetic kidney disease; CRP, C-reactive protein; HD, haemodialysis; PD, peritoneal dialysis; QoL, quality of life; RCT, randomized controlled trial; Scr, serum creatinine; SR, systematic review; WEU, well-established use. *—Lack of preferred reporting items for systematic reviews and meta-analyses statement (PRISMA).

Figure 2 summarizes the progression from randomized controlled trials through systematic reviews to regulatory-relevant evidence grading. Although consistent adjunctive clinical benefits are observed across renal, pulmonary, and oncologic indications, limitations in methodological quality, preparation heterogeneity, and lack of documented long-term EU medicinal use prevent fulfillment of EMA criteria for well-established use (WEU), which requires: (i) recognized therapeutic efficacy, (ii) acceptable safety, (iii) sufficient clinical evidence, (iv) use for at least 10 years within the European Union, and (v) a well-defined herbal substance or preparation.

Across these reviews, consistent improvements were reported in surrogate renal and inflammatory outcomes, including reductions in serum creatinine, blood urea nitrogen, C-reactive protein, and proteinuria, as well as improvements in albumin and hemoglobin levels in dialysis populations. Preventive use before contrast exposure was associated with a reduced incidence of contrast-associated acute kidney injury in several trials. However, all reviews identified substantial methodological limitations, including: (i) predominantly open-label RCTs, (ii) inadequate reporting of allocation concealment and blinding, (iii) short treatment duration and follow-up, and (iv) reliance on surrogate rather than hard clinical endpoints (e.g., mortality, progression to end-stage kidney disease). Certainty of evidence was graded as low to very low using the grading of recommendations assessment, development and evaluation (GRADE) methodology [147] in the original reviews, primarily due to risk of bias, indirectness, and imprecision.

https://doi.org/10.3390/ph19030519

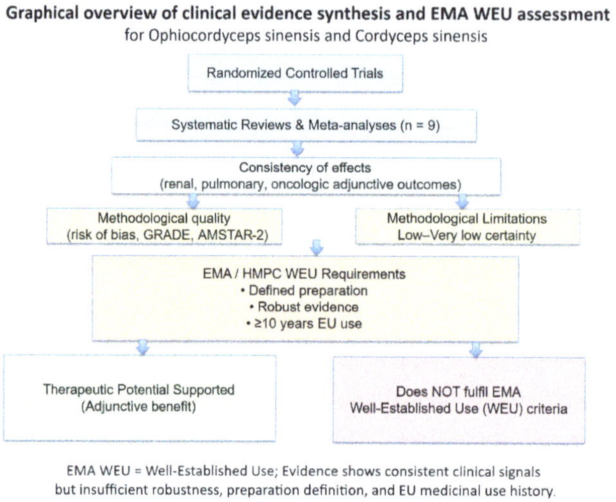

Figure 2. Graphical overview of clinical evidence synthesis and EMA-oriented grading of *O. sinensis*.

A critical limitation for *O. sinensis* is the heterogeneity of preparations. Most clinical trials investigated fermented mycelial products (e.g., Bailing, Jinshuibao, Zhiling) rather than the wild fungus, and variability in fungal strains, manufacturing processes, and dosing regimens was observed. This heterogeneity limits the extrapolation of findings to a single, well-defined herbal substance or preparation.

Systematic reviews of *O. sinensis* evaluated its adjunctive use in COPD, lung cancer, and renal dysfunction. Across COPD studies, adjunctive use was associated with improvements in lung function parameters (e.g., FEV_1), exercise tolerance, and quality-of-life scores. In lung cancer, meta-analyses reported improved tumor response rates, immune markers, and reduced treatment-related adverse reactions when *O. sinensis* was added to chemo- or radiotherapy. In renal dysfunction, consistent improvements in biochemical markers were observed.

Despite these positive signals, the evidence base shared several limitations:

- Trials were almost exclusively conducted in China;
- Most studies were small and short-term;
- Blinding and placebo control were largely absent;
- Outcomes were frequently surrogate or supportive rather than definitive clinical endpoints.

Accordingly, the certainty of evidence ranged from low to moderate, with significant downgrading for risk of bias and indirectness.

Many reviews used the name *O. sinensis* to describe commercial mycelial preparations that are taxonomically closer to *O. sinensis* or other related fungi. This taxonomic and pharmaceutical ambiguity represents a major obstacle for regulatory classification and evidence consolidation.

Overall, across nine systematic reviews, both *O. sinensis* preparations demonstrate biologically plausible and clinically consistent adjunctive benefits, particularly in renal disease and chronic pulmonary conditions. However, when assessed against the EMA criteria relevant to well-established herbal medicinal products, the current body of evidence does not meet the requirements for WEU, as outlined in Table 3.

This conclusion is driven not by lack of efficacy signals, but by:

- Insufficient methodological robustness;
- Absence of EU-based medicinal use documentation;
- Lack of a single, standardized herbal substance or preparation;
- Predominant reliance on surrogate outcomes.

https://doi.org/10.3390/ph19030519

From a scientific perspective, the evidence supports potential therapeutic value and justifies further high-quality clinical research. From an EMA regulatory perspective, the findings are more consistent with traditional herbal medicinal products rather than well-established use.

2.3.2.2. Clinical Evidence for Anti-Fatigue Effects of *O. sinensis* and *C. militaris*: Implications for EMA Well-Established Use

Early placebo-controlled clinical studies examined the effects of *O. sinensis* (cordymax™ Cs-4) therapy in elderly patients with fatigue and other aging-related symptoms [148–150]. Compared with placebo-treated patients who showed no improvement in symptoms, most *O. sinensis* (Cs-4)-treated patients reported overall clinical improvement [149]. The subjective improvements included promotion to endurance capacity [150] and alleviation of fatigue, cold intolerance, dizziness, frequent nocturia, tinnitus, hyposexuality, and amnesia [13,149].

The results of some studies of *O. sinensis* in a limited number of healthy subject athletes suggest that it can increase exercise performance [151,152], tolerance to high-intensity exercise [153], and alleviate muscle injury [154], maintain the hemoglobin and hematocrit levels [154], while the results of a few other placebo-controlled randomized studies were not reproducible and do not show health benefits [154,155].

Two review articles summarized the effects of *O. sinensis* on aerobic performance and fitness in human studies [144,145].

Supplementation with *O. sinensis* was expected to exhibit a potential physical performance-enhancing (ergogenic) effect by increasing time to exhaustion when administered regularly for 2 to 16 weeks before exercise, although its effects on improving aerobic fitness remain inconsistent [145]. Most studies involved active, young participants; however, the ergogenic potential of *O. sinensis* in aging and sedentary populations remains poorly understood, as few studies have examined it [145].

In summary, the potential benefits of *O. sinensis* supplementation are supposed to: (i) improve aerobic performance, (ii) enhance oxygen utilization, (iii) increase maximal oxygen consumption (VO_2max, a key indicator of aerobic fitness), and (iv) delay fatigue. However, the problems and challenges are: (i) some studies do not exhibit improvements, and the effects are inconsistent, (ii) the benefits may depend on the dosage used. Overall, while promising, more high-quality human studies are needed to fully understand its effects, especially across different populations such as older adults and sedentary individuals.

Welch et al., (2023) [144] reviewed 29 full texts of the 4308 potentially relevant articles selecting seven randomized trials of *O. sinensis* conducted with a total of 286 healthy human subjects [150,154–160] and applying PRISMA, the Cochrane risk-of-bias tool, the Jadad's quality scale, and the Checklist score of Items for Reporting Trials of Chinese Herbal Medicine Formulas from CONSORT extension for Chinese herbal medicine. Formulas were applied to the data with the purpose of critically assessing the current evidence for or against the effectiveness or efficacy of *O. sinensis*. Their evaluation highlights the need to conduct high-quality, low-bias clinical trials [144]. The authors conclude that supplementation with *O. sinensis* may affect aerobic performance and could have implications for various athletic events; however, insufficient reporting of the details of the *O. sinensis* preparation used was a common issue across the included studies. Of the included studies, five reported significant pre- and post-intergroup differences in the effect of *O. sinensis* supplementation on aerobic performance [144].

Importantly, between-group analysis showed no significant changes in VO_2max, work rate at the metabolic threshold, or work rate at the ventilatory threshold between the treatment and placebo groups [144].

In some studies, baseline (before treatment) primary outcome measures differ significantly between the placebo and *O. sinensis* groups [150], suggesting a lack of randomisation. A fatal methodological flaw in other studies was that between-group changes from baseline over time (before and after treatment) were not assessed to exclude the placebo effect. The products and their method of

https://doi.org/10.3390/ph19030519

preparation were insufficiently characterized to demonstrate reproducibility and consistency in the results of various clinical trials.

Table A8 summarizes results of meta-analysis of randomized placebo-controlled clinical trials of *O. sinensis* in athletes [152–154] and healthy adults [150,158,161,162], as well as in other human subjects with symptoms of long COVID [163], mild COVID-19 [164], asthma [165], exercise fatigue [152], and *C. militaris* in mild liver dysfunction [166], depression with insomnia [167] and fatigue [153,154,161,162].

Clinical trials of *O. sinensis* include traditional extracts and cultivated mycelial products. The majority of fatigue-related trials of *O. sinensis* investigated fermented mycelial preparations, most commonly Cs-4®. Randomized, double-blind, placebo-controlled trials in healthy older adults demonstrated improvements in exercise tolerance, VO_2max, ventilatory threshold, and perceived exertion, outcomes that are directly relevant to physical fatigue. Early Japanese double-blind trials demonstrated reductions in subjective fatigue scores and improved tolerance during graded exercise tests in healthy adults. Additional studies in athletes and physically active individuals reported improved exercise tolerance and oxygen-related biomarkers, although findings were inconsistent across studies. Null results were frequently observed in highly trained populations, suggesting a limited ergogenic ceiling effect and reinforcing the notion that fatigue-modulating effects may be most relevant in sub-optimally conditioned or aging individuals.

This section critically reviews fatigue-specific clinical trials of *O. sinensis* in healthy adults, older adults, and individuals with post-COVID-19 conditions. It assesses the strength of the evidence against the European Medicines Agency (EMA) criteria for well-established use (WEU). EMA WEU requirements include recognized efficacy, acceptable safety, consistent clinical evidence, a well-defined herbal preparation, and at least 10 years of medicinal use within the European Union. Species are analyzed separately due to regulatory and pharmacognostic relevance.

Appendix A Table A9 is focused exclusively on long COVID/post-COVID fatigue. As summarized in the table, direct clinical evidence for the use of *O. sinensis* in long COVID-related fatigue is currently limited but emerging. A recent randomized, waitlist-controlled trial in patients with long COVID demonstrated that Cs-4® significantly improved fatigue severity, functional capacity, and health-related quality of life compared with usual care [163]. This study represents the most direct clinical evidence for an anti-fatigue effect of *O. sinensis* in a post-viral population. However, the trial was limited by regional recruitment, short follow-up, and reliance on patient-reported outcomes. Evidence on COVID-19-related fatigue is emerging but remains limited. An industry-sponsored randomized study reported improvements in fatigue and recovery time during acute COVID-19 when *O. sinensis* capsules were used as add-on therapy. However, the lack of peer review and methodological transparency substantially reduces the evidentiary weight.

Fatigue-specific clinical trials of *O. sinensis* demonstrate biologically plausible and clinically observable benefits, particularly in aging and post-viral populations. However, when evaluated against EMA/HMPC standards, the evidence base remains insufficient for WEU designation, primarily due to methodological limitations and heterogeneity in preparation.

Overall, across healthy, aging, and post-infectious populations, *O. sinensis* demonstrates biologically plausible and clinically observable anti-fatigue effects, with the strongest signals seen in older adults and long COVID patients. However, under EMA/HMPC standards, the current evidence base is insufficient to support well-established use due to methodological limitations, evidence quality (most trials are small, short-term, and use heterogeneous or surrogate fatigue endpoints); GRADE certainty would be low to moderate: downgrading was primarily due to risk of bias (blinding, allocation concealment), inconsistency across populations, indirectness (exercise performance vs. validated fatigue scales), and imprecision (small sample sizes), preparation heterogeneity (fermented mycelium, different strains, combination products), preventing the definition of a single herbal preparation, and a lack of documented long-term EU medicinal use. From a scientific perspective, the evidence justifies further high-quality trials using validated fatigue endpoints. From a

https://doi.org/10.3390/ph19030519

regulatory perspective, the data align more closely with traditional use of herbal medicinal products than with well-established use (WEU) status, and emerging clinical signals warrant further confirmatory trials using validated fatigue instruments. Future studies should prioritize validated fatigue scales, longer follow-up, and standardized preparations to strengthen both scientific and regulatory credibility.

2.4. Systems-Level Mechanisms of O. sinensis, C. militaris, and Cordycepin: An Integrative Network Pharmacology and Experimental Evidence Review

Caterpillar Fungus and Orange Cordyceps are medicinal fungi traditionally valued for their restorative, endurance-enhancing, and homeostasis-supporting properties. These attributes align with the modern concept of adaptogenic activity, characterized by improved resistance to physical, chemical, and biological stressors [26,28,134].

Both fungi contain diverse bioactive metabolites, including nucleosides (adenosine, 3-deoxy-adenosine/cordycepin), sterols, peptides, and polysaccharides. The pharmacological breadth of *O. sinensis* suggests multi-target effects rather than classical single-receptor drug actions. Network pharmacology provides a systematic approach to deciphering these complex interactions, integrating predicted targets, signaling pathways, molecular docking, and multi-omics data.

Network pharmacology, combining computational target prediction, pathway enrichment, and systems biology, has become a significant framework for elucidating the complex multi-target actions of such herbal [168–173], including *O. sinensis, C. militaris*, and cordicepin and other fungi preparations [68,174,175]. Many network pharmacology studies of *O. sinensis* employ a so-called "reverse pharmacology" approach [176], based on plants described in ancient texts or on the empirical knowledge of traditional healers, and are focused on elucidating their mechanisms of action, which is typical of TCM. However, most reports remain scattered, disease-specific, or lacking integration with wet-lab validation. Despite numerous studies [57,60,103,140,144,174,175,177–208], no comprehensive synthesis has unified the mechanistic insights across species, compounds, and disease contexts. A unified synthesis is needed to understand the core pharmacological principles of *O. sinensis* and *C. militaris*.

This section provides the most comprehensive overview to date of network pharmacology analyses of *O. sinensis, C. militaris*, and cordycepin, integrating computational predictions and experimental evidence to derive a consolidated mechanistic model. This study integrates 37 network pharmacology investigations, including 22 experimental validation studies, along with Appendix A Tables A10 and A11 [177–206], to define the adaptogenic potential and systems-level pharmacology of Caterpillar Fungus, Orange Cordyceps, and cordycepin.

Across the studies, the workflow is similar: selection of active constituents of Cordyceps → predict molecular targets → build protein–protein interaction/pathway networks → dock key compounds to target proteins → sometimes validate in cells/animals. Importantly, these are hypothesis-generating in silico, so their strength depends on follow-up experiments (Appendix A Tables A10 and A11).

Across fungal species and study designs, highly consistent mechanistic hubs emerged: inflammatory cytokines (TNF, IL-6, IL-1β), stress-activated kinases (MAPK1/3/8), survival pathways (AKT1), mitochondrial regulators (FOXO3, HIF-1), apoptotic mediators (CASP3, BAX/BCL2), transcriptional co-regulators (CREBBP, EP300, FOXO3), and metabolic enzymes (IDH1, CYP19A1), Figure 3, Tables A12 and A13.

https://doi.org/10.3390/ph19030519

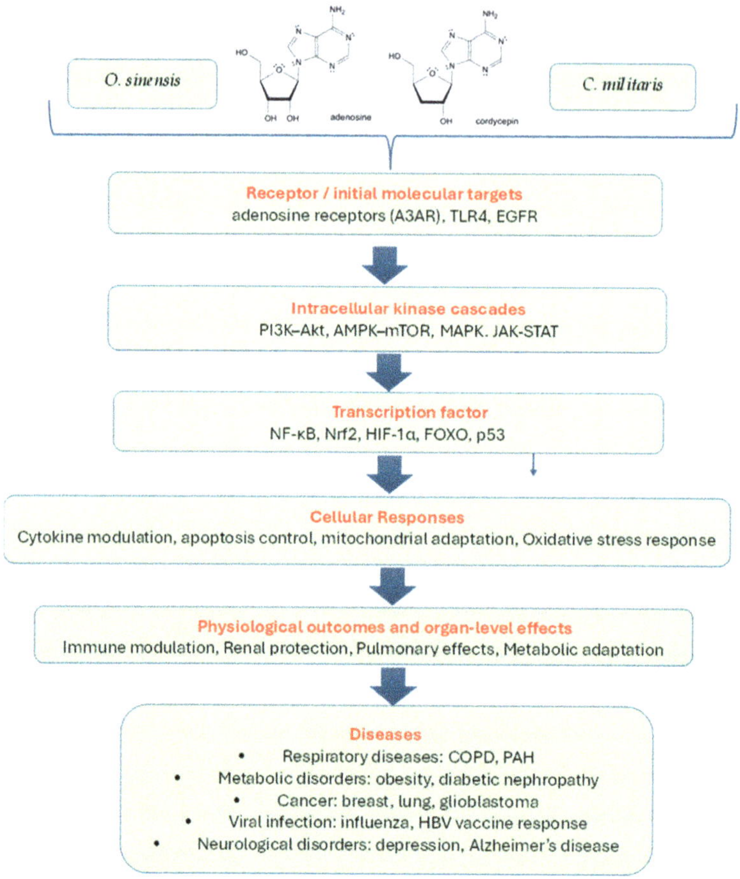

Figure 3. Hierarchical mechanistic integration of network-derived targets of *O. sinensis*, adenosine, *C. militaris*, and cordycepin-induced adaptive stress response, network signaling pathways, and biological functions, which are summarized in Appendix A Table A13, including primary function related to: (i) PI3K–AKT/FOXO–SIRT metabolic survival axis, (ii) AMPK–mTOR–autophagy axis, (iii) NRF2–KEAP1 antioxidant axis, (iv) TLR4–MyD88–NF-κB/MAPK inflammatory axis, (v) NLRP3 Inflammasome/Pyroptosis, and (vi) HIF-1 hypoxia response. *O. sinensis*, adenosine, *C. militaris*, and cordycepin act as multi-target modulators converging on integrated adaptive stress-response signaling, immunometabolic, and mitochondrial pathways.

The most frequently enriched recurrent pathways included PI3K–Akt, MAPK, NF-κB, apoptosis, oxidative-stress regulation, and AMPK–SIRT1–PGC-1α, the latter closely linked to metabolic and mitochondrial adaptation, Appendix A Table A12. This convergence indicates that *O. sinensis* and *C. militaris* metabolites act not through a single canonical receptor but through a broad network modulation that affects immunity, metabolism, mitochondrial function, and cell-survival signaling—consistent with the systems-level pharmacology expected of adaptogenic botanicals.

Experimental evidence validated predicted mechanisms in obesity, COPD, pulmonary hypertension, cancer, influenza, and vaccine immunogenicity (Appendix A Table A10), Figure 3.

Experimental validation studies evidence confirmed network predictions in:

- Immune modulation via TLR4/TNF-α [182];
- Cancer apoptosis via PI3K–Akt and caspase regulation [187];
- Apoptotic pathway activation in cancer [178,187];
- Cytokine normalization and lung restoration in COPD [174];

https://doi.org/10.3390/ph19030519

- PAH through apoptosis and vascular remodeling repair [191];
- Obesity/metabolic syndrome via AKT1/MAPK14/GSK3B [192];
- HBV vaccine response enhancement [177].

The integrative analysis of network pharmacology data combined with experimentally validated studies demonstrates that *O. sinensis*, *C. militaris*, and cordycepin share a convergent mechanistic architecture centered on immune modulation, stress-kinase regulation, metabolic adaptation, mitochondrial support, and apoptosis control. The repeated identification and validation of PI3K–Akt, MAPK, NF-κB, and AMPK–SIRT1–PGC-1α pathways indicate that *O. sinensis*, *C. militaris*, and cordycepin are systems-level adaptogenic agents capable of normalizing physiological functions across multiple organ systems. These findings support the therapeutic potential of standardized preparations and justify further translational research, particularly in immunometabolic and chronic inflammatory diseases.

Table 4 presents the key findings of network pharmacology studies and the characteristic differences between *O. sinensis* [139,197,198,208] and *C. militaris* preparations [182,183,185,206] (Appendix A Tables A10 and A11).

The implications and predictions for health claims inferred from the network pharmacology studies, Table 4, can be summarized as follows:

- *O. sinensis* exhibits broad-spectrum organ support and multi-pathway modulation, especially in chronic diseases and viral infections. The most defensible, network-anchored claims are around kidney support/adjunct in chronic kidney disease, inflammation/oxidative stress, and respiratory immune modulation—with some clinical meta-analytic support but still needing higher-quality trials [136,139].
- *C. militaris* shows targeted cytotoxicity and immune activation, making it more suitable for oncology and immunotherapy applications. *C. militaris* preparations, explicitly characterized by high content of cordycepin, have the strongest network-mechanistic case for anticancer mechanisms, immune modulation (TLR4–TNF, macrophage polarization), and metabolic/urate axes. The evidence is growing, but disease-specific clinical endpoints remain limited [182,183,185].

Pathways are stratified according to an evidence-tier framework:

- Tier 1 (Prediction Only): Identified through in silico network modeling and enrichment analysis without biological confirmation.
- Tier 2 (Experimental Validation): Supported by in vitro or in vivo mechanistic studies.
- Tier 3 (Clinical Alignment): Mechanistic pathways supported by human clinical biomarker modulation or RCT endpoints.

https://doi.org/10.3390/ph19030519

Table 4. Characteristic differences in in silico prediction-only (Tier 1) * and experimentally validated (Tier 2) network pharmacology studies and clinical alignment (Tier 3) of *O. sinensis*, *C. militaris* preparations, and cordycepin.

Feature	*O. sinensis*	*C. militaris*	Cordycepin
Main bioactive constituents	Adenosine/2′-deoxyadenosine, ergosterol, adenosine, glutamine, diverse peptides	Cordycepin (3′-deoxyadenosine), adenosine, polysaccharides, ergosterol	Cordycepin
Dominant validated indications (Tier 2)	COPD, lung cancer, CKD, ischemic stroke, diabetic nephropathy, UV injury, vaccine adjuvant (Tier 3)	Immune modulation, lung cancer, COPD, gouty nephropathy, SARS-CoV-2	Cancer, obesity, depression, PAH, immunosuppression, glioblastoma
Main predicted indications (Tier 1)	Liver cancer, DN, hypoxia, depression, PCOS, influenza	COVID-19 inflammation	Cancer, Alzheimer's, kinase inhibition
Signature pathways (Tier 2)	PI3K-Akt, TNF, AGE-RAGE, IL-17, chemokine, apoptosis, lipid metabolism	TLR, inflammatory lipid pathways, apoptosis, oxidative stress, metabolic regulation	Apoptosis, AMPK-mTOR, PI3K-Akt, Nrf2, Wnt/β-catenin, metabolic reprogramming
Predicted pathways (Tier 1)	AGE-RAGE, VEGF, PI3K-Akt, FOXO, neurotrophic, inflammatory	A3AR, JNK, AMPK, AKT, MAPKs, FOXO3	Apoptosis, neurodegeneration, and kinase inhibition
Core hubs repeatedly validated (Tier 2)	AKT1, CASP3, PTGS2, HIF1A, NFKB1, VEGFA, PTEN, STING, CXCR4,	TLR4, TNF, EGFR, IDH1, PTGS2, ABCG2, p53	AKT1, CASP3, EGFR, Nrf2, GSK3β, β-catenin, FOXO, MAPKs
Core predicted hubs (Tier 1)	TNF, MAPK1, EGFR, IL6, VEGFA, ACE, CASP3	NR3C1, thrombin, inflammatory kinases	A3AR, JNK, AMPK, AKT, MAPKs, FOXO3
Key validated differences (Tier 2)	immune-pulmonary-renal axis, lipid/steroid mediation, inflammatory microenvironment remodeling (Tier 3)	immune activation, metabolic enzymes, antiviral/anticancer lipid-nucleoside networks	intracellular stress signaling, kinase control, apoptosis, metabolic rewiring

(*)—Tier 1 studies expand hypothesis space but lack biological confirmation, Appendix A Table A11.

This structured presentation reduces target inflation bias and visually distinguishes hypothesis-generating predictions from experimentally or clinically supported mechanisms.

Convergent evidence from network pharmacology, experimental studies, and multi-omics analyses demonstrates that *O. sinensis*, *C. militaris*, and cordycepin share a unified mechanistic architecture centered on immune modulation, stress-kinase regulation, mitochondrial adaptation, and metabolic homeostasis. This integrated systems pharmacology supports their classification as adaptogenic natural products with relevance to chronic inflammatory, metabolic, and immunological diseases. Future work prioritizing standardized preparations and mechanistically powered clinical studies will be essential for therapeutic translation.

Table A14 presents an evidence-tier framework that distinguishes Tier 1 (in silico prediction), Tier 2 (experimental validation), and Tier 3 (clinical alignment). Figure 4 and Table 4 reflect validation levels and reduce potential target inflation bias.

Figure 4 presents frequency heatmaps summarizing the recurrence of predicted and validated targets and enriched pathways across 37 independent network pharmacology studies involving *O. sinensis*, *C. militaris*, and cordycepin. Heatmaps were generated using AI to visualize the frequency of reported targets and enriched pathways across 37 network pharmacology studies. For each entity (*O. sinensis*, *C. militaris*, cordycepin), the number of independent publications reporting a given target or pathway was counted. Color intensity represents recurrence frequency, with warmer colors indicating higher convergence across studies.

Table 5 shows the effects of cordycepin on adaptive stress–response signaling pathways and physiological roles [36,209–217]. Appendix A Table A13 presents the major adaptive stress response pathways modulated by cordycepin, highlighting key genes, their biological roles, and the primary supporting studies.

https://doi.org/10.3390/ph19030519

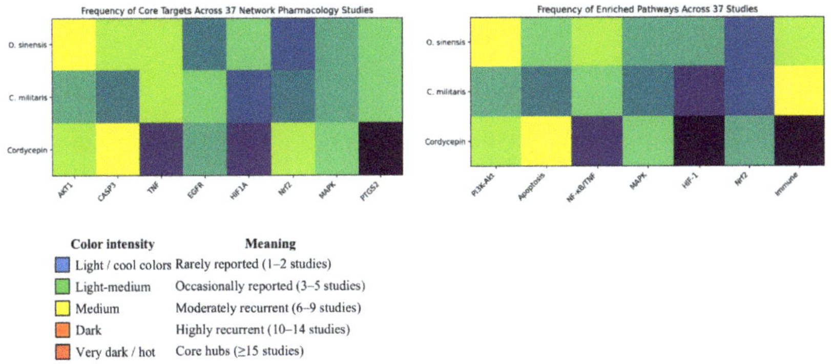

Figure 4. The heatmaps are frequency heatmaps, not expression heatmaps. They visualize how often a given target or pathway appears across your 37 network pharmacology studies, separated by: *O. sinensis*, *C. militaris*, and cordycepin. Each cell indicates the number of independent publications reporting a given target or pathway. Highly frequent targets and pathways may reflect research prevalence and database structure rather than relative biological importance. Color intensity reflects convergence level: (i) warmer/darker colors = higher recurrence across studies (high-confidence hubs), (ii) cooler/lighter colors = lower recurrence (hypothesis-generating pathways). Functional modules are grouped into: (i) Immunoinflammatory signaling (e.g., NF-κB, TNF, TLR pathways), (ii) metabolic and mitochondrial regulation (e.g., AMPK–mTOR, SIRT1–PGC-1α), (iii) apoptosis and cell-survival signaling (e.g., PI3K–Akt, CASP3), (iv) oxidative stress response (e.g., Nrf2–KEAP1 axis).

Caterpillar Fungus, Orange Cordyceps, and 3-deoxyadenosine exhibit a unified adaptogenic pharmacology that involves immune modulation, mitochondrial enhancement, stress-signal regulation, and metabolic homeostasis. These effects arise through multi-target synergy across PI3K–Akt, MAPK, NF-κB, apoptosis, and AMPK–SIRT1–PGC-1α pathways. The strong convergence of network and experimental evidence supports their potential in immunometabolic and stress-related disorders.

Our findings align with a recent review providing evidence-based rationale for Chinese traditional medicinal mushrooms, which demonstrate multi-target anti-inflammatory activity by modulating key cellular mediators (macrophages, regulatory T cells, natural killer cells) and signaling pathways (NF-κB, MAPK, NLRP3 inflammasome, Nrf2/HO-1) of mushrooms for chronic inflammation management [68].

Table 5. Adaptive stress–response signaling pathways and physiological role modulated by cordycepin.

Pathway/Module	Key Genes/Molecules	Physiological Roles	Representative Publications
AMPK–mTOR–Autophagy Axis	PRKAA1/2 (AMPKα), RPTOR, RICTOR, MTOR, ULK1, BECN1, LC3B, ATG5/7, SQSTM1	Cellular energy sensor; promotes autophagy, ATP conservation, and repair during stress.	Hawley et al., 2020 [36] Marcelo et al., 2019 [209] Li et al., 2017 [210].
NRF2–KEAP1 Antioxidant Axis	NFE2L2 (NRF2), KEAP1, HMOX1, NQO1, GCLC, GCLM, SOD2, CAT, GPX1	Regulates antioxidant enzymes, detoxification, redox homeostasis, and cytoprotection.	Wang Z et al., 2019 [211]
TLR4–MyD88–NF-κB/MAPK Inflammatory Axis	TLR4, MYD88, NFKB1, RELA, IKBKB, MAPK14, MAPK8, MAPK1/3, TNF, IL6, PTGS2, NOS2	Controls innate immune activation; cordycepin suppresses pro-inflammatory cytokines and iNOS/COX-2 expression.	Choi YH et al., 2014 [212] Yang J et al., 2017 [213] Sun Y et al., 2020 [214]
NLRP3 Inflammasome/Pyroptosis Regulation	NLRP3, CASP1, GSDMD, IL1B, IL18	Limits pyroptotic cell death and IL-1β release; anti-inflammatory and neuroprotective effects.	Liu Z et al., 2025 [215] Zhang X et al., 2021 [216]
PI3K–AKT/FOXO–SIRT Pathway	PIK3CA/B, AKT1, FOXO3, SIRT1, TP53	Balances survival vs. repair; mediates stress resistance, longevity, and metabolic adaptation.	Li T et al., 2019 [217]

Table 6 summarizes key genes involved in cordycepin-induced adaptive stress–response signaling pathways and their physiological roles [33–38].

https://doi.org/10.3390/ph19030519

Table 6. Key genes involved in cordycepin-induced adaptive stress–response signaling pathways and their physiological roles.

Signaling Pathway	Key Genes Involved	Physiological Role
AMPK pathway	AMPK, SIRT1, MTOR	Energy sensing, lifespan extension
Sirtuin signaling	SIRT1, FOXO3, PARP1	Regulates stress response, aging,
mTOR signaling	MTOR, AMPK, SIRT1, TP53	Nutrient sensing, autophagy, and protein synthesis
DNA damage response	TP53, PARP1	Genomic stability, cancer prevention

2.5. Food and Drug Regulation of *O. sinensis* and *C. militaris* in Western and Oriental Worlds

Wild *O. sinensis* has medicinal rather than culinary use in TCM, traditionally as a tonic, and is not classified as an edible mushroom in food codes. Cultured mycelium of *O. sinensis* can be food-grade or supplement-grade, depending on the strain and national registration (Appendix A Table A15). *C. militaris*, by contrast, is generally recognized as edible and is widely cultivated as a functional food mushroom. Table 7 summarizes the regulatory/edible/novel-food status of *O. sinensis* vs. *C. militaris* across major regions, with key references to support claims. Data derived from peer-reviewed studies [16,218], official food and drug regulatory websites, and Rapid Alert System for Food and Feed (RASFF) notifications [219–228].

Table 7. Regulatory classification of "Cordyceps" mushroom in the EU, USA, China, Japan, and the Republic of Korea.

Region	*O. sinensis* *	*C. militaris*	Notes
China	Traditionally medicinal, wild OS is not a general everyday food. Listed in the Chinese *Pharmacopeia* as a traditional medicinal material (TCM drug), not a general food. *Ophiocordyceps sinensis* mycelium and fermented products (some strains) may appear as approved food ingredients if separately registered.	Approved as a "new resource food" (novel food ingredient) since 2009; widely used in foods/health foods in China.	Used in decoctions, capsules, and medicinal soups. Only specific strains of cultivated mycelium (e.g., Cs-HK1) are allowed as food supplements. Contemporary reviews of the Chinese regulatory framework note *C. militaris* approval as novel/new resource food (2009) [218].
Japan/Republic of Korea	Classified as a traditional medicinal material, used in Kampo or functional foods under regulatory oversight.	In Asian countries, the cultural and historical use supports a more permissive edible status for *C. militaris*	In Asian countries, the cultural and historical use supports a more permissive edible status for *C. militaris*
USA	Marketed mainly as dietary supplements (mycelium/extracts). No GRAS (Generally Recognized As Safe) listing for wild *O. sinensis*; marketed forms are dietary supplements under DSHEA, typically using cultivated mycelium (e.g., *O. sinensis* Cs-4).	Marketed as dietary supplements, enforcement actions are taken when drug-like claims are made.	The U.S. classifies many mushroom extracts as dietary supplements. If a product claims to treat a disease, the FDA may treat it as a drug. U.S. Food and Drug Administration. FDA warning letters show Cordyceps products can be challenged if marketed with disease claims. There is no public GRAS for wild OS itself.
EU	Considered a novel food if intended as a food ingredient, wild *O. sinensis* itself is not authorized under general edible mushroom lists. Not novel in food supplements (entry in the EU Novel Food status catalog).	"Not yet authorized–novel food."	Authorization required under the Novel Foods Regulation. The European Commission's Novel Food portal lists *C. militaris* (mycelium and fruiting body) as not yet authorized; multiple RASFF alerts flag unauthorized use of *C. militaris* in supplements. *O. sinensis* is shown as "not novel in food supplements."
Sweden	Follows EU Novel Food rules.	Follows EU Novel Food rules.	In the EU, Novel Food law is harmonized; Sweden applies the EU stance. Check the EC catalog and consult the Swedish National Food Agency if you need product-specific confirmation.

* Safety considerations: (i) Natural wild *O. synensis* may accumulate arsenic and heavy metals from high-altitude soils; limits have been noted in Chinese safety advisories, (ii) cultured mycelium (fermentation products) avoids this risk and is the basis of most approved "Cordyceps" food supplements (e.g., Cs-4 strain), (iii) no known severe allergic risks at standard doses, but data remain limited.

In China, *C. militaris* has a new resource-food status (since 2009) [218], so it is widely used in domestic foods/health foods. In the Republic of Korea and Japan, *C. militaris* is regarded as edible/medicinal under functional food or Kampo frameworks, whereas *O. sinensis* is used as a medicinal fungus rather than a culinary mushroom. In the USA, both are typically sold as dietary supplements, avoiding disease claims to stay out of the "new drug" category. Overall, in the EU, *O. sinensis* (mycelium and fruiting body) is used as a food supplement without a novel food authorisation (other

https://doi.org/10.3390/ph19030519

food uses may still be novel). *C. militaris* (mycelium and fruiting body) is novel and not yet authorized; placing supplements with *C. militaris* on the EU market requires a successful novel food authorisation or an exemption that does not currently exist and can be expected at the Rapid Alert System for Food and Feed (RASFF) alerts portal, see Appendix A [225–228], Table A15. The Appendix A Tables A16–A20 show characteristic features of *O. sinensis* and *C. militaris* across key pharmacopeias and regulatory frameworks, including health claims and medicinal uses.

2.6. Resilience Biology, Inflammation, and Adaptogens: An Umbrella Review of Biological Evidence and Regulatory Frameworks Across Europe, the United States, and Asia

Stress responses and inflammation are evolutionarily conserved adaptive processes essential for survival and recovery, restoring homeostasis following injury or challenge [229–236], as shown in Appendix A Table A21. While inflammation is firmly established as a pathological and regulatory target in Western medicine [237,238], stress adaptation and resilience biology remain poorly integrated into regulatory frameworks, particularly within the European Union [239–241]. Adaptogens are proposed to enhance adaptive capacity and nonspecific recovery in various diseases and disorders [26,28,134,242]. Despite accumulating biological evidence, adaptogens lack regulatory recognition in the EU [241], while receiving broader acceptance in the United States [237,243], and Asia [244].

This umbrella review section synthesizes evidence from systematic reviews, narrative reviews, and regulatory documents to compare (i) biological definitions of inflammation, stress, and adaptive stress responses; (ii) their physiological roles and resolution mechanisms; and (iii) regulatory acceptance of adaptogenic botanicals across the European Union (EU), United States (US), and selected Asian jurisdictions. A structured umbrella review approach was applied to peer-reviewed reviews (2000–2024) addressing inflammation, stress physiology, adaptogens, and regulatory science. Regulatory guidance from EFSA, EMA, FDA, and Asian authorities was examined. Findings were narratively synthesized.

Stress and inflammation share common adaptive purposes and resolution dynamics (Table 8). Both stress and inflammation are beneficial in acute settings and harmful in chronic settings (Appendix A Table A20). Chronic stress drives chronic inflammation, and chronic inflammation feeds back into stress circuits.

Table 8. Similarities and differences between inflammation and stress responses.

Aspect	Inflammation	Stress Response
Purpose	Restore homeostasis	Restore homeostasis
Nature	Protective, adaptive	Protective, adaptive
Mediators	Cytokines, eicosanoids	Hormones, neurotransmitters
Resolution	Actively regulated	Actively regulated
Pathology arises when	Chronic, unresolved	Chronic, dysregulated
Localization	Primarily local	Systemic
Primary system	Immune system	Neuroendocrine system
Measurability	Clear biomarkers (CRP, IL-6)	Context-dependent biomarkers (cortisol variability)
Disease framing	Recognized pathological entity	Often framed as a risk factor
Consequences of failed resolution	Chronic inflammation: Cardiovascular disease Autoimmune disorders Neurodegeneration Cancer progression	Chronic stress/inflammaging: Depression and anxiety Metabolic syndrome Immune suppression or hyperactivation Accelerated aging

Unfortunately, terms such as stress, fatigue, and adaptation have not been formally recognized as a regulatable pathological entity in the EU. The reason lies in the basic concepts of health and fatigue in Western and Oriental medical paradigms, as reflected in the food and drug regulatory authorities in Europe, the USA, China, India, and Japan. Key conflict: traditional systems intervene upstream of disease, whereas EU drug regulators say "no disease exists yet" (Tables 9 and 10).

https://doi.org/10.3390/ph19030519

Table 9. Regulatory acceptance of adaptogens: EU vs. US vs. Asia.

Dimension	European Union	United States	Asia (China, Japan, the Republic of Korea, India)
Adaptogen term	Not recognized	Informally tolerated	Explicitly recognized
Regulatory model	Disease- & nutrient-centric	Risk-based consumer access	Systems & functional medicine
Acceptable claim style	Narrow, mechanistic	Structure–function	Functional, pattern-based
Stress-related claims	Rejected	Allowed with disclaimer	Allowed
Traditional use	Secondary	Optional	Central

Why is the "anti-inflammatory" effect a recognized regulatory term, but "antistress", "anti-fatigue", and "stress-protective" are not recognized in Europe? Regulatory reasoning is that: inflammation is a defined pathological process, established clinical biomarkers exist, precise pharmacological mechanisms are known, and historical drug precedents exist (NSAIDs, corticosteroids). Consequently, the European Medicines Agency accepts anti-inflammatory mechanism-based claims and botanical medicines with demonstrated effects on inflammatory mediators.

Meanwhile, the terms "antistress", "anti-fatigue", and "stress-protective" are not accepted by EMA because of regulatory concerns, including: (i) "Stress" is considered a normal life experience, not a disease, (ii) claims imply psychological or psychiatric effects, and (iii) risk of unsubstantiated or exaggerated health claims. Scientific challenges include: (i) stress is considered contextual and subjective, (ii) no single, validated disease definition, and (iii) biomarkers are indirect, variable, and situation-dependent. Thus, authorities avoid approving terms that: (i) lack precise physiological targets, (ii) cannot be consistently quantified, and (iii) blur boundaries between food, supplements, and medicines.

A core regulatory paradox is that vitamins and antioxidants are recognized, but adaptogens are not. The reason is that EU Regulation favors selected target, single-pathway, disease-linked, measurable mechanisms, while adaptogenic effects are systems-level and contextual. While adaptogens aim to normalize stress responses rather than inhibit a specific pathological pathway, this does not fit the reductionist regulatory model.

EU drug authorities consider stress as an adaptive life process, but not a disease target, and adaptogens as a regulatory misfit, but not a scientific invalidity. Adaptogens fail not scientifically, but structurally. EU drugs regulators lack a legal category for resilience enhancers. Adaptogens challenge regulatory frameworks because they support resilience rather than treat disease.

In 2007, EMEA's "Reflection paper on the adaptogens concept" clarified that the term "adaptogen" is applied to different herbal medicinal products (including preparations derived from Eleutherococcus, Ginseng, and Rhodiola) that have the capacity to normalize bodily functions and strengthen systems compromised by stress [241]. They are reported to have a protective effect on health against a wide variety of environmental assaults and emotional conditions [241]. EMA approved EU Community Monographs for Rhodiola, Eleutherococcus, and Ginseng as traditional herbal medicinal products for the relief of stress-related symptoms, such as fatigue and exhaustion [245]. EMEA "Reflection paper on the adaptogens concept" concluded "*The concept of adaptogens is sufficient to be considered in the assessment of traditional herbal medicinal products (e.g., monograph on Eleutherococcus root). As the term "adaptogen" is considered not appropriate for a marketing authorisation, more clinical studies, and data on the efficacy in a well-defined clinical condition would be necessary*" [241]. When the second sentence is taken out of context from the EMA conclusion, e.g., on Wikipedia, it creates a misleading impression of the scientific validity of the adaptogenic concept. Over the last two decades, our understanding of the mechanisms of action and clinical conditions of adaptogens has been substantially enriched through network pharmacology and molecular biology studies [26,28,134,171,173,246,247], whereas the clinical evidence of their efficacy remains insufficient due to various methodological shortcomings and limited characterization of study products [241].

Adaptogens are rejected in the EU not because they lack biological validity, but because European regulation has no legal concept of resilience. In contrast, Asia is built on it, and the US pragmatically tolerates it (Table 10).

Table 10. Western regulatory vs. traditional medical paradigms: core worldview difference.

Dimension	Western Regulatory Paradigm (EFSA/EMA)	Traditional Medical Paradigms (TCM, Ayurveda, etc.)
Primary goal	Treat or prevent a defined disease	Restore balance and resilience
Model	Reductionist, mechanistic	Systems-based, integrative
Body concept	Sum of organs and pathways	Dynamic, interconnected whole
Health	Absence of pathology	Capacity to adapt and recover
Evidence	Isolated endpoints, biomarkers	Pattern recognition, outcomes over time
Disease vs. dysfunction	Requires: A defined pathological condition Clear causal pathway Measurable, reproducible endpoints Works well for: Inflammation Deficiency diseases Infections	Focuses on: Functional imbalance before disease Fatigue, low vitality, stress intolerance Recovery capacity
Evidence hierarchy mismatch	Standardized extracts Dose–response relationships Single or narrow endpoints	Multi-target effects Long-term use Context-dependent outcomes Synergistic formulations

Adaptogens demonstrate modulatory effects on immune, inflammatory, neuroendocrine, and metabolic pathways consistent with resilience biology [26,28,134,242,246] yet lack a regulatory category in Europe. The US adopts a permissive structure–function approach, while Asian systems explicitly integrate adaptogens within traditional and functional medicine paradigms.

This review clarifies conceptual and regulatory barriers to recognizing resilience-supporting interventions and informs future regulatory innovation. Adaptogens are not rejected due to insufficient biology, but because current regulatory frameworks lack concepts for resilience and adaptive capacity. Establishing a regulatory category for resilience-supporting physiological modulators could align regulation with contemporary systems biology.

3. Discussion

3.1. An Integrative Network Pharmacology and Systems-Level Mechanisms of Ophiocordyceps sinensis, Cordyceps militaris, and Cordycepin

The quantitative synthesis of 37 network pharmacology studies reveals a highly convergent and biologically coherent systems-level pharmacological architecture underlying the activities of *O. sinensis*, *C. militaris*, and cordycepin. Rather than supporting isolated, disease-specific mechanisms, aggregated networks consistently converge on a limited set of high-centrality molecular hubs and signaling modules that govern cellular stress adaptation, immunometabolic homeostasis, inflammatory tone, and survival–death decisions.

3.1.1. Convergence on a Conserved Stress-Adaptive Signaling Core

Across species and preparations, the most frequently identified hubs—including AKT1, CASP3, TNF/NF-κB, MAPKs, HIF-1α, and Nrf2—define a conserved stress-adaptation core network. These nodes integrate metabolic sensing (PI3K–Akt, AMPK–mTOR), redox regulation (Nrf2), inflammatory control (TNF/NF-κB, TLR signaling), and apoptotic regulation (caspase cascades), Appendix A Table A20. The repeated emergence of this hub constellation across heterogeneous disease

https://doi.org/10.3390/ph19030519

models indicates that *O. sinensis* and *C. militaris*-derived products function as coordinated regulators of cellular resilience systems rather than as single-target agents.

This convergence provides a mechanistic foundation for the traditional classification of Cordyceps mushroom as tonic or adaptogenic medicines and is consistent with contemporary network-medicine models, in which therapeutic benefit arises from distributed modulation of interacting stress-response circuits rather than maximal perturbation of isolated molecular targets.

3.1.2. Species-Level Pharmacology Reflects Network Breadth, Not Redundancy

Although *O. sinensis* and *C. militaris* share substantial overlaps in their predicted and validated networks, their frequency profiles reveal distinct pharmacological emphases. *O. sinensis* shows preferential enrichment in immune–pulmonary–renal metabolic networks, with frequent involvement of HIF-1, AGE–RAGE, VEGF, chemokine, and inflammatory lipid pathways. This pattern suggests dominant engagement of hypoxia adaptation, vascular regulation, tissue microenvironment remodeling, and chronic inflammatory control, aligning closely with its traditional and contemporary investigation in respiratory, renal, ischemic, and fatigue-associated disorders.

In contrast, *C. militaris* demonstrates stronger relative representation of immune receptor signaling, oxidative-stress pathways, and metabolic enzymes, consistent with a mechanistic orientation toward immune modulation, antiviral and anticancer responses, and metabolic regulation. The prominence of TLR-associated and lipid-inflammatory pathways supports its emerging positioning as an immune-functional and anticancer medicinal fungus.

Thus, while the two species occupy overlapping regions of pharmacological network space, they exhibit distinct systems-level biases rather than functional redundancy.

3.1.3. Cordycepin Acts as a Dominant Molecular Effector Within Broader Fungal Networks

Cordycepin-centered networks display a distinct topological signature, characterized by high-centrality intracellular signaling hubs that control apoptosis, kinase cascades, and metabolic checkpoints. Compared with whole-fungus preparations, cordycepin exhibits a disproportionately strong action of caspase signaling, AMPK–mTOR, PI3K–Akt, Wnt/β-catenin, and Nrf2 pathways, indicating a more targeted regulation of intracellular stress integration, metabolic reprogramming, and survival–death switching.

These patterns support a model in which cordycepin acts as a dominant molecular effector that drives a subset of *C. militaris* pharmacology. However, the broader immunological, vascular, and lipid–steroid signaling observed for whole-fungus preparations likely reflects synergistic contributions from additional nucleosides, polysaccharides, sterols, peptides, and secondary metabolites. Consequently, cordycepin recapitulates but does not fully reproduce the systems-level pharmacology of *C. militaris*.

3.1.4. Validated Versus Predicted Networks Define Evidence Tiers

Stratification of validated and prediction-only studies demonstrates that the most frequently recurring hubs and pathways—PI3K–Akt, NF-κB/TNF, apoptosis, MAPKs, HIF-1, Nrf2, and immune signaling—are robust to evidence filtering and consistently supported by experimental data. In contrast, lower-frequency pathways are concentrated in prediction-only studies, representing hypothesis-generating extensions rather than confirmed pharmacological cores.

This separation establishes an evidence-tier framework that may guide translational prioritization: validated networks provide mechanistic foundations suitable for biomarker development and clinical positioning, whereas prediction-only networks identify directions for targeted experimental expansion.

3.1.5. Implications for Natural-Product Systems Pharmacology

Collectively, these findings position Caterpillar Fungus, Orange Cordyceps-derived products as archetypal systems-level natural therapeutics whose biological activities arise from coordinated

https://doi.org/10.3390/ph19030519

regulation of adaptive stress-response networks. The consistent involvement of immunometabolic, redox, hypoxia, and apoptosis modules underscores their potential relevance not only for disease intervention but also for functional resilience, recovery support, and maintenance of physiological function during aging.

Moreover, the alignment between traditional tonic indications and modern network-level convergence highlights network pharmacology as a translational bridge between ethnopharmacology and molecular systems medicine, enabling rational development, standardization, and positioning of medicinal fungi.

The integrative analysis of network pharmacology data, combined with experimentally validated studies, demonstrates that Caterpillar Fungus, Orange Cordyceps, and cordycepin share a convergent mechanistic architecture centered on immune modulation, stress-kinase regulation, metabolic adaptation, mitochondrial support, and apoptosis control. The repeated identification and validation of PI3K–Akt, MAPK, NF-κB, and AMPK–SIRT1–PGC-1α pathways indicate that Orange Cordyceps acts as a systems-level adaptogenic agent, capable of normalizing physiological functions across multiple organ systems. These findings support the therapeutic potential of standardized preparations of Caterpillar Fungus and Orange Cordyceps and justify further translational research, particularly in immunometabolic and chronic inflammatory diseases.

The striking convergence across species, compounds, and diseases indicates that Caterpillar Fungus, Orange Cordyceps, and cordicepin operate as network-level adaptogens. Their actions modulate: immune homeostasis, mitochondrial resilience, redox balance, stress-kinase signaling, and metabolic efficiency. These domains correspond to the core characteristics of adaptogenic botanicals.

Although 3-deoxyadenosine undergoes rapid metabolism and has low plasma concentrations, these levels are compatible with hormetic activation of AMPK, SIRT1, and FOXO pathways—mechanisms central to metabolic and mitochondrial adaptation.

Alignment of network predictions with experimental data across diverse disease models strongly supports the robustness of the mechanistic model.

3.1.6. Limitations

Limitations of these studies include heterogeneity of extracts, target inflation bias, uneven experimental validation, and overrepresentation of cancer/inflammation models. Variability in fungal strains, extraction methods, and analytical techniques remains a challenge. More standardized preparations and human mechanistic trials are required.

As a matter of fact, all the network pharmacology studies of *O. sinensis* were conducted on a limited number of one (cordicepin) to 13 bioactive constituents/compounds (Tables A10 and A11) in the total of 84 compounds identified in *O. sinensis*, Figures A1–A5, and Table A3. Many other bioactive fungi secondary metabolites (Tables A3–A6), specifically alkaloids, flavonoids, sterols, cyclodipeptides, and other bioactive *O. sinensis* secondary metabolites, were not included in the network analysis. That is an essential omission that may affect the outcomes of these studies, and the overall evidence supporting health claims, and medical use in drug authorities' assessments. Most network pharmacology studies analyze only a subset of fungal metabolites because compound selection is typically based on overlap between known molecular targets and disease-associated targets. Consequently, many primary and secondary metabolites listed in Section 2.1 remain outside current network analyses because their targets are unknown. The proposed core network in these studies reflects the subset of metabolites currently under study rather than responses to the full chemical diversity of *O. sinensis* and *C. militaris*. The lack of knowledge can be overcome in future studies using various molecular biology methodologies, including transcriptome-wide microarray profiling of gene expression experiments on extracts containing all extractive constituents of *O. sinensis* or *C. militaris*, in a non-targeted study design discussed in Section 3.1.7.

https://doi.org/10.3390/ph19030519

3.1.7. Future Perspectives

Network pharmacology is a relatively new, biology-based interdisciplinary field that combines principles of pharmacology and systems biology to study the complex interactions between drugs, their targets (e.g., receptors or enzymes), pathological processes, and diseases within integrated, holistic systems, exploring the polypharmacology and toxicology of drugs by utilizing the computational tools and network analysis algorithms.

Depending on the aims, the design and methodology of NP studies can be specific disease-targeted or non-targeted studies, where

- Disease-targeted bioinformatic-based network analysis reveals the molecular mechanisms of action, common molecular targets of active compounds, and stimulus-response coupling signaling pathways [57,60,103,140,144,174,175,177–208]. Such study design and methodology do not account for synergistic and antagonistic interactions in networks induced by various constituents of the complex, multi-component extracts, which can lead to unexpected outcomes, e.g., [246,247].
- Non-targeted transcriptome-wide microarray profiling of gene expression-based experiments following integrated metabolomics and network analysis, revealing all molecular targets of active compounds and their response, coupling signaling pathways. The results of these studies can predict unknown physiological functions, health consequences, and therapeutic indications due to synergistic and antagonistic interactions [171,173,246,247].
- Currently, all conducted network pharmacology studies on Caterpillar Fungus, Orange Cordyceps, and cordicepin are limited to disease-targeted investigations of Chinese TCM prescriptions for the treatment of kidney diseases and related disorders. Non-targeted transcriptome-wide microarray profiling of gene expression-based experiments can lead to the discovery of new therapeutic indications and functional claims.

All published network pharmacology studies of *O. sinensis* have a targeted design focused on a specific disease. The search for unknown therapeutic uses can be pursued by exploring alternative study designs based on gene expression, and by using transcriptomics, proteomics, and metabolomics (omics-wide array) methodologies to discover new targets associated with potential pathologies and diseases.

Further perspectives include integration of multi-omics, AI-driven causal inference, pharmacokinetic–network modeling, and biomarker-guided trials.

3.2. Nucleosides Adenosine and Cordycepin as Mediators of Adaptive Stress Response and Anti-Fatigue Activity of O. sinensis, and C. militaris

Published pharmacokinetic studies of cordycepin and adenosine show remarkable variability, with rapid metabolism, low oral bioavailability, and plasma concentrations often in the low nanomolar range [127,128,131,132]. These levels are insufficient to activate classical high-affinity adenosine receptors or produce direct pharmacological effects via receptor agonism or antagonism (Section 2.2). Purinergic receptors are important for regulating inflammation, muscle contraction, neurotransmission, and nociception. Extracellular ATP and its metabolites are the main ligands for these receptors. ATP supplementation in healthy subjects for 4 weeks did not change blood or plasma ATP concentrations. Of all ATP metabolites, only plasma uric acid levels increased significantly after the administration of 5000 mg of ATP [85]. A single oral dose of ATP is not bioavailable in healthy human subjects, which may explain why several studies failed to detect ergogenic effects of oral ATP supplementation. On the other hand, increases in uric acid after release of ATP in the proximal part of the small intestine suggest that ATP or one of its metabolites is absorbed and metabolized [84]. This implies that extensive metabolism has no effect on the bioactivity of accumulated ATP in intracellular processes, and particularly on the AMPK-mediated signaling pathway, which plays an essential role in stress response, cellular senescence, apoptosis, autophagy, angiogenesis, protein and glycogen synthesis, steroids biosynthesis, mTOR signaling, etc. [59,248]

https://doi.org/10.3390/ph19030519

(Appendix A Figures A6–A8). Similarly, 3-deoxyadenosine (cordycepin), even at physiological concentrations, may compete with adenosine for receptors, thereby triggering AMPK- and AKT (protein kinase B)-mediated intracellular signaling pathways. Some predicted kinase interactions may not be directly achievable at physiological concentrations, and indirect or systems-level mechanisms may contribute to biological activity. Further studies are required, as physiological concentrations of cordycepin are essential for experimental evidence supporting our hypothesis. For comparison, Ginsenoside Rg5 in physiological concentrations (nM-pM-fM) significantly deregulates gene expressions in brain cell culture [173].

These nucleosides fall within the range where hormetic activation of metabolic stress-response pathways, such as AMPK, SIRT1, TIGAR, and PGC-1α, occurs. Thus, the inconsistencies in pharmacokinetic and pharmacodynamic characteristics of cordycepin are not contradictory but relatively entirely consistent with the concept that cordycepin functions as a metabolic adaptogen with a biphasic hormetic dose–response. Cordycepin may act as a driver, triggering the organism's adaptive stress response in stress-induced and aging-related diseases.

The lack of correlation between plasma cordycepin concentration and biological outcomes indicates that it does not act through linear, dose-dependent pharmacology but rather through multi-target metabolic adaptation, characteristic of adaptogenic botanicals. In this context, even low, transient, and variable systemic exposures can induce stable improvements in transcription and mitochondrial function.

Cordycepin exhibits a genuine adaptogenic profile driven by low-dose hormetic activation of metabolic resilience pathways, particularly AMPK, SIRT1, PGC-1α, and TIGAR. Although it lacks CNS stimulant effects and does not act via adenosine receptors, cordycepin enhances mitochondrial efficiency, improves ATP production, and increases resistance to physical and metabolic stress. Within *C. militaris* or *O. sinensis* extracts, synergistic interactions among multiple constituents amplify these effects, providing a biologically plausible explanation for the anti-fatigue and performance-enhancing outcomes observed in animal and human studies.

Cordycepin exerts effects through peripheral metabolic enhancement, mitochondrial biogenesis, and hormetic stress adaptation rather than through central adenosinergic stimulation. Cordycepin acts as a low-dose metabolic hormetic agent, while Orange Cordyceps and Caterpillar Fungus extracts display multi-target synergy that cannot be explained by nucleosides alone. This framework resolves the apparent contradictions between cordycepin's limited CNS pharmacology and the robust anti-fatigue outcomes observed in animals and humans.

3.3. Western Regulatory vs. Traditional Medical Paradigms

TCM and Ayurveda are based on a holistic and integrative approach, multi-target and polyvalent action [134], but they rely on archaic theories. In contrast, Western conventional medicine, based on a reductional approach, selective targeting, and specific action in the treatment of diseases, relies on another archaic theory of galenic preparations that ignores interactions and overlaps among regulatory systems and the effects of other constituents in multi-component plant extracts. In fact, both approaches are complementary, particularly in the treatment of diseases of complex pathology associated with the stress system interacting with other regulatory systems. The concomitant administration of several Western conventional medicines that selectively act on various receptors provides more effective treatment in hypertension, post-stroke rehabilitation, viral infections, etc. The "ready for use" of complex botanicals and botanical hybrid products used in the Eastern world acts similarly. The challenge is to understand the mechanisms of action and scientifically validate their efficacy, quality, and safety by strengthening the integration of TCM into European health systems, improving quality control, conducting randomized clinical trials, and improving regulatory standards [249].

The concept of adaptogens originated in Eastern medical and pharmacological traditions and describes natural products that increase an organism's capacity to maintain physiological home-

https://doi.org/10.3390/ph19030519

ostasis under conditions of stress [28,135]. In this framework, stress is understood as a multisystem challenge that affects neuroendocrine regulation, energy metabolism, immune competence, and cognitive and physical performance, particularly in aging and stress-exposed populations [229,230,250–256].

While adaptogens are commonly recognized as a pharmacological category in several non-European regulatory and medical systems [256–264], they are not formally acknowledged within EFSA or EMA frameworks. The term “adaptogen” is considered not appropriate for a marketing authorization within EFSA or EMA frameworks [241], which require substantiation of discrete, well-defined physiological endpoints and do not evaluate systems-level concepts such as adaptation or stress resilience [238–240]. As a consequence, holistic or systems-level constructs such as “adaptation”, “stress resilience”, or “anti-fatigue” cannot be evaluated as such under current EU food or medicinal product legislation.

Importantly, the lack of regulatory recognition does not imply scientific invalidity of the adaptogen concept but rather reflects methodological constraints of existing regulatory paradigms.

In summary, the adaptogen concept represents a systems-level interpretation of complex physiological responses, whereas EFSA evaluation operates at the level of single, well-defined functional outcomes. By translating adaptive effects into EFSA-recognized physiological functions—such as physical performance or perceived exertion—it is possible to preserve scientific validity while remaining compliant with regulatory requirements.

This translational framework enables constructive dialogue between scientific innovation and regulatory practice, without forcing premature or inappropriate reclassification of complex biological concepts.

3.4. Resilience Biology as the Missing Regulatory Construct

The findings of this review indicate that the regulatory marginalization of adaptogens in Europe does not arise from a lack of biological plausibility, but from a structural gap in regulatory concepts. Inflammation and stress responses are both evolutionarily conserved adaptive systems with active resolution mechanisms [229–236]; however, only inflammation is formally recognized as a regulatable pathological entity within European frameworks [238].

Adaptogenic botanicals consistently demonstrate modulatory effects across immune, inflammatory, neuroendocrine, and metabolic systems [26,28,134]. These effects are bidirectional, context-dependent, and primarily aimed at restoring homeostasis rather than suppressing specific pathways. Such characteristics align poorly with disease-centric regulatory logic but are fully consistent with contemporary systems biology, allostasis, and resilience theory [232,265].

Asian medical systems have long operationalized this concept by framing health as adaptive capacity rather than the absence of disease [244]. In contrast, European regulation—despite recognizing allostasis, inflammation resolution, and psychoneuroimmunology at the scientific level—lacks a functional category that allows these principles to be translated into health claims or product classifications [238–240]

3.4.1. Why a Hybrid EU–Asia Model Is Scientifically Justified

A hybrid EU–Asia regulatory model reconciles two complementary strengths: the European emphasis on safety, standardization, and evidentiary rigor, and the Asian emphasis on functional balance, recovery, and resilience embedded in traditional medical systems [26,28,134,244,264,265].

This review demonstrates that adaptogens act upstream of pathology by supporting recovery kinetics, physiological flexibility, and stress-response resolution—features increasingly recognized as determinants of long-term health outcomes [232,265]. These effects are not adequately captured by current EU categories, such as vitamins, antioxidants, or anti-inflammatory agents, which are anchored in deficiency-correction or pathway-inhibition models [238–240]. Nevertheless, adapto-

https://doi.org/10.3390/ph19030519

genic effects can be measured using non-disease endpoints, including return-to-baseline time, performance maintenance under load, and immune homeostasis markers [26,28].

Importantly, the proposed hybrid model does not dilute regulatory rigor. Rather, it reallocates evidentiary focus from disease endpoints to functional adaptation metrics, maintaining consumer protection while enabling scientific innovation consistent with systems biology.

3.4.1.1. Resilience-Supporting Physiological Modulators as a Regulatory Bridge

The proposed category of resilience-supporting physiological modulators (RSPMs) offers a legally conservative yet biologically modern solution. By explicitly excluding disease prevention or treatment claims, this category preserves the boundary between food supplements and medicines while legitimizing claims related to recovery, homeostasis, and adaptive capacity. Such a category would be compatible with the existing institutional roles of the European Food Safety Authority—responsible for safety evaluation and health-claim substantiation—and the European Medicines Agency, which oversees the boundary between functional and pharmacological activity [238–241]. Asian regulatory frameworks would serve as functional reference models rather than direct validation pathways, allowing integration without undermining EU legal coherence.

Further expert consensus guidelines can be developed to focus on the selection and justification of outcome measures and endpoints across various stress-induced and aging-related health conditions, and to propose measurable resilience-related biomarkers as candidate endpoints to operationalize the proposed resilience-supporting physiological modulator (RSPM) framework. The criteria for resilience and the biomarker set are similar to those summarized in a recent review on adaptogens [26], including recovery indices in chronic unpredictable stress (CUS) animal models, which induce affective behaviors in mice and, once established, measure stress-related alterations in the intrinsic excitability and synaptic regulation of the medial prefrontal cortex layer pyramidal neurons, cortisol recovery kinetics, cytokine balance ratios, and adaptive stress–response signaling pathways markers, e.g., G-protein coupled (GPCR), tyrosine, toll-like receptors, and I3PK-AKT, AMPK-mediated pathways known to promote survival in response to stress, suggesting neuroprotective activity and the potential benefits of adaptogens in neurodegenerative diseases.

3.4.1.2. Regulatory Language as a Determinant of Scientific Visibility

One of the essential points of this review is that language—not evidence—is the principal barrier to adaptogen acceptance for marketing authorization in Europe. Terms such as anti-stress or adaptogenic for marketing authorization are rejected not because stress biology is unrecognized, but because stress is classified as a normal life condition rather than a regulatable physiological domain [238–241]. The hybrid model resolves this tension by shifting the claim architecture toward supporting normal physiological function during periods of increased demand, a formulation already consistent with European health-claim jurisprudence. This reframing allows resilience biology to be communicated without encroaching on medical or psychological claims, thereby increasing regulatory acceptability while preserving scientific meaning.

3.4.2. Outlook and Future Directions

3.4.2.1. From Disease Regulation to Health Maintenance

European regulatory systems are approaching a conceptual inflection point. As chronic, lifestyle-associated conditions increasingly dominate healthcare burden, the inability to regulate interventions that support recovery and adaptive capacity represents a growing limitation (Furman et al., 2019) [265]. Resilience biology provides a scientifically grounded framework to address this gap.

The hybrid EU–Asia model outlined here offers a pathway to transition from a purely disease-reactive paradigm toward health-maintenance regulation, without compromising evidentiary standards or public safety.

https://doi.org/10.3390/ph19030519

3.4.2.2. Implications for Regulatory Science

Future regulatory development should prioritize:

- Formal recognition of homeostasis and recovery as legitimate physiological outcomes;
- Acceptance of systems-level functional endpoints alongside classical biomarkers;
- Development of claim guidance specific to resilience-supporting functions.

Pilot implementation through emerging-science claim pathways, limited botanical lists, and post-market monitoring would allow regulatory learning while maintaining risk control [238–240].

3.4.2.3. Implications for Research and Industry

Adoption of a resilience-focused regulatory category would incentivize improved human study designs using load-and-recovery paradigms, better standardization of complex botanical preparations, and closer integration of traditional knowledge with modern clinical research [26,244]. This would reduce the current disconnect between scientific evidence, regulatory acceptance, and consumer communication.

3.4.2.4. Concluding Perspective

The regulatory challenge posed by adaptogens is not an anomaly but a signal: modern biology has outgrown purely disease-centric regulation. A hybrid EU–Asia regulatory model integrating resilience biology would align policy with science, recognize health as a dynamic adaptive process, and provide a coherent framework for interventions that maintain function rather than treat pathology.

Resilience is not an alternative to medicine; it is the biological foundation upon which medicine succeeds.

4. Materials and Methods

This mixed-methods review explores evidence from 9 systematic clinical and 37 network pharmacology studies on *O. sinensis*, *C. militaris*, and cordycepin, extracting active compounds, disease indications, predicted targets, enriched signaling pathways, and mechanistic conclusions to elucidate their molecular actions in diseases treated in TCM. A systematic review of meta-analyses of randomized controlled trials (RCTs) was conducted to evaluate the efficacy, safety, quality control practices, and compliance with EMA criteria for well-established herbal medicinal products. Data synthesis included pooled effect-size estimation and risk-of-bias assessment using Cochrane methods. A structured umbrella review approach was applied to peer-reviewed reviews addressing inflammation, stress physiology, adaptogens, and regulatory science. Regulatory guidance from EFSA, EMA, FDA, and Asian authorities was examined, and findings were narratively synthesized.

4.1. Literature Search

This review thoroughly explores the current evidence on the network pharmacology studies of *O. synensis*, *C. militaris*, and cordycepin, covering publications from 2010 to 2025 and addressing inflammation, stress physiology, adaptogens, and regulatory science. Regulatory guidance from EFSA, EMA, FDA, and Asian authorities was examined. Findings were narratively synthesized. A search was conducted using several major databases and platforms, including PubMed, Google Scholar, ScienceDirect, Scopus, CNKI, and Web of Science, as well as the Google search engine, the National Library of Medicine, regulatory documents from EFSA, EMA, FDA, and Asian health authorities, and the ChatGPT AI technology.

The search strategy involved targeted use of keywords such as "*Ophiocordyceps sinensis*", "*Cordyceps militaris*" (L.), "network pharmacology," "randomized" AND "health claims", "indications" AND "pharmacopeia", AND "dietary supplements". The search was limited to English-language publications within the specified period. The review process adhered to EMA guidelines, and the quality of the studies was evaluated using CONSORT and Cochrane standards.

https://doi.org/10.3390/ph19030519

4.2. Inclusion and Exclusion Criteria

4.2.1. Inclusion Criteria

For network pharmacology synthesis:

- Studies explicitly performing target prediction and pathway enrichment analyses.
- Studies identifying protein–protein interaction (PPI) networks.
- Studies reporting enriched KEGG/GO pathways.
- Studies involving *O. sinensis*, *C. militaris*, or cordycepin as primary exposure.

For experimental validation:

- In vitro or in vivo confirmation of predicted targets/pathways.
- Clear reporting of biological endpoints.
- Mechanistic linkage to predicted signaling hubs.

For clinical evaluation:

- Randomized controlled trials (RCTs).
- Systematic reviews or meta-analyses.
- Clearly defined preparation type.

4.2.2. Exclusion Criteria

- Reviews without primary mechanistic data.
- Studies lacking explicit pathway enrichment methods.
- Case reports without mechanistic evaluation.

4.3. Data Extraction

Data extraction covered: major active compounds/ligands, disease indications, predicted molecular targets, enriched signaling pathways, docking scores, and presence of experimental validation. Target convergence and pathway frequency analyses were performed to identify core mechanistic hubs.

Included studies employed network pharmacology tools such as target prediction algorithms, KEGG/GO pathway enrichment, molecular docking, transcriptomics, metabolomics, or integrated multi-omics. Ten studies with experimental validation—including cellular assays, animal disease models, and clinical observations—were also included.

Reviews addressing inflammation resolution, stress biology, adaptogens, or regulatory frameworks were also included. Findings were narratively integrated across biological, clinical, and regulatory domains.

4.4. Data Integration and Evidence Integration Strategy

All AI-assisted frequency aggregation was manually verified against original publications to prevent duplication or misclassification.

Thirty-seven network pharmacology studies were identified. For each study:

- Predicted targets were extracted.
- Enriched pathways were recorded.
- Frequency of pathway recurrence across independent studies was counted.

To reduce "target inflation bias," predicted targets were stratified according to validation level:

- In silico prediction only;
- Experimentally validated (cellular or animal models);
- Clinically supported endpoints.

Targets and pathways were aggregated across studies. Mechanistic convergence was assessed by frequency. Experimental studies were cross-mapped onto predicted networks. Heatmaps (Fig-

https://doi.org/10.3390/ph19030519

ure 4) represent recurrence frequency across independent publications, not gene expression magnitude.

AI-assisted tools were used exclusively for structured aggregation and visualization of manually extracted data. Literature identification, study selection, and data extraction were performed manually from full-text publications. Extracted variables (intervention, targets, enriched pathways, validation status, and study identifiers) were compiled into standardized tables (Tables A10 and A11) prior to AI processing. AI was subsequently used only to compute recurrence frequencies, stratify findings by evidence tier, and generate graphical heatmaps (Figure 4). No automated literature screening, target prediction, or mechanistic interpretation was performed by AI. All aggregated outputs were manually cross-verified against the original dataset to prevent duplication or misclassification.

5. Conclusions

Many reviews on various aspects of the medical mushroom *O. sinensis*, which has historically been recognized in Asian traditional medical systems for its ability to enhance vitality, describe pleiotropic therapeutic applications. However, the polyvalent adaptogenic potential of *O. sinensis* has not been systematically proven, and a consolidated mechanistic synthesis integrating both network predictions and experimental validation is lacking. This review, for the first time, shows that:

- *O. sinensis*, *C. militaris*, and cordycepin share a common adaptogenic mechanism of maintenance of cellular and integrated biology system functions homeostasis.
- The systems-level adaptogenic mechanism of these fungi is characterized by their ability to modulate multiple interconnected biological networks rather than acting on a single target.
- This is in line with TCM and Ayurveda holistic concepts and the modern concept of pleiotropic therapeutic activity of adaptogens and particularly of *O. sinensis*.
- The review reveals controversy regarding the bioavailability of cordycepin in vivo and its concentration in vitro studies, raising the hypothesis that cordycepin may act as a driver, triggering the organism's adaptive stress response in stress-induced and aging-related diseases.
- Nucleosides, adenosine and cordycepin, along with other adaptogenic botanical metabolites (steroids and phenolics), contribute to the maintenance of cellular and integrated biology system functions homeostasis.
- Network pharmacology studies identify multi-target pathways, including convergent hubs, such as PI3K-Akt, AMPK–mTOR, MAPK, apoptosis, Nrf2 and AMPK–SIRT1–PGC-1α pathways.
- By influencing pathways associated with immune regulation, mitochondrial function, and metabolic adaptation, they orchestrate a holistic response that enhances the organism's resilience to various stressors.
- This integrative effect is especially significant in the context of complex disorders, where multifactorial interventions are necessary for effective therapeutic outcomes.
- This is the first comparative meta-analysis of validated vs. predicted effects of *O. sinensis*, *C. militaris* and species-level versus cordycepin-driven mechanisms.
- Validation studies confirm predictions across chronic obstructive pulmonary disease, pulmonary arterial hypertension, cancer, obesity, influenza, and immunogenicity.

Caterpillar Fungus, Orange Cordyceps, and 3-deoxyadenosine exhibit a unified adaptogenic pharmacology that involves immune modulation, mitochondrial enhancement, stress-signal regulation, and metabolic homeostasis. These effects arise through multi-target synergy across PI3K–Akt, MAPK, NF-κB, apoptosis, and AMPK–SIRT1–PGC-1α pathways. The meta-analysis of network pharmacology studies suggests that *O. sinensis* and *C. militaris* act as multi-compound immunometabolic regulators, while cordycepin functions as a dominant molecular effector controlling apoptosis, metabolism, and adaptive stress signaling. The strong convergence of network and ex-

https://doi.org/10.3390/ph19030519

perimental evidence supports their potential in immunometabolic and stress-related disorders. Distinguishing validated from predicted networks is essential for translational reliability.

Results of network pharmacological studies of OS, CM, and CC that demonstrate activation of adaptive extracellular and intracellular signaling pathways, key mediators, and physiological functions are associated with pleiotropic health effects.

Clinical efficacy of OS, CM, and CC is noticed in stress-induced physical and cognitive fatigue, mental and immune disorders; these studies are limited to physical fatigue in healthy individuals, chronic kidney disease, respiratory conditions, and cancer adjunct therapy.

The effects of cordycepin were demonstrated in micromolar concentrations in vitro cell models. Clinical and pharmacokinetic studies show that high concentrations of cordycepin, adenosine, and their bioactive metabolites, ATP and CTP, in blood circulation cannot be achieved with therapeutic doses of *O. sinensis* and *C. militaris* due to intensive enzymatic metabolism and renal clearance. However, since ATP, adenosine, cordycepin, and other purine metabolites are involved in numerous physiological processes and exert pharmacological effects, we can hypothesize that they trigger these effects at physiological nanomolar concentrations. Cordycepin may function as a systems-level metabolic trigger rather than as a classical high-affinity receptor ligand.

The adaptogenic concept represents a systems-level interpretation of complex physiological responses characteristic of holistic TCM and Ayurvedic concepts, whereas European Food Safety Authority regulatory frameworks lack concepts for resilience and adaptive capacity and operate at the level of single, well-defined functional outcomes, which raises regulatory issues for food and drugs in Western countries.

This review clarifies conceptual and regulatory barriers to recognizing resilience-supporting interventions and informs future regulatory innovation. The review for the first time suggests establishing a regulatory category for resilience-supporting physiological modulators that could align food and drug regulation in the EU with contemporary systems biology, thereby complementing EFSA, EMA, FDA, and Asian authorities.

Numerous critical appraisals and limitations were discussed above in detail across the sections on clinical and network pharmacology, as well as in the regulatory framework. Future perspectives of primary importance include integrating TCM into European health systems, improving quality control, conducting randomized clinical trials effectively, strengthening regulatory standards, and the wide implementation of network pharmacology study design and methodology, which account for synergistic and antagonistic interactions by various constituents of the complex, multi-component extracts, which can lead to unexpected outcomes. They include transcriptome-wide microarray profiling of gene-expression-based experiments, integrated with metabolomics and network analyses, revealing all molecular targets of active compounds and coupling signaling pathways to final outcomes. The results of these studies can reveal unknown health consequences and therapeutic indications, leading to new drug discoveries.

Funding: This research received no external funding.

Institutional Review Board Statement: Not applicable.

Informed Consent Statement: Not applicable.

Data Availability Statement: No new data were created or analyzed in this study.

Acknowledgments: The authors acknowledge the use of artificial intelligence (AI) technology (ChatGPT for iOS, version 1.202, model 2025, OpenAI, L.L.C.) as an assistive tool for language refinement and drafting support. All scientific interpretation, synthesis, and final editorial decisions remain the responsibility of the authors. The author used AI tools (ChatGPT-5, Microsoft MS365 Copilot) strictly as assistive tools to suggest references and surface alternative methodological formulations. References were partly suggested by AI and partly selected by the author; all citations and formatting were reviewed, curated, and approved by the author. AI-proposed methodological options were critically assessed and either adopted or rejected by the author. All concepts and interpretations are solely the author's, originating from practical observations.

https://doi.org/10.3390/ph19030519

Conflicts of Interest: The author was self-employed by Phytomed AB, being the founder and owner of this Research & Development company. The author declares that the research was conducted in the absence of any commercial or financial relationships that could be construed as a potential conflict of interest.

Appendix A.

Appendix A.1. Taxonomy, Scientific and Vernacular Names of Ophiocordyceps sinensis and Cordyceps militaris

Ophiocordyceps sinensis is a species of ascomycete fungi in the family Ophiocordycipitaceae.
Cordyceps militaris is a species of ascomycete fungi in the family Cordycipitaceae.

Table A1. Scientific and vernacular names of *Ophiocordyceps sinensis* and *Cordyceps militaris*.

Accepted Scientific Name	***Ophiocordyceps sinensis* (Berk.) G.H. Sung, J.M. Sung, Hywel-Jones & Spatafora, 2007**	***Cordyceps militaris* (L.) Fr., 1818**
Synonims	*Cordyceps sinensis* (Berk.) Sacc. (1878), *Sphaeria sinensis* Berk. (1843)	*Clavaria militaris* L., 1753
Language	Vernacular names	
Sanskrit	Yarsagumba	
Tibetan	Yarsa gumba, Yarcha gumba (དབྱར་རྩ་དགུན་འབུར་)	
Nepali	Keera jhar, Jeevan buti, Keeda ghass, Chyou kira, Sanjeevani bhooti (यार्सागुम्बा)	
Chinese (Mandarin)	Dong chong xi cao (冬蟲夏草, or 冬虫夏草, meaning “winter worm, summer grass”)	Běi chóng cǎo (北虫草) Northern Cordyceps
Japanase	Tocheikasa, Tochyuka-sou	冬虫夏草 (Tōchūkasō)
Korean	동충하초 (Dong Chung Ha Cho)	북충초 (Buk chung cho)
Vietnamese	Đông trùng hạ thảo	Đông trùng hạ thảo quân đội
Thai	ถั่งเช่า (Thungchao)	ถั่งเช่าเหนือ (Thungchao nuea)
French	cordyceps, champignon chenille	
German	Cordyceps, Chinesischer Raupenpilz, Tibetischer, Raupenpilz, Tibetischer Raupenkeulenpilz	
Italian	cordyceps, fungo del bruco	
Spanish	cordyceps	
English	Caterpillar fungus, Cordyceps mushroom, Winter Worm—Summer Grass	Scarlet Caterpillar Club, Orange Cordyceps

Etymology: Ophiocordyceps = from Greek ophio- (“snake-like”) + cordyle (“club”) + ceps (“head”). Refers to the slender, serpentine fruiting body; sinensis = Latin for “from China,” where the species was first described (Berkeley, 1843). The traditional phrase “冬虫夏草” (Dōng chóng xià cǎo) encapsulates its dual nature as both animal (insect larva) and plant-like (fungal fruiting body). Cordyceps = from Greek kordyle (club) + ceps (head), militaris = Latin for “military”—a reference to its upright, orange, “soldier-like” appearance.

Table A2. Taxonomy of *Ophiocordyceps sinensis* and *Cordyceps militaris*.

Scientific Name	***Ophiocordyceps sinensis* (Berk.) G.H. Sung, J.M. Sung, Hywel-Jones & Spatafora, 2007**	***Cordyceps militaris* (L.) Fr., 1818**
Domain	Eukaryota (eukaryotes)	Eukaryota (eukaryotes)
Kingdom	Fungi	Fungi
Phylum	Ascomycota (ascomycete fungi)	Ascomycota (ascomycete fungi)
Class	Sordariomycetes	Sordariomycetes
Order	Hypocreales	Hypocreales
Family	Ophiocordycipitaceae	Cordycipitaceae
Genus	*Ophiocordyceps*	*Cordyceps*
Species	*Ophiocordyceps sinensis*	*Cordyceps militaris*

https://doi.org/10.3390/ph19030519

Appendix A.2. Chemical Composition, Bioactive Compounds, and Pharmacological Activity of Ophiocordyceps sinensis and Cordyceps militaris Species

Overall, 110 primary and secondary metabolites of *O. sinensis* and *C. militaris* fungi were identified in several comprehensive reviews of their traditional uses, chemical composition, and pharmacological activity [16,18,19,69–71]. Figures A1–A5 and Tables A3–A6.

Table A3. Chemical bioactive constituents of *O. sinensis* [21,29,65] and *C. militaris* [23,66,67].

C. sinensis	*C. militaris*
Cordycepic acid, glutamic acid, amino acids (phenylalnine, praline, histidine, valine, oxyvaline, arginine): polyamines (1,3-diamino propane, cadaverine, spermidine, spermine, homospermidine, and purtescine): cyclic dipeptides (cyclo-(gly-pro), cyclo-(leu-pro), cyclo-(val-pro), cyclo-(ala-leu), cyclo-(alaval), and cyclo-(thr-leu), saccharides and sugar derivatives (d-mannitol, oligosaccharides, and polysaccharides); sterols (ergosterol, delta-3 ergosterol, ergosterol peroxide, 3-sistosterol, daucosterol and campesterol); nucleotides, and nucleosides, including adenine, adenosine, inosine, cytidine, cytosine, guanine, uridine, thymidine, uracil, hypoxanthine, guanosine, uracil, uridine, guanosine, and deoxyuridine and cordycepia; saturated and unsaturated fatty acids, their derivatives and other organic acids (oleic, linoleic, palmitic and stearic acids); vitamins (B1, B2, B12, E, and K); and inorganic elements (K, Na, Ca, Mg, Fe, Ca, Mn, Zn, Pi, Se, Al, Si, Ni, Si, Ti, Cr, Ga, V, and Zr).	cordycepin, cordycepic acid, pentostatin, carotenoids (lutein, zeaxanthin, cordyxanthins), L-ergothioneine, ergosterol, polysaccharides, glycoproteins, 5-Methyltryptamine Lovastatin 5-Hydroxy-L-tryptophan L-Tryptophan Serotonine L-Phenylalanine

Table A4. The pharmacological activity of bioactive compounds of *O. sinensis* and *C. militaris* *).

Classification	Compound, the Pharmacological Activity, and the Reference
Nucleoside and *bases*	Adenosine: Neuroprotection, immunomodulatory [266,267]
	Cordycepin: Neuroprotection, anti-metastatic, anti-platelet aggregation, anti-inflammatory activity, anticancer [62,129,268]
	Dimethylguanosine: Antioxidant and HIV-1 protease [269]
	Guanosine: Immunomodulatory [266,267]
	Cordysinin B: Anti-inflammatory activity [71]
Sterols	Ergosteryl-3-O-β-D-glucopyranoside: Anti-inflammatory, antioxidant [71,81]
	5α,8α-epidioxy-22E-ergosta-6,9-(11)-22-trien-33β-ol: Cytotoxic against HL-60 cell line [270]
	5α,6α-epoxy-5α-ergosta-7,22-dien-3β-ol: Cytotoxic against HL-60 cell line [270]
	5α,8α-epidioxy-24(R)-methylcholesta-6,22-dien-3β-Dglucopyranoside: Antitumor [81]
	Ergosta-4,6,8(14),22-tetraen-3-one: Antitumor [81]
	22-dihydro-ergosteryl-3-O-β-D-glucopyranoside: Antitumor [81]
Cyclodipeptides	Cordyceamide A: Cytotoxicity against L929, A375 and Hela cell lines [271]
	Cordyceamide B: Cytotoxicity against L929, A375 and Hela cell lines [271]
	Cycloaspeptide A: Cytotoxicity against HeLa and MCF7 cell lines [272]
	Cycloaspeptide C: Cytotoxicity against HeLa and MCF7 cell lines [272]
	Cycloaspeptide F: Cytotoxicity against HeLa and MCF7 cell lines [272]
	Cycloaspeptide G: Cytotoxicity against HeLa and MCF7 cell lines [272]
	Cyclo(L-Pro-L-Val): Antioxidant, anti-inflammatory [71]
	Cyclo(L-Phe-L-Pro): Antioxidant, anti-inflammatory [71]
	Cyclo(L-Pro-L-Tyr): Antioxidant, anti-inflammatory [71]
Alkaloids	Cordysinin A: Anti-inflammatory, antioxidant [16,19]
	Cordysinin C: anticancer [16,70]
	Cordysinin D: anticancer [16,70]
	Flazin: Antioxidant, anti-inflammatory [70]
	Perlolyrine (100) Antioxidant, anti-inflammatory, anticancer [70]
	α-methoxy-α-trifluoro-methylphenylacetyl chlorides: Anti-inflammatory [71]
	1-acetyl-β-carboline: Anticancer [70,71]
	gliocladicillins A: antitumor cell proliferation inhibitors and apoptosis inducers [16,69]
	gliocladicillin B: antitumor cell proliferation inhibitors and apoptosis inducers [16,69]
	11,11′-dideoxyverticillin: antitumor cell proliferation inhibitors and apoptosis inducers [16,69]
Flavonoids	3′,4′,7-trihydroxyisoflavone: Antioxidant [71]
	Diadzein: Antioxidant, anti-inflammatory [71]
	6,7,2′,4′,5′-pentamethoxyflavone: Antioxidant activity, anti-HIV-1 protease [269]
	Glycitein-7-O-β-D-glucoside-4′-O-methylate: Anti-inflammatory [273]
	Iso-sinensetin (120) Antioxidant activity, anti-HIV-1 protease [269]
Miscellaneous	Ophicordin: Antifungal [274]
	2-Furancarboxylic acid: Anti-inflammatory, antioxidant [71]
	3-hydroxy-2-methyl-4-pyrone: Anti-inflammatory, antioxidant [71]
	Cordycerebroside A: Anti-inflammatory [275]
	Soyacerebroside I: Anti-inflammatory [275]
	Glucocerebroside: Anti-inflammatory [275]

*—Data extracted from the review Olatunji et al., 2018 [19].

https://doi.org/10.3390/ph19030519

Table A5. Summary of biomarkers and pharmacological activity used for quality control of Cordyceps [18].

Nucleosides	
	Anti-tumor activities; Ca2+ antagonist; depresses the excitability of CNS neurons, inhibits release of various neurotransmitters presynaptically and anticonvulsant activity [72–74] stimulate axon growth in vitro and in the adult central nervous system [75]
Polysaccharides	
	Anti-oxidation, immuno-potentiation, anti-tumor, and hypoglycemic activity [76–79]; anti-inflammatory activity and suppresses the humoral immunity in mice [80]
Ergosterol and its analogs	
	Cytotoxic activity, anti-viral activity, and anti-arrhythmia effect [81,82]; suppress the activated human mesangial cells and alleviate immunoglobulin A nephropathy (Berger's disease) [83]
Mannitol	
	Diuretic, anti-tussive, and anti-free radical activities [18]
Peptides	
	Anti-tumor and immuno-potentiation activities [18]

Table A6. Pharmacological activity of total extracts of *Ophiocordyceps sinensis* and *Cordyceps militaris* in experimental study models [19,97].

O. sinensis	***C. militaris***
Anti-arteriosclerosis: Rats	Acetylcholinesterase inhibition
Anticancer Mice	Anti-allergic Mice
Anti-diabetic Rats	Anticancer A 4T1, SMMC-7721, BGC-823,MCF-7 cells
Anti-fatigue Rats	Anti-HCV
Anti-fibrotic HK-2, HLFS cells	Anti-HCV
Anti-hypertensive Rats	Antihyperglycemic Mice
Anti-inflammatory HM cells	Antihyperlipidemic Mice
Antioxidant	Anti-inflammatory human ADMSC cells
Anti-thrombotic Humans	Antimicrobial
Antitumor S-180 cells	Anti-obesity C58BL/6 J mice
Hepatoprotective HepG2 cells	Antioxidant
Immunomodulatory RAW 264.7 cells	Antitumor J6/JFH1-huh 7.5 cells
Radio-protective Mice	Hepatoprotective Mice
Renoprotective Rats	HIV-1 protease inhibiting
	HuH-7-derived OR6, AH1R cells
	Hypouricemic Mice
	Immunomodulatory Sea Cucumbers

Table A7. Dietary uses of *O. sinensis* in medicinal dishes.

Dishes	**Indications for Use**
Cooked with an old duck	For patients with cancer, asthenia, or after severe illness
Cooked with hen	For hyposexuality (especially emission)
Cooked with black-bone hen	For asthenia (especially Qi-Yin asthenia)
Cooked with lean pork	For fatigue, male impotence, and "kidney" asthenia
Cooked with sparrow	For antiaging/senescence
Cooked with quail	For fatigue, poor appetite, "kidney" asthenia, and tuberculosis
Cooked with steamed turtle	For male/female hyposexuality
Cooked with baked abalone	For chronic bronchitis, COPD, tuberculosis, arteriosclerosis, cataracts, and for healthy individuals in any season

Data adapted from Jiang (1994) [135] and Zhu et al. (1998) [13].

https://doi.org/10.3390/ph19030519

Appendix A.3. Clinical Studies

Table A8. Summary of Randomized Placebo-Controlled Clinical Trials of *O. sinensis* and *C. militaris*.

Species	Botanical Material/ Product	Comparator	Daily Dose	Duration	Population/ Condition	Sample Size	Study Design (GCP) *	Primary Endpoints	Outcome Measures	Key Clinical Results	Effect Size (reported/ Calculable)	Risk of Bias (Cochrane)	Citation
O. sinensis	Cs-4 mycelium (Paecilomyces hepiali)	Placebo	999 mg/day (333 mg TID)	12 weeks	Healthy elderly (50–75 y)	n = 20	DB-PC RCT	Exercise performance	VO_2max, ventilatory threshold, VT, MT	↑ ventilatory & metabolic thresholds; no VO_2max change	VO_2max SMD ≈ 0	Low	Chen et al., 2010 [150]
O. sinensis	Mycelium extract	Placebo	2 g/day	12 weeks	Amateur marathoners	n = 12	DB-PC RCT	Aerobic performance	CPET, HR	↓ HR at submax load; ↑ aerobic performance	SMD small–moderate	Moderate	Savioli et al., 2022 [159]
O. sinensis	Cs-4	Placebo	3 g/day	12 weeks	Healthy elderly	n = 37	Randomized DB-PC	Aerobic capacity	VO_2max, FEV_1	Significant ↑ VO_2max	SMD ≈ 0.54	Moderate	Xiao et al., 2004 [158]
O. sinensis	Cs-4 (CordyMax)	Placebo	3 g/day	5 weeks	Trained cyclists	n = 25	Randomized DB-PC	Endurance	Time-to-exhaustion	No difference	SMD ≈ 0.00	Low	Parcell et al., 2004 [156]
O. sinensis	Herbal formulation	Standard asthma care	NR	3 months	Moderate–severe asthma	n = 120	RCT	QoL	AQLQ, FEV_1	Significant QoL improvement	MD (AQLQ) +0.8	Moderate	Wang et al., 2016 [165]
O. sinensis	Cs-4 mycelium, capsule	Placebo "Wait-list group."	1.6 g (4 caps 0.4 g/caps daily)	12 weeks, follow-up at week 24	Long COVID	n = 110 (55/55}	Waitlist-controlled RCT	Change in the symptom severity, COVID-19 Yorkshire Rehabilitation Scale (C19-YRSm **) at 12 weeks	Long Covid symptoms severity (C19-YRSm&), Fatigue, sleep, QoL, depression, anxiety,	Significant multi-domain improvement. Improved Long COVID severity symptoms, fatigue & QoL	Moderate, Significant change from baseline between-group difference (adjusted for duration and vaccine doses)	Low Some concerns	Chen et al., 2025 [163]
O. sinensis	Mycelium extract	Standard care	NR	≥8 weeks	Diabetic kidney disease	>13,000 (meta-analysis)	Systematic review of RCTs	Renal surrogates	Proteinuria, Cr	↓ proteinuria, ↓ Cr	Pooled MD significant	High	Xue et al., 2024 [140]
O. sinensis	Mycelium extract	Standard care	NR	NR	Dialysis patients	n = 2914	Meta-analysis	Inflammation, anemia	CRP, Hb, Alb	Improvements in surrogates	Low certainty	High	Liu et al., 2024 [136]
O. sinensis	Mycelium extract	Placebo	NR	Peri-procedure	CA-AKI risk	n = 1271	Systematic review	AKI incidence	Serum Cr	↓ CA-AKI incidence	RR <1	Moderate	Pu et al., 2024 [138]
O. sinensis	Mycelium	Placebo	1 g (3.5 mg of adenosine and 40 mg polysaccharide)	Single dose	Healthy young adults	n = 14	DB crossover RCT	Muscle recovery	$CD34^+$/$Pax7^+$ cells	Accelerated stem-cell recruitment	Not pooled	Low	Dewi et al., 2024 [276]
O. sinensis	Cordyceps capsules	Placebo	1.5 g (3 × 500 mg)	15 days	Mild-moderate COVID-19	65 (32/33)	Double-blind RCT	Recovery time	Viral load days at hospital; Serum biomarkers	Faster recovery vs placebo	Moderate	Some concerns	ANM Health (2023) [164]
O. sinensis	*Cordyceps sinensis*	Chemo alone		6 months	NSCLC	60	RCT		Survival, QoL	Improved survival, QoL	Moderate	Some concerns	Hao et al. (2008) [277]

https://doi.org/10.3390/ph19030519

Table A8. *Cont.*

Species	Botanical Material/ Product	Comparator	Daily Dose	Duration	Population/ Condition	Sample Size	Study Design (GCP) *	Primary Endpoints	Outcome Measures	Key Clinical Results	Effect Size (reported/ Calculable)	Risk of Bias (Cochrane)	Citation
O. sinensis	Cordyceps + NP regimen	NP regimen		6 months	Advanced NSCLC	80	RCT		Tumour response	Improved response rate	Moderate	Some concerns	Hao et al. (2007) [278]
O. sinensis	CBG-CS-2 mycelium	Placebo		8 weeks	Healthy adults	80	Double-blind RCT		Immune markers	↑ immune markers	Moderate	Low	Jung et al. (2019) [279]
O. sinensis	Cordyceps + anthocyanin	Placebo		8 weeks	Middle-aged adults	40	Double-blind RCT		Mental condition	Improved mood	Small	Some concerns	Morikubo et al. (2005) [280]
O. sinensis	Cordyceps extract	Placebo		6 weeks	Asthma	120	Double-blind RCT		HRQoL	Improved HRQoL	Moderate	Some concerns	Wang et al. (2016) [165]
O. sinensis	*C. sinensis* capsules	Placebo	2400 mg in 6 capsules	8 weeks	Healthy young adults	30	Double-blind RCT		Testosterone, strength	No effect	None	Low	Hsu et al. (2011) [155]
O. sinensis	Extract powder	Placebo	0.5 g	2 weeks	Exhaustive running exercise	36	Double-blind RCT	Recovery time	Respiratory variables, heart rate, and lactate,	↓ fatigue ↓ recovery time	Significant difference vs. placebo	Some concerns	Nagata et al., 2006 [152]
C. militaris	*C. militaris*	Placebo		3 weeks	Healthy adults	28	Double-blind RCT		Exercise tolerance	↑ tolerance	Small	Low	Hirsch et al. (2017) [153]
C. militaris	Fruiting body extract (standardised)	Placebo	NR	8 weeks	Healthy adults	n = 40	DB-PC RCT	Immune response	NK activity	Significant ↑ NK activity	SMD moderate	Low	Ontawong et al., 2024 [162]
C. militaris	Mycelium extract	Placebo	1.5 g/day	8 weeks	Mild liver dysfunction	n = 57	Randomized DB-PC	Liver enzymes	ALT, AST	Significant ↓ ALT & AST vs. placebo	MD −12 U/L Moderate	Low	Heo et al., 2015 [166]
C. militaris (dominant)	PeakO_2 mushroom blend	Placebo	1.0–2.0 g/day) and 12 g/day	28 days	Healthy adults	n = 40 + 43	DB-PC RCT	Endurance	VO_2peak, Time-to-fatigue	↑ VO_2peak in subgroups: Improved tolerance vs. baseline	ES not calculable (no control SD), Heterogeneous	Moderate	Dudgeon et al., 2018 [161]
C. militaris	Fruiting body extract	Placebo	1.8 g/day	16 weeks	Endurance athletes	n = 11	DB-PC RCT	Hematology	Hb, CK	↑ Hb, ↓ muscle damage	MD clinically relevant	Low	Nakamura et al., 2024 [154]
C. militaris	Mycelium capsules+ duloxetine	Placebo + duloxetine	4 g/day	6 weeks	Depression with insomnia	n = 59	Double-blind RCT	Changes in the Athens Insomnia Scale (AIS) score Sleep quality	Sleep quality PSQI, ISI	*C. militaris* did not improve sleep symptoms in patients with depression; no superiority over placebo.	0.6	Low–Moderate	Zhou et al., 2021 [167]

*—DB-PC = double-blind placebo-controlled, RCT = randomized controlled trial, ES = effect size, RoB = Risk of Bias (Cochrane domains, summary judgment); **—C19-YRSm—modified COVID-19 Yorkshire Rehabilitation Scale including the following symptoms in the symptom severity subscale: breathlessness; cough/throat sensitivity/voice change; fatigue; smell/taste; pain/discomfort; cognition; palpitations/dizziness; post-exertional malaise; anxiety/mood; and sleep. Each item was scored on a scale from 0–3 to indicate severity.

https://doi.org/10.3390/ph19030519

Table A9. Clinical trials evaluating *O. sinensis* for fatigue and related outcomes in COVID-19 and Long COVID.

Study, Year	Preparation/ Dose	Population	Study Design	Duration	Fatigue-Related Outcomes	Meta-Analysis Results	Main Findings	Key limitations	GRADE-Style Certainty *
Chen et al., 2025 [163]	*O. sinensis* Cs-4® (fermented mycelium)	Long COVID patients	Randomized, waitlist-controlled clinical trial	12 weeks	Fatigue severity scales, exercise tolerance, HRQoL	No meta-analysis available (single RCT); aligns with pooled post-viral fatigue effects of adaptogens	Significant reduction in fatigue severity and improvement in functional capacity and QoL compared with usual care	Single-region study; short follow-up; patient-reported outcomes	Moderate (exploratory) ●●●○
ANM Health, 2023 [164]	*O. sinensis* Capsules (add-on therapy)	Mild–moderate COVID-19 patients	Randomized, double-blind, placebo-controlled	14–28 days	Fatigue, recovery time, QoL	Not pooled; excluded from formal meta-analyses due to reporting limitations	Faster symptom resolution and reduced fatigue compared with placebo	Industry-sponsored; non–peer-reviewed; limited methodological transparency	Low ●●○○

* Level of evidence reflects EMA/HMPC-oriented qualitative grading, not formal regulatory classification. Abbreviations: HRQoL, health-related quality of life. DB-RCT, double-blind randomized controlled trial.

GRADE-Style Certainty Explanation (Adapted for Frontiers):

- ●●●● **High:** Very unlikely to change confidence
- ●●●○ **Moderate:** Likely to have an important impact on confidence
- ●●○○ **Low:** Further research is very likely to change the estimate
- ●○○○ **Very low:** Evidence uncertainty

Appendix A.4. Network Pharmacology/Systems Pharmacology

The 22 studies in which network pharmacology/systems pharmacology was combined with wet-lab or clinical validation (animal models, cell experiments, or RCTs) are listed in Table A10. The 15 in-silico prediction studies by network pharmacology analysis are listed in Table A11.

https://doi.org/10.3390/ph19030519

Table A10. Overview of network-pharmacology studies of *O. sinensis*, *C. militaris* preparations, and cordycepin, supported by experimental validation.

Study (Year)	Dose/Concentration Main Bioactive Compounds	Disease or Physiological Function	Key Targets/Nodes Validated	Signaling Pathways	Type of Validation & Main Mechanistic Outcome
Jiang et al., 2023 [175]	*O. sinensis*; arachidonic acid, lysergol, glycitein; stigmasterol, sitosterol, linoleic acetate, karanjin, aurantiamide acetate, and berberine. 1000 mg/kg in rats,	Ischemic stroke	CASP3, PTGS2, and PPARG, AR, NOS2, PTGS2, PTGS1, CYP17A1, ADRB2, CHRM2, ESR1, RXRA, and SCN5A	IL-17, AGE-RAGE, and TNF signaling pathways	The mechanism of action of *O. sinensis* is related to the regulation of blood lipids, anti-apoptotic effects, and anti-inflammatory effects. The results of the docking analysis suggest that sitosterol, lysergol, and stigmasterol have high affinities to some core proteins (CASP3, PTGS2, PPARG, JUN, and ESR1.
Wang et al., 2017 [177]	*O. sinensis*, Cordycepin. 0.2, 1 or 2 mg/kg In mice	Hepatitis B vaccine adjuvant	Immune-response targets related to B- and T-cell activation and cytokine signaling	Immune & vaccine-response pathways (e.g., T-cell receptor, cytokine signaling)	Systems pharmacology predicted cordycepin as an adjuvant; BALB/c mouse vaccination showed enhanced humoral and cellular HBV responses without apparent toxicity. Effects of cordycepin (C) on serum HBV antibodies, lymphocyte proliferation and cytokine levels in spleen cell supernatants.
Zhang X et al., 2023 [178]	*O. sinensis* extract A total of 54 active ingredients which are not specified for their name and chemical structure. 300, 600, 1200 mg/kg in mice	Lung adenocarcinoma	Breast cancer type 1 susceptibility protein (BRCA1) and G1/S-specific cyclin-E1 (CCNE1) and oxidative-stress regulators	PI3K–Akt, HIF-1 signaling, apoptosis pathways	Bioinformatics + network analysis predicted anti-Lung adenocarcinoma targets; in vivo validation showed *O. sinensis* inhibits tumor growth and modulates these pathways.
Ma and Jin, 2024 [143]	*O. sinensis* 121 bioactive compounds, including cordycepin	Chronic obstructive pulmonary disease (COPD)	CXCR4, PDGFRB, PARP1, SRC, HIF1A, NFKB1, HDAC 2, and PKACA	Chemokine signaling	The target analysis of the Bailing capsule's effects revealed interactions with multiple targets. The study suggested that the mechanism might involve interactions with chemokines, tyrosine kinase receptors, and other related molecular signaling pathways.
Zhou et al., 2025 [174]	*C. sinensis* Sphingolipid. 0.405 g/kg/day (L-CS), 0.81 g/kg/day (M-CS), and 1.62 g/kg/day (H-CS); in rats	Chronic obstructive pulmonary disease (COPD)	PLA2G4E and B4GALT4 proteins AKT1, ESR1, TLR4, and MMP9; TNF-α, IL-8, and multiple metabolic proteins	PI3K-AKT signaling pathway Inflammatory and metabolic pathways	*O. sinensis* alleviated lung injury, cytokine profiles, and inflammation in the COPD model of rats; Proteomics + metabolomics + network analysis connected altered proteins/metabolites to COPD-relevant pathways including PI3K-AKT signaling pathway in COPD rats, potentially affecting glycerophospholipid metabolism and sphingolipid metabolism by targeting PLA2G4E and B4GALT4 proteins, thereby alleviating the inflammatory response and mitigating lung tissue damage caused by COPD.
Zhang Y et al., 2023 [179]	*O. sinensis*; arachidonic acid, linoleyl acetate, cerevisterol, beta-sitosterol, peroxyergosterol, cholesterol, and cholesteryl palmitate. 50 µg/mL fermented *O. sinensis* (in vitro a proximal tubular HK-2 cell line derived from normal human kidney)	diabetic kidney disease	RELA, JNK1, PTEN, VEGFA, EGF, ERK2, CASP3, AKT1, MMP9. *O. synensis* downregulated the expressions of Bax, Caspase-3, VEGFA, P-AKT, and P-ERK, and upregulated the expression of PTEN	AKT and ERK signaling pathway	*O. synensis* has nephroprotective effects, which functions via promoting proliferation and inhibiting apoptosis of renal proximal tubular cells, likely by targeting Caspase-3, Bax, VEGFA and PTEN.
Li et al., 2024 [180]	*O. sinensis* adenosine; 2′deoxyadenosine; cordycepin; adenine; uracil; hypoxanthine; uridine; guanosine hydrate; thymidine. CS extract (150 mg/kg in mice; 2′-deoxyadenosine The dose is Not specified	acute kidney injury (AKI)	STING, Irf3, Perforin, IFN-γ, GAPDH	STING/IRF3 pathway	2′-deoxyadenosine treatment significantly alleviated FA-induced renal damage in vivo and alleviated the renal injury in NK cells by activating the STING/IRF3 pathway to inhibit perforin release in vitro. 2′-deoxyadenosine could mitigate AKI by downregulating NK cell activity (by decreasing perforin and IFN-γ expression) and inhibiting the stimulator of interferon genes and phosphorylated IFN regulatory factor 3.

https://doi.org/10.3390/ph19030519

Table A10. *Cont.*

Study (Year)	Dose/Concentration Main Bioactive Compounds	Disease or Physiological Function	Key Targets/Nodes Validated	Signaling Pathways	Type of Validation & Main Mechanistic Outcome
Tao et al., 2024 [139]	*O. sinensis* mycelial preparation (Bailing capsules), including arachidonic acid, linoleoyl acetate, cerevisterol, beta-sitosterol, peroxyergosterol, cholesteryl palmitate, and cholesterol 0.8–5 g/day in humans	Chronic kidney disease (CKD), human RCT	Inflammatory & metabolic renal function markers including: PTPN1, HSD11B1, HSD11B2, HMGCR, AR, NR1H3, NR3C1, CNR2, CYP19A1, CYP17A1, and DRD2	Neuroactive ligand-receptor interaction, Chemical carcinogenesis receptor activation, Diabetic cardio-myopathy, cAMP signaling, Inflammatory mediator regulation of TRP channels, Insulin resistance, Proteoglycans, Serotonergic synapse, AGE-RAGE signaling, EGFR tyrosine kinase inhibitor resistance, Prolactin signaling, Endocrine resistance, C-type lectin receptor, ErbB, VEGF, Arachidonic acid metabolism, and Adipocytokine signaling pathways.	Network pharmacology analysis identified 190 common targets of *O. synensis* (Bailing Capsule) and chronic kidney disease associated with immune response, inflammatory response, vascular endothelial damage, cell proliferation, and fibrosis. Clinical trials showed improved renal indices and reduced inflammation when the Bailing capsule was added to standard CKD therapy. Mechanistic validation is indirect but consistent.
He et al., 2020 [181]	*O. sinensis* Adenosine exopolysaccharide, amino acid, mannitol human keratinocyte line HaCaT (50, 250, and 500 µg/mL extract	UVB-induced damage in human keratinocytes	Aquaporin 3 (AQP3)	PPAR signaling pathway, cholesterol metabolism, and ovarian steroidogenesis.	Cordyceps significantly decreased intracellular UVB-induced oxidative stress, including ROS production and intracellular H2O2 content. Besides, AQP3, which mediates intracellular signaling and transports H2O2 into cells, was significantly increased in the presence of Cordyceps extract under UVB irradiation. In addition, the DNA repair effect of Cordyceps extract after UV irradiation was proven to be effective by the comet assay.
Pei et al., 2023 [182]	*C. militaris* polysaccharides	Immune modulation (non-specific, innate/adaptive immunity)	TNF, MAPK3, CASP3, VEGFA, STAT3; TLR4	Toll-like receptor (TLR4), TNF-α signaling; macrophage M1↔M2 polarization and immune activation, apoptosis, cytokine pathways	Network analysis identified immune targets enriched in TLR pathways; in vitro macrophage assays showed altered polarization, and in vivo mouse experiments confirmed TLR4/TNF-α activation by *C. militaris* polysaccharides consistent with predictions.
Kim et al., 2025 [183]	*C. militaris* extracts (cordycepin, adenosine) Lung cancer cell lines (LLC1, H460, H1299	Lung cancer	p53, EGFR, apoptosis-related targets	PI3K–Akt, p53, apoptosis	Network pharmacology/docking indicated cordycepin and adenosine as key ligands targeting EGFR/p53-related networks; cell experiments showed enhanced apoptosis and anticancer activity, particularly after optimizing extraction/drying procedures to enrich key actives.
Wang et al., 2025 [184]	*C. militaris* fruiting body; nucleosides (uridine, guanosine, adenosine, cordycepin, N^6-(2-hydroxyethyl)adenosine);	Chronic obstructive pulmonary disease (COPD)	IDH1, CYP19A1, lipid-metabolism targets	Linoleic acid metabolism, inflammatory and oxidative pathways	HPLC fingerprinting + metabolomics + network pharmacology; COPD mouse model demonstrated improved lung function and pathology; docking supported strong binding of CM components to IDH1/CYP19A1.
Zhou et al., 2024 [185]	*C. militaris* (cordycepin, ergosterol) 100 and 200 mg/kg/d *C. militaris* extract;	Gouty nephropathy/hyperuricemia	cyclooxygenase-2 (COX-2); renal transport proteins ABCG2, GLUT9, and URAT1; Xanthine oxidase (XO),	Inflammation (PTGS2, NLRP3, etc.) signaling pathway and uric acid metabolic pathway (XDH, ADA, UMOD).	Network pharmacology suggested cordycepin + ergosterol as core ligands; in vivo data show anti-hyperuricemic effect via XO inhibition and modulation of renal urate transporters.
Gandhale et al., 2024 [186]	*C. militaris* adenosine, cinnamic acid, citric acid, cordycepin, dipicolinic acid, ergosterol, fumaric acid, hypoxanthine, N-acetylgalactosamine, p-hydroxybenzoic acid, β-sitosterol, and δ-tocopherol Vero E6 cells (25, 50, 75, 100 µg/mL) *C. militaris* aqueous extract in-vitro	SARS-CoV-2	Multiple targets	Numerous interactions	Cordycepin, Cicadapeptin-I, Cicadapeptin-II, Cordycerebroside-B, and N-Acetyl galactosamine were found to be top scorers To assess the anti-SARS-CoV-2 activity of the *C. militaris* aqueous extract in-vitro, at 80% confluency, Vero E6 cells were infected in triplicate with SARS-CoV-2
Lee et al., 2019 [187]	Cordycepin and *C. militaris* extract constituents MCF-7 human breast cancer cell line, treatment with *C. militaris* (100 µg/mL) and cordycepin (25, 50 µM).	Breast cancer (MCF-7 cells)	Apoptosis-related proteins: CASP3, BAX, BCL2, X-linked inhibitor of apoptosis protein (XIAP) Caspases; p53, Hedgehog signaling components	Apoptosis, p53, Hedgehog, estrogen, PI3K–Akt, pathways	Cordycepin exhibited the ability to induce apoptotic cell death by increasing the cleavage of caspase-7, -8, and -9, increasing the Bax/Bcl-2 protein expression ratio, and decreasing the protein expression of X-linked inhibitor of apoptosis protein (XIAP) in MCF-7 cells. Consequently, the *C. militaris* concentrate and cordycepin exhibited significant anticancer effects through their ability to induce apoptosis in breast cancer cells.

https://doi.org/10.3390/ph19030519

Table A10. *Cont.*

Study (Year)	Dose/Concentration Main Bioactive Compounds	Disease or Physiological Function	Key Targets/Nodes Validated	Signaling Pathways	Type of Validation & Main Mechanistic Outcome
Chen et al., 2024 [57]	Cordycepin (10 μM, 20 μM, 50 μM, 100 μM, or 200 μM) in The human breast cancer cell lines MCF7 and MDA-MB-231, as well as the human monocyte cell line THP-1.	breast cancer	Alumin gene ALB	protein tetramerization, regulation of protein complex disassembly, and somatic diversification of immunoglobulin signaling	Cordycepin regulates tumor immune suppression by upregulating the downregulated ALB, thereby playing an anti-tumor role.
Qui et al., 2025 [188]	Cordycepin	Fibrosarcoma	AKT1	Akt1 (protein kinase B) and disruption of protein phosphorylation pathways	Cordycepin significantly inhibited cell activity at an effective concentration of 100 μmol/L. Key observations included changes in cell morphology, reduced migration, inhibited proliferation, cell cycle arrest at the G0/G1 and G2/M phases, and induction of apoptosis. Western blot analysis further confirmed that cordycepin simultaneously downregulated both the expression and phosphorylation levels of Akt in a dose-dependent manner.
Zhong et al., 2025 [189]	Cordycepin 50 mg/kg/d, 100 mg/kg/d, 200 mg/kg/d of cordycepin in mice	Cancer immunosuppression	EGFR, upregulated the protein expression of Nrf2, NQO1 and HO-1 in the spleens	metabolic and immune pathways	Cordycepin ameliorated cyclophosphamide-induced immunosuppression of mice by reversing metabolic dysfunction and activating the Nrf2 pathway through regulating EGFR, indicating its potential as a therapeutic agent for immunosuppression.
Chen et al., 2022 [190]	Cordycepin (alone and in combination) 80 mM of cordycepin in Human glioblastoma cells (LN-229, U251, T98G)	Glioblastoma (GBM)	Multiple tumor and apoptosis targets (predicted network)	PI3K-Akt, apoptosis, cell proliferation pathways	Network pharmacology predicted synergy; in vitro assays supported enhanced cytotoxicity when cordycepin combined with doxorubicin; docking suggested binding to targets involved in GBM survival.
Wang et al., 2025 [102]	Cordycepin 20 mg/kg and 40 mg/kg In rats	Chronic unpredictable mild stress (CUMS) induced depression	Cordycepin increased protein levels of p-GSK3β, β-catenin, and nuclear β-catenin, and enhanced transcription of downstream genes PKM, LDHA, Cyclin D1 and C-myc in brains of CUMS-induced rats	GSK3β/β-catenin signaling	Cordycepin exerted an antidepressant effect by modulating the GSK3β/β-catenin pathway. Western blot and Real-time PCR were applied to validate the signaling pathway.
Lin et al., 2024 [191]	Cordycepin	Pulmonary arterial hypertension (PAH)	TP53, AKT1, CASP3, BAX, BCL2L1	Apoptosis, PI3K–Akt, vascular remodeling pathways	Network analysis and docking identified PAH-core genes; in MCT-induced PAH rats, cordycepin reduced RVSP and vascular remodeling and modulated PASMC proliferation/apoptosis,
Liao et al., 2025 [192]	Cordycepin (±5′-monophosphate) 40 mg/kg in mice.	Western-diet–induced obesity	CPS1, HRAS, MAPK14, AKT1, GSK3B, EGFR, CASP3, APOA1/2/3, APOM, etc.	Metabolic pathways, insulin signaling, HIF-1, FOXO, lipid & atherosclerosis, TNF, IL-17, Toll-like receptor signaling, inflammatory pathways	Integrated network pharmacology, transcriptomics, and docking analysis identified 244 potential targets and core hubs; cordycepin improved obesity and metabolic parameters in animal experiments: core targets and pathways involved in obesity were validated by gene expression and phenotypic changes. The authors uncover a potential mechanism of action of cordycepin against obesity through network pharmacology and quantitative transcriptomics, providing evidence for obesity pathogenesis and suggesting that cordycepin is a potential lead compound for anti-obesity treatment.

https://doi.org/10.3390/ph19030519

Table A11. Overview of network-pharmacology studies on *Ophiocordyceps sinensis*, *Cordyceps militaris*, and cordycepin, in-silico predictions without experimental validation.

Study (Year)	Main Bioactive Compounds	Disease or Physiological Function	Key Targets/Nodes Validated	Signaling Pathways	Type of Mechanistic Outcome
Li J. et al., 2021 [193]	*O. sinensis*, 6 main active ingredients, including adenosine, ergosterol,	Liver cirrhosis,	MAPK1, CASP8, TNF, VEGFA	Hepatitis B, cancer, apoptosis, and inflammation signaling	Modulation of inflammatory and apoptotic pathways.
Mu et al., 2023 [194]	*O. sinensis*; arachidonic acid, sitosterol, berberine, Higenamine, Cordycepin, Uralene. Crachidonic aci Caffeine	Liver cancer	TNF, CASP3, BCL2, IL6, VEGF-A, NF, Caspase 3 (CASP3), B-Cell Lymphoma 2 (BCL2), Interleukin-6 (IL-6), Vascular Endothelial Growth Factor-A (VEGF-A), and Prostaglandin-endoperoxide Synthase 2 (PTGS2)	hepatitis B, cancer, Advanced Glycation Endproducts-Receptor for Advanced Glycation Endproducts (AGE-RAGE) signaling pathway, non-alcoholic fatty liver disease, hepatitis C, alcoholic liver disease, and IL-17 signaling pathway, Nucleotide-binding Oligomerization Domain (NOD)-like receptor signaling pathway, and TNF signaling pathway	The authors suggest that the antitumor effect of *O. sinensis* primarily in hepatocellular carcinoma originates from its intricate influence on the target proteins through a complex interplay of its constituents.
Gonzalez-Llerena et al., 2025 [195]	129 compounds, including cordycepsidone A, jiangxienone, and flazin, exhibiting binding affinity comparable or superior to clinically used inhibitors across the Cordyceps genus (including *C. militaris*, *O. sinensis*)	Cancer (broad anticancer potential)	Hub proteins such as TYMS, AURKA, and CDK1 were identified as primary targets, Multi-target lists across cancer biology (eg. EGFR, AKT, CASP families)	PI3K-Akt, MAPK, apoptosis, cell cycle, immune pathways; Oncogenic pathways, including cell cycle regulation, DNA replication, and apoptosis.	Systematic identification of putative multitarget anticancer agents in Cordyceps genus; suggests prioritized compounds for further testing.
Ma et al., 2022 [60]	*O. sinensis*, adenosine, ergosterol, nucleosides	Oral lichen planus (OLP)	TNF, IL6, CD4, EGFR, IL1B	PI3K–Akt, MAPK, apoptosis, T-cell activation	Predicted multi-target action; docking supported ligand-target interactions; authors propose anti-inflammatory/immunomodulatory mechanism.
Long et al., 2021 [196]	*O. sinensis* Including daucosterol, vitamin A, inosine, peroxyergosterol, vitamin B1, cerevisterol, linoleic acid, alpha-trehalose, and galactomannan	Hypoxia	O. cordyceps inctrease the expression of MAPK1,MAPK3, VEGFA, and decrease the expression of AKT1, PIK3CA, and RAC1 under hypoxic conditions	VEGF signaling pathway	*O. sinensis* promotes angiogenesis by regulating the VEGF signaling pathway, which might be one of the mechanisms of hypoxia adaptation, and improves the survival rate of H9C2 cells.
Zhang et al., 2022 [197]	*O. sinensis*, 7 main active ingredients: arachidonic acid, linoleyl acetate, beta-sitosterol, peroxyergosterol, cerevisterol, cholesteryl palmitate, and cholesterol	Depression Antidepressant, serotonergic, Anti-neuroinflammatory	Catalase (CAT), CREB binding protein (CREBBP), epidermal growth factor (EGF), and E1A binding protein P300.	The FOXO, the hypoxia-inducible factor 1 (HIF-1), and Huntington's disease signaling pathways, oxidative stress response, and neurotrophic signaling	Authors propose antioxidant and epigenetic (CREB/EP300) modulation as potential antidepressant mechanisms; docking supports several compound–target interactions.
Zhou et al., 2023 [198]	*O. sinensis* D-glutamine 2,3-dihydroxypropyl hexadecanoate 4-(2-aminopropyl) − 2-methoxyphenol Caffeine	Influenza infection	SRC, RHOA, HSP90AA1, VEGFA, EGFR	PI3K-Akt, HIF-1, Influenza A, COVID-19 Innate immunity, cytokine signaling, and antiviral response. Butanoate, thiamine, amino-acid metabolism, TCA, arginine biosynthesis	Predicted immunomodulatory and antiviral host-target modulation and maintain respiratory immune balance via NF κB/IL-17 signaling and PI3K–AKT–linked survival pathways.; docking supported interactions with immune signaling proteins. UPLC-MS metabolomics + network pharmacology + molecular pharmacology; differential metabolites mapped to antiviral pathways, and pharmacological assays supported the anti-influenza effects of selected components by network mapping and glutamine docking to SRC and EGFR, targeting viral/airway targets.
Li Y. et al., 2021a [199]	*O. sinensis*, Seven active ingredients including arachidonic acid, linoleyl acetate, cerevisterol, beta-sitosterol, peroxyergosterol, cholesterol, and cholesteryl palmitate	Diabetic nephropathy (DN)	TNF, MAPK1, EGFR, ACE, CASP3	AGE-RAGE signaling pathway in diabetic complications, TNF signaling pathway, PI3K-Akt signaling pathway, and IL-17 signaling pathway	The mechanism of multicomponent, multitarget, and multichannel action of *O. sinensis* in treating diabetic nephropathy is due to targeting TNF, MAPK1, EGFR, ACE, and CASP3 signaling pathways, which are involved in the inflammatory response, apoptosis, oxidative stress, and insulin resistance.

https://doi.org/10.3390/ph19030519

Table A11. *Cont.*

Study (Year)	Main Bioactive Compounds	Disease or Physiological Function	Key Targets/Nodes Validated	Signaling Pathways	Type of Mechanistic Outcome
Xi et al., 2024 [200]	Bailing capsules (*O. sinensis* preparations), various metabolites	Diabetic nephropathy	TNF, IL6, TGF-β–related nodes, oxidative stress targets	AGE-RAGE, PI3K–Akt, inflammatory and fibrotic signaling	Network-pharmacology synthesis suggests Bailing capsules act via anti-inflammatory, anti-oxidative and anti-fibrotic multi-target effects in DN.
Guan et al., 2023 [201]	*O. sinensis*; 106 compounds including linoleyl acetate, cholesteryl palmitate, arachidonic acid, and	Polycystic ovary syndrome	JAK2, PPARG, PI3K, and AKT1 were upregulated, whereas those of ESR1 and IRS1 were downregulated in PCOS model mice.	JAK-STAT and PI3K-Akt signaling pathways	qPCR findings indicated that BL exerted anti-PCOS effects via PIK3CA, ESR1, AKT, PPARG, and IRS1 targets affecting PI3K-Akt signaling pathways
Singh et al., 2024 [202]	16 steroids including beta-sitosterol, cholest-5-en-3β-ol, 3β, and 7α-Dihydroxycholest-5-ene Cholest-4-en-3-one	SARS-CoV-2	Glucocorticoid receptor (NR3C1), thrombin (F2),	17 inflammatory pathways	*Cordyceps militaris* as an add-on therapy that may reduce the progression of inflammatory co-morbidities among patients infected with SARS-CoV-
Chen et al., 2025 [203]	Cordycepin	Colorectal Cancer	24 drug targets	activates the p53 signaling	Cordycepin inhibits the proliferation of SW480 cells and suppresses tumor growth by modulating the apoptotic pathway.
Li et al., 2025 [204]	Cordycepin	Cancer	A3 adenosine receptor (A3AR),	MAPK, AMPK, mTOR, and Wnt/β-catenin	
Khan and Tania, 2023 [205]	Cordycepin	Cancer	JNK, MAPK, AMPK, PI3K/Akt, ERK, mTOR, GSK-3b, FAK kinases	the c-Jun N-terminal kinase (JNK), mitogen-activated protein kinase (MAPK), AMP kinase (AMPK), phosphoinositide 3-kinase (PI3K)/Akt, extracellular signal-regulated kinase (ERK), mammalian target of rapamycin (mTOR), glycogen synthase kinase (GSK)-3b, and focal adhesion kinase (FAK) pathways	kinase inhibitors can have crucial roles in cancer treatment, targeting tyrosine kinases might be one of the molecular mechanisms involved in the anticancer potential of cordycepin
Ma X. et al., 2022 [206]	Cordycepin	Alzheimer's disease	AKT1, MAPK8, BCL2L1, FOXO3, and CTNNB1 associated with pathogenic genes APP, MAPT, and PSEN2 and with longevity in Alzheimer's Disease	PI3K-Akt, MAPK, apoptosis, neuroinflammation pathways. Lipid and atherosclerosis,	Network/docking predicted cordycepin interacts with AD-relevant targets and signaling pathways targeting MAPK8, FOXO3, and CTNNB1, which may have significant clinical and treatment implications. The authors present cordycepin as a multi-target candidate for neurodegeneration (with in silico support).

https://doi.org/10.3390/ph19030519

Table A12. Abbreviations of proteins.

Abbreviations	Full Name, and Description
AKT1	Protein Kinase B—regulates survival and metabolism
AMPK	AMP-activated protein kinase (PRKAA1/2/PRKAG1)—cellular energy sensor
BECN1	Beclin-1—core autophagy regulator
CASP1	Caspase 1—cleaves IL-1b/IL-18 and activates pyroptosis
FOXO3	Forkhead Box O3—transcription factor promoting stress resistance
GSDMD	Gasdermin D—effector of pyroptosis
HIF1A	Hypoxia-Inducible Factor 1 Alpha—transcription factor for hypoxia response
HMOX1	Heme Oxygenase 1—cytoprotective enzyme against oxidative stress
KEAP1	Kelch-Like ECH-Associated Protein 1—NRF2 inhibitor
LC3B	Microtubule-Associated Protein 1 Light Chain 3 Beta—autophagosome marker
MAPK1/3	Mitogen-Activated Protein Kinase 1/3—cell proliferation & stress signaling
MAPK14/p38	Mitogen-Activated Protein Kinase 14—controls cytokine response
MAPK8/JNK1	Mitogen-Activated Protein Kinase 8—stress-activated kinase
mTOR	Mechanistic Target of Rapamycin—regulator of growth and autophagy
MYD88	Myeloid Differentiation Primary Response 88—adaptor protein for TLR signaling
NF-kB	Nuclear Factor kappa-light-chain-enhancer of activated B cells—inflammation regulator
NLRP3	NOD-Like Receptor Family Pyrin Domain Containing 3—inflammasome component
NQO1	NAD(P)H Quinone Dehydrogenase 1—detoxification enzyme
NRF2	Nuclear Factor Erythroid 2-Related Factor 2—antioxidant transcription factor
PDK1	Pyruvate Dehydrogenase Kinase 1—reduces oxygen consumption by blocking PDH
PGC-1-α	Peroxisome proliferator-activated receptor gamma coactivator 1-alpha—transcriptional coactivator that regulates the genes involved in energy metabolism.
PI3K	Phosphatidylinositol 3-Kinase—upstream activator of AKT
SIRT1	Sirtuin 1—NAD-dependent deacetylase regulating metabolism and aging
SLC2A1	Glucose Transporter 1—mediates glucose uptake under hypoxia
TLR4	Toll-Like Receptor 4—innate immune sensor for LPS
ULK1	Unc-51 Like Autophagy Activating Kinase 1—initiates autophagy
VEGFA	Vascular Endothelial Growth Factor A—angiogenesis mediator

https://doi.org/10.3390/ph19030519

Table A13. Cordycepin-induced adaptive stress Response Network signaling pathways and biological functions.

Abbreviation	Full Name	Primary Function
PI3K–AKT/FOXO–SIRT Metabolic Survival Axis		
PIK3CA/PIK3CB	Phosphatidylinositol-4,5-Bisphosphate 3-Kinase Catalytic Subunits	Generate PIP3 for AKT activation.
AKT1	Serine/Threonine Kinase 1	Promotes cell survival and metabolism.
FOXO3	Forkhead Box O3	Transcription factor inducing stress resistance and repair genes.
SIRT1	NAD-Dependent Deacetylase Sirtuin 1	Regulates metabolism, stress resistance, and longevity.
TP53 (p53)	Tumor Protein p53	DNA damage response and apoptosis regulator.
AMPK–mTOR–Autophagy Axis		
AMPK	AMP-activated protein kinase (subunits PRKAA1, PRKAA2, PRKAG1)	Cellular energy sensor; activates catabolic pathways to restore ATP.
mTOR	Mechanistic Target of Rapamycin	Regulates growth, protein synthesis, and autophagy.
ULK1	Unc-51 Like Autophagy Activating Kinase 1	Initiates autophagy signaling downstream of AMPK.
BECN1	Beclin-1	Core autophagy regulator; nucleates autophagosome formation.
LC3B (MAP1LC3B)	Microtubule-Associated Proteins 1A/1B Light Chain 3B	Marker of autophagosome membrane formation.
SQSTM1/p62	Sequestosome 1	Cargo receptor linking ubiquitinated proteins to autophagy machinery.
ATG5, ATG7	Autophagy Related 5 and 7	Essential enzymes for autophagosome membrane elongation.
NRF2–KEAP1 Antioxidant Axis		
NRF2 (NFE2L2)	Nuclear Factor Erythroid 2–Related Factor 2	Transcription factor controlling antioxidant and detoxification genes.
KEAP1	Kelch-Like ECH-Associated Protein 1	Cytoplasmic inhibitor of NRF2; targets it for degradation.
HMOX1 (HO-1)	Heme Oxygenase 1	Degrades heme; produces cytoprotective metabolites.
NQO1	NAD(P)H Quinone Dehydrogenase 1	Detoxifies quinones and prevents redox cycling.
SOD2	Superoxide Dismutase 2, mitochondrial	Converts superoxide radicals to hydrogen peroxide.
CAT	Catalase	Converts hydrogen peroxide to water and oxygen.
GPX1	Glutathione Peroxidase 1	Reduces lipid and hydrogen peroxides using glutathione.
TLR4–MyD88–NF-κB/MAPK Inflammatory Axis		
TLR4	Toll-Like Receptor 4	Pattern-recognition receptor sensing bacterial LPS.
MYD88	Myeloid Differentiation Primary Response 88	Adaptor protein mediating TLR/IL-1 receptor signaling.
IKBKB	Inhibitor of NF-κB Kinase Subunit Beta	Phosphorylates IκB, enabling NF-κB nuclear translocation.
NFKB1/RELA (p50/p65)	Nuclear Factor κB Subunits	Master regulators of inflammation, immunity, and apoptosis.
MAPK1/3 (ERK1/2)	Mitogen-Activated Protein Kinases 1/3	Regulate cell proliferation, inflammation, and stress responses.
MAPK8 (JNK1)	c-Jun N-terminal Kinase 1	Mediates apoptosis and stress signaling.
MAPK14 (p38 MAPK)	Mitogen-Activated Protein Kinase 14	Controls cytokine production and inflammatory response.
TNF	Tumor Necrosis Factor Alpha	Proinflammatory cytokine.
IL6	Interleukin 6	Cytokine linking inflammation to metabolism and stress.
PTGS2 (COX-2)	Prostaglandin-Endoperoxide Synthase 2	Catalyzes prostaglandin synthesis in inflammation.
NOS2 (iNOS)	Inducible Nitric Oxide Synthase	Produces nitric oxide in immune defense and inflammation.
NLRP3 Inflammasome/Pyroptosis		
NLRP3	NOD-Like Receptor Family Pyrin Domain Containing 3	Sensor forming inflammasome complexes in response to stress.
CASP1	Caspase 1	Cleaves pro–IL-1β/IL-18 and activates pyroptosis.
GSDMD	Gasdermin D	Executes pyroptotic cell death upon cleavage.
IL1B	Interleukin 1 Beta	Proinflammatory cytokine processed by inflammasome.
IL18	Interleukin 18	Enhances immune and inflammatory responses.
HIF-1 Hypoxia Response		
HIF1A	Hypoxia-Inducible Factor 1 Alpha	Master regulator of hypoxia responses and metabolic adaptation.
VEGFA	Vascular Endothelial Growth Factor A	Promotes angiogenesis and oxygen delivery.

Table A14. Evidence-Tier Framework for Mechanistic Integration.

Evidence Tier	Definition	Data Source	Strength	Limitation
Tier 1: In Silico Prediction	Targets/pathways identified by network pharmacology, molecular docking, and enrichment analysis	KEGG/GO enrichment, PPI networks	Hypothesis-generating	Risk of target inflation; no biological confirmation
Tier 2: Experimental Validation	Predicted pathways confirmed in vitro or in vivo	Cell models, animal studies	Mechanistic support	Often, supra-physiological concentrations, species differences
Their 3: Clinical Evidence	Mechanisms aligned with RCT endpoints or biomarker modulation in humans	RCTs, meta-analyses	Highest relevance	Heterogeneity of preparations; surrogate endpoints

https://doi.org/10.3390/ph19030519

Appendix A.5. Food and Drug Regulation of Cordyceps Mushroom

Table A15. Regulatory status of *O. sinensis* and *C. militaris* worldwide.

Region/Jurisdiction	*O. sinensis*	*C. militaris*	Notes/Caveats/References
China (as food/health-food regulation)	*O. sinensis* is historically used as a medicinal fungus; in China, the wild form is not a regular food, but specific cultivated strains/preparations may have food or "medicine-food homologous" (药食同源) status in some local jurisdictions	*C. militaris* is approved in China as a "new resource food" (新资源食品) (i.e., allowed for food/health food use) since 2009	The Chinese "new resource food" system permits certain traditionally medicinal fungi and their derivatives for official consumption under controlled conditions.
Japan/Korea/East Asia	Often regulated under traditional medicine/health food frameworks, not as general food	*C. militaris* is regarded as an edible and medicinal fungus; considered safe and edible in many Asian settings (used in cuisine and supplements)	In Asian countries, the cultural and historical use supports a more permissive edible status for *C. militaris*.
United States	*O. sinensis* per se is not Generally Recognized As Safe (GRAS)/food-approved; typical marketplace status is as a dietary supplement (mycelium cultures, etc.).	*C. militaris* is generally sold as a dietary supplement; the FDA has issued warning letters when Cordyceps products are marketed as treatment for diseases (i.e., considered new drugs) [233].	The U.S. classifies many mushroom extracts as dietary supplements. If a product claims to treat a disease, the FDA may treat it as a drug.
European Union (Novel Food Regulation)	Mycelium and fruiting body of *O. sinensis* "not novel in food supplements" per updated Novel Food Catalogue (i.e., recognized in supplement use)	*C. militaris* (mycelium and fruiting body) remains classified as unauthorized/novel food in supplements (i.e., not yet accepted)	A February 2025 update clarified that *O. sinensis* mycelium and fruiting bodies are not novel (for supplements), but *C. militaris* is still subject to novel food approval.
EU Food Use beyond supplements	Use of *O. sinensis* outside of supplements (e.g., in foods, beverages) may be treated as Novel and require pre-market authorization under Regulation (EU) 2015/2283	For *C. militaris*, any use (mycelium, fruiting body) in foods or supplements is under novel food control until approved	The non-novel status currently applies only to "food supplements" of *O. sinensis*; other forms may still be novel.

Data derived from peer-reviewed study (Chen 2013 [16]), official food and drug regulatory websites, and Rapid Alert System for Food and Feed (RASFF) notifications [225–235]. The RASFF page shows the alert and the product name. This is robust evidence that *C. militaris* is being flagged by EU member authorities as unauthorized in supplements.

Tables A16–A20 were generated by artificial intelligence (AI) technology (ChatGPT for IOS, version 1202, model, 2025 OpenAI, L.L.C.)

Table A16. Characteristic feature of *Ophiocordyceps sinensis* and *Cordyceps militaris* across key pharmacopoeias and regulatory frameworks.

O. sinensis	*C. militaris*
• Chinese Pharmacopoeia (ChP) ○ ✅ Official monograph for wild *O. sinensis*. ○ Quality markers include adenosine, polysaccharides, and mannitol. Adenosine is considered a key quality indicator. ○ Cordycepin is present only in trace amounts in wild specimens (~0.006–0.075 mg/g), so not a standard assay marker. • Korean Pharmacopoeia (KP) ○ ✅ Official monograph for *C. sinensis*. ○ Standards emphasize adenosine and, likely, polysaccharide content. • Vietnamese & Thai Pharmacopoeias ○ ✅ Often include *C. sinensis* (limited detail available). ○ Typically regulated as herbal supplements or medicinal fungi. • European Union ○ ✅ Recognized as a novel food/dietary supplement. ○ No formal inclusion in the European Pharmacopoeia, but officially permitted under EC/EFSA frameworks. • USA ○ ✅ Included in American Herbal Pharmacopoeia (AHP). ○ ⚠️ Not yet in the USP–NF official drug compendium. Regulated as a dietary supplement.	• Chinese & Korean Pharmacopoeias ○ Historically focused on *C. sinensis*, but *C. militaris* is increasingly recognized in herbal/pharma spheres, especially cultivated strains. • Thai & Vietnamese Pharmacopoeias ○ ✅ Often include *C. militaris*, especially for research and supplement use; however, formal monograph details are sparse. • European Union ○ ⚠️ Not yet listed as a novel food or in Pharm Eur. Products containing *C. militaris* typically require novel-food approval or fall under THMPD (traditional herbal medicinal products) regulations. • USA ○ ✅ Included in AHP. ○ ⚠️ Not yet in the USP–NF official compendia, but prevalent in supplement market.

Table A17. Health Claims (Supplements & Traditional Use) *.

Claim Category	*O. sinensis*	*C. militaris*
Energy and stamina	Traditional use for fatigue, high-altitude sickness	Claimed for fatigue and endurance, supported by more experimental data
Lung health/Respiratory health	Strong traditional use (asthma, COPD, bronchitis)	Similar claims; modern support based on anti-inflammatory effects
Kidney health/Tonic	Major use in Traditional Chinese Medicine (TCM)	Less emphasized traditionally, but included in general tonic claims
Libido/Sexual function	Used as an aphrodisiac and reproductive tonic	Also claimed, with more cordycepin-driven studies
Improving respiratory health	Broad claims in both systems	Often marketed more actively for immune health due to extract standardization
Anti-aging/Longevity	Central to its traditional appeal	Also marketed for longevity, supported by antioxidant research

*—Common Health Claims. Both species are marketed for: Acting as adaptogens to reduce fatigue and stress, enhancing energy and stamina, supporting immune function, and improving respiratory health.

https://doi.org/10.3390/ph19030519

Table A18. Use as Traditional Medicine and as Modern Dietary Supplements.

Category	*O. sinensis*	*C. militaris*
Traditional Chinese Medicine (TCM)	Used for chronic kidney disease, lung weakness, impotence, wasting diseases	Used in similar contexts, but less prestigious historically
Modern Supplements/Functional Foods	Rare, expensive; used in elite or luxury wellness products	Widely available; found in capsules, powders, drinks, etc.
Availability	Wild harvesting leads to scarcity and high prices; may contain contaminants or adulterants	Cultivated industrially; standardized extracts available; more sustainable
Research Base	Historically revered, but limited due to cost/availability	Extensive modern pharmacological studies due to ease of cultivation
Regulatory approval	Limited due to sourcing and consistency	More amenable to standardization and functional food use worldwide

Table A19. Indications for Use as medicines.

Indication	*O. sinensis*	*C. militaris*
Athletic performance	Traditional use	Supported by modern studies
Anti-aging & vitality	Strong cultural use	
Respiratory conditions	Common in TCM	Supported by modern studies
Cancer adjunct therapy	Limited evidence	Supported by modern studies
Immune modulation	Traditional use	Supported by modern studies
Chronic kidney disease	Traditional use	Supported by modern studies
lung weakness	Traditional use	
impotence	Traditional use	
Other chronic wasting diseases	Traditional use	

Table A20. Essential features.

Feature	*O. sinensis*	*C. militaris*
Cordycepin content	Minimal	High
Tradition (TCM)	Considered a superior tonic	Less traditional prestige
Cost	Extremely high	Affordable
Sustainability	Not sustainable	Fully cultivable
Main health focus	Lung, kidney, and general tonic	Immunity, energy, anti-cancer

Table A21. Definitions and Description of Essential Terms.

Term	Definitions and Description
Stress.	Stress is a systemic neuroendocrine response to perceived or actual challenges that threaten homeostasis. Stress is triggered by physical, psychological, metabolic, or social stressors, and mediated primarily by: (i)—Hypothalamic–pituitary–adrenal (HPA) axis (cortisol) and (ii)—Sympathetic nervous system (adrenaline, noradrenaline). The physiological role of stress is to mobilize energy, enhance alertness, and prioritize survival functions. Resolution: Stress hormones return to baseline after the threat passes and require intact feedback mechanisms.
Inflammation.	Inflammation is a localized, innate immune response to tissue injury, infection, or danger signals. Inflammation is triggered by pathogens, tissue damage, or toxins, mediated by immune cells, cytokines, and prostaglandins, and produces classic signs: redness, heat, swelling, pain, and loss of function. The physiological role of inflammation is to eliminate the cause of injury, remove damaged tissue, and initiate tissue repair. Resolution: inflammation is actively terminated by pro-resolving mediators (lipoxins, resolvins), returning tissue to baseline or near-baseline function.
The adaptive stress response.	The adaptive stress response is the organism's capacity to respond to stressors efficiently and recover without damage. Adaptive stress response is characterised by: (i)—flexible activation and deactivation of stress pathways, (ii)—Involves cellular stress responses (heat shock proteins, antioxidant enzymes, autophagy), and (iii)—Maintains allostasis (stability through change). Physiological role: (i)—improves resilience, (ii)—enhances tolerance to future stressors, (iii)—prevents progression to pathology.
Pleiotropic activity.	In medicine, pleiotropic activity refers to a drug's ability to produce multiple effects beyond its primary therapeutic purpose. This phenomenon, known as pleiotropy, can manifest as both additional therapeutic benefits and unwanted side effects. Understanding pleiotropic activity is crucial for drug repurposing, in which an existing drug is used to treat a new, distinct condition. It also influences the development of targeted therapies, as a treatment designed to address the root genetic cause of a condition could potentially alleviate several symptoms simultaneously. This approach offers a holistic method for managing complex genetic disorders, addressing the underlying biological defect rather than just symptoms.

Figures A1–A5 below show the chemical structures of primary and secondary metabolites of *O. sinensis* and *C. militaris*.

https://doi.org/10.3390/ph19030519

Primary metabolites of *O. sinensis* and *C. militaris*

Nucleosides and nucleotides

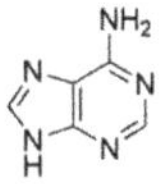

Adenine

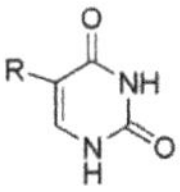

Tiamine R=CH_3

Uracil R=H

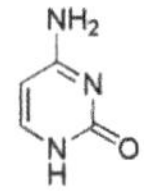

Cytosine

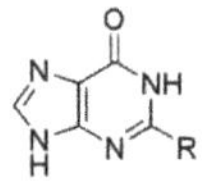

Guanine R=NH_2

Hypoxanthine R=H

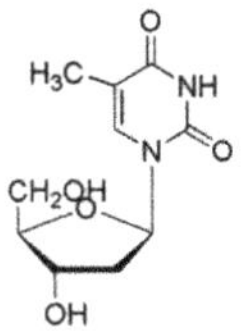

Thymidine

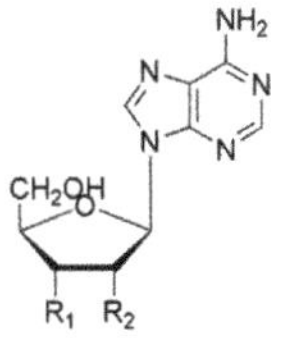

Adenosine R_1=R_2=OH

2'-deoxyadenosine R_1=OH, R_2=H

Cordycepin R_1=H, R_2=OH

3'-amino-2'-deoxyadenosine R_1= NH_2, R_2=OH

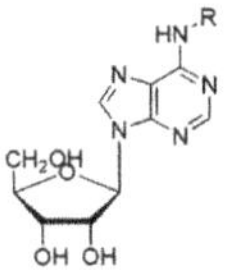

N[6]-methyladenosine R=CH_3

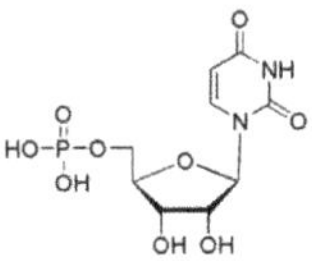

Uridine-5'-monophospate

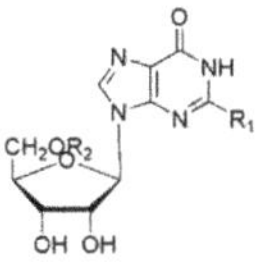

Inosine R_1=R_2=H

Guanosine R_1=NH_2, R_2=H

Guanosine R_1=NH_2, R_2=HPO_4-

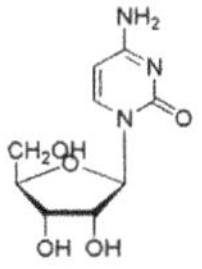

Cytidine

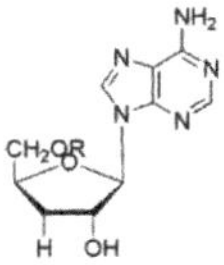

Adenosine-5'-monophosphate R=HPO_4-

O5'-acetylcordycepin R=$COCH_3$

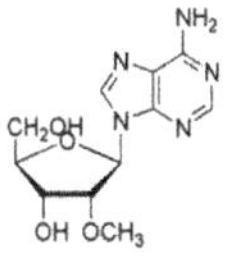

Cordysinin B

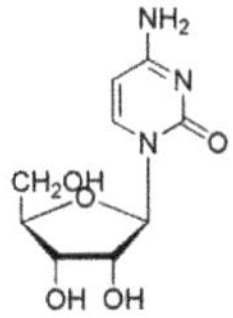

Cytidine

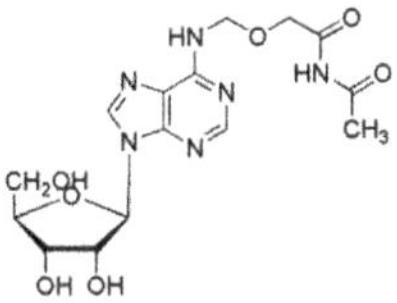

N6-[β-(acetycarbamoyloxy)ethyl]-adenosine

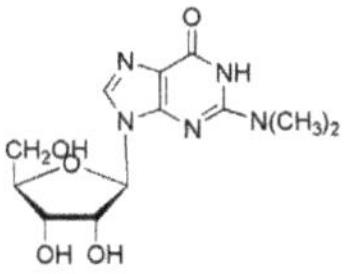

Tiamine

Uracil

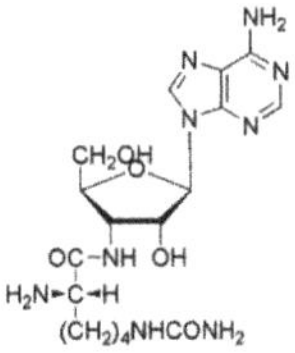

Homocitrullylaminoadenosine

Figure A1. Primary metabolites: nucleosides and nucleotides.

https://doi.org/10.3390/ph19030519

Primary metabolites of *O. sinensis* and *C. militaris*

Sterols

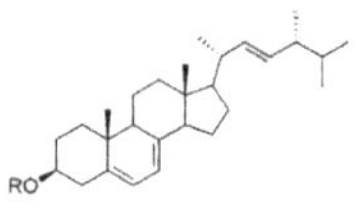

Ergosterol R=H
Ergosteryl-3-O-β-D-glucopyranoside R=Glu

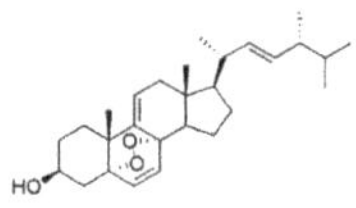

5α,8α-epidioxy-22E-ergosta-6,9-(11)-22-trien-33β-ol

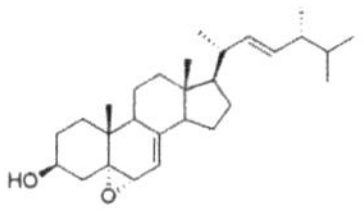

5α,6α-epoxy-5α-ergosta-7,22-dien-3β-ol

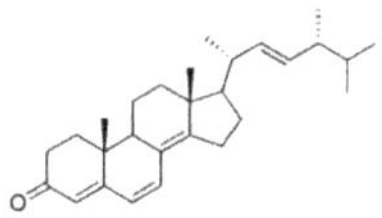

Ergosta-4,6,8(14),22-tetraen-3-one

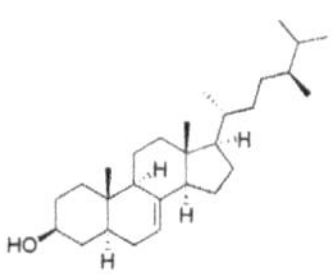

Fungisterol

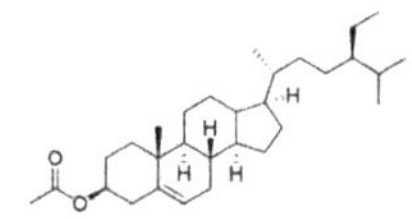

β-sitosterol-3-O-acetate

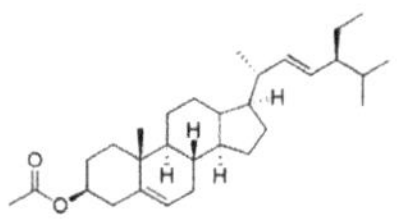

Stigmasterol-3-O-acetate

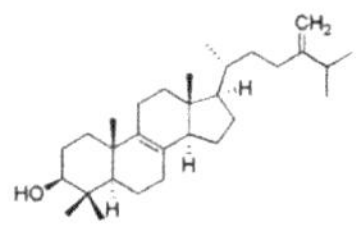

4,4-dimethyl-5α-ergosta-8,24(28)-dien-3β-ol

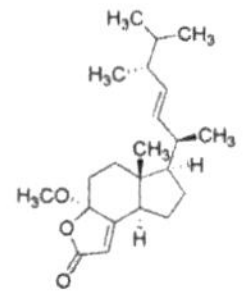

17(R)-17-methyl-lincisterol

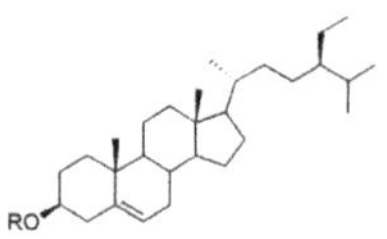

β-sitosterol R=H
Daucosterol R=Glu

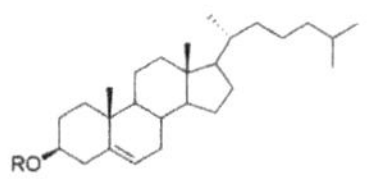

Cholesterol R=H
Cholesteryl palmitate $R=CO(CH_2)_{14}CH_3$

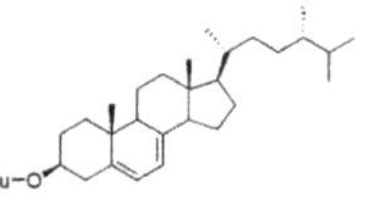

22-dihydro-ergosteryl-3-O-β-D-glucopyranoside

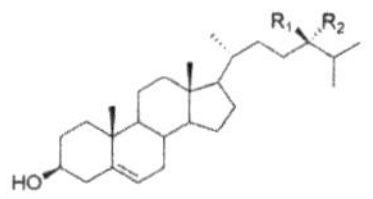

Campesterol $R_1=CH_3$, $R_2=H$
Dihydrobrassicasterol $R_1=H$, $R_2=CH_3$

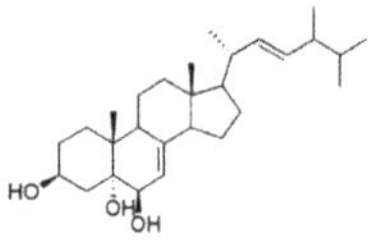

Ergosta-7,22-diene-3,5,6-triol

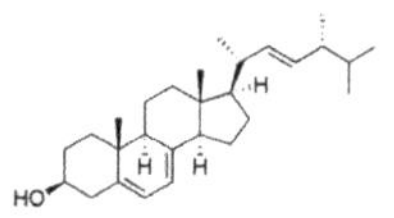

δ-3-Ergosterol

Figure A2. Primary metabolites: sterols.

https://doi.org/10.3390/ph19030519

Secondary metabolites of *O. sinensis*

Alkaloids

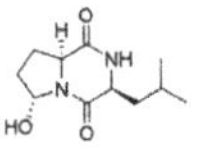

Cordysinin A

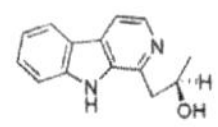

Cordysinin C

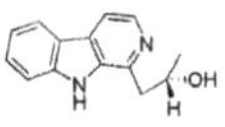

Cordysinins D

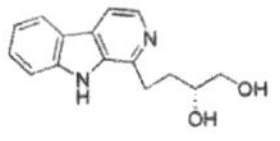

Cordysinins E

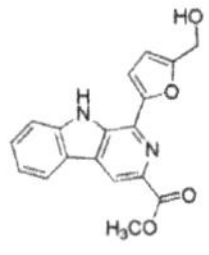

Flazin

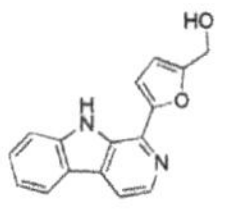

100

Perlolyrine

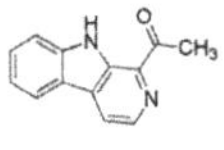

101

1-acetyl-β-carboline

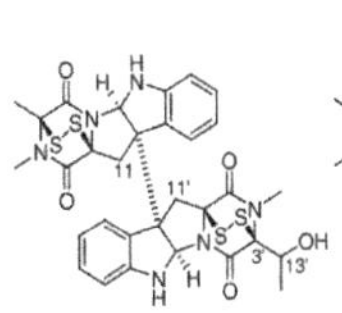

gliocladicillin A

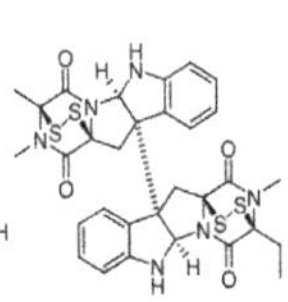

gliocladicillin B

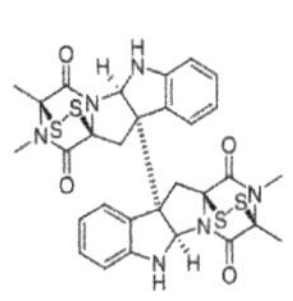

11,11'- dideoxyverticillin

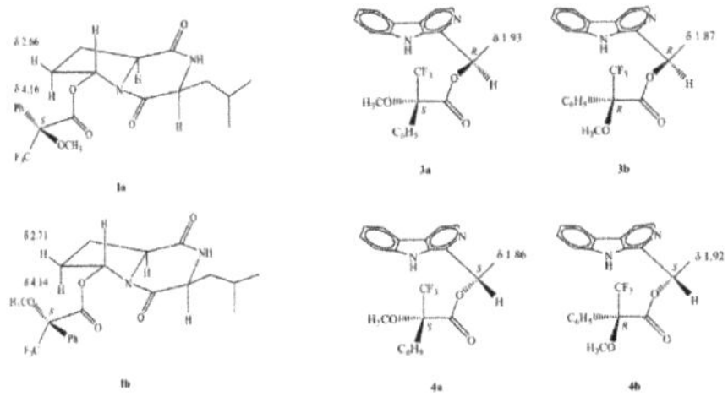

α-methoxy-α-trifluoro-methylphenylacetyl (MTPA) chlorides

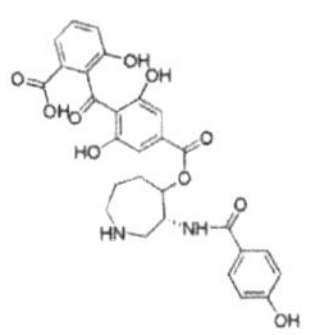

Ophicordin

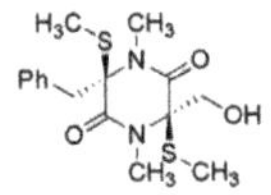

Bisdethiodimethylthio-hyalodendrin

1,3-diaminopropane

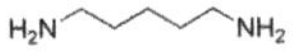

Cadaverine

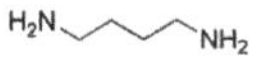

Putrescine

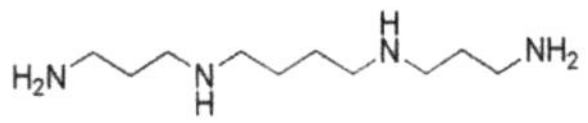

Spermine

Alkaloid cyclopeptides

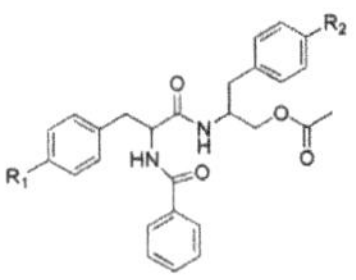

Cordyceamide A R_1=OH, R_2=H

Cordyceamide B R_1=OH, R_2=OH

Aurantamide acetate R_1= R_2=H

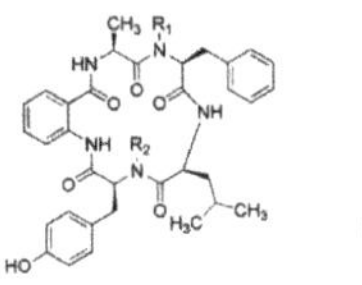

Cycloaspeptide A R_1=CH_3, R_2=CH3

Cycloaspeptide C R_1=H, R_2=CH_3

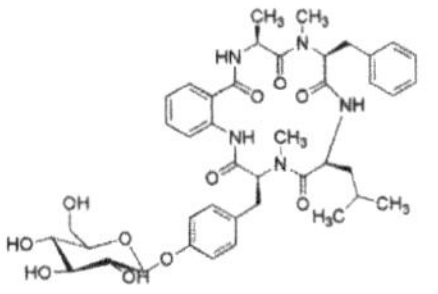

Cycloaspeptide F

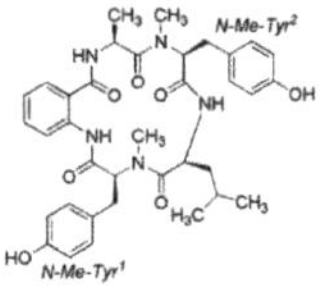

Cycloaspeptide G

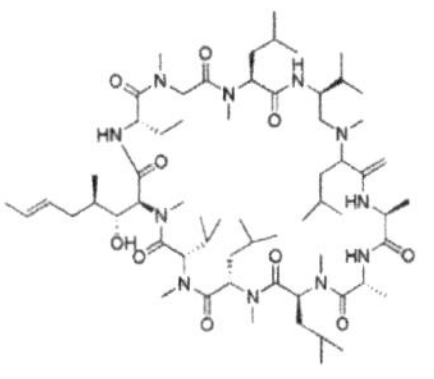

Cyclosporin

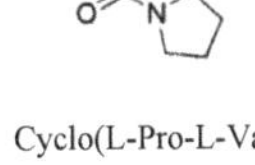

Cyclo(L-Pro-L-Val)

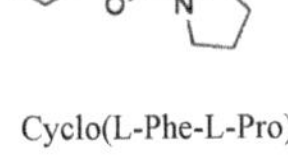

Cyclo(L-Phe-L-Pro)

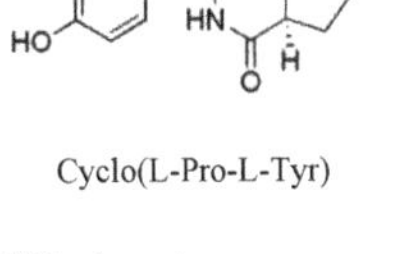

Cyclo(L-Pro-L-Tyr)

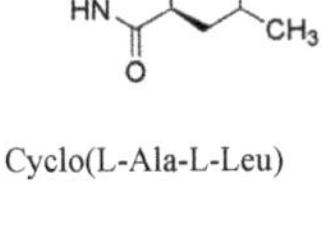

Cyclo(L-Ala-L-Leu)

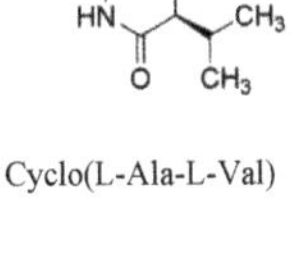

Cyclo(L-Ala-L-Val)

Figure A3. Secondary metabolites of *O. sinensis*.

https://doi.org/10.3390/ph19030519

Secondary metabolites of *O. sinensis*

Flavonoids

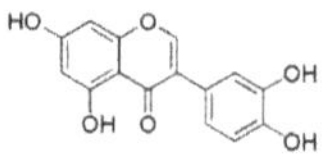

Orobol

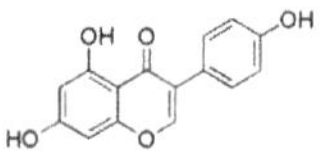

Genistein

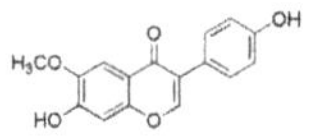

Glycitein

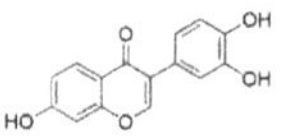

3′,4′,7-trihydroxyisoflavone

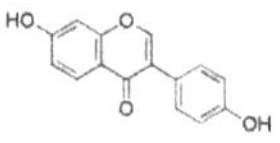

Diadzein

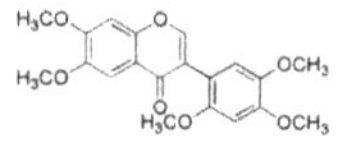

6,7,2′,4′,5′-pentamethoxyflavone

Phenolics

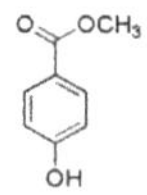

4-Hydroxy-acetophenone

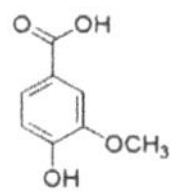

Vanillic acid

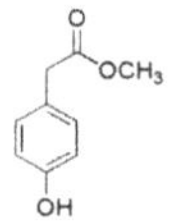

Methyl-p-hydroxy phenylacetate

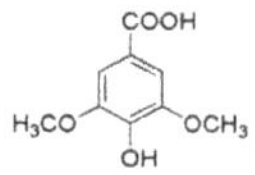

Syringic acid

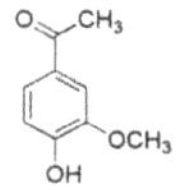

Acetovanillone

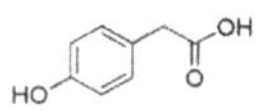

p-hydroxy-phenylacetic acid

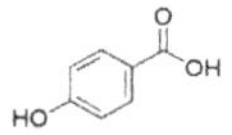

p-hydroxy-benzoic acid

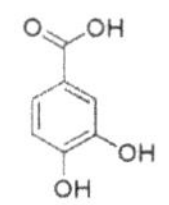

Protocatechuic acid

Miscellaneous

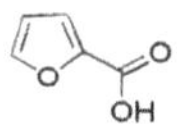

2-Furan-carboxylic acid

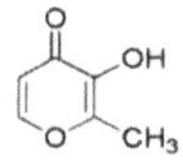

3-hydroxy-2-methyl-4-pyrone

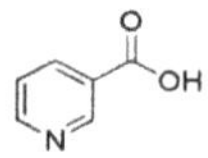

Nicotinic acid

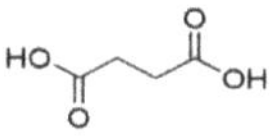

Succinic acid

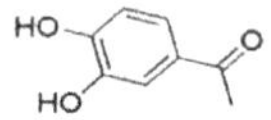

3,4 -dihydroxy-acetophenone

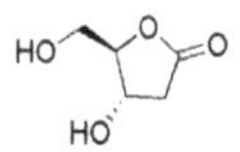

2-Deoxy-D-ribono-1,4-lactone

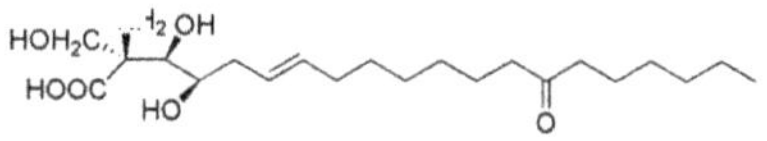

1-Methylpyrimidine-2,4-dione

Figure A4. Secondary metabolites of O. sinensis (continued).

https://doi.org/10.3390/ph19030519

Secondary metabolites of *C. militaris*

Alkaloids

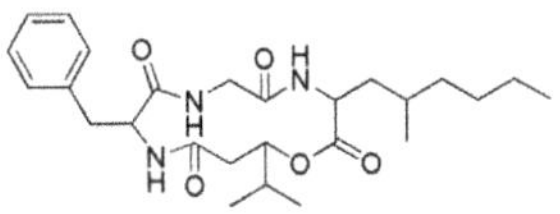

Cordyceptide A

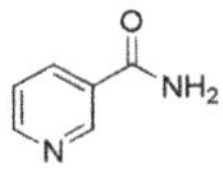

Nicotinic amide

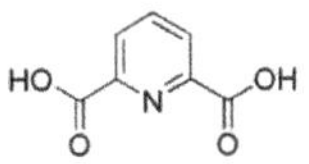

Pyridine-2,6-dicarboxylic acid

Macrolides

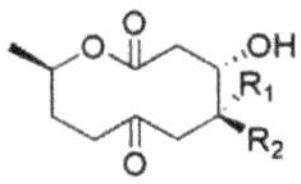

Cepharosporolides C R_1=H, R_2=OH

Inactive Compound R_1=H, R_2=OCH_3

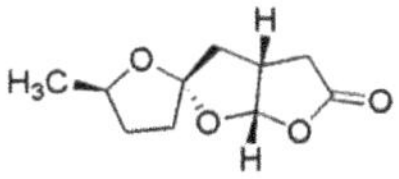

Cepharosporolide E

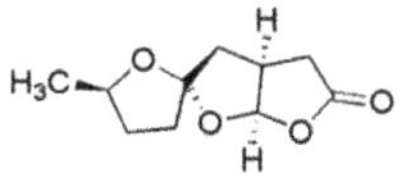

Cepharosporolide E

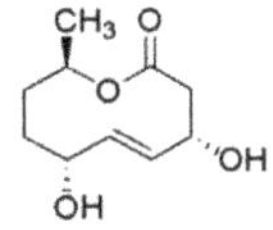

Inactive Compound

Miscellaneous

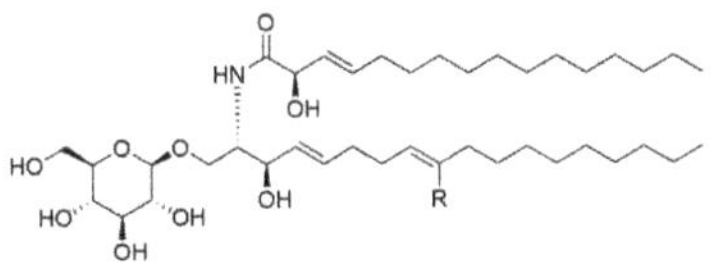

Cordycerebroside A R=CH_3

Soyacerebroside I R=H

Glucocerebroside R=CH_3

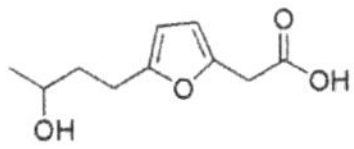

2-Carboxymethyl-4-(3′-hydroxybutyl)furan

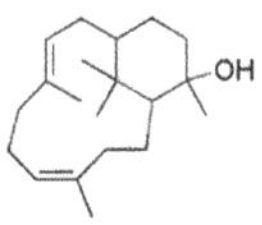

Verticiol

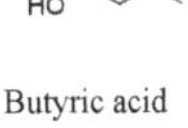

Butyric acid

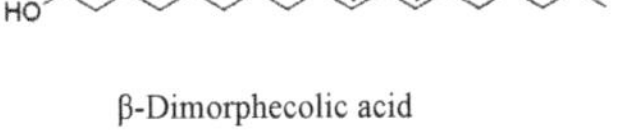

β-Dimorphecolic acid

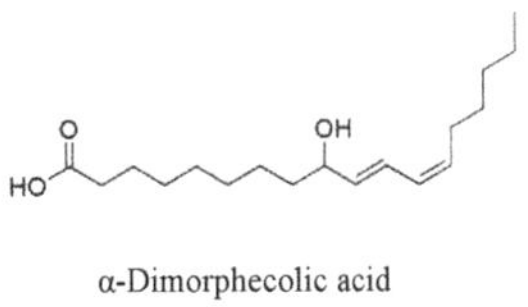

α-Dimorphecolic acid

Figure A5. Secondary metabolites of *C. militaris*.

https://doi.org/10.3390/ph19030519

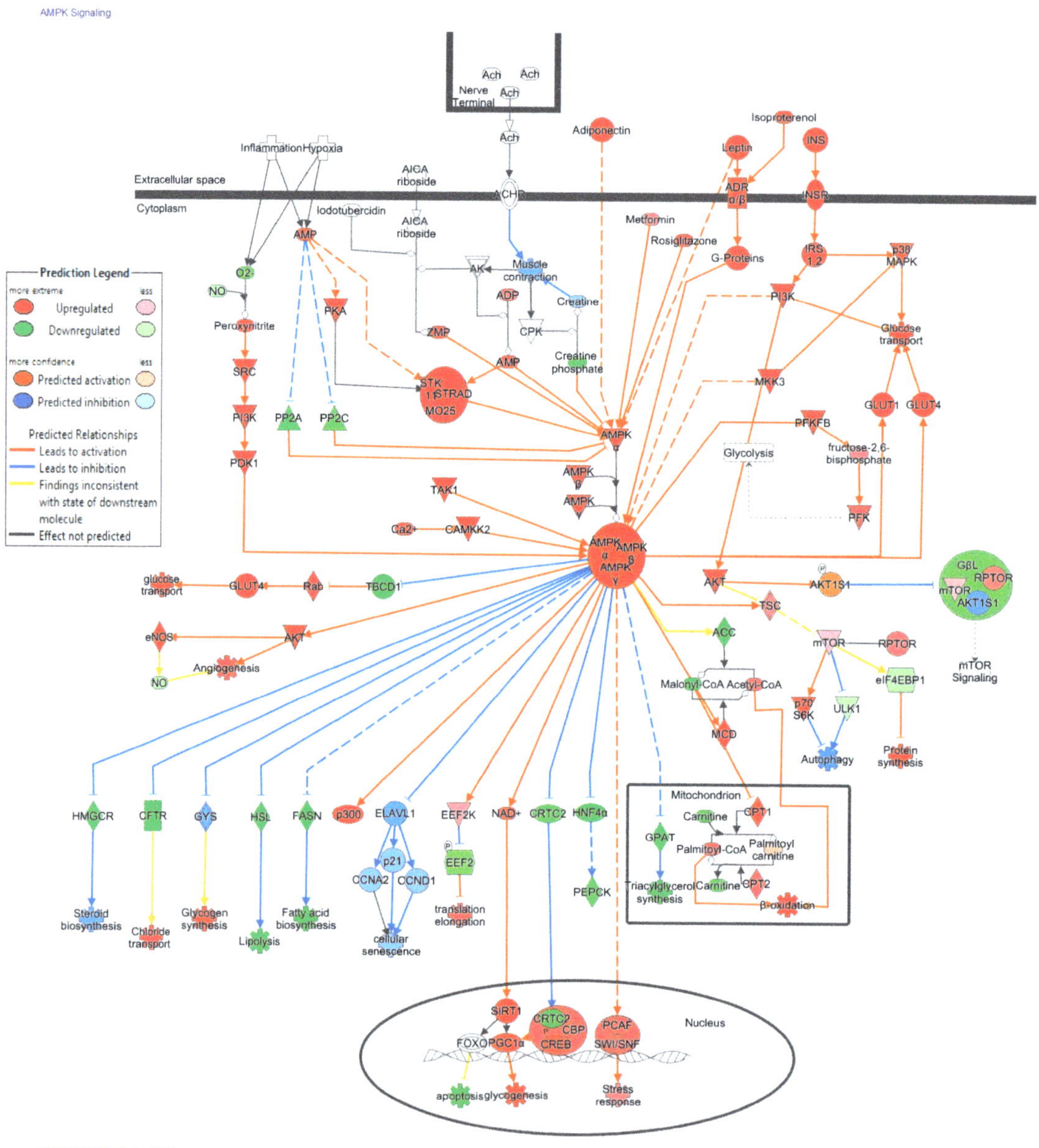

Figure A6. Activation of the AMPK signaling pathways and multiple effects on stress response, cellular senescence, apoptosis, autophagy, angiogenesis, protein and glycogen synthesis, steroids biosynthesis, mTOR signaling, and other canonical adaptive signaling pathways [246].

https://doi.org/10.3390/ph19030519

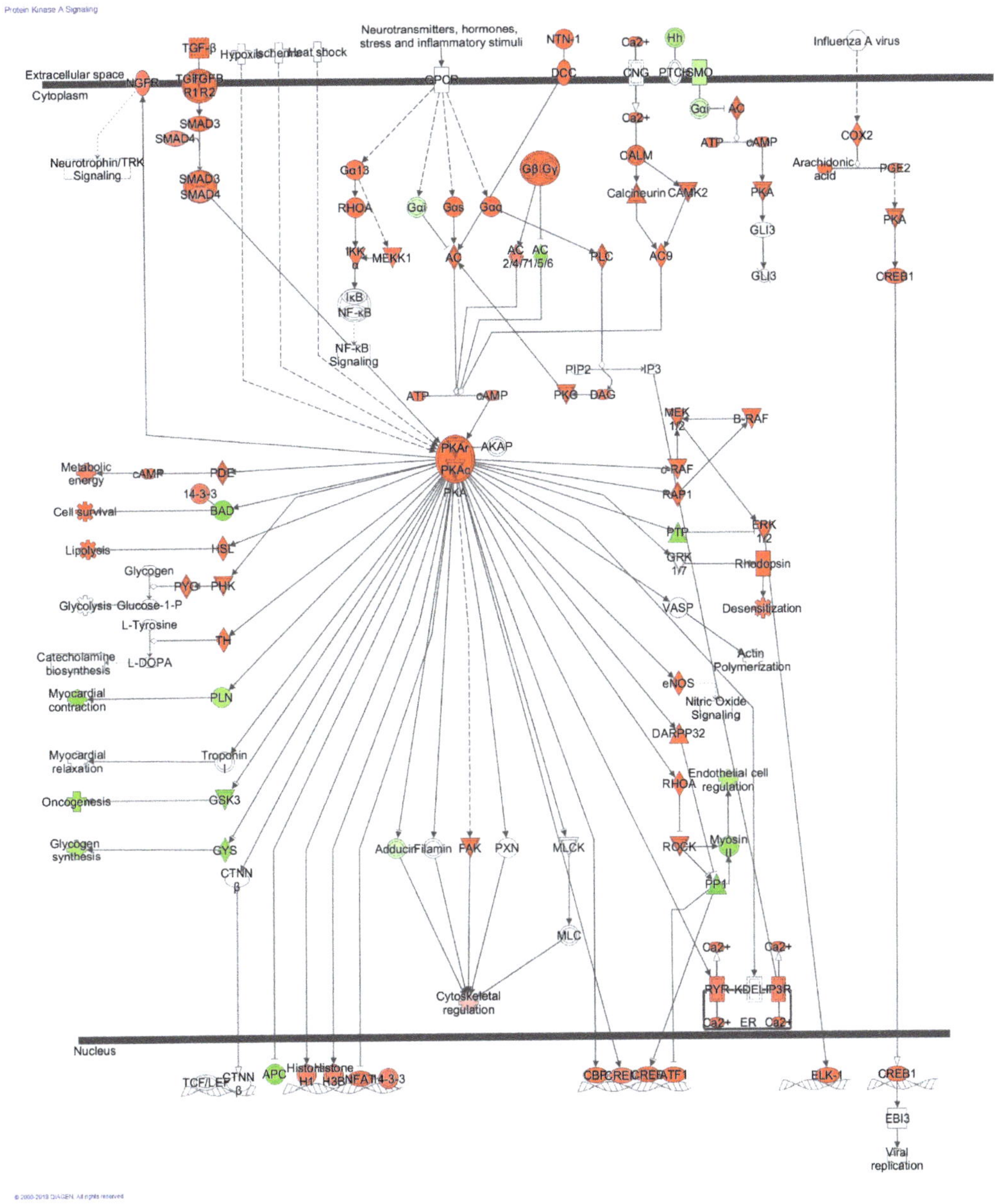

Figure A7. The neurotrasmitters, hormones, stress, and inflammatory stimulus induced activation of protein kinase A (PKA) signaling pathways and multiple effects on metabolic energy, lipolisis, glycogen synthesis, oncogenesis, cell survival, and other canonical adaptive signaling pathways [246].

https://doi.org/10.3390/ph19030519

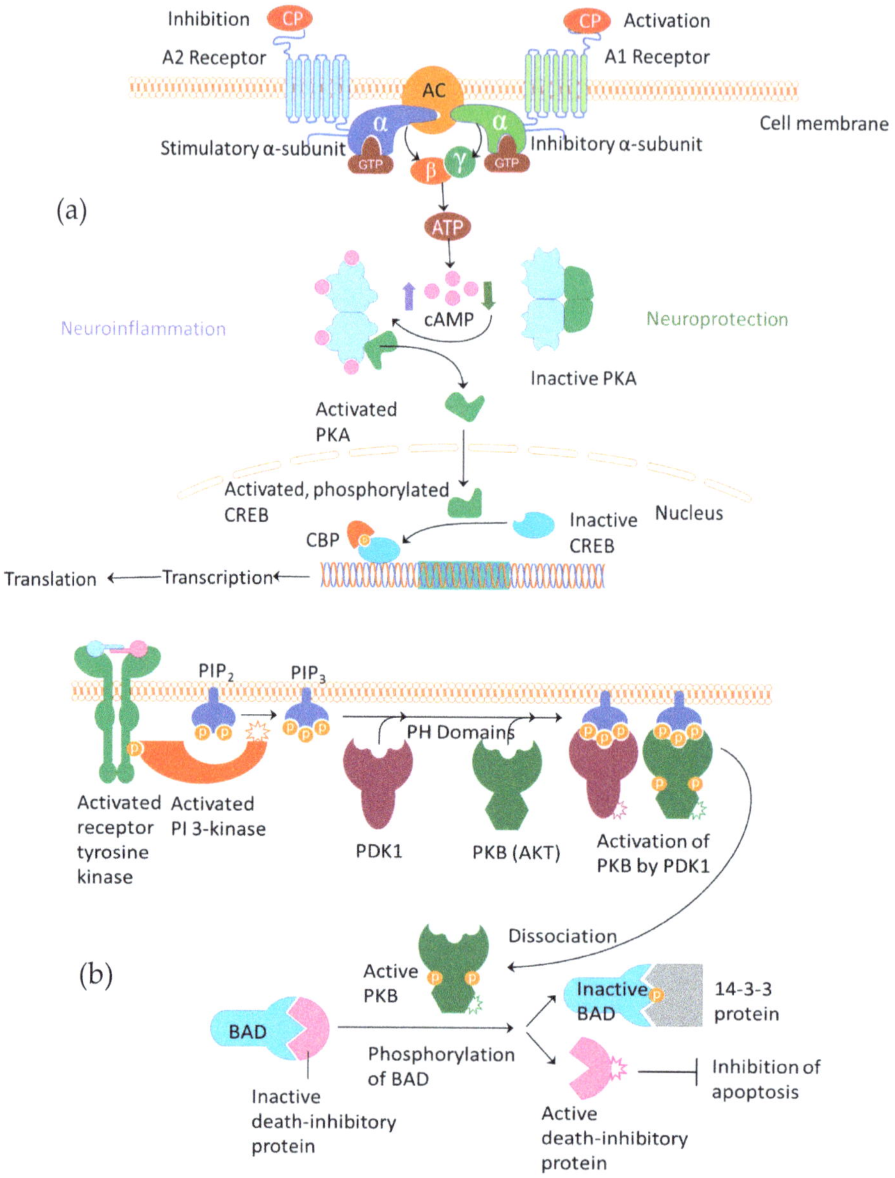

Figure A8. (**a**) Neuroprotective effects of cordycepin on activation of cAMP, PKA and cAMP-response element binding protein (CREB) in neuroinflammation [59,248], and (**b**) PI3-kinase and PKB (AKT) signaling of inhibition of apoptosis that promotes cell survival.

References

1. *Taxonomy Browser: Ophiocordyceps sinensis*; NCBI, National Library of Medicine: Bethesda, MD, USA. Available online: https://www.ncbi.nlm.nih.gov/Taxonomy/Browser/wwwtax.cgi?mode=Info&id=72228 (accessed on 21 January 2026).
2. *Taxonomy Browser: Cordyceps militaris*; NCBI, National Library of Medicine: Bethesda, MD, USA. Available online: https://www.ncbi.nlm.nih.gov/Taxonomy/Browser/wwwtax.cgi?command=show&mode=node&id=73501&lvl= (accessed on 21 January 2026).
3. Botanical Drug Development. *Guidance for Industry*; FDA: Silver Spring, MD, USA, 2016. Available online: https://www.fda.gov/files/drugs/published/Botanical-Drug-Development--Guidance-for-Industry.pdf (accessed on 21 January 2026).

https://doi.org/10.3390/ph19030519

4. Ahmadjian, V.; Alexopoulos, C.J.; Moore, D. Fungus. Encyclopaedia Britannica. 2025. Available online: https://www.britannica.com/science/fungus (accessed on 21 January 2026).
5. Moore, D.; Encyclopaedia Britannica. Outline of Classification of Fungi. 2025. Available online: https://www.britannica.com/science/fungus/Outline-of-classification-of-fungi (accessed on 21 January 2026).
6. Petruzzello, M.; Encyclopaedia Britannica. Cordyceps. 2025. Available online: https://www.britannica.com/science/cordyceps (accessed on 21 January 2026).
7. Winkler, D. *Cordyceps sinensis* (Berk.) Sacc.: Economy, Ecology, and Ethno-Mycology of Yartsa Gunbu, a Medicinal Fungus Endemic for the Tibetan Plateau. *Int. J. Med. Mashrooms* **2005**, *7*, 481–482. [CrossRef]
8. Winkler, D. Caterpillar Fungus production and sustainability on the Tibetan Plateau and in the Himalayas. *Asian Med.* **2009**, *5*, 291–316. [CrossRef]
9. Dong, C.; Yao, Y.-J. Comparison of some metabolites among cultured mycelia of medicinal fungus, *Ophiocordyceps sinensis* (Ascomycetes) from different geographical regions. *Int. J. Med. Mushrooms* **2010**, *12*, 287–297. [CrossRef]
10. Kunwar, R.M.; Mahat, L.; Acharya, R.P.; Bussmann, R.W. Medicinal plants, traditional medicine, markets and management in far-west Nepal. *J. Ethnobiol. Ethnomed.* **2013**, *9*, 24. [CrossRef]
11. Liu, D.; Cheng, H.; Bussmann, R.W.; Guo, Z.; Liu, B.; Long, C. An ethnobotanical survey of edible fungi in Chuxiong City, Yunnan, China. *J. Ethnobiol. Ethnomed.* **2018**, *14*, 42. [CrossRef]
12. Wei, Y.; Zhang, L.; Wang, J.; Wang, W.; Niyati, N.; Guo, Y.; Wang, X. Chinese caterpillar fungus (*Ophiocordyceps sinensis*) in China: Current distribution, trading, and futures under climate change and overexploitation. *Sci. Total Environ.* **2021**, *755*, 142548. [CrossRef]
13. Zhu, J.S.; Halpern, G.M.; Jones, K. The scientific rediscovery of an ancient Chinese herbal medicine: *Cordyceps sinensis*: Part I. *J. Altern. Complement. Med.* **1998**, *4*, 289–303. [CrossRef]
14. Zhu, J.S.; Halpern, G.M.; Jones, K. The scientific rediscovery of a precious ancient Chinese herbal regimen: *Cordyceps sinensis*: Part II. *J. Altern. Complement. Med.* **1998**, *4*, 429–457. [CrossRef]
15. Wang, S.Y.; Shiao, M.S. Pharmacological functions of Chinese medicinal fungus *Cordyceps sinensis* and related species. *Food Drug Anal.* **2000**, *8*, 15. [CrossRef]
16. Chen, P.X.; Wang, S.; Nie, S.; Marcone, M. Properties of *Cordyceps sinensis*: A review. *J. Funct. Foods* **2013**, *5*, 550–569. [CrossRef]
17. Yue, K.; Ye, M.; Zhou, Z.; Sun, W.; Lin, X. The genus Cordyceps: A chemical and pharmacological review. *J. Pharm. Pharmacol.* **2013**, *65*, 474–493. [CrossRef] [PubMed]
18. Li, S.P.; Yang, F.Q.; Tsim, K.W.K. Quality control of *Cordyceps sinensis*. *J. Pharm. Biomed. Anal.* **2006**, *41*, 1571–1584. [CrossRef] [PubMed]
19. Olatunji, O.J.; Tang, J.; Tola, A.; Auberon, F.; Oluwaniyi, O.; Ouyang, Z. The genus Cordyceps: An extensive review. *Fitoterapia* **2018**, *129*, 293–316. [CrossRef] [PubMed]
20. Das, S.K.; Masuda, M.; Sakurai, A.; Sakakibara, M. Medicinal uses of *Cordyceps militaris*. *Fitoterapia* **2010**, *81*, 961–968. [CrossRef]
21. Panda, A.K.; Swain, K.C. Traditional uses and medicinal potential of *Cordyceps sinensis*. *J. Ayurveda Integr. Med.* **2011**, *2*, 9–13. [CrossRef]
22. Jędrejko, K.J.; Lazur, J.; Muszyńska, B. *Cordyceps militaris*: Chemical constituents and biological activity. *Foods* **2021**, *10*, 2634. [CrossRef]
23. Phull, A.R.; Ahmed, M.; Park, H.J. *Cordyceps militaris* as a biofunctional food source. *Microorganisms* **2022**, *10*, 405. [CrossRef]
24. Abdullah, S.; Kumar, A. A brief review on the medicinal uses of *Cordyceps militaris*. *Pharmacol. Res. Mod. Chin. Med.* **2023**, *7*, 100228. [CrossRef]
25. Hasnain, M.; Jamsheed, R.A.; Hussain, Z.; Latif, R. A Comparative study on *Cordyceps militaris* and *Ophiocordyceps sinensis*. *Int. J. Nat. Med. Health Sci.* **2023**, *2*, 1–6.
26. Panossian, A.; Lemerond, T. Two Sides of the Same Coin for Health: Adaptogenic Botanicals as Nutraceuticals for Nutrition and Pharmaceuticals in Medicine. *Pharmaceuticals* **2025**, *18*, 1346. [CrossRef]
27. Brekhman, I.I.; Dardymov, I.V. New Substances of Plant Origin which Increase Nonspecific Resistance. *Annu. Rev. Pharmacol.* **1969**, *9*, 419–430. [CrossRef] [PubMed]
28. Panossian, A.; Lemerond, T.; Efferth, T. Adaptogens in Long-Lasting Brain Fatigue: An Insight from Systems Biology and Network. *Pharmaceuticals* **2025**, *18*, 261. [CrossRef] [PubMed]
29. Shashidhar, M.G.; Giridhar, P.; Sankar, K.U.; Manohar, B. Bioactive principles from Cordyceps sinensis: A potent food supplement—A review. *J. Funct. Foods* **2013**, *5*, 1013–1030. [CrossRef] [PubMed]
30. Sharma, P.; Tulsawani, R. Efficacy of Aqueous Extract of Chinese Caterpillar Mushroom *Ophiocordyceps sinensis* (Ascomycota) Against Simulated Altitude Stress and Subacute Toxicity Studies. *Int. J. Med. Mushrooms* **2022**, *24*, 21–34. [CrossRef]
31. Rajput, R.; Sharma, P.; Mishra, J.; Bhardwaj, A.; Sharma, R.K.; Singh, K.; Bansal, A.; Misra, K. Bioactive Fractions from the Chinese Caterpillar Mushroom, *Ophiocordyceps sinensis* (Ascomycetes), Elucidate Adaptogenic Role against Hypoxia Stress. *Int. J. Med. Mushrooms* **2020**, *22*, 1121–1133. [CrossRef]
32. Di Lorenzo, R.; Falanga, D.; Ricci, L.; Colantuono, A.; Greco, G.; Angelillo, M.; Nugnes, F.; Di Serio, T.; Costa, D.; Tito, A.; et al. NAD-Driven Sirtuin Activation by *Cordyceps sinensis* Extract: Exploring the Adaptogenic Potential to Promote Skin Longevity. *Int. J. Mol. Sci.* **2024**, *25*, 4282. [CrossRef]

https://doi.org/10.3390/ph19030519

33. Wang, Z.; Wang, X.; Qu, K.; Zhu, P.; Guo, N.; Zhang, R.; Abliz, Z.; Yu, H.; Zhu, H. Binding of cordycepin monophosphate to AMP-activated protein kinase and its effect on AMP-activated protein kinase activation. *Chem. Biol. Drug Des.* **2010**, *76*, 340–344. [CrossRef]
34. Wang, M.; Han, Z.; Fan, B.; Qu, K.; Zhang, W.; Li, W.; Li, J.; Li, L.; Li, J.; Li, H.; et al. Discovery of Oral AMP-Activated Protein Kinase Activators for Treating Hyperlipidemia. *J. Med. Chem.* **2024**, *67*, 7870–7890. [CrossRef]
35. Wu, C.; Guo, Y.; Su, Y.; Zhang, X.; Luan, H.; Zhang, X.; Zhu, H.; He, H.; Wang, X.; Sun, G.; et al. Cordycepin activates AMP-activated protein kinase (AMPK) via interaction with the γ1 subunit. *J. Cell. Mol. Med.* **2014**, *18*, 293–304. [CrossRef]
36. Hawley, S.A.; Ross, F.A.; Russell, F.M.; Atrih, A.; Lamont, D.J.; Hardie, D.G. Mechanism of Activation of AMPK by Cordycepin. *Cell Chem. Biol.* **2020**, *27*, 214–222. [CrossRef]
37. Radhi, M.; Ashraf, S.; Lawrence, S.; Tranholm, A.A.; Wellham, P.A.D.; Hafeez, A.; Khamis, A.S.; Thomas, R.; McWilliams, D.; de Moor, C.H. A Systematic Review of the Biological Effects of Cordycepin. *Molecules* **2021**, *26*, 5886. [CrossRef] [PubMed]
38. Chueaphromsri, P.; Kunhorm, P.; Phonchai, R.; Chaicharoenaudomrung, N.; Noisa, P. Cordycepin Enhances SIRT1 Expression and Maintains Stemness of Human Mesenchymal Stem Cells. *In Vivo* **2023**, *37*, 596–610. [CrossRef] [PubMed]
39. Hobbs, C.; Upton, R.; Gafner, S. *Cordyceps Botanical Adulterants Prevention Bulletin*; ABC-AHP-NCNPR Botanical Adulterants Prevention Program: Austin, TX, USA, 2024. Available online: https://www.herbalgram.org/resources/botanical-adulterants-prevention-program/adulterants-bulletins/new-cordyceps-bulletin-october-2024/ (accessed on 16 March 2026).
40. Sung, G.H.; Hywel-Jones, N.L.; Sung, J.M.; Luangsa-Ard, J.J.; Shrestha, B.; Spatafora, J.W. Phylogenetic classification of Cordyceps and the clavicipitaceous fungi. *Stud. Mycol.* **2007**, *57*, 5–59. [CrossRef] [PubMed]
41. Islam, W.; Adnan, M.; Shabbir, A.; Naveed, H.; Abubakar, Y.S.; Qasim, M.; Tayyab, M.; Noman, A.; Nisar, M.S.; Khan, K.A.; et al. Insect-fungal interactions: A detailed review of entomopathogenic fungi's pathogenicity to combat insect pests. *Microb. Pathog.* **2021**, *159*, 105122. [CrossRef]
42. Ashraf, S.A.; Elkhalifa, A.E.O.; Siddiqui, A.J.; Patel, M.; Awadelkareem, A.M.; Snoussi, M.; Ashraf, M.S.; Adnan, M.; Hadi, S. Cordycepin for Health and Wellbeing: A Potent Bioactive Metabolite of an Entomopathogenic Cordyceps Medicinal Fungus and Its Nutraceutical and Therapeutic Potential. *Molecules* **2020**, *25*, 2735. [CrossRef]
43. Boddy, L. Chapter 9. Interactions with humans and other animals. In *The Fungi*, 3rd ed.; Elsevier: London, UK, 2016; pp. 293–336. Available online: https://www.sciencedirect.com/science/article/pii/B9780123820341000098 (accessed on 16 March 2026).
44. Lin, W.J.; Lee, Y.I.; Liu, S.L.; Lin, C.C.; Chung, T.Y.; Chou, J.Y. Evaluating the tradeoffs of a generalist parasitoid fungus, Ophiocordyceps unilateralis, on different sympatric ant hosts. *Sci. Rep.* **2020**, *10*, 6428. [CrossRef]
45. Qiu, X.; Cao, L.; Han, R. Analysis of Volatile Components in Different *Ophiocordyceps sinensis* and Insect Host Products. *Molecules* **2020**, *25*, 1603. [CrossRef]
46. Sen, S.; Karati, D.; Priyadarshini, R.; Dua, T.K.; Paul, P.; Sahu, S.; Nandi, G. *Cordyceps sinensis* (yarsagumba): Pharmacological properties of a mushroom. *Pharmacol. Res. Mod. Chin. Med.* **2023**, *8*, 100294. [CrossRef]
47. Watanabe, T.; Rajbhandari, K.K.; Malla, K.J.; Yahara, S. *Cordyceps synensis* (Berk.) Sacc. In *A Handbook of Medicinal Plants of Nepal*; Kobfa Publishing Project: Bangkok, Thailand, 2005; pp. 72–73. Available online: https://www.researchgate.net/publication/259973143_A_Hand_Book_of_Medicinal_Plants_of_Nepal#fullTextFileContent (accessed on 24 April 2025).
48. Wei, P.; Wang, K.; Luo, C.; Huang, Y.; Misilimu, D.; Wen, H.; Jin, P.; Li, C.; Gong, Y.; Gao, Y. Cordycepin confers long-term neuroprotection via inhibiting neutrophil infiltration and neuroinflammation after traumatic brain injury. *J. Neuroinflamm.* **2021**, *18*, 137. [CrossRef]
49. Lin, B.; Li, S. Cordyceps as an Herbal Drug. In *Herbal Medicine: Biomolecular and Clinical Aspects*, 2nd ed.; Benzie, I.F.F., Wachtel-Galor, S., Eds.; CRC Press/Taylor & Francis: Boca Raton, FL, USA, 2011; Chapter 5. Available online: https://www.ncbi.nlm.nih.gov/books/NBK92758/ (accessed on 16 March 2026).
50. National Pharmacopoeia Committee. Cordyceps (Dongchongxiacao), Chinese Caterpillar Fungus. In *Pharmacopoeia of the People's Republic of China*; English ed. Chemical Industry Press: Beijing, China, 2011; p. 129. Available online: https://books.google.se/books/about/Pharmacopoeia_of_the_People_s_Republic_o.html?id=Z49IXwAACAAJ&redir_esc=y (accessed on 3 September 2025).
51. Ma, Z.; Liu, Q.; Hong, Y.; Chen, J.; Tang, J.; Tang, Y.; Wang, L. Comparative analysis of bioactive ingredients of natural and cultivated *Ophiocordyceps sinensis*. *Future Integr. Med.* **2024**, *3*, 251–261.
52. Wang, M.; Meng, X.Y.; Yang, R.L.; Qin, T.; Wang, X.Y.; Zhang, K.Y.; Fei, C.Z.; Li, Y.; Hu, Y.L.; Xue, F.Q. *Cordyceps militaris* polysaccharides can enhance the immunity and antioxidation activity in immunosuppressed mice. *Carbohydr. Polym.* **2012**, *89*, 461–466. [CrossRef] [PubMed]
53. Jędrejko, K.; Kała, K.; Sułkowska-Ziaja, K.; Krakowska, A.; Zięba, P.; Marzec, K.; Szewczyk, A.; Sękara, A.; Pytko-Polończyk, J.; Muszyńska, B. *Cordyceps militaris*-Fruiting Bodies, Mycelium, and Supplements: Valuable Component of Daily Diet. *Antioxidants* **2022**, *11*, 1861. [CrossRef] [PubMed]
54. Jędrejko, K.; Kała, K.; Sułkowska-Ziaja, K.; Krakowska, A.; Szewczyk, A.; Guśpiel, K.; Muszyńska, B. Analysis of bioactive compounds in *Cordyceps militaris* fruiting bodies and dietary supplements: In vitro bioaccessibility determination in artificial digestive juices. *Int. J. Food Sci. Technol.* **2024**, *59*, 4011–4019. [CrossRef]
55. Sun, H.; Wei, S.; Gong, Y.; Ding, K.; Tang, S.; Sun, W.; Yuan, C.; Huang, L.; Liu, Z.; Chen, C.; et al. Neuroprotective effects of cordycepin inhibit glutamate-induced apoptosis in hippocampal neurons. *Cell Stress Chaperones* **2024**, *29*, 10–20. [CrossRef]

https://doi.org/10.3390/ph19030519

56. Chai, X.; Pan, M.; Wang, J.; Feng, M.; Wang, Y.; Zhang, Q.; Sun, Y. Cordycepin exhibits anti-fatigue effect via activating TIGAR/SIRT1/PGC-1α signaling pathway. *Biochem. Biophys. Res. Commun.* **2022**, *637*, 127–135. [CrossRef]
57. Chen, L.; Wei, W.; Sun, J.; Sun, B.; Deng, R. Cordycepin enhances anti-tumor immunity in breast cancer by enhanceing ALB expression. *Heliyon* **2024**, *10*, e29903. [CrossRef]
58. Cheng, Z.; He, W.; Zhou, X.; Lv, Q.; Xu, X.; Yang, S.; Zhao, C.; Guo, L. Cordycepin protects against cerebral ischemia/reperfusion injury in vivo and in vitro. *Eur. J. Pharmacol.* **2011**, *664*, 20–28. [CrossRef]
59. Govindula, A.; Pai, A.; Baghel, S.; Mudgal, J. Molecular mechanisms of cordycepin emphasizing its potential against neuroinflammation: An update. *Eur. J. Pharmacol.* **2021**, *908*, 174364. [CrossRef]
60. Ma, X.; Zhao, Y.; Yang, T.; Gong, N.; Chen, X.; Liu, G.; Xiao, J. Integration of network pharmacology and molecular docking to explore the molecular mechanism of Cordycepin in the treatment of Alzheimer's disease. *Front. Aging Neurosci.* **2022**, *14*, 1058780. [CrossRef]
61. Ramesh, T.; Yoo, S.K.; Kim, S.W.; Hwang, S.Y.; Sohn, S.H.; Kim, I.W.; Kim, S.K. Cordycepin (3′-deoxyadenosine) attenuates age-related oxidative stress and ameliorates antioxidant capacity in rats. *Exp. Gerontol.* **2012**, *47*, 979–987. [CrossRef]
62. Tuli, H.S.; Sandhu, S.S.; Sharma, A.K. Pharmacological and therapeutic potential of Cordyceps with special reference to Cordycepin. *3 Biotech* **2014**, *4*, 1–12. [CrossRef] [PubMed]
63. Cunningham, K.G.; Manson, W.; Spring, F.S.; Hutchinson, S.A. Cordycepin, a metabolic product isolated from cultures of *Cordyceps militaris* (Linn.) link. *Nature* **1950**, *166*, 949–954. [CrossRef] [PubMed]
64. Radwan, M.A.; Willson, H.R. The Structure of Cordycepin. *Acta Crystallogr. B* **1980**, *36*, 2185–2187. [CrossRef]
65. Maľučká, L.U.; Uhrinová, A.; Lysinová, P. Medicinal mushrooms *Ophiocordyceps sinensis* and *Cordyceps militaris*. Liečivé huby *Ophiocordyceps sinensis* a *Cordyceps militaris*. *Ceska Slov. Farm.* **2022**, *71*, 259–265. [CrossRef]
66. Lee, C.T.; Huang, K.S.; Shaw, J.F.; Chen, J.R.; Kuo, W.S.; Shen, G.; Grumezescu, A.M.; Holban, A.M.; Wang, Y.T.; Wang, J.S.; et al. Trends in the Immunomodulatory Effects of *Cordyceps militaris*: Total Extracts, Polysaccharides and Cordycepin. *Front. Pharmacol.* **2020**, *11*, 575704. [CrossRef]
67. Kała, K.; Cicha-Jeleń, M.; Hnatyk, K.; Krakowska, A.; Sułkowska-Ziaja, K.; Szewczyk, A.; Lazur, J.; Muszyńska, B. Coffee with *Cordyceps militaris* and *Hericium erinaceus* Fruiting Bodies as a Source of Essential Bioactive Substances. *Pharmaceuticals* **2024**, *17*, 955. [CrossRef]
68. Xiaoying, M.; Peng, Z.; Hong, W.; Na, G.; Jun, X.; Ying, Z.; Xun, C.; Guoli, L. From functional foods to immunotherapeutic agents: Mechanistic insights into medicinal mushroom bioactives in chronic inflammation management. *Front. Nutr.* **2025**, *12*, 1725297. [CrossRef]
69. Chen, Y.; Guo, H.; Du, Z.; Liu, X.Z.; Che, Y.; Ye, X. Ecology-based screen identifies new metabolites from a Cordyceps-colonizing fungus as cancer cell proliferation inhibitors and apoptosis inducers. *Cell Prolif.* **2009**, *42*, 838–847. [CrossRef]
70. Tshikhudo, P.P.; Mabhaudhi, T.; Koorbanally, N.A.; Mudau, F.N.; Avendaño Caceres, E.O.; Popa, D.; Calina, D.; Sharifi-Rad, J. Anticancer Potential of β-Carboline Alkaloids: An Updated Mechanistic Overview. *Chem. Biodivers.* **2024**, *21*, e202301263. [CrossRef]
71. Yang, M.L.; Kuo, P.C.; Hwang, T.L.; Wu, T.S. Anti-inflammatory principles from *Cordyceps sinensis*. *J. Nat. Prod.* **2011**, *74*, 1996–2000. [CrossRef]
72. Corradetti, R.; Lo Conte, G.; Moroni, F.; Passani, M.B.; Pepeu, G. Adenosine decreases aspartate and glutamate release from rat hippocampal slices. *Eur. J. Pharmacol.* **1984**, *104*, 19–26. [CrossRef] [PubMed]
73. Schmidt, C.; Bellingham, M.C.; Richter, D.W. Adenosinergic modulation of respiratory neurones and hypoxic responses in the anaesthetized cat. *J. Physiol.* **1995**, *483*, 769–781. [CrossRef] [PubMed]
74. Ballarin, M.; Herrera-Marschitz, M.; Casas, M.; Ungerstedt, U. Striatal adenosine levels measured 'in vivo' by microdialysis in rats with unilateral dopamine denervation. *Neurosci. Lett.* **1987**, *83*, 338–344. [CrossRef] [PubMed]
75. Benowitz, L.I.; Goldberg, D.E.; Irwin, N. Inosine stimulates axon growth in vitro and in the adult CNS. *Prog. Brain Res.* **2002**, *137*, 389–399. [CrossRef]
76. Li, S.P.; Su, Z.R.; Dong, T.T.; Tsim, K.W. The fruiting body and its caterpillar host of *Cordyceps sinensis* show close resemblance in main constituents and anti-oxidation activity. *Phytomedicine* **2002**, *9*, 319–324. [CrossRef]
77. Yamaguchi, Y.; Kagota, S.; Nakamura, K.; Shinozuka, K.; Kunitomo, M. Antioxidant activity of the extracts from fruiting bodies of cultured *Cordyceps sinensis*. *Phytother. Res.* **2000**, *14*, 647–649. [CrossRef]
78. Kiho, T.; Ookubo, K.; Usui, S.; Ukai, S.; Hirano, K. Structural features and hypoglycemic activity of a polysaccharide (CS-F10) from the cultured mycelium of *Cordyceps sinensis*. *Biol. Pharm. Bull.* **1999**, *22*, 966–970. [CrossRef]
79. Li, S.P.; Zhao, K.J.; Ji, Z.N.; Song, Z.H.; Dong, T.T.; Lo, C.K.; Cheung, J.K.; Zhu, S.Q.; Tsim, K.W. A polysaccharide isolated from *Cordyceps sinensis*, a traditional Chinese medicine, protects PC12 cells against hydrogen peroxide-induced injury. *Life Sci.* **2003**, *73*, 2503–2513. [CrossRef]
80. Yu, R.; Song, L.; Zhao, Y.; Bin, W.; Wang, L.; Zhang, H.; Wu, Y.; Ye, W.; Yao, X. Isolation and biological properties of polysaccharide CPS-1 from cultured *Cordyceps militaris*. *Fitoterapia* **2004**, *75*, 465–472. [CrossRef]
81. Bok, J.W.; Lermer, L.; Chilton, J.; Klingeman, H.G.; Towers, G.H. Antitumor sterols from the mycelia of *Cordyceps sinensis*. *Phytochemistry* **1999**, *51*, 891–898. [CrossRef]
82. Lindequist, U.; Lesnau, A.; Teuscher, E.; Pilgrim, H. Untersuchungen zur antiviralen Wirksamkeit von Ergosterol-peroxid [The antiviral action of ergosterol peroxide]. *Pharmazie* **1989**, *44*, 579–580. [PubMed]

https://doi.org/10.3390/ph19030519

83. Lin, C.Y.; Ku, F.M.; Kuo, Y.C.; Chen, C.F.; Chen, W.P.; Chen, A.; Shiao, M.S. Inhibition of activated human mesangial cell proliferation by the natural product of *Cordyceps sinensis* (H1-A): An implication for treatment of IgA mesangial nephropathy. *J. Lab. Clin. Med.* **1999**, *133*, 55–63. [CrossRef] [PubMed]
84. Arts, I.C.; Coolen, E.J.; Bours, M.J.; Huyghebaert, N.; Stuart, M.A.; Bast, A.; Dagnelie, P.C. Adenosine 5′-triphosphate (ATP) supplements are not orally bioavailable: A randomized, placebo-controlled cross-over trial in healthy humans. *J. Int. Soc. Sports Nutr.* **2012**, *9*, 16. [CrossRef] [PubMed]
85. Coolen, E.J.; Arts, I.C.; Bekers, O.; Vervaet, C.; Bast, A.; Dagnelie, P.C. Oral bioavailability of ATP after prolonged administration. *Br. J. Nutr.* **2011**, *105*, 357–366. [CrossRef]
86. Chatnarin, S.; Thirabunyanon, M. Potential bioactivities via anticancer, antioxidant, and immunomodulatory properties of cultured mycelial enriched β-D-glucan polysaccharides from a novel fungus *Ophiocordyceps sinensis* OS8. *Front. Immunol.* **2023**, *14*, 1150287. [CrossRef]
87. Huang, L.; Li, Q.; Chen, Y.; Wang, X.; Zhou, X. Determination and analysis of cordycepin and adenosine in the products of *Cordyceps* spp. *Afr. J. Microbiol. Res.* **2009**, *3*, 953–961.
88. Zhou, Y.; Wang, M.; Zhang, H.; Huang, Z.; Ma, J. Comparative study of the composition of cultivated, naturally grown *Cordyceps sinensis*, and stiff worms across different sampling years. *PLoS ONE* **2019**, *14*, e0225750. [CrossRef]
89. Li, Q.; Liao, H.; Zhang, C. Comparative HPLC Determination of Cordycepin in *Cordyceps militaris* from Different Locations. *Food Sci.* **2014**. [CrossRef]
90. Su, Y.; Li, P.; Zhang, H.; Lin, M.; Liu, W.; Xu, R.; Hu, H.; Liu, Y.M. Simultaneous Quantification of Adenosine and Deoxyadenosine Isomers in Foods with High Sensitivity. *Anal. Methods* **2019**, *11*, 4946–4950. [CrossRef]
91. Gu, C.; Zhang, D.; Zhai, W.; Zhang, H.; Wang, S.; Lv, S.; Bao, Y.; Zhu, D.; Feng, S.; Guo, S.; et al. Research progress on *Cordyceps militaris* polysaccharides. *Food Biosci.* **2022**, *45*, 101503. [CrossRef]
92. Chen, L.H.; Wu, Y.; Guan, Y.M.; Jin, C.; Zhu, W.F.; Yang, M. Analysis of the High-Performance Liquid Chromatography Fingerprints and Quantitative Analysis of Multicomponents by Single Marker of Products of Fermented *Cordyceps sinensis*. *J. Anal. Methods Chem.* **2018**, *2018*, 5943914. [CrossRef] [PubMed]
93. Zhang, J.; Zhang, W.; Wu, X.; Fu, W.; Yang, C.; Long, N. Insights into the Mycosphere Fungal Community and Its Association with Nucleoside Accumulation in *Ophiocordyceps sinensis*. *J. Fungi* **2025**, *11*, 696. [CrossRef] [PubMed]
94. Yuan, J.P.; Wang, J.H.; Liu, X.; Kuang, H.C.; Zhao, S.Y. Simultaneous determination of free ergosterol and ergosteryl esters in *Cordyceps sinensis* by HPLC. *Food Chem.* **2007**, *105*, 1755–1759. [CrossRef]
95. Hu, D.; Yang, X.; Hu, C.; Feng, Z.; Chen, W.; Shi, H. Comparison of Ergosterol and Vitamin D2 in Mushrooms *Agaricus bisporus* and *Cordyceps militaris* Using Ultraviolet Irradiation Directly on Dry Powder or in Ethanol Suspension. *ACS Omega* **2021**, *6*, 29506–29515. [CrossRef]
96. Zhao, J.; Shi, T.; Zhu, W.; Chen, L.; Guan, Y.; Jin, C. Quality control method of sterols in fermented *Cordyceps sinensis* based on combined fingerprint and quantitative analysis of multicomponents by single marker. *J. Food Sci.* **2020**, *85*, 2994–3002. [CrossRef]
97. Lo, H.C.; Hsieh, C.; Lin, F.Y.; Hsu, T.H. A Systematic Review of the Mysterious Caterpillar Fungus *Ophiocordyceps sinensis* in DongChongXiaCao (Dōng Chóng Xià Cǎo) and Related Bioactive Ingredients. *J. Tradit. Complement. Med.* **2013**, *3*, 16–32. [CrossRef]
98. Suhadolnik, R.J. Naturally occurring nucleoside and nucleotide antibiotics. *Prog. Nucleic Acid Res. Mol. Biol.* **1979**, *22*, 193–291. [CrossRef]
99. Hueng, D.Y.; Hsieh, C.H.; Cheng, Y.C.; Tsai, W.C.; Chen, Y. Cordycepin inhibits migration of human glioblastoma cells by affecting lysosomal degradation and protein phosphatase activation. *J. Nutr. Biochem.* **2017**, *41*, 109–116. [CrossRef]
100. Wang, Z.; Wu, X.; Liang, Y.N.; Wang, L.; Song, Z.X.; Liu, J.L.; Tang, Z.S. Cordycepin Induces Apoptosis and Inhibits Proliferation of Human Lung Cancer Cell Line H1975 via Inhibiting the Phosphorylation of EGFR. *Molecules* **2016**, *21*, 1267. [CrossRef]
101. Zhang, J.; Yang, Z.; Zhao, Z.; Zhang, N. Structural and pharmacological insights into cordycepin for neoplasms and metabolic disorders. *Front. Pharmacol.* **2024**, *15*, 1367820. [CrossRef]
102. Wang, Y.; Deng, Y.; Feng, M.; Chen, J.; Zhong, M.; Han, Z.; Zhang, Q.; Sun, Y. Cordycepin extracted from *Cordyceps militaris* mitigated CUMS-induced depression of rats via targeting GSK3β/β-catenin signaling pathway. *J. Ethnopharmacol.* **2025**, *340*, 119249. [CrossRef] [PubMed]
103. Kopalli, S.R.; Cha, K.M.; Lee, S.H.; Hwang, S.Y.; Lee, Y.J.; Koppula, S.; Kim, S.K. Cordycepin, an Active Constituent of Nutrient Powerhouse and Potential Medicinal Mushroom *Cordyceps militaris* Linn., Ameliorates Age-Related Testicular Dysfunction in Rats. *Nutrients* **2019**, *11*, 906. [CrossRef] [PubMed]
104. Takahashi, S.; Tamai, M.; Nakajima, S.; Kato, H.; Johno, H.; Nakamura, T.; Kitamura, M. Blockade of adipocyte differentiation by cordycepin. *Br. J. Pharmacol.* **2012**, *167*, 561–575. [CrossRef] [PubMed]
105. National Pharmacopoeia Committee. Bailing Jiaonang, Bailing capsule. In *Pharmacopoeia of the People's Republic of China*; English ed. Chemical Industry Press: Beijing, China, 2010; pp. 540–541. Available online: https://books.google.se/books/about/Pharmacopoeia_of_the_People_s_Republic_o.html?id=Z49IXwAACAAJ&redir_esc=y (accessed on 3 September 2025).
106. Latini, S.; Pedata, F. Adenosine in the central nervous system: Release mechanisms and extracellular concentrations. *J. Neurochem.* **2001**, *79*, 463–484. [CrossRef]

107. Porkka-Heiskanen, T.; Kalinchuk, A.V. Adenosine, energy metabolism, and sleep homeostasis. *Sleep Med. Rev.* **2011**, *15*, 123–135. [CrossRef]
108. Eltzschig, H.K.; Thompson, L.F.; Karhausen, J.; Cotta, R.J.; Ibla, J.C.; Robson, S.C.; Colgan, S.P. Endogenous adenosine produced during hypoxia attenuates neutrophil accumulation: Coordination by extracellular nucleotide metabolism. *Blood* **2004**, *104*, 3986–3992. [CrossRef]
109. Eltzschig, H.K.; Carmeliet, P. Hypoxia and inflammation. *N. Engl. J. Med.* **2011**, *364*, 656–665. [CrossRef]
110. Rau, A.R.; Ariwodola, O.J.; Weiner, J.L. Presynaptic adenosine A_1 receptors modulate excitatory transmission in the rat basolateral amygdala. *Neuropharmacology* **2014**, *77*, 465–474. [CrossRef]
111. Brambilla, D.; Chapman, D.; Greene, R. Adenosine mediation of presynaptic feedback inhibition of glutamate release. *Neuron* **2005**, *46*, 275–283. [CrossRef]
112. Dobson, G.P.; Arsyad, A.; Letson, H.L. The Adenosine Hypothesis Revisited: Modulation of Coupling between Myocardial Perfusion and Arterial Compliance. *Front. Physiol.* **2017**, *8*, 824. [CrossRef]
113. Görlach, A. Control of adenosine transport by hypoxia. *Circ. Res.* **2005**, *97*, 1–3. [CrossRef] [PubMed]
114. Tune, J.D.; Gorman, M.W.; Feigl, E.O. Matching coronary blood flow to myocardial oxygen consumption. *J. Appl. Physiol.* **2004**, *97*, 404–415. [CrossRef] [PubMed]
115. Hori, M.; Kitakaze, M. Adenosine, the heart, and coronary circulation. *Hypertension* **1991**, *18*, 565–574. [CrossRef] [PubMed]
116. Casey, D.P.; Madery, B.D.; Pike, T.L.; Eisenach, J.H.; Dietz, N.M.; Joyner, M.J.; Wilkins, B.W. Adenosine receptor antagonist and augmented vasodilation during hypoxic exercise. *J. Appl. Physiol.* **2009**, *107*, 1128–1137. [CrossRef]
117. Dengler, F. Activation of AMPK under Hypoxia: Many Roads Leading to Rome. *Int. J. Mol. Sci.* **2020**, *21*, 2428. [CrossRef]
118. Bowser, J.L.; Phan, L.H.; Eltzschig, H.K. The Hypoxia-Adenosine Link during Intestinal Inflammation. *J. Immunol.* **2018**, *200*, 897–907. [CrossRef]
119. Decking, U.K.; Schlieper, G.; Kroll, K.; Schrader, J. Hypoxia-induced inhibition of adenosine kinase potentiates cardiac adenosine release. *Circ. Res.* **1997**, *81*, 154–164. [CrossRef]
120. Hardie, D.G. AMP-activated protein kinase: An energy sensor that regulates all aspects of cell function. *Genes Dev.* **2011**, *25*, 1895–1908. [CrossRef]
121. Jeon, S.M. Regulation and function of AMPK in physiology and diseases. *Exp. Mol. Med.* **2016**, *48*, e245. [CrossRef]
122. Melani, A.; Pugliese, A.M.; Pedata, F. Chapter Thirteen—Adenosine Receptors in Cerebral Ischemia. In *International Review of Neurobiology*; Mori, A., Ed.; Academic Press: London, UK, 2014; Volume 119, pp. 309–348. [CrossRef]
123. Jacobson, K.A.; Gao, Z.G. Adenosine receptors as therapeutic targets. *Nat. Rev. Drug Discov.* **2006**, *5*, 247–264. [CrossRef]
124. Willson, C. The clinical toxicology of caffeine: A review and case study. *Toxicol. Rep.* **2018**, *5*, 1140–1152. [CrossRef] [PubMed]
125. Fernández-Dueñas, V.; Gómez-Soler, M.; López-Cano, M.; Taura, J.J.; Ledent, C.; Watanabe, M.; Jacobson, K.A.; Vilardaga, J.P.; Ciruela, F. Uncovering caffeine's adenosine A2A receptor inverse agonism in experimental Parkinsonism. *ACS Chem. Biol.* **2014**, *9*, 2496–2501. [CrossRef] [PubMed]
126. Ishibashi, K.; Miura, Y.; Wagatsuma, K.; Toyohara, J.; Ishiwata, K.; Ishii, K. Adenosine A2A Receptor Occupancy by Caffeine After Coffee Intake in Parkinson's Disease. *Mov. Disord.* **2022**, *37*, 853–857. [CrossRef] [PubMed]
127. Qi, S.; Guan, H.; Wang, Y.; Fang, Q.; Cheng, X.; Liu, P.; Wei, H.; Liu, W.; Wang, C. Simultaneous determination of cordycepin and its metabolite 3′-deoxyinosine in rat whole blood by ultra-high-performance liquid chromatography coupled with Q Exactive hybrid quadrupole orbitrap high-resolution accurate mass spectrometry and its application to accurate pharmacokinetic studies. *J. Sep. Sci.* **2023**, *46*, e2200602. [CrossRef]
128. Li, M.; Liu, F.; Guo, L.; Fan, W.; Wang, J.; Lu, B.; Hong, G.; Zhang, W.; Tian, S.; Mao, J.; et al. Distribution and Pharmacokinetic Characteristics of Cordycepin in Rat: Investigated by UHPLC-HRMS/MS and Blood-Brain Synchronous Microdialysis. *Biomed. Chromatogr.* **2025**, *39*, e70038. [CrossRef]
129. Nakamura, K.; Shinozuka, K.; Yoshikawa, N. Anticancer and antimetastatic effects of cordycepin, an active component of *Cordyceps sinensis*. *J. Pharmacol. Sci.* **2015**, *127*, 53–56. [CrossRef]
130. Chang, W.K.; Chen, Y.T.; Lin, C.P.; Wang, C.J.; Shieh, H.R.; Chi, C.W.; Tsai, T.H.; Chen, Y.J. Cordycepin Augments the Efficacy of Anti-PD1 against Colon Cancer. *Biomedicines* **2024**, *12*, 1568. [CrossRef]
131. Lee, J.B.; Radhi, M.; Cipolla, E.; Gandhi, R.D.; Sarmad, S.; Zgair, A.; Kim, T.H.; Feng, W.; Qin, C.; Adrower, C.; et al. A novel nucleoside rescue metabolic pathway may be responsible for therapeutic effect of orally administered cordycepin. *Sci. Rep.* **2019**, *9*, 15760. [CrossRef]
132. Tsai, Y.J.; Lin, L.C.; Tsai, T.H. Pharmacokinetics of adenosine and cordycepin, a bioactive constituent of *Cordyceps sinensis* in rats. *J. Agric. Food Chem.* **2010**, *58*, 4638–4643. [CrossRef]
133. Kaptchuk, T.J. *The Web That Has No Weaver*; Congdon and Weed: New York, NY, USA, 1983; pp. 55–65. Available online: https://books.google.se/books/about/The_Web_That_Has_No_Weaver.html?id=6BiGl562OgEC&redir_esc=y (accessed on 16 March 2026).
134. Panossian, A.G.; Efferth, T.; Shikov, A.N.; Pozharitskaya, O.N.; Kuchta, K.; Mukherjee, P.K.; Banerjee, S.; Heinrich, M.; Wu, W.; Guo, D.A.; et al. Evolution of the adaptogenic concept from traditional use to medical systems: Pharmacology of stress- and aging-related diseases. *Med. Res. Rev.* **2021**, *41*, 630–703. [CrossRef]
135. Jiang, S.J. A tonic application of *Cordyceps sinensis* in medicinal diets. *J. Chin. Med. Mater.* **1994**, *17*, 47–48.

https://doi.org/10.3390/ph19030519

136. Liu, M.; Cui, C.; Chang, T.; Zhou, Q.; Cui, Y.; Zhang, S.; Liao, X. Effects and safety of *Ophiocordyceps sinensis* preparation in the adjuvant treatment for dialysis patients: A systematic review and meta-analysis. *Front. Pharmacol.* **2024**, *15*, 1360997. [CrossRef] [PubMed]
137. Wu, F.; Xu, C.; Si, X.; He, F.; Xu, K.; Zhang, Y.; Lin, S. Efficacy of traditional Chinese medicine *Cordyceps sinensis* as an adjunctive treatment in patients with renal dysfunction: A systematic-review and meta-analysis. *Front. Med.* **2025**, *11*, 1477569. [CrossRef] [PubMed]
138. Pu, F.; Li, T.; Shen, C.; Wang, Y.; Tang, C.; Zhang, X.; Yan, L.; Xu, Q.; Liu, J. Fermented *Ophiocordyceps sinensis* mycelium products for preventing contrast-associated acute kidney injury: A systematic review of randomized controlled trials. *Ren. Fail.* **2024**, *46*, 2300302. [CrossRef]
139. Tao, Y.; Luo, R.; Xiang, Y.; Lei, M.; Peng, X.; Hu, Y. Use of bailing capsules (cordyceps sinensis) in the treatment of chronic kidney disease: A meta-analysis and network pharmacology. *Front. Pharmacol.* **2024**, *15*, 1342831. [CrossRef]
140. Xue, X.; Jin, X.Y.; Ye, X.L.; Li, K.Y.; Li, J.X.; Liu, X.H.; Bai, J.; Liu, Q.; Zhang, B.R.; Zou, X.R.; et al. *Ophiocordyceps sinensis* preparations combined with the renin-angiotensin system inhibitor for diabetic kidney disease treatment: An umbrella review of systematic reviews and network meta-analysis. *Front. Pharmacol.* **2024**, *15*, 1360633. [CrossRef]
141. Wang, C.; Wang, J.; Qi, Y. Adjuvant treatment with *Cordyceps sinensis* for lung cancer: A systematic review and meta-analysis of randomized controlled trials. *J. Ethnopharmacol.* **2024**, *327*, 118044. [CrossRef]
142. Yu, X.; Mao, Y.; Shergis, J.L.; Coyle, M.E.; Wu, L.; Chen, Y.; Zhang, A.L.; Lin, L.; Xue, C.C.; Xu, Y. Effectiveness and Safety of Oral *Cordyceps sinensis* on Stable COPD of GOLD Stages 2-3: Systematic Review and Meta-Analysis. *Evid. Based Complement. Altern. Med.* **2019**, *2019*, 4903671. [CrossRef]
143. Ma, G.; Jin, Y. Therapeutic efficacy and pharmacological mechanism of Bailing capsule on chronic obstructive pulmonary disease: A meta-analysis and network pharmacology. *Pharm. Biol.* **2024**, *62*, 803–817. [CrossRef]
144. Welch, J.; Kole, R.; Daniels, S. The effectiveness and efficacy of *Ophiocordyceps sinensis* supplementation: A systematic review of randomized clinical trials on healthy humans. *Int. J. Herb. Med.* **2023**, *11*, 15–22. [CrossRef]
145. Dewi, L.; Khemtong, C. Ergogenic Aid by Cordyceps: Does It Work?? *Curr. Nutr. Rep.* **2025**, *14*, 97. [CrossRef] [PubMed]
146. European Medicines Agency. *Guideline on the Assessment of Clinical Safety and Efficacy in the Preparation of EU Herbal Monographs for Well-Established and Traditional Herbal Medicinal Products EMA/HMPC/104613/2005—Rev. 1*; EMA: London, UK, 2017. Available online: https://www.ema.europa.eu/en/documents/scientific-guideline/guideline-assessment-clinical-safety-and-efficacy-preparation-eu-herbal-monographs-well-established-and-traditional-herbal-medicinal-products_en.pdf (accessed on 16 March 2026).
147. Brennan, S.E.; Johnston, R.V. Research Note: Interpreting findings of a systematic review using GRADE methods. *J. Physiother.* **2023**, *69*, 198–202. [CrossRef] [PubMed]
148. Cao, Z.; Wen, Y. Therapeutic effect analysis of JinShuiBao capsule in treatment of 33 elderly senescent XuZheng patients. *J. Appl. Tradit. Chin. Med.* **1993**, *1*, 32–33.
149. Zhang, Z.; Huang, W.; Liao, S.; Li, J.; Lei, L.; Lui, J.; Leng, F.; Gong, W.; Zhang, H.; Wan, L.; et al. Clinical and laboratory studies of JinShuiBao in scavenging oxygen free radicals in elderly senescent XuZheng patients. *J. Admin. Tradit. Chin. Med.* **1995**, *5*, 14–18.
150. Chen, S.; Li, Z.; Krochmal, R.; Abrazado, M.; Kim, W.; Cooper, C.B. Effect of Cs-4® (*Cordyceps sinensis*) on exercise performance in healthy older subjects: A double-blind, placebo-controlled trial. *J. Altern. Complement. Med.* **2010**, *16*, 585–590. [CrossRef]
151. Nagata, A.; Tajima, T.; Moriyasu, S. Cordyceps drinks and running performance. *J. Exerc. Sports Physiol.* **2002**, *9*, 85–92.
152. Nagata, A.; Tajima, T.; Uchida, M. Supplemental anti-fatigue effects of *Cordyceps sinensis* (Tochu-Kaso) extract powder during three stepwise exercise of human. *Jpn. J. Phys. Fit. Sports Med.* **2006**, *55*, S145–S152. [CrossRef]
153. Hirsch, K.R.; Smith-Ryan, A.E.; Roelofs, E.J.; Trexler, E.T.; Mock, M.G. *Cordyceps militaris* Improves Tolerance to High-Intensity Exercise After Acute and Chronic Supplementation. *J. Diet. Suppl.* **2017**, *14*, 42–53. [CrossRef]
154. Nakamura, A.; Shinozaki, E.; Suzuki, Y.; Santa, K.; Kumazawa, Y.; Kobayashi, F.; Nagaoka, I.; Koikawa, N. Effect of the Administration of *Cordyceps militaris* Mycelium Extract on Blood Markers for Anemia in Long-Distance Runners. *Nutrients* **2024**, *16*, 1835. [CrossRef]
155. Hsu, C.C.; Lin, Y.A.; Su, B.; Li, J.H.; Huang, H.Y.; Hsu, M.C.P. No effect of *Cordyceps sinensis* supplementation on testosterone level and muscle strength in healthy young adults for resistance training. *Biol. Sport.* **2011**, *28*, 107–110. [CrossRef]
156. Parcell, A.C.; Smith, J.M.; Schulthies, S.S.; Myrer, J.W.; Fellingham, G. *Cordyceps sinensis* (CordyMax Cs-4) supplementation does not improve endurance exercise performance. *Int. J. Sport Nutr. Exerc. Metab.* **2004**, *14*, 236–242. [CrossRef] [PubMed]
157. Nicodemus, J.K.; Hagan, R.D.; Zue, J.S.; Baker, C. Supplementation with cordyceps cs-4 fermentation product promotes fat metabolism during prolonged exercise. *Med. Sci. Sports Exerc.* **2001**, *33*, S164. [CrossRef]
158. Xiao, Y.; Huang, X.; Zhu, J. Randomized double-blind placebo-controlled clinical trial and assessment of fermentation product of *Cordyceps sinensis* (Cs-4) in enhancing aerobic capacity and respiratory function of the healthy elderly volunteers. *Chin. J. Integr. Med.* **2004**, *10*, 187–192.
159. Savioli, F.P.; Zogaib, P.; Franco, E.; AlvesDe Salles, F.C.; Giorelli, G.V.; Andreoli, C.V. Effects of *Cordyceps sinensis* supplementation during 12 weeks in amateur marathoners: A randomized, double-blind placebo-controlled trial. *J. Herb. Med.* **2022**, *34*, 100570. [CrossRef]
160. Zhou, X.; Gong, Z.; Su, Y.; Lin, J.; Tang, K. Cordyceps fungi: Natural products, pharmacological functions and developmental products. *J. Pharm. Pharmacol.* **2009**, *61*, 279–291. [CrossRef]

161. Dudgeon, W.D.; Thomas, D.D.; Dauch, W.; Scheett, T.P.; Webster, M.J. The effects of high and low-dose *Cordyceps militaris*-containing mushroom blend supplementation after seven and twenty-eight days. *Am. J. Sports Sci.* **2018**, *6*, 1–7. [CrossRef]
162. Ontawong, A.; Pengnet, S.; Thim-Uam, A.; Munkong, N.; Narkprasom, N.; Narkprasom, K.; Kuntakhut, K.; Kamkeaw, N.; Amornlerdpison, D. A randomized controlled clinical trial examining the effects of *Cordyceps militaris* beverage on the immune response in healthy adults. *Sci. Rep.* **2024**, *14*, 7994. [CrossRef]
163. Chen, Y.; Chen, G.; Zhang, C.; Tang, G.; Chan, Y.; Wang, N.; Feng, Y. Randomized, waitlist-controlled trial of *Cordyceps sinensis* mycelium culture extract (Cs4) for long COVID patients in Hong Kong. *Acta Mater. Med.* **2025**, *4*, 250–261.
164. ANM Health. A Randomized, Double-Blind, Placebo-Controlled Study to Evaluate the Efficacy and Safety of Cordyceps Capsules as an Add-On Therapy in Patients with Mild to Moderate COVID-19 Infection. Available online: https://anm.health/wp-content/uploads/2023/08/Annexure-i-Clinical-Trials-Research-Summry.pdf (accessed on 16 March 2026).
165. Wang, N.; Li, J.; Huang, X.; Chen, W.; Chen, Y. Herbal Medicine *Cordyceps sinensis* Improves Health-Related Quality of Life in Moderate-to-Severe Asthma. *Evid. Based Complement. Altern. Med.* **2016**, *2016*, 6134593. [CrossRef]
166. Heo, J.Y.; Baik, H.W.; Kim, H.J.; Lee, J.M.; Kim, H.W.; Choi, Y.S.; Won, J.H.; Kim, H.M.; Park, W.I.; Kim, C.Y. Efficacy and Safety of *Cordyceps militaris* in Korean adults with mild liver dysfunction. *J. Clin. Nutr.* **2015**, *7*, 81–86. [CrossRef]
167. Zhou, J.; Chen, X.; Xiao, L.; Zhou, J.; Feng, L.; Wang, G. Efficacy and Safety of *Cordyceps militaris* as an Adjuvant to Duloxetine in the Treatment of Insomnia in Patients With Depression: A 6-Week Double- Blind, Randomized, Placebo-Controlled Trial. *Front. Psychiatry* **2021**, *12*, 754921. [CrossRef]
168. Ru, J.; Li, P.; Wang, J.; Zhou, W.; Li, B.; Huang, C.; Li, P.; Guo, Z.; Tao, W.; Yang, Y.; et al. TCMSP: A database of systems pharmacology for drug discovery from herbal medicines. *J. Cheminform.* **2014**, *6*, 13. [CrossRef] [PubMed]
169. Cui, G.; Li, M.; Guo, W.; Gao, M.; Zhu, Q.; Liao, J. AI-driven network pharmacology: Multi-scale mechanisms of traditional Chinese medicine from molecular to patient analysis. *Comput. Struct. Biotechnol. J.* **2025**, *27*, 5087–5104. [CrossRef] [PubMed]
170. Barth, S.W.; Efferth, T. Network pharmacology to elucidate the role of phytotherapy in neurocognitive disorders. *Phytomedicine* **2025**, *148*, 157031. [CrossRef] [PubMed]
171. Panossian, A.; Efferth, T. Network Pharmacology of Adaptogens in the Assessment of Their Pleiotropic Therapeutic Activity. *Pharmaceuticals* **2022**, *15*, 1051. [CrossRef]
172. Panossian, A. Trends and Pitfalls in the Progress of Network Pharmacology Research on Natural Products. *Pharmaceuticals* **2025**, *18*, 538. [CrossRef]
173. Panossian, A.; Abdelfatah, S.; Efferth, T. Network Pharmacology of Red Ginseng (Part I): Effects of Ginsenoside Rg5 at Physiological and Sub-Physiological Concentrations. *Pharmaceuticals* **2021**, *14*, 999. [CrossRef]
174. Zhou, W.; Liu, Y.; Gao, Y.; Suonanlamao; Ma, Y.; Xiao, Y.; Wei, L. Integrating proteomics, metabolomics, and network pharmacology to investigate the mechanism of *Cordyceps sinensis* in the treatment of COPD rats. *J. Pharm. Biomed. Anal.* **2025**, *266*, 117076. [CrossRef]
175. Jiang, Y.; Liu, Z.; Hu, J.; Sun, S.; Xie, X.; Kong, X.; Tang, Y. Pharmacodynamic evaluation of *Cordyceps sinensis* (Berk.) Sacc. for ischemic stroke in rats and potential mechanism through network pharmacology and molecular docking. *J. Tradit. Chin. Med. Sci.* **2023**, *10*, 196–207. [CrossRef]
176. Butterweck, V.; Nahrstedt, A. What is the best strategy for preclinical testing of botanicals? A critical perspective. *Planta Medica* **2012**, *78*, 747–754. [CrossRef]
177. Wang, J.; Liu, R.; Liu, B.; Yang, Y.; Xie, J.; Zhu, N. Systems Pharmacology-based strategy to screen new adjuvant for hepatitis B vaccine from Traditional Chinese Medicine *Ophiocordyceps sinensis*. *Sci. Rep.* **2017**, *7*, 44788. [CrossRef]
178. Zhang, X.; Wang, M.; Liang, X.; Wang, J.; Zhang, M.; Li, C.; Wei, L.; Bi, H. Bioinformatics analysis and in vivo validation study of *Ophiocordyceps sinensis* (Berk.)G.H.Sungetal against lung adenocarcinoma. *J. Ethnopharmacol.* **2023**, *317*, 116739. [CrossRef] [PubMed]
179. Zhang, Y.; Xu, L.; Lu, Y.; Zhang, J.; Yang, M.; Tian, Y.; Dong, J.; Liao, L. Protective effect of *Cordyceps sinensis* against diabetic kidney disease through promoting proliferation and inhibiting apoptosis of renal proximal tubular cells. *BMC Complement. Med. Ther.* **2023**, *23*, 109. [CrossRef] [PubMed]
180. Li, S.; Pang, W.; Wang, Y.; Zhang, Y. *Cordyceps sinensis* extract protects against acute kidney injury by inhibiting perforin expression in NK cells via the STING/IRF3 pathway. *Aging* **2024**, *16*, 5887–5904. [CrossRef] [PubMed]
181. He, H.; Tang, J.; Ru, D.; Shu, X.; Li, W.; Li, J.; Ma, L.; Hu, X.; Xiong, L.; Li, L. Protective effects of Cordyceps extract against UVB-induced damage and prediction of application prospects in the topical administration: An experimental validation and network pharmacology study. *Biomed. Pharmacother.* **2020**, *121*, 109600. [CrossRef]
182. Pei, H.; He, Z.; Chen, W.; Zhao, Y.; Li, J.; Wang, R.; Zong, Y.; Du, R. Network pharmacology and molecular docking analysis on the mechanism of *Cordyceps militaris* polysaccharide regulating immunity through TLR4/TNF-α pathways. *J. Biochem. Mol. Toxicol.* **2023**, *37*, e23345. [CrossRef]
183. Kim, H.L.; Park, J.; Kim, H.I.; Boo, M.; Sim, J.H.; Kim, H.; Choi, H.; An, S.; Yang, H.; Shin, S.; et al. Integrating Network Pharmacology and Optimization of Preparation Methods to Enhance the Anticancer Effect of *Cordyceps militaris* on Lung Cancer. *Anticancer Res.* **2025**, *45*, 2963–2984. [CrossRef]

https://doi.org/10.3390/ph19030519

184. Wang, P.; Zong, Y.; Huang, X.; Zhang, W.; Di, L. Study on the potential mechanism of *Cordyceps militaris* in chronic obstructive pulmonary disease via integrating metabolomics and network pharmacology. *J. Pharm. Pharmacol.* **2025**, *78*, rgaf114. [CrossRef]
185. Zhou, H.B.; Feng, L.J.; Liang, X.D.K.; Zhou, Z.X.; Li, M.; Zhang, J.L.; Su, G.H. Mechanism of *Cordyceps militaris* in gouty nephropathy explored using network pharmacology and molecular docking technology. *Food Biosci.* **2024**, *60*, 104299. [CrossRef]
186. Gandhale, P.; Chikhale, R.; Khanal, P.; Biswa, V.; Ali, R.; Khan, M.S.; Gurav, N.; Ayyanar, M.; Das, S.; Gurav, S. Quest for Anti-SARS-CoV-2 antiviral therapeutics: In-silico and in-vitro analysis of edible mushroom- *Cordyceps militaris*. *J. Ayurveda Integr. Med.* **2024**, *15*, 100979. [CrossRef]
187. Lee, D.; Lee, W.-Y.; Jung, K.; Kwon, Y.S.; Kim, D.; Hwang, G.S.; Kim, C.-E.; Lee, S.; Kang, K.S. The Inhibitory Effect of Cordycepin on the Proliferation of MCF-7 Breast Cancer Cells, and Its Mechanism: An Investigation Using Network Pharmacology-Based Analysis. *Biomolecules* **2019**, *9*, 414. [CrossRef] [PubMed]
188. Qiu, X.; Li, C.; Wang, J.; Yu, H.; Wang, R.; Wang, L.; Zhang, S.; Tang, Y.; Li, Z.; Li, Q. Cordycepin Inhibits Proliferation, Migration, and Promotes Apoptosis in Fibrosarcoma HT1080 Cells by Targeting Akt1 and Kinase Activity Through Network Pharmacology Analysis. *Cell Biochem. Funct.* **2025**, *43*, e70103. [CrossRef] [PubMed]
189. Zhong, M.; Feng, M.; Chen, X.; Zhang, Y.; Wang, Y.; Yuan, P.; Zhang, T.; Han, Z.; Tang, C.; Zhang, Q.; et al. Cordycepin attenuated cyclophosphamide (CTX)-induced immunosuppression in mice via EGFR/Nrf2 antioxidant signaling pathway. *Int. Immunopharmacol.* **2025**, *163*, 115235. [CrossRef] [PubMed]
190. Chen, J.; Zhuang, Y.D.; Zhang, Q.; Liu, S.; Zhuang, B.B.; Wang, C.H.; Liang, R.S. Exploring the mechanism of cordycepin combined with doxorubicinin treating glioblastoma based on network pharmacology and biological verification. *PeerJ.* **2022**, *10*, e12942. [CrossRef]
191. Lin, J.; Zhang, Y.; Lin, S.; Ding, H.; Liu, W. Integrating Network Pharmacology and Experimental Verification to Explore the Pharmacological Mechanisms of Cordycepin against Pulmonary Arterial Hypertension in Rats. *Comb. Chem. High Throughput Screen.* **2024**, *27*, 2776–2789. [CrossRef]
192. Liao, Y.; Wang, M.; Qin, F.; Liu, T.; Chen, J. Integrating network pharmacology, quantitative transcriptomic analysis, and experimental validation revealed the mechanism of cordycepin in the treatment of obesity. *Front. Pharmacol.* **2025**, *16*, 1571480. [CrossRef]
193. Li, J.; Chen, Y.; Li, J.; Chen, L.; Wang, J.; Jiang, Y.; Zhang, B. Study on the Mechanism of *Ophiocordyceps sinensis* in Treating Liver Cirrhosis Based on Network Pharmacology. *J. Dali Univ.* **2021**, *6*, 16–21.
194. Mu, Y.; Zheng, D.; Peng, D.H.; Wang, E.C.; Ye, F.; Wang, J. *Cordyceps sinensis* for the Treatment of Liver Cancer: A Network Pharmacology and Molecular Docking Study. *Indian J. Pharm. Sci.* **2023**, *85*, 119–128. [CrossRef]
195. Gonzalez-Llerena, J.L.; Treviño-Almaguer, D.; Leal-Mendez, J.A.; Garcia-Valdez, G.; Balderas-Moreno, A.G.; Heya, M.S.; Balderas-Renteria, I.; Camacho-Corona, M.D.R.; Espinosa-Rodriguez, B.A. The Cordyceps Genus as a Potential Source of Bioactive Compounds for Adjuvant Cancer Therapy: A Network Pharmacology Approach. *Pharmaceuticals* **2025**, *18*, 667. [CrossRef]
196. Long, H.; Qiu, X.; Cao, L.; Han, R. Discovery of the signal pathways and major bioactive compounds responsible for the anti-hypoxia effect of Chinese cordyceps. *J. Ethnopharmacol.* **2021**, *277*, 114215. [CrossRef]
197. Zhang, X.; Wang, M.; Qiao, Y.; Shan, Z.; Yang, M.; Li, G.; Xiao, Y.; Wei, L.; Bi, H.; Gao, T. Exploring the mechanisms of action of *Cordyceps sinensis* for the treatment of depression using network pharmacology and molecular docking. *Ann. Transl. Med.* **2022**, *10*, 282. [CrossRef] [PubMed]
198. Zhou, J.; Wang, M.; Sun, T.; Zhou, X.; Wang, J.; Wang, Y.; Zhang, R.; Luo, R.; Yu, H. Uncovering anti-influenza mechanism of *Ophiocordyceps sinensis* using network pharmacology, molecular pharmacology, and metabolomics. *Medicine* **2023**, *102*, e34843. [CrossRef] [PubMed]
199. Li, Y.; Wang, L.; Xu, B.; Zhao, L.; Li, L.; Xu, K.; Tang, A.; Zhou, S.; Song, L.; Zhang, X.; et al. Network pharmacology investigation of *Cordyceps sinensis* in diabetic nephropathy. *J. Diabetes Res.* **2021**, *2021*, 8891093. [CrossRef] [PubMed]
200. Xi, W.; Zhao, X.; Wang, B.; Zhu, Y.; Li, H. A Review of the Mechanism of Bailing for Diabetic Nephropathy Based on ChatGPT and Network Pharmacology. *Int. J. Clin. Pract.* **2024**, *2024*, 1432594. [CrossRef]
201. Guan, H.R.; Li, B.; Zhang, Z.H.; Wu, H.S.; He, X.L.; Dong, Y.J.; Su, J.; Lv, G.Y.; Chen, S.H. Network pharmacology of Bailing capsule in polycystic ovary syndrome. *BMC Complement. Med. Ther.* **2023**, *23*, 458. [CrossRef]
202. Singh, M.; Verma, H.; Gera, N.; Baddipadige, R.; Choudhary, S.; Bhandu, P.; Silakari, O. Evaluation of *Cordyceps militaris* steroids against COVID-19 cytokine storm. *J. Biomol. Struct. Dyn.* **2024**, *42*, 5159–5177. [CrossRef]
203. Chen, Y.; Wang, P.; Zhang, M.; Yang, H.; Liang, B. Cordycepin against colorectal cancer via network pharmacology. *Comb. Chem. High Throughput Screen*, 2025; *in press*. [CrossRef]
204. Li, Y.; Han, Y.; Wang, N.; Bi, Y.; Yang, W.; Yang, Y.; Ren, X. Cordycepin as an anticancer compound. *Am. J. Chin. Med.* **2025**, *53*, 2137–2165. [CrossRef]
205. Khan, M.A.; Tania, M. Cordycepin and kinase inhibition in cancer. *Drug Discov. Today* **2023**, *28*, 103481. [CrossRef]
206. Ma, H.; Wang, G.; Guo, X.; Yao, Y.; Li, C.; Li, X.; Xin, M.; Xu, X.; Zhang, S.; Sun, Z.; et al. Network pharmacology of *Cordyceps sinensis* in oral lichen planus. *J. Oncol.* **2022**, *2022*, 3156785. [CrossRef]
207. Yang, L.; Yin, T.; Li, Y. Cordyceps preparations in chronic kidney disease. *Integr. Med. Nephrol. Androl.* **2025**, *12*, e24-00030. [CrossRef]

208. Liu, Y.; Guo, Z.J.; Zhou, X.W. Chinese cordyceps: Bioactive components and antitumor mechanisms. *Molecules* **2022**, *27*, 6576. [CrossRef] [PubMed]
209. Marcelo, A.; Brito, F.; Carmo-Silva, S.; Matos, C.A.; Alves-Cruzeiro, J.; Vasconcelos-Ferreira, A.; Koppenol, R.; Mendonça, L.; de Almeida, L.P.; Nóbrega, C. Cordycepin activates autophagy in Machado-Joseph disease. *Hum. Mol. Genet.* **2019**, *28*, 51–63. [CrossRef] [PubMed]
210. Li, X.; Zhou, Y.; Zhang, X.; Cao, X.; Wu, C.; Guo, P. Cordycepin prevents atherosclerosis via autophagy. *Oncotarget* **2017**, *8*, 94726–94737. [CrossRef] [PubMed]
211. Wang, Z.; Chen, Z.; Jiang, Z.; Luo, P.; Liu, L.; Huang, Y.; Wang, H.; Wang, Y.; Long, L.; Tan, X.; et al. Cordycepin prevents radiation ulcer via NRF2/AMPK. *Nat. Commun.* **2019**, *10*, 2538. [CrossRef]
212. Choi, Y.H.; Kim, G.Y.; Lee, H.H. Anti-inflammatory effects of cordycepin. *Drug Des. Dev. Ther.* **2014**, *8*, 1941–1953. [CrossRef]
213. Yang, J.; Li, Y.Z.; Hylemon, P.B.; Zhang, L.Y.; Zhou, H.P. Cordycepin modulates NLRP3 inflammasome. *Biomed. Pharmacother.* **2017**, *95*, 1777–1788. [CrossRef]
214. Sun, Y.; Huang, W.; Tang, P.; Zhang, X.; Yu, B.; Fan, Y.; Ge, X. Neuroprotective effects of cordycepin in Parkinson's disease. *J. Funct. Foods* **2020**, *75*, 104274. [CrossRef]
215. Liu, Z.; Lv, L.; Wei, J.; Xie, Y.; Jili, M.; Huang, Y.; Yang, R.; Luo, Y. Cordycepin attenuates macrophage pyroptosis. *Front. Pharmacol.* **2025**, *16*, 1526616. [CrossRef]
216. Zhang, X.L.; Huang, W.M.; Tang, P.C.; Sun, Y.; Qiu, L.; Yu, B.C.; Hong, Y.X.; He, Y.; Ge, X.Q. Cordycepin inhibits mitochondrial fission. *Neurotoxicology* **2021**, *84*, 1–13. [CrossRef]
217. Li, T.; Wen, L.; Cheng, B. Cordycepin alleviates hepatic lipid accumulation. *Biochem. Biophys. Res. Commun.* **2019**, *516*, 632–638. [CrossRef]
218. Hu, Y.; Wu, Y.; Song, J.; Ma, M.; Xiao, Y.; Zeng, B. Advancing *Cordyceps militaris* industry. *Bioengineering* **2024**, *11*, 783. [CrossRef]
219. European Commission. Novel Food Status Catalogue. Available online: https://food.ec.europa.eu/food-safety/novel-food/novel-food-status-catalogue_en (accessed on 20 January 2026).
220. European Commission. Food and Feed Information Portal. Available online: https://ec.europa.eu/food/food-feed-portal/screen/novel-food-catalogue/updates (accessed on 20 January 2026).
221. European Commission. RASFF Notification 2024.6020. Available online: https://webgate.ec.europa.eu/rasff-window/screen/notification/703657 (accessed on 20 January 2026).
222. European Commission. RASFF Notification 2022.4226. Available online: https://webgate.ec.europa.eu/rasff-window/screen/notification/559027 (accessed on 20 January 2026).
223. European Commission. RASFF Notification 2024.2611. Available online: https://webgate.ec.europa.eu/rasff-window/screen/notification/674503 (accessed on 20 January 2026).
224. Functional Mushrooms Simplified. EU Regulations Guide. Available online: https://functionalmushrooms.eu/novel-food-and-functional-mushrooms/ (accessed on 20 January 2026).
225. Nutra Compliance. EU Novel Food Catalogue Update. Available online: https://nutracompliance.com/EU-novel-food-catalogue-updates-february-2025 (accessed on 20 January 2026).
226. European Food Safety Authority. Navigating Novel Foods. Available online: https://www.efsa.europa.eu/en/news/navigating-novel-foods-what-efsas-updated-guidance-means-safety-assessments (accessed on 20 January 2026).
227. U.S. Food and Drug Administration. Mushroom Revival Warning Letter. Available online: https://www.fda.gov/inspections-compliance-enforcement-and-criminal-investigations/warning-letters/mushroom-revival-inc-610361-12012020 (accessed on 20 January 2026).
228. Antion Consulting. China Novel Food Ingredients System. Available online: https://www.antion.net/En/Blog/view/id/36Ul9no000opK4Da6QEXKVkzxQO0O0OO0O0O.html (accessed on 20 January 2026).
229. McEwen, B.S.; Stellar, E. Stress mechanisms. *Arch. Intern. Med.* **1993**, *153*, 2093–2101. [CrossRef] [PubMed]
230. McEwen, B.S. Stress mediators. *N. Engl. J. Med.* **1998**, *338*, 171–179. [CrossRef] [PubMed]
231. McEwen, B.S. Neurobiology of stress. *Physiol. Rev.* **2007**, *87*, 873–904. [CrossRef] [PubMed]
232. McEwen, B.S.; Wingfield, J.C. Homeostasis and stress. *Horm. Behav.* **2010**, *57*, 105–111. [CrossRef]
233. Medzhitov, R. Origin of inflammation. *Nature* **2008**, *454*, 428–435. [CrossRef]
234. Nathan, C.; Ding, A. Nonresolving inflammation. *Cell* **2010**, *140*, 871–882. [CrossRef]
235. Serhan, C.N.; Levy, B.D. Resolvins in inflammation. *J. Clin. Investig.* **2018**, *128*, 2657–2669. [CrossRef]
236. Serhan, C.N.; Gupta, S.K.; Perretti, M.; Godson, C.; Brennan, E.; Li, Y.; Soehnlein, O.; Shimizu, T.; Werz, O.; Chiurchiù, V.; et al. Atlas of inflammation resolution. *Mol. Asp. Med.* **2020**, *74*, 100894. [CrossRef]
237. U.S. Food and Drug Administration. Dietary Supplement Health and Education Act. Available online: https://ods.od.nih.gov/About/DSHEA_Wording.aspx (accessed on 20 January 2026).
238. European Food Safety Authority. Antioxidant health claims guidance. *EFSA J.* **2012**, *10*, 2474. Available online: https://www.efsa.europa.eu/sites/default/files/consultation/nda110426a,0.pdf (accessed on 20 January 2026).

https://doi.org/10.3390/ph19030519

239. European Food Safety Authority. Health claim applications guidance. *EFSA J.* **2011**, *9*, 2170. Available online: https://efsa.onlinelibrary.wiley.com/doi/pdf/10.2903/j.efsa.2016.4367https://efsa.onlinelibrary.wiley.com/doi/pdf/10.2903/j.efsa.2016.4367 (accessed on 20 January 2026).
240. European Food Safety Authority. Physical performance health claims. *EFSA J.* **2012**, *10*, 2817. Available online: https://efsa.onlinelibrary.wiley.com/doi/epdf/10.2903/j.efsa.2012.2817https://efsa.onlinelibrary.wiley.com/doi/epdf/10.2903/j.efsa.2012.2817 (accessed on 20 January 2026).
241. European Medicines Agency. Reflection Paper on Adaptogens. Available online: https://www.ema.europa.eu/en/documents/scientific-guideline/reflection-paper-adaptogenic-concept_en.pdf (accessed on 20 January 2026).
242. Panossian, A. Understanding adaptogenic activity: Specificity of the pharmacological action of adaptogens and other phytochemicals. *Ann. N. Y. Acad. Sci.* **2017**, *1401*, 49–64. [CrossRef] [PubMed]
243. Cohen Healthcare. Adaptogens and FDA/FTC Compliance. Available online: https://cohenhealthcarelaw.com/adaptogens-and-fda-ftc-compliance/ (accessed on 20 January 2026).
244. World Health Organization. *WHO Traditional Medicine Strategy 2014–2023*; WHO Press: Geneva, Switzerland, 2013. Available online: https://www.who.int/publications/i/item/9789241506096 (accessed on 20 January 2026).
245. European Medicines Agency. EU Herbal Monograph on Rhodiola Rosea. Available online: https://www.ema.europa.eu/en/documents/herbal-monograph/final-european-union-herbal-monograph-rhodiola-rosea-l-rhizoma-et-radix-revision-1_en.pdf (accessed on 20 January 2026).
246. Panossian, A.; Seo, E.J.; Efferth, T. Novel molecular mechanisms for the adaptogenic effects of herbal extracts on isolated brain cells using systems biology. *Phytomedicine* **2018**, *50*, 257–284. [CrossRef]
247. Panossian, A.; Lemerond, T.; Efferth, T. State-of-the-Art Review on Botanical Hybrid Preparations in Phytomedicine and Phytotherapy Research: Background and Perspectives. *Pharmaceuticals* **2024**, *17*, 483. [CrossRef]
248. Qin, P.; Li, X.; Yang, H.; Wang, Z.-Y.; Lu, D. Therapeutic Potential and Biological Applications of Cordycepin and Metabolic Mechanisms in Cordycepin-Producing Fungi. *Molecules* **2019**, *24*, 2231. [CrossRef]
249. Efferth, T. Establishing traditional Chinese medicine in Europe. *Chin. Herb. Med.* **2025**, *17*, 409–413. [CrossRef]
250. Chrousos, G.P. Stress and disorders of the stress system. *Nat. Rev. Endocrinol.* **2009**, *5*, 374–381. [CrossRef]
251. Dhabhar, F.S. Effects of stress on immune function: The good, the bad, and the beautiful. *Immunol. Res.* **2014**, *58*, 193–210. [CrossRef]
252. Segerstrom, S.C.; Miller, G.E. Psychological stress and the human immune system: A meta-analytic study. *Psychol. Bull.* **2004**, *130*, 601–630. [CrossRef]
253. Lupien, S.J.; McEwen, B.S.; Gunnar, M.R.; Heim, C. Effects of stress throughout the lifespan on the brain, behaviour and cognition. *Nat. Rev. Neurosci.* **2009**, *10*, 434–445. [CrossRef] [PubMed]
254. Arnsten, A.F.T. Stress signalling pathways that impair prefrontal cortex structure and function. *Nat. Rev. Neurosci.* **2009**, *10*, 410–422. [CrossRef] [PubMed]
255. Ferrucci, L.; Fabbri, E. Inflammageing: Chronic inflammation in ageing, cardiovascular disease, and frailty. *Nat. Rev. Cardiol.* **2018**, *15*, 505–522. [CrossRef] [PubMed]
256. World Health Organization. *WHO Monographs on Selected Medicinal Plants*; WHO Press: Geneva, Switzerland, 1999; Volume 1, pp. 168–182.
257. World Health Organization. *WHO Monographs on Selected Medicinal Plants*; WHO Press: Geneva, Switzerland, 2002; Volume 2, pp. 82–96.
258. World Health Organization. *WHO Monographs on Selected Medicinal Plants*; WHO Press: Geneva, Switzerland, 2007; Volume 3, pp. 296–313.
259. World Health Organization. *WHO Monographs on Selected Medicinal Plants*; WHO Press: Geneva, Switzerland, 2009; Volume 4, pp. 373–391.
260. World Health Organization. *WHO Monographs on Selected Medicinal Plants in the Newly Independent States (NIS)*; WHO Press: Geneva, Switzerland, 2010; Volume 5, pp. 141–159.
261. Samuelsson, G.; Bohlin, L. *Drugs of Natural Origin*, 6th ed.; Swedish Academy of Pharmaceutical Sciences: Stockholm, Sweden, 2009. Available online: https://www.routledge.com/Drugs-of-Natural-Origin-ATreatiseof-Pharmacognosy-Seventh-Edition/Samuelsson-Bohlin/p/book/9789198094251 (accessed on 10 February 2025).
262. British Herbal Medicine Association. *British Herbal Pharmacopoeia*; BHMA: Exeter, UK, 1996; pp. 89–90.
263. Bradley, P.R. (Ed.) *British Herbal Compendium*; BHMA: Exeter, UK, 1996; Volume 1, pp. 89–91, 115–118.
264. Li, S.; Xiao, W. General expert consensus on the application of network pharmacology in the research and development of new traditional Chinese medicine drugs. *Chin. J. Nat. Med.* **2025**, *23*, 129–142. [CrossRef]
265. Furman, D.; Campisi, J.; Verdin, E.; Carrera-Bastos, P.; Targ, S.; Franceschi, C.; Ferrucci, L.; Gilroy, D.W.; Fasano, A.; Miller, G.W.; et al. Chronic inflammation in the etiology of disease across the life span. *Nat. Med.* **2019**, *25*, 1822–1832. [CrossRef]
266. Cheng, W.; Zhang, X.; Song, Q.; Lu, W.; Wu, T.; Zhang, Q.; Li, C. Determination and comparative analysis of 13 nucleosides and nucleobases in natural fruiting body of *Ophiocordyceps sinensis* and its substitutes. *Mycology* **2017**, *8*, 318–326. Available online: https://www.tandfonline.com/doi/full/10.1080/21501203.2017.1385546 (accessed on 16 March 2026). [CrossRef]

https://doi.org/10.3390/ph19030519

267. Yu, L.; Zhao, J.; Zhu, Q.; Li, S.P. Macrophage biospecific extraction and high perf ormance liquid chromatography for hypothesis of immunological active components in *Cordyceps sinensis*. *J. Pharm. Biomed. Anal.* **2007**, *44*, 439–443. Available online: https://www.sciencedirect.com/science/article/abs/pii/S0731708507000234 (accessed on 16 March 2026). [CrossRef]
268. Tuli, H.S.; Sharma, A.K.; Sandhu, S.S.; Kashyap, D. Cordycepin: A bioactive metabolite with therapeutic potential. *Life Sci.* **2013**, *93*, 863–869. Available online: https://www.sciencedirect.com/science/article/abs/pii/S0024320513005845 (accessed on 16 March 2026). [CrossRef]
269. Jiang, Y.; Wong, J.H.; Fu, M.; Ng, T.B.; Liu, Z.K.; Wang, C.R.; Li, N.; Qiao, W.T.; Wen, T.Y.; Liu, F. Isolation of adenosine, iso-sinensetin and dimethylguanosine with antioxidant and HIV-1 protease inhibiting activities from fruiting bodies of *Cordyceps militaris*. *Phytomedicine* **2011**, *18*, 189–193. [CrossRef]
270. Matsuda, H.; Akaki, J.; Nakamura, S.; Okazaki, Y.; Kojima, H.; Tamesada, M.; Yoshikawa, M. Apoptosis-inducing effects of sterols from the dried powder of cultured mycelium of *Cordyceps sinensis*. *Chem. Pharm. Bull.* **2009**, *57*, 411–414. [CrossRef]
271. Jia, J.M.; Tao, H.H.; Feng, B.M. Cordyceamides A and B from the Culture Liquid of *Cordyceps sinensis* (B ERK.) S ACC. *Chem. Pharm. Bull.* **2009**, *57*, 99–101. [CrossRef]
272. Zhang, Y.; Liu, S.; Liu, H.; Liu, X.; Che, Y. Cycloaspeptides F and G, cyclic pentapeptides from a cordyceps-colonizing isolate of *Isaria farinosa*. *J. Nat. Prod.* **2009**, *72*, 1364–1367. Available online: https://pubs.acs.org/doi/10.1021/np900205m (accessed on 16 March 2026). [CrossRef]
273. Kim, J.H.; Park, D.K.; Lee, C.H.; Yoon, D.Y. A New Isoflavone Glycitein 7-O-beta-d-Glucoside 4″-O-methylate, isolated from *Cordyceps militaris* grown on Germinated Soybeans Extract, Inhibits EGF-induced Mucus Hypersecretion in the Human Lung Mucoepidermoid Cells. *Phytother. Res.* **2012**, *26*, 1807–1812. [CrossRef] [PubMed]
274. Kneifel, H.; König, W.A.; Loeffler, W.; Müller, R. Ophiocordin, an antifungal antibiotic of Cordyceps ophioglossoides. *Arch. Microbiol.* **1977**, *113*, 121–130. [CrossRef] [PubMed]
275. Chiu, C.P.; Liu, S.C.; Tang, C.H.; Chan, Y.; El-Shazly, M.; Lee, C.L.; Du, Y.C.; Wu, T.Y.; Chang, F.R.; Wu, Y.C. Anti-inflammatory cerebrosides from cultivated *Cordyceps militaris*. *J. Agric. Food Chem.* **2016**, *64*, 1540–1548. [CrossRef] [PubMed]
276. Dewi, L.; Liao, Y.C.; Jean, W.H.; Huang, K.C.; Huang, C.Y.; Chen, L.K.; Nicholls, A.; Lai, L.F.; Kuo, C.H. Cordyceps sinensis accelerates stem cell recruitment to human skeletal muscle after exercise. *Food Funct.* **2024**, *15*, 4010–4020. [CrossRef]
277. Hao, L.; Wang, Q.; Kobayashi, M.; Tamesada, M.; Wang, H.J. Effectiveness of *Cordyceps sinensis* alone or in combination with chemotherapy in patients with non-small cell lung cancer. *Biotherapy* **2008**, *22*, 345–349.
278. Hao, L.; Wang, Q.; Wang, B.; Wang, H.J. Clinical observation of cordyceps combined with NP regimen in treatment of advanced non-small cell lung cancer. *J. Dalian Med. Univ.* **2007**, *29*, 563–565. Available online: https://journal.dmu.edu.cn/en/article/doi/10.11724/jdmu.2007.06.14 (accessed on 16 March 2026).
279. Jung, S.J.; Jung, E.S.; Choi, E.K.; Sin, H.S.; Ha, K.C.; Chae, S.W. Immunomodulatory effects of a Cordyceps mycelium extract (Paecilomyces hepiali; CBG-CS-2): Randomized double-blind clinical trial. *BMC Complement. Altern. Med.* **2019**, *19*, 77. [CrossRef]
280. Morikubo, K.; Uchida, M.; Kume, A.; Tsunoo, H.; Tajima, T.; Nagata, A. Cordyceps and mental condition. *Jpn. Pharmacol. Ther.* **2005**, *33*, 729–734.

pharmaceuticals

MDPI

Review

Two Sides of the Same Coin for Health: Adaptogenic Botanicals as Nutraceuticals for Nutrition and Pharmaceuticals in Medicine

Alexander Panossian [1,*] and Terrence Lemerond [2]

[1] Phytomed AB, Sjöstadsvägen 6, 59344 Västervik, Sweden
[2] EuroPharma USA Inc., Green Bay, WI 54311, USA; terryl@europharmausa.com
* Correspondence: ap@phytomed.se

Abstract: Background: Adaptogens, commonly used as traditional herbal medicinal products for the relief of symptoms of stress, such as fatigue and exhaustion, belong to a category of physiologically active compounds related to the physiological process of adaptability to stressors. They are used both as pharmaceuticals in medicine and as dietary supplements or nutraceuticals in nutrition, depending on the doses, indications to treat diseases, or support health functions. However, such a dual-faced nature of adaptogens can lead to inconsistencies and contradictory outcomes from Food and Drug regulatory authorities in various countries. **Aims:** This narrative literature review aimed to (i) specify five steps of pharmacological testing of adaptogens, (ii) identify the sources of inconsistencies in the assessment of evidence the safety, efficacy, and quality of multitarget adaptogenic botanicals, and (iii) propose potential solutions to address some food and drug regulatory issues, specifically adaptogenic botanicals used for prevention and treatment of complex etiology diseases including stress-induced, and aging-related disorders. **Overview:** This critically oriented narrative review is focused on (i) five steps of pharmacological testing of adaptogens are required in a sequential order, including appropriate in vivo and in vitro models in animals, in vitro model, and mechanisms of action by a proper biochemical assay and molecular biology technique in combination with network pharmacology analysis, and clinical trials in stress-induced and aging-related disorders; (ii) the differences between the requirements for the quality of pharmaceuticals and dietary supplements of botanical origin; (iii) progress, trends, pitfalls, and challenges in the adaptogens research; (iv) inadequate assignment of some plants to adaptogens, or insufficient scientific data in case of *Eurycoma longifolia*; (v) inconsistencies in botanical risk assessments in the case of *Withania somnifera*. **Conclusions:** This narrative review highlights the importance of harmonized standards, transparent methodologies, and a balanced, evidence-informed approach to ensure consumers receive effective and safe botanicals. Future perspectives and proposed solutions include (i) establish internationally harmonized guidelines for evaluating botanicals based on their intended use (e.g., pharmaceutical vs. dietary supplement), incorporating traditional use data alongside modern scientific methods; (ii) encourage peer review and transparency in national assessments by mandating public disclosure of methodologies, data sources, and expert affiliations; (iii) create a tiered evidence framework that allows differentiated standards of proof for traditional botanical supplements versus pharmaceutical candidates; (iv) promote international scientific dialogs among regulators, researchers, and industry to develop consensus positions and avoid unilateral bans that may lack scientific rigor; (v) formally recognize adaptogens a category of natural products for prevention stress induced brain fatigue, behavioral, and aging related disorders.

Keywords: botanicals; dietary supplements; pharmaceuticals; adaptogens; network pharmacology; food and drug regulation

1. Introduction

Adaptogens belong to a category of physiologically active compounds or botanicals that trigger physiological processes of adaptability to stressors [1–3]. More than 110 medicinal plants were found to exhibit adaptogenic activity [2]. The number of plants reported as being adaptogenic has increased exponentially during the past decades. However, only a few of them comply with the most characteristic features, as shown in Table 1, an upgrade from [2].

In the first definition of adaptogens dated 1958, a toxicologist, Lasarev, focused on the so-called "state of non-specific resistance of organism" [4,5] that is associated with the notions of "adaptability" [6,7] defined by Georges Cunghilaim in 1943 and "stress", Cannon [8] and Hans Selye [9,10]. In 1967, Brekhman and Dadimov implemented the term adaptogens in pharmacognosy, postulating that adaptogens are innocuous medicinal plants, normalizing body functions in response to various harmful environmental conditions [11,12], as shown in Table 1. The first adaptogens extensively studied were Ginseng, probably its reputation as a panacea for all diseases [13,14], Eleutherococcus (Siberian ginseng), and later *Rhodiola rosea* (Golden root) due to their tonic effects [15–22]. These postulates were supported by numerous publications during the last decades [1–3], resulting in updated definitions of adaptogens, see Tables 1 and 2 [2,23], included in textbooks of pharmacognosy and phytotherapy [24–32], due to tremendous progress in biomedical sciences. However, new evidence is required to support the safety of some adaptogens, e.g., Withania, Bryonia, and some other putative adaptogens, such as Sideris, Eurocoma, Hypericum, etc., supporting Brekhmans' postulations and current definitions of adaptogens.

Table 1. Summary of characteristics of adaptogens *.

Definition: Adaptogens are natural compounds or plant extracts that enhance the adaptability and survival of living organisms in response to stress. *Therapeutic category and action*: adaptogens, tonic, immunomodulatory [4,15–22,24–49], *Chemical class*: predominantly tetracyclic triterpene, phenethyl- and phenylpropanoid glycosides, lignans, etc. *Pharmacological activity*: adaptogenic, tonic, stress-protective, stimulating *Mechanism of action*: multitarget effects on the neuroendocrine-immune system; adaptogens are adaptive stress response modifiers of cellular and organismal defense systems, activating intracellular and extracellular adaptive signaling pathways, expression of stress-activated proteins, neuropeptides, antioxidant enzymes, and anti-apoptotic proteins of an organism, resulting in nonspecific resistance to various stressors and increased survival [1–3,14,23,33–36].

*—Reproduced from Panossian et al. [2] with minor modifications.

Depending on indications for their use to treat diseases, or health-supporting functional claims, they can be classified both as drugs in medicine and as dietary supplements or nutraceuticals in nutrition, e.g., *Panax ginseng* C.A.Mey. roots [47,48], Schisandra chinensis (Turcz.) Baill., fruit [38], *Sedum roseum* (L.) Scop. (syn. *Rhodiola rosea* L.) [48]. In this context, adaptogens occupy a unique and complex position at the intersection of food and pharmaceutical regulation [50,51], different from other categories of physiological compounds like vitamins, minerals, or antioxidants, which are essential for various physiological processes in the human organism.

A concept underlying preventive treatment for "subhealth" conditions ("*fu zheng*" in TCM for strengthening body resistance and "vital energy"—*qi*) by adaptogens was implemented in the USSR under the names Medical Fitness, Pharmacomacia, and Valeology [2,50,51]. The dual-faced nature of some botanicals used as pharmaceuticals and dietary supplements for nutrition can lead to inconsistencies and contradictory outcomes from the Food and Drug regulatory authorities in various countries. For instance, reports from Danish and Indian food authorities on the safety of Ashwagandha [52–55] reveal inconsistencies and controversial conclusions. As a result, this can raise conflicts of interest between the pharmaceutical and food industry and the Food and Drug regulatory authorities [56].

This narrative overview is an extension to our previous review articles on adaptogens, aiming to identify the sources of inconsistencies in the assessment of evidence, ensure the safety, efficacy, and quality of botanicals, and propose potential solutions to address the issues, particularly in the field of multi-component Botanicals and Botanical Herbal Products dealing predominantly with complex etiology, e.g., fatigue, adaptation in stress-induced, and aging-related disorders and diseases, see Table 1. These reviews provided comprehensive information on adaptogens' research [1–3,15,33–36,41–49], including results of clinical studies. In this critically oriented narrative literature review, we raised two simple questions:

- How to distinguish adaptogens from other herbs that are claimed as putative adaptogens, e.g., *Eurycoma longifolia* [57]?
- What are the sources of controversial conclusions from the assessment of efficacy and safety of the same plant in various countries, e.g., *Withania somnifera* in India and Denmark [52–56]?

We also hypothesized that this is due to insufficient evidence and differences in the criteria for assessing the quality, efficacy, and safety of botanicals, which may lead to inconsistent results, particularly in clinical studies.

2. Progress, Trends, Pitfalls, and Challenges in the Adaptogens Research

Adaptogens are botanicals that enhance adaptability, resilience, resistance, and survival in response to stress-induced and aging-related disorders [2,3].

The term adaptogen is derived from adaptation, which is coined for the physiological process of adaptability [6,7], Figure 1, of the organism to repeated action of the botanical that triggers adaptive stress response via intracellular and extracellular adaptive signaling pathways and networks in neuroendocrine-immune, cardiovascular, and gastrointestinal systems and resulting in increased adaptability, resilience, resistance, and survival in stress-induced and aging-related disorders [1–3].

Adaptogens play a similar role in defending the plant against environmental challenges, including viruses, harmful bacteria, insect-borne diseases, excessive UV rays, and the physiological ravages of chronic stress [3].

Initially, the postulated definition of adaptogens was modified several times (Table 2), as our understanding of their mode and mechanisms of action, and the progress in biomedical sciences over the last few decades, improved [1–3]. Witnessing the progress in stress research, the evolution of the adaptogen concept and milestones of adaptogen research [59,60] reflects scientific knowledge to new findings over time: from discoveries of hormones, neurotransmitters, molecular chaperones (heat shock proteins), neuropeptide NPY, eicosanoids, and other mediators of intracellular and extracellular communications in response to adaptive hormetic response, to network pharmacology of OMICs and systems biology concepts [1–3].

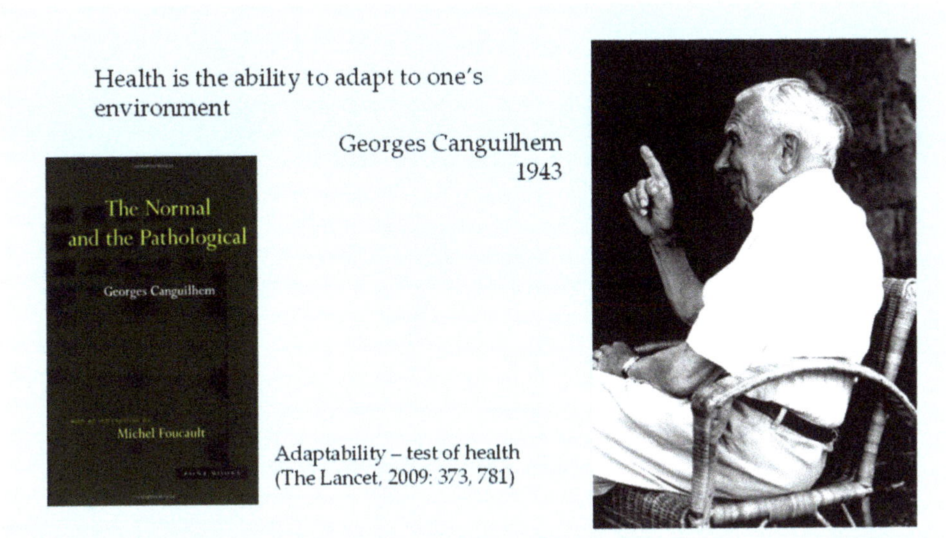

Figure 1. Georges Canguilhem introduced the term adaptability in 1943, who defined adaptability as the ability of an organism to alter itself or its responses to the changed environment or circumstances and assumed that adaptability shows the ability to learn and improve from experience—repeated mild exposure or low doses of stress result in the increased resistance of cells and organisms to subsequent stress exposure, resulting in an adaptation that favors survival [6,7]. According to the WHO definition, "health is the state of complete physical, mental, and social well-being and not merely the absence of disease or infirmity" [58]. Notably, that is formally different from the definition of health distinct by George Canguilhem as "the ability to adapt to one's environment", but in line with the WHO.

Table 2. Definitions of adaptogens *.

• Adaptogens are medicinal substances causing the "state of nonspecifically increased resistance" of the organism.
• Only those preparations that meet the following requirements may be included in the group of adaptogens: (a) An adaptogen should be innocuous and cause minimal disorders in the physiological functions of an organism; (b) The action of an adaptogen should be nonspecific, i.e., it should increase resistance to adverse influences of a wide range of factors of physical, chemical, and biological nature, (c) An adaptogen may possess normalizing action irrespective of the direction of the foregoing pathologic changes.
• The adaptogens are nontoxic compounds with polyvalent mechanisms of action and pharmacological effects related to adaptability and survival.
• Adaptogens are substances that elicit in an organism a state of nonspecifically raised resistance, allowing them to counteract stressor signals and to adapt to exceptional strain.
• Adaptogens are metabolic regulators that increase the ability of an organism to adapt to environmental factors and to avoid damage from such factors.
• Plant adaptogens are agents that reduce the damaging effects of various stressors due to the reduction in the reactivity of the host defense system. They adapt organisms to stress and have a curative impact on stress-induced disorders
• Adaptogenic substances have the capacity to normalize body functions and strengthen systems compromised by stress. They have a protective effect on health against a wide variety of environmental assaults and emotional conditions.

Table 2. *Cont.*

• Adaptogens comprise a pharmacotherapeutic group of herbal preparations used to: increase attention and endurance in fatigue and prevent/mitigate/reduce stress-induced impairments and disorders related to neuro-endocrine and immune systems. • Botanical adaptogens are plant extracts, or specific constituents of plant extracts, which function to increase survival in animals and humans by stimulating their adaptability to stress by inducing adaptive responses. • Adaptogens are stress-response modifiers that increase an organism's nonspecific resistance to stress by increasing its ability to adapt and survive. • Botanical adaptogens are metabolic regulators that increase survival by increasing adaptability in stress. • Adaptogens are natural compounds or plant extracts that increase the adaptability and survival of living organisms to stress. • Adaptogen—any of various natural substances used in herbal medicine to normalize and regulate the systems of the body. https://www.dictionary.com/browse/adaptogen (assessed on 3 September 2025). • Adaptogens are currently defined as a therapeutic category/ pharmacological group of herbal medicines or/and nutritional products, increasing adaptability, survival, and resilience in stress and aging by triggering intracellular and extracellular adaptive signaling pathways of cellular and organismal defense systems (stress system, e.g., neuroendocrine-immune complex • Adaptogens act as chronic eustress, activating adaptive stress response, resilience, and overall survival. Adaptogens trigger the defense adaptive stress response of the organism to stressors, leading to the extension of the limits of resilience to overload, brain fatigue, and mental and aging disorders [3] • The term "adaptogen" refers to a time-dependent physiological adaptation process of the organism in response to the repeated administration of a plant substance that activates intracellular and extracellular adaptive signaling pathways and triggers an adaptive stress response [23].

*—Reproduced from Panossian et al. [2] with additions.

Overall, the mechanism of action of adaptogens remains largely unexplored, despite significant progress in brain and endocrine research, particularly in the regulation of biorhythms, which are closely linked to senescence and aging processes (Figures 2 and 3) [1–3]. Several hypothetical models of time [1–3,12,61–66] and dose [3] dependent relationship effects of adaptogens were considered based on adaptive stress response and homeostasis concepts [1–3].

Considering the chemical structure of adaptogenic compounds, they were distinguished into three groups, suggesting that their pharmacological activity is associated with effects on the neuroendocrine immune complex and multitarget pleiotropic effects [1–3,15]. They include

(i) Steroids-like tetracyclic and pentacyclic triterpenes, such as ginsenosides, withanolides, cucurbitacines, and andrographolides, which structurally resemble the catabolic hormones corticosteroids that inactivate the stress system to protect against overreaction to stressors; and anabolic-androgenic steroids structurally related to testosterone and estrogen androgenic steroid hormones which regulate lipids and sugar metabolism via hypothalamus–pituitary–adrenal hypothalamus–pituitary–adrenal (HPA)-axis = hypothalamus–pituitary–adrenal axis [1–3,15,67,68].

(ii) Catecholamine-like phenolic compounds such as phenylpropanoids, phenylethane derivatives, and lignans, having similar to neurotransmitter hormones pharmacophores and suggesting an effect on the sympathetic nervous system, possibly implying an impact in the early stages of the stress response [1–3],

(iii) Oxylipins [2,15,69] (unsaturated C-18 trihydroxy and epoxy polyhydroxylated unsaturated fatty acids), homologous to anti-inflammatory resolvins and pro-inflammatory leukotrienes [70], which are involved in the pathogenesis of Alzheimer's disease. *Rhodiola rosea*, *Withania somnifera*, and *Eleutherococcus senticosus* downregulate the expression of key genes (ALOX5AP, DPEP2, LTC4S) involved in the biosynthesis of leukotrienes A, B, C, D, and E, resulting in inhibition of the leukotriene signaling pathway, suggesting their potential benefits in Alzheimer's disease [3,71].

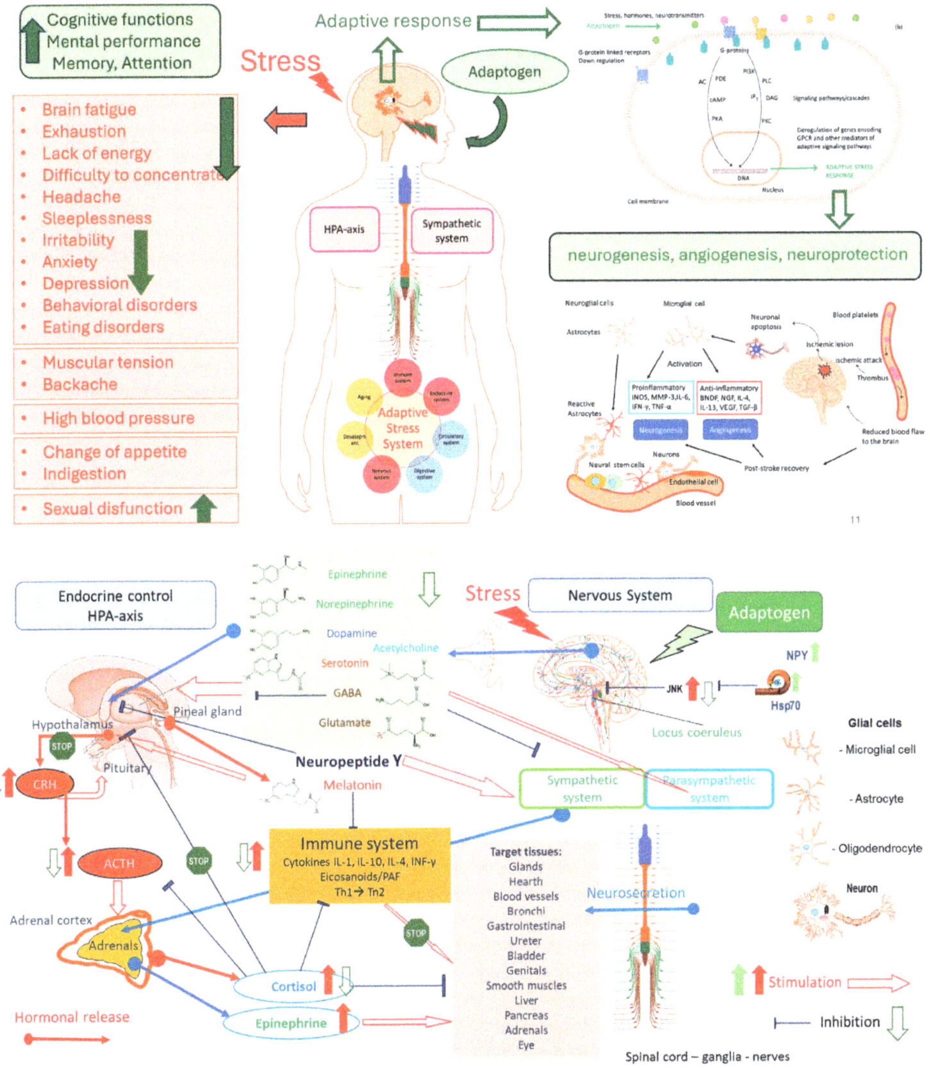

Figure 2. Chronic stress-induced symptoms, as well as the effects of adaptogens on key mediators and effectors of the adaptive stress response, result in neuroprotection, leading to improved cognitive function and enhanced mental and physical performance. Brain cells respond adaptively by enhancing their ability to function and resist stress, as demonstrated by an update from the authors' free-access publication, along with their accompanying drawings. Simplified overview of the stress system (central nervous system, CNS, and peripheral tissues/organs in the periphery) and reciprocal connections of elements of the neuroendocrine-immune complex to mobilize an adaptive response against the stressor [3].

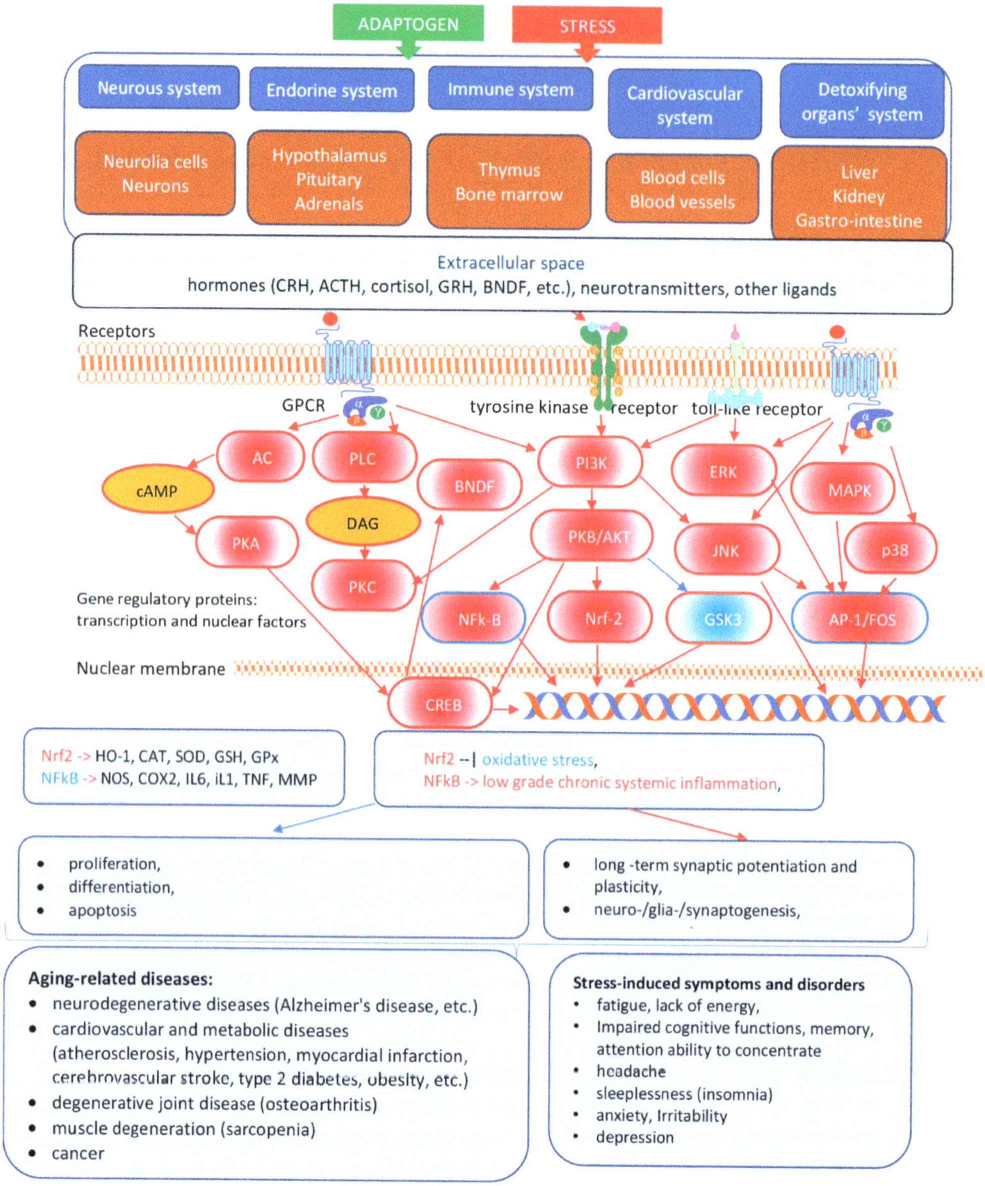

Figure 3. The hypothetical molecular mechanisms and modes of pharmacological action of adaptogens on key mediators of the neuroendocrine-immune complex, cardiovascular, and detoxifying systems that regulate the adaptive stress response to stressors/pathogens in stress- and aging-induced diseases and disorders [3,19]. Reproduced from the authors' free-access publication [66] and the authors' drawings. Activation is shown in red, while the inhibition is in blue (effect of ginseng/ginsenosides), cycles/ellipses, arrows, and clouds. BDNF, brain-derived neurotrophic factor; cAMP, cyclic adenosine monophosphate; CREB, cAMP-responsive element-binding protein; ERK, extracellular signal-regulated kinase; GSK-3, glycogen synthase kinase-3; JNK, the c-Jun N-terminal kinase (JNK)/stress-activated protein kinase (SAPK MAPK, mitogen-activated protein kinase; NF-kB, nuclear factor-kappa B; Nrf2, nuclear factor E2-related factor 2; PI3K, phosphatidylinositol 3-kinase; PKA, protein kinase A; PKB, protein kinase B; PLC, phospholipase C.

Figure 3 illustrates the effects of adaptogens on key mediators of the neuroendocrine-immune complex, cardiovascular, and detoxification systems that regulate the adaptive stress response to stressors/pathogens in stress- and aging-induced diseases and disorders. CRH- and ACTH-induced stimulation of GPCR receptors activates the cAMP-dependent protein kinase (PKA) signaling pathway, regulating energy balance and metabolism across multiple systems, including adipose tissue (lipolysis), liver (gluconeogenesis and glucose tolerance), pancreas, and gut (insulin exocytosis and sensitivity). The key molecules involved in the PI3K-Akt signaling pathway are receptor tyrosine kinases. Activating the PI3K-Akt signaling pathway promotes cell proliferation and growth, stimulates cell cycle, vascular remodeling, and cell survival, and inhibits cell apoptosis in response to extracellular signals. The nonspecific antiviral action of adaptogens is associated with the activation of innate immunity by upregulation of the expression of the pathogen's pattern recognition receptors, specifically toll-like receptors and TLR-mediated signaling pathways. The protein kinase C (PKC) family of enzymes, with its various isoforms, plays a cell-type-specific and essential role, particularly in the immune system, through NF-κB activation [3].

Three stress-activated MAPK signaling pathways, which play crucial roles in cell proliferation, differentiation, survival, and death, have been implicated in the pathogenesis of numerous human diseases, including Alzheimer's disease, Parkinson's disease, and cancer.

- The stress factors inducing the activation of the c-Jun N-terminal kinase (JNK)/stress-activated protein kinase (SAPK)-mediated adaptive signaling pathway are heat shock, irradiation, reactive oxygen species, cytotoxic drugs, inflammatory cytokines, hormones, growth factors, and other stresses. Activating the JNK/MAPK10 signaling pathway promotes cell death and apoptosis by upregulating proapoptotic genes.
- The activation of the extracellular-signal-regulated kinase (ERK) pathway is initiated by hormones and stresses to trigger endothelial cell proliferation during angiogenesis, T cell activation, long-term potentiation in hippocampal neurons, phosphorylation of the transcription factor p53, activation of phospholipase A2 in mast cells, followed by activation of biosynthesis of leukotrienes and inflammation/allergy, etc.
- The third major stress-activated p38 signaling pathway contributes to the control of inflammation, the release of cytokines by macrophages and neutrophils, apoptosis, cell differentiation, and cell cycle regulation [3].

2.1. *Stress-Protective, Stimulating, and Tonic Activity of Adaptogens*

The stress-protective effect is a result of feedback downregulation mechanisms following single-dose stimulation of an adaptogen (a mild pro-stressor) and repeated administration of plant adaptogens or physical exercise (tonic effect). One of the adaptive stress-response mechanisms of feedback regulation in organisms is the HPA-mediated loop of feedback down-regulation in anti-inflammatory response, as shown in Figure 2, where the key regulator is cortisol [61,63,65,68]. Adaptogens trigger various alternative signaling pathways via stress-adaptive feedback networks (see Figure 3, refs. [1–3]).

Stress as a defense response of an organism to external factors (strain) stimulates the formation of endogenous activating messengers, such as catecholamines, prostaglandins (PG), cytokines, nitric oxide (NO), and PAF ("switch on"-system), which in turn activate energy and metabolic resources of the organism. For example, NO is produced in large quantities during host defense and immunologic reactions. Corticosteroids, CRF, Heat shock proteins (Hsp), and PGE2 are endogenous mediators of cellular communications, which protect cells and whole organisms from overreacting to the activating messengers ("switch off" system) [61,68].

The balance between the activities of the "switch on" and "switch off" systems—"reactivity"—reflects the organism's sensitivity to stressors and its level of protection against their damaging effects, "homeostasis". It appears that, in the process of adapting to the impact of stressors, this balance is shifted to a higher level of equilibrium and homeostasis. Adaptogens increase the production of both activating and deactivating messengers of the stress system. In other words, adaptogens increase the capacity of the stress system to respond to external signals at the higher level of equilibrium-heterostasis [61,68].

Thus, a single administration of an adaptogen primarily produces a challenging (stimulating or stress-agonizing) effect, a fact that is utilized in sports medicine, where a single dose of an adaptogen can enhance athletes' performance by making them more alert [62–65,72]. The stimulating effects of a single dose of adaptogens are primarily due to interactions within the central nervous system (CNS) and hypothalamic–pituitary–adrenal (HPA) axis but do not require prolonged processes such as gene and protein expression, neurogenesis, cell proliferation, and differentiation [1–3,62–65]. The tonic effect of adaptogens is due to their repeated administration at multiple doses [3,15,63].

Plant adaptogens stimulate the nervous system through mechanisms that are quite different from those of conventional stimulants. Depending on the mediators of the stress system involved in the adaptogen-induced stress response, an immediate (single-dose effect) or a long-term (following multiple administrations) stimulating effect may be observed [65,73].

There are essential differences between adaptogens and conventional stimulants of the CNS, such as caffeine, nicotine, amphetamines, and cocaine, which produce a sense of euphoria and can be used to increase alertness and the ability to concentrate on mental tasks, boosting endurance and productivity [2,24,65]. However, long-term stimulant abuse can impair cognitive function and lead to psychotic symptoms and drug dependence. In contrast, adaptogens which exhibit high rate of recovery process after exhaustive physical load, low energy depletion, increased performance in stress and survival in stress, good quality of arousal, lack of senescence, rare side effects, upregulation of expression DNA/RNA and proteins, increased Hsp70 synthesis, and activation of NPY production, which activate HPA -axis [2,65,74,75].

Adaptogens exhibit stress-protective and tonic effects [15–18,62,65], as shown in Figure 4a. After repeated dose administration, they trigger adaptive stress response signaling pathways and mediate gene expression in the HPA axis and other body tissues [1–3,61,65,74,75], as shown in Figures 2 and 3. The stress-protective effect achieved by multiple administrations of adaptogens is not the result of inhibiting the stress response of an organism but rather of adaptive changes in the organism in response to the repeated stress-agonistic effect of the adaptogens [1–3,62,68,76–78]. Importantly, adaptogens exhibit anti-stress effects by activating cellular adaptive mechanisms, acting as eustressors or challengers (i.e., "good stressors"), mild stress mimetics, agonists, or "stress vaccines" that induce stress-protective responses, but not stress antagonists [1–3,24,68,76–78].

Adaptogens-induced outcomes and changes in various endpoints from the baseline over time (Figure 4a) depend on the baseline: (i) a state of rest, and (ii) under various stressors. Under rest, they exhibit a stimulating impact on a single dose and a tonic effect with repeated multiple administration (preconditioning), similar to physical exercise (preconditioning). Against the background of stress (physical exertion or mental stress, preconditioning), adaptogens exhibit a stress-protective effect by reducing the threshold of sensitivity to the stressor and thereby extending the duration of the protective effect in time until the fatigue phase, until complete exhaustion or damaging effect (distress) of continuous stressful exposure, e.g., in stroke [3].

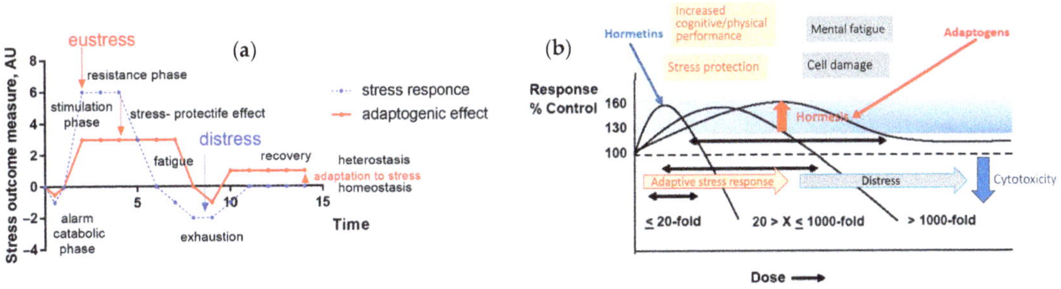

Figure 4. (**a**)—Simplified pattern of adaptive stress response over time (blue color dot line) and stress protective effect of an adaptogen (red color line) increasing resistance and decreasing sensitivity to a conditional stressor, extending the duration of the resistance anabolic phase to fatigue, and preventing the onset of the exhaustion phase (distress), leading to adaptation to stress and increasing the level of homeostasis. AU—an arbitrary unit of an outcome measure of a stress response, e.g., increasing the number of errors over time detected in Conner's computerized cognitive performance test for attention and impulsivity, biochemical markers (cortisol, nitric oxide, etc.) [79]. It is reproduced and modified from [3,61,66]. (**b**)—Simplified hypothetical description of the hormetic dose–response relationship of toxic hormetins and adaptogens; author's drawings reproduced from the authors' free access publication [3].

The dose-effect relationship of adaptogens is typically characterized by a bell-shaped curve in many pharmacological models, and in some models, a biphasic curve emerges at excessively high doses [3] (Figure 4b). This aligns somewhat with the hormesis concept, characterized by a biphasic reversal effect, where positive (stimulating) effects at low doses transition to negative (toxic/harmful) effects at high doses. The drug-response interactions model has several other limitations regarding biphasic dose–response. The primary mechanism common to both conditioning a hormetic and adaptive response is that it activates molecular signaling pathways, enhancing the cell and organism's ability to tolerate more severe stress. The optimal range of doses for adaptogens or conditioning treatments corresponds to the hormetic zone dose–response pattern. The underlying molecular mechanisms of hormesis are not fully understood. The theoretical background of hormesis is related to the hypothesis of interactions between biologically active compounds (ligands, interventions, or drugs) and two target proteins (receptors) that exhibit functionally opposite responses at different concentrations. It was proposed that a drug acting as a competitive antagonist at either or both of the receptors changes the relationship between the two opposing concentration-effect curves, resulting in potentiation, antagonism, or reversal of the observed effect; the theoretical model suggested that the total impact on the system can be obtained by the algebraic summation of the two effects resulting from the activation of the two opposing receptor populations, providing a classical hormesis biphasic curve. However, in practice, dose–response patterns are significantly complicated due to many other interactions, including: (i)—multiple targets (receptors) of different affinity to the active compound, (ii)—other regulatory proteins or mediators in the networks involved in the adaptive stress response, (iii)—feedback downregulations in the molecular signaling pathways and/or; (iv)—the metabolic transformation of active ligands into metabolites, a secondary ligand, has different affinities to various receptors of the adaptive stress response [35]. These observations demonstrate that a specific plant extract, characterized by a product-specific quantitative and qualitative composition, as well as an HPLC fingerprint/pharmaceutical profile, can exhibit varying pharmacological activity, profiles, and signatures depending on the dose, resulting in a dual response in the organism, ranging from positive to inactive or even negative [3,35].

2.2. What Is Necessary and Sufficient to Be Classified as an Adaptogenic Plant?

Five steps of pharmacological testing of adaptogens are required in a sequential order:

- An appropriate in vivo model in animals
- An appropriate in vitro model
- Mechanism of action by a proper biochemical assay
- Mechanism of action by an appropriate molecular biology technique in combination with network pharmacology analysis
- Clinical trials in stress-induced and aging-related disorders

Pharmacologic assessment of adaptogenic activity is commonly used in various animal stress tests involving exposure to cold, heat, altered atmospheric pressure and oxygen content, radiation, toxic substances, starvation, fear, and chronic diseases. It has been demonstrated that the primary feature of adaptogens is their ability to enhance resistance to both physical and emotional stress [15]. The most suitable pharmacological methods for assessing adaptogenic activity are chronic unpredictable stress (CUS) animal models, which induce affective behaviors in mice and, once established, measure stress-related alterations in the intrinsic excitability and synaptic regulation of the medial prefrontal cortex layer 5/6 pyramidal neurons. Adult male mice received 2 weeks of 'less intense' stress or 2 or 4 weeks of 'more intense' CUS, followed by assessment of sucrose preference for anhedonia and the elevated plus maze for anxiety. They forced a swim test for evaluation of depressive-like behaviors. An intense CUS exposure results in increased anhedonia, anxiety, and depressive behaviors, while less intense stress results in no measured behavioral phenotypes [80].

Adaptogens activate multiple cytoprotective mechanisms that increase cell survival (antioxidant, immune modulation, Hsp70 modulation [1–3]), and trigger the generation of hormones (e.g., corticotropin, cortisol, gonadotropin-releasing hormones, urocortin, melatonin [33]), neuropeptide N [75], and neurohormones, and neurotransmitters playing a key role in metabolic regulation and homeostasis [3], Figure 2.

Adaptogens trigger an adaptive stress response, activating adaptive signaling pathways, e.g., G-protein coupled (GPCR), tyrosine, toll-like receptors, and I3PK-mediated pathways that are known to promote survival in response to stress, suggesting neuroprotective activity and potential benefits of adaptogens in neurodegenerative diseases, Figure 4 [1–3,33].

Overall, adaptogens are active in numerous conditions and diseases associated with stress and aging-related impairments of the neuroendocrine-immune complex, as well as energy and fatigue, which must be tested clinically in human subjects [2,3].

2.3. Progress and Trends in Adaptogens Research

Breakthroughs in our knowledge of the mechanisms of action of adaptogens are usually associated with the discovery of previously unknown mediators of intracellular and intercellular communications and their physiological functions and mechanisms of action, such as molecular chaperones of neuropeptide Y and many new proteins involved in the regulation of homeostasis and the development of various diseases and their symptoms. For instance, in post-stroke and traumatic long-lasting brain or mental fatigue associated with impaired angiogenesis and neurogenesis during recovery [3]. An invaluable breakthrough was the application of network pharmacology methods, leveraging the latest techniques in molecular biology, metabolomics, proteomics, transcriptomics, genomics, and microbiomics to study interactions.

Adaptogens are characterized as botanicals with polyvalent action and pleiotropic activity, often referred to as a "Ginseng-like panacea for all diseases [13,14]." Progress in biomedical science, particularly in network pharmacology, metabolomics, proteomics, transcriptomics, genomics, and microbiomics—collectively known as omics—and systems biology, has significantly contributed to uncovering the mechanisms of action of adaptogens and enhancing our understanding of their effects [3,14,23,33–36,81–87].

Network pharmacology is an emerging discipline that integrates systems biology, bioinformatics, and pharmacology to understand the actions of drugs on a systemic, network level. Instead of the traditional "one drug–one target" model, network pharmacology employs the "multitarget, multi-component" paradigm, which is particularly useful for complex diseases and multi-herbal medicines, Table 3 [3,14,33,35,81].

Table 3. Basic Principles of Network Pharmacology: Traditional vs. Network Pharmacology.

Feature	Traditional Pharmacology	Network Pharmacology
Philosophy	Reductionist—targets one gene/protein	Systems-oriented—considers multitarget interactions
Target Focus	Single molecule	Multiple targets, often in networks
Drug Design Goal	High specificity	Modulation of networks/pathways
View of Disease	Caused by the dysfunction of a single entity	Disease as a network perturbation
Data Used	Experimental pharmacokinetics/dynamics	Multi-omics, PPI networks, computational modeling
Mechanism Identification	Binding affinity and downstream effects	Topological influence on biological networks
Predictive Capacity	Limited to known targets	Broader scope; includes off-targets, repurposing, synergy predictions
Herbal/TCM Suitability	Not applicable	Especially suitable due to the multi-component nature
Validation	Strong experimental support	Requires computational and experimental integration
Limitations	Ignores complexity and off-target effects	Data noise, oversimplified networks, context-ignorant models

Network pharmacology offers a robust systems-level framework for understanding drug mechanisms, especially in complex, multitarget conditions. While it introduces a more realistic model of pharmacological action, it must overcome limitations like data incompleteness, lack of dynamism, and validation gaps. For mechanistic insights, it should ideally be integrated with experimental biology and temporal models to achieve both predictive power and clinical relevance [81].

The advancement of integrative omics network pharmacology and artificial intelligence in natural products has opened new avenues for the following areas:

- elucidation of the mechanisms of action of medicinal plants [3,14,33–36,71,81–83,85,88–91];
- understanding the synergistic therapeutic actions of complex bioactive components in medicinal plants [3,33–35,92,93];
- providing a rationale for traditional Chinese medicine, as well as enhancing the quality of TCM drug research and the speed and efficiency of developing new TCM products [94–99];
- discovering and developing new botanical hybrid combinations [3,14,35];
- predict drug–herb interactions [100], adverse events [101], and potential toxic effects [102–105].

Unlike conventional medicines, botanical adaptogens comprise multi-component active compounds and phytochemicals, whose interactions lead to novel and unexpected pharmacological activities due to their synergistic and antagonistic effects [14,33,35,81,106]. Emerging research also highlights how extraction methods can significantly influence the physicochemical and functional characteristics of bioactive plant-derived components, such as dietary fibers from *Rubus chingii* Hu., suggesting that extraction processes may similarly impact the efficacy and bioavailability of botanicals [107].

Similarly, the pharmacological activity of a combination of several plants or herbal extracts, such as those in botanical hybrid preparations (e.g., TCM formulas), results in a new biologically active substance with unique pharmacological characteristics [35].

Primary outcomes from gene expression studies of adaptogens in isolated brain cells indicate that adaptogens activate adaptive stress-response canonical pathways, modulating numerous physiological processes and the progression of stress-induced and aging disorders [3]. In addition, various adaptogens regulate the expression of many other genes involved in neurogenesis, angiogenesis, innate immunity, and inflammaging, which play a crucial role in stress-induced and aging-related disorders [2,93].

Network pharmacology provides a possible mechanism of action. Network analysis must be conducted in combination with bioinformatic databases and experimental pharmacology, based on the results of gene expression and transcriptomics arrays obtained in vitro or in vivo studies, and validated, e.g., by PCT technique.

Molecular docking approaches in silico studies are not a stand-alone technique. Without functional assays (e.g., enzymatic inhibition) and binding studies (e.g., surface plasmon resonance, isothermal calorimetry, or microscale thermophoresis), there is no evidence to support the accuracy of in silico results. Otherwise, they remain hypothetical.

Various challenges in network pharmacology for natural products and phytotherapy research, which should be addressed [81,106].

2.4. Pitfalls in Adaptogen Research: Inadequate Assignment of Some Plants to Adaptogens or Insufficient Scientific Data

Polyvalence of some medicinal plants often leads to unsupported claims that they are adaptogens, as is the case with *Eurycoma longifolia*. While it is recognized in traditional medicine across Southeast Asia and regulated in markets like the EU, the official pharmacopeial status appears to be limited to three countries: Malaysia, Indonesia, and Vietnam. Several publications claim that *Eurycoma longifolia* Jack is an adaptogen [108–114]. However, there is no scientific evidence supporting these statements. The authors refer to:

- Traditional use of "Malaysian Ginseng" as an aphrodisiac that stimulates sexual desire, antimalarial, anti-diabetic, antimicrobial, and antipyretic activities, and its polyvalent activity in various diseases [115,116],
- Gonadotropin-induced increase in testosterone in vitro studies and elevated blood testosterone in animals and human studies [57,110,117,118], possibly associated with an increase in male fertility and ergogenic activity [109,110,112,113,119–121].

However, that is not a sufficient characteristic criterion to classify Eurycoma as an adaptogen. See the definition and characteristics of adaptogens in the Amendment below.

Furthermore, the quality of clinical trials in humans, preclinical studies in animals, and in vitro studies is not satisfactory, making it difficult to draw robust conclusions on the efficacy and safety of Eurocoma products.

E.g., Talbott et al., 2013 [111] state that:

- Active compounds of Eurycoma are 4300 dalton glycopeptides consisting of 36 amino acids.

> *"Eurycoma contains a group of small peptides referred to as "eurypeptides" with 4300 dalton glycopeptides 36 amino acids that are known to have effects in improving energy status and sex drive in studies of rodents. Animal studies have shown that many of the effects of the extract are mediated by its glycoprotein components. Typical dosage recommendations, based on traditional use and on the available scientific evidence in humans, including dieters and athletes, call for 50–200 mg/day of a water-extracted tongkat ali root standardized to 22% eurypeptides."*

However, the publication does not contain any information about the analytical methods used for quantification, accuracy, precision, selectivity, or purity of the analytical markers, which are essential for ensuring reproducible quality and efficacy. There is nothing in that study [111] about numerous biological active plant secondary metabolites isolated from *E. longifolia* various extracts, e.g., quassinoids eurycomanone, 13α(21)-epoxyeurycomanone, 13,21-dihydroeurycomanone, 14,15 β -dihydroxy-klaineanone, longilactone and eurycomalacton, 9-methoxycanthin-6-one; Laurycolactone; Eurycolactone B; Eurycomalide A; Eurylactone; Longilactone; Eurycomalactone; Eurycomanone; Eurycomanol; Pasakbumin B; Hydroxyklaineanone; Biphenyl-neolignan; Quassin etc., which are known as poorly water-soluble compounds [115,116,120–123].

- According to the authors Talbott et al., 2013 [111], the mechanism of action is related to *"the bioactive complex 4300 dalton glycopeptides ("eurypeptides" with 36 amino acids) has been shown to activate the CYP17 enzyme (17 alphahydroxylase and 17,20 lyase) to enhance the metabolism of pregnenolone and progesterone to yield more DHEA (dehydroepiandrosterone) and androstenedione, respectively [114]. This glycoprotein water-soluble extract of Eurycoma longifolia has been shown to deliver anti-aging and antistress benefits subsequent to its testosterone balancing effects"*.

The effects of tongkat ali in restoring normal testosterone levels appear to be less due to actually "stimulating" testosterone synthesis, but rather by increasing the release rate of "free" testosterone from its binding hormone, sex-hormone-binding-globulin (SHBG).

In this way, eurycoma may be considered not so much a testosterone "booster" (such as an anabolic steroid), but rather a "maintainer" of normal testosterone levels and a "restorer" of normal testosterone levels (from "low" back "up" to normal ranges). This would make eurycoma particularly beneficial for individuals with sub-normal testosterone levels, including those who are dieting for weight loss, middle-aged individuals suffering with fatigue or depression, and intensely training athletes who may be at risk for overtraining."

That is not related to the known mechanisms of action of adaptogens on the neuroendocrine-immune complex; see Amendment below.

Furthermore, the results of a clinical study of *Eurycoma longifolia* (Physta®) water extract plus multivitamins show a lack of activity when *Eurycoma longifolia* (Physta®) was compared with placebo [109]: Results: *"there were no significant between-group differences, within-group improvements were observed in the SF-12 QoL, POMS and MMSQ domains", which is associated with CNS activity of Eurycoma longifolia (Physta®) water extract plus multivitamins on quality of life, mood and stress"*.

This clearly shows a lack of effect of *Eurycoma longifolia* (Physta®) on the CNS, suggesting that Eurycoma is not an adaptogen.

There are many shortcomings in conducted randomized, placebo-controlled, double-blind clinical trials [109,110,112,119–121,124], which are not in line with CONSORT recommendations [125,126], including insufficient information regarding:

- Insufficient description of the study medication (see above),
- Randomization (a method used to generate the random allocation sequence, including details of restriction)
- Implementation (who generated the allocation sequence, enrolled participants, assigned participants to their groups, etc.)
- Blinding (preparation had the same appearance, test, and odor as placebo; how care providers, those assessing outcomes, were blinded; how the success of blinding was evaluated)
- Allocation concealment (the mechanism used to implement the random allocation sequence, such as sequentially numbered containers, describing any steps taken to

conceal the sequence until interventions were assigned; it is not clear whether the sequence was concealed until interventions were assigned),

- Procedure for treatment compliance (how measurements of compliance of individual patients with the treatment regimen under study were documented).
- Monitoring,
- Settings and locations where the data were collected,
- Quality assurance and quality control,
- Deviations from the protocol
- Selective reporting
- The trial was conducted per ICH guidelines for GCP.
- Voucher specimen (i.e., retention sample was retained and, if so, where it is kept or deposited).
- The role of the study sponsor/funder,
- Inappropriate statistical tools and statistical analysis (e.g., lack of between-groups comparison of changes from the baseline by two-way ANOVA, etc.).

Other limitations of the studies, e.g., Muniandy et al., 2023 [124]:

⇒ a purposive sampling in a randomized, double-blinded, placebo-controlled, parallel-group study.

⇒ lost to follow-up and missing data points

⇒ the lack of nutritional intake information, which can be a limitation for a comprehensive analysis of the potential influence of dietary factors on the observed outcomes.

Overall, there is no convincing evidence yet to support the claim that Eurocoma is an adaptogen.

2.5. Dual-Use Dilemma and Inconsistencies in Botanical Risk Assessments in the Case of Withania somnifera

Below is an insight into *"the two sides of the same coin"* and double standards in the assessment of the safety of *Withania somnifera* (L.) Dunal (Ashwagandha/Winter cherry root), resulting in controversial conclusions in India and Denmark [52–54,56,127,128].

Ashwagandha is the most popular plant in India and has been used in the traditional medical system (Ayurveda) to treat many diseases and health conditions for thousands of years. Due to its polyvalent pharmacological and adaptogenic activity, it is also known as Indian Ginseng [129–132]. Numerous preclinical and clinical studies have been conducted with several Ashwagandha preparations to provide evidence on their efficacy and safety in various conditions [133–153]. However, in most clinical studies, the authors typically conclude that *"The findings from the included studies indicate that Ashwagandha formulations have beneficial effects on stress and anxiety. The adverse effects associated with Ashwagandha are limited; however, further information is required to determine its safety with long-term administration"* [139].

Withania somnifera (L.) Dunal. is recognized in several national pharmacopeias and regulatory frameworks worldwide, though its status varies by country, including:

- In India, *Withania somnifera* is officially included in the Indian Herbal Pharmacopeia [154] where the monograph outlines: (i)—the plant names, (ii)—geographical distribution, (iii)—macroscopic and microscopic description of the roots, (iv)—chemical constituents (steroidal lactones including withanone, withaferin A, withanolides I, II, III, A, D, E, F, G, H, I, J, K, L, M, WS-L, P, and S, withasomnidienone, withanolide C, and alkaloids viz., cuscohygrine, anahygrine, tropine, pseudotropine, anaferine, isopellatierine, 3-tropyltigloate), (v)—Assays/analytical methods including HPLC conditions fingerprints, identifying withaferin A in extracts and withanolide J in vitro culture, (v)—quantitative standards (including total alkaloids (in total about0,2%), (vi)—adulteration, (vii)—pharmacology section, (viii)—reported activities including antistress, immunomodulatory, anticancer, antioxidant, an-ticonvulsive, anthelminthic, antiarthritic, chemopreventive, antibacterial, cardiopro-tective, antidepressant, anti-toxic, hypoglycemic, diuretic, hypercholesterolemic, im-munosuppressive, antiradical, and adaptogenic activities, and (ix)—therapeutic category: adaptogen.

- In Europe, EMEA conducted a comprehensive literature search and reviewed available data, including information on the market in the European Union obtained from HMPC members. This review concluded that the requirements for establishing a Community herbal monograph on traditional herbal medicinal products containing *Withania somnifera* (L.) are met. Dunal, radix are not fulfilled since:
    - the requirement of the definition of the 'herbal preparation' as the HMPC has not been able to find adequate evidence allowing a description of the herbal preparations (insufficient extract specification according to pharmaceutical requirements,
    - lack of adequate evidence allowing a demonstration of at least 30 years of medicinal use, including at least 15 years in the European Union.

The public statement dated 9 July 2013 claims that HMPC claims that a Community herbal monograph on *Withania somnifera* (L.) Dunal, radix cannot be established at present [155,156].

- Denmark has banned Ashwagandha, citing safety concerns. This decision has been criticized by various scientific communities advocating for evidence-based evaluations [52,53].
- In Sweden, the regulation of Ashwagandha is decentralized, allowing local authorities to make decisions regarding its use. This approach permits its availability under certain conditions [157,158].
- In the U.S., Ashwagandha is permitted as a dietary supplement. The United States Pharmacopeia (USP) provides guidelines for its quality control, including High-Performance Liquid Chromatography (HPLC) methods to assess total withanolide content USP [159,160].
- Ashwagandha is allowed as a food supplement in the UK. The Medicines and Healthcare Products Regulatory Agency (MHRA) has approved clinical trials involving Ashwagandha, indicating its acceptance within specific regulatory frameworks [161].
- Ashwagandha is available as a dietary supplement in Germany. However, the Federal Institute for Risk Assessment (BfR) has recommended its inclusion in the EU's list of substances for which safety has not been conclusively established, suggesting caution in its use [162].
- Ashwagandha is included in the Australian Register of Therapeutic Goods (ARTG), with over 320 listed medicines containing it, reflecting its acceptance in therapeutic products [163]
- Within the Association of Southeast Asian Nations (ASEAN), Ashwagandha is not uniformly included in national pharmacopeias. However, efforts are underway to harmonize traditional medicine regulations across member states. The ASEAN Common Technical Document (ACTD) framework is being utilized to standardize quality, safety, and efficacy requirements for herbal products, such as Ashwagandha [55].

A recent case in point is the Danish Technical University (DTU) Food Institute's risk assessments of *Withania somnifera* (Ashwagandha) root [52,53], in which DTU identified possible thyroid and reproductive effects at high doses. These reports, which contributed to national-level restrictions and influenced regulatory positions in other countries, have been widely criticized by scientific and regulatory communities for methodological shortcomings and a lack of transparency [56,127]. The Danish agency cited concerns about hormonal effects and lack of a well-defined safe dose, and then concluded that this focus was controversial. As noted by the Danish Veterinary and Food Administration, its report argued no safe dose could be proven with existing data, a conclusion some experts find unconvincing [56,164]. Meanwhile, neither the EFSA [165] nor the FDA has taken similar actions; Ashwagandha remains a permitted supplement in both regions [164].

The views, scientific opinions, and conclusions drawn by Food and Drug authorities [52–54,165,166], dietary supplement manufacturers [167,168], experts in the field [169,170], distributors [171], independent reviewers [164], and researchers [3,35] differ and are somewhat contradictory.

2.5.1. Food and Drug Authorities

- In April 2023, Denmark banned Withania, stating that it is impossible to find a safe dose given the current data. The ban was based on a finding in 2020 by the Danish Technical University (DTU) that ashwagandha may induce abortions and has a possibly harmful effect on thyroid and sex hormones [52]. This decision was based on only one study in rodents, which found that ashwagandha reduced sperm quality and quantity [172], and one trial in humans suggested that ashwagandha might increase thyroid hormone levels [173], which could potentially cause delirium, heart failure, and dehydration [173].
- In Report of the Expert Committee constituted by the Ministry of Ayush, Govt. of India. The Central Council for Research in Ayurvedic Sciences, the experts state that "*Numerous safety studies consistently demonstrate that standardized Ashwagandha (Withania somnifera) root extract is safe for human consumption. The scientific data reveal that Ashwagandha root is well-tolerated across a wide range of doses, with no adverse outcomes reported in diverse demographic and clinical cohorts. Thus, the Expert Committee holds a strong view that the current evidence supporting the safety and efficacy of Ashwagandha root is robust, allowing it to be safely recommended and integrated into global health practices. This reinforces its standing as a safe herb in both traditional and contemporary health contexts; nevertheless, using correctly identified species is crucial, and stringent quality control should be carried out suitably in accordance with applicable regulatory norms. In view of its scientifically proven safety, the globally available and popular Indian herb Ashwagandha (Withania Somnifera) can be judiciously prescribed by the Ayurvedic physicians for its health benefits in humans* [54]. *The report by the DTU Food Institute (published in May 2020) needs a reconsideration due to two main reasons:*
    - *The report is not taking into consideration the different properties concerning function and safety between different plant parts of Ashwagandha*
    - *There is evolving evidence on the safety and efficacy of Ashwagandha published since 2020 (more than 400 papers), DTU report* [52], *there are glaring instances of a lack of rigorous scientific scrutiny in the DTU risk assessment report, including conclusions drawn from publications of predatory journals*" [54].
- The National Institute for Public Health and the Environment (RIVM) studied whether herbal preparations containing *Withania somnifera* are harmful to health, concluding that the herb can induce harmful effects in individuals who are sensitive to it. It is unknown which individuals are sensitive to *Withania somnifera*. As a precaution, RIVM advises consumers not to use herbal preparations containing *Withania somnifera*, especially during pregnancy [165].
- In contrast, the EFSA assessment report and scientific opinion support the safety of ashwagandha [166]. As quoted, "*In addition to its historical uses and pre-clinical studies, in the multiple published human clinical studies, ashwagandha and its preparations have been investigated in healthy adults, children, the elderly, and diseased populations. Although the*

primary objective of the majority of these trials was to investigate efficacy for health benefits, these studies provide insight into the potential safety and 'tolerability' of ashwagandha and its preparations in a diverse population. In healthy adults and children, Ashwagandha root has been used at doses of up to 5000 mg/day without adverse effects. Of the over 60 human clinical studies identified, more than 30 were placebo-controlled, double-blind clinical trials. As double-blind placebo-controlled trials are least likely to result in bias, these trials provide an opportunity to assess safety. Adverse effects of ashwagandha root or its preparations are rarely reported in humans. In some clinical trials, adverse effects were reported; however, the incidence was similar to that of the placebo group. A majority of the adverse events were transient and minor, and the frequency of these events was not related to the duration of intake. The findings from all of these studies support the safety-in-use of Ashwagandha root preparations [166].

2.5.2. Dietary Supplement Manufacturers

- All Ashwagandha are not the same. All studies are product-specific, meaning they are conducted exclusively on the extract contained in KSM66. In all studies, the dose of 2 × 300 mg has been used, i.e., one capsule in the morning and one in the evening. Experience, combined with safety studies, shows that in cases of increased need, the dose can be doubled [168].
- In response to the DTU report, an expert report of the World Ashwagandha Council and Ixoreal Biomed Inc., Los Angeles, California, USA, and Heyderabad, India, presented data from 79 human clinical studies, 29 Toxicity studies, and 130 preclinical studies. The report also discusses observations by DTU Food Institute and presents data-driven responses to the comments. The results suggest that Ashwagandha root extract) It is clinically beneficial for reducing stress and anxiety by balancing cortisol levels, enhancing memory and cognition, increasing sex drive, endurance, and strength, as well as promoting muscle growth and recovery, and improving sleep quality and overall quality of life. The data assure its safety, as no serious adverse events have been reported in any of the clinical trials. Animal studies include acute and long-term toxicity assessment, including reproductive and developmental toxicity. The authors claim that KSM-66 Ashwagandha extract is safe and conclude that the report by the DTU Food Institute needs a reconsideration due to two main reasons:
    - The report does not take into consideration the different properties concerning function and safety between different plant parts of Ashwagandha
    - There is evolving evidence on the safety and efficacy of Ashwagandha published since 2020 [167].

2.5.3. Independent Reviewers

While these side effects are frightening, the report does not present a clear case for ashwagandha's impact on hormones and fertility. The cases mentioned by the authors are rare, and many studies have found no evidence of thyroid problems. As far as abortion is concerned, the report presents no clinical evidence of ashwagandha as an abortifacient. Reference is made to the World Health Association's advice that people should not consume ashwagandha during pregnancy or breastfeeding because "there is information that the root has been used as an abortifacient." The origin of this information is unclear, but it was likely passed down as part of the Ayurvedic medical system. On the other hand, some journal articles state that ashwagandha is safe to use during pregnancy and was even used to boost health before and after birth. Without clear evidence, Demark took the most cautious option and banned ashwagandha altogether [164]. Whether or not consumers should follow Denmark's ban is unclear. The concerns brought up by the DTU's report are significant but not backed by substantial clinical evidence—especially the claims about ashwagandha inducing abortions. The European Medicines Agency and the FDA, two of the largest pharmaceutical regulating agencies, have yet to follow in Denmark's footsteps by restricting or prohibiting ashwagandha. While this does not necessarily mean that Denmark is wrong about the potential side effects of ashwagandha, it does mean that the clinical data is limited enough that big pharmaceutical government agencies are not considering it [164].

Such a contradictory response to the regulatory requirements of the same plant products and their use in medicine is not surprising due to many objective and subjective reasons, including:

- Dose-dependent reversal effect of Withania demonstrated in gene-expression study on cultivated brain cell culture, suggesting inhibition of corticotropin-releasing hormone CRH signaling pathways and inflammation in the concentration of 1.5 mg/L, and opposite effect—activation of CRH signaling pathway leading to the pro-inflammatory impacts in higher concentration of 5 mg/L [3,35]. A similar dose-dependent reversal effect of Withania was observed on the Electrophysiological Activity in Hippocampal Long-Term Potentiation, a Synaptic Model of Memory in the hippocampus slice model in vitro. In concentrations of 0.5–1.0 mg/L, Withania extract significantly increases pyramidal cell activity; however, at a higher dose of 2.5–10 mg/L, the effect decreases (Supplement S1, Figure S12).
- Inconsistencies result from studies dealing with diverse Withania extracts of diverse chemical composition, depending on numerous factors during harvesting, cultivation, methods of extraction of herbal substance, processing of herbal product, etc., ensuring sustainable quality and reproducible effects in pharmacological and clinical studies can lead to contradictory results.
- Surprisingly, the quality of the studies of Withania, which raised concerns about the safety, was not scrupulously assessed in the DPU report. For example, the reporting of the clinical trial (registered at ClinicalTrials.gov, Identifier: NCT00761761) of Ashwagandha on thyroid and sex hormones [173–175] does not meet the CONSORT and ICH GCP requirements and cannot be taken into account for warning and banning Ashwagandha in Denmark and the Netherlands. The placebo/verum blinding and assignment procedures were not sufficiently described. Assessment criteria must be consistent across all studies.

Similar conclusions were drawn in a comprehensive review of preclinical and clinical studies examining the neuropsychiatric effects of WS, specifically its application in stress, anxiety, depression, and insomnia [176]. While benefits were seen in the reviewed studies, significant variability in the Withania root extracts examined prevents a consensus on the optimum Withania preparation or dosage for treating neuropsychiatric conditions. Withania generally appears safe for human use; however, it will be essential to investigate potential herb-drug interactions involving Withania if used alongside pharmaceutical interventions. Further elucidation of the active compounds of WS is also needed [176].

In summary, the incorporation of Ashwagandha into national pharmacopeias and its regulatory acceptance vary globally. While countries like India, the United States, and Australia have established standards or included it in official registers, others, such as France and Denmark, approach it with caution or restrictions. Ongoing efforts, particularly within ASEAN, aim to harmonize regulations for traditional herbal medicines, which could potentially influence Ashwagandha's status in the future [55].

2.6. Key Issues Identified

1. Blurring of Pharmacological and Nutritional Frameworks

Withania somnifera L. is traditionally consumed as a root extract in dietary supplements to support stress management, sleep, and hormonal balance. However, the DTU assessments failed to distinguish between its pharmacological and nutritional uses, applying pharmaceutical-level toxicological expectations to a botanical widely regarded as safe under traditional and evidence-based guidelines. That is a critical point in DTU assessment, as the study of question [172] involved dry steam of *Withania somnifera* dried 50% ethanol extract, which is a significantly different preparation of roots specified in the Indian and UK Pharmacopeias and used for other indications and health claims.

2. Inappropriate Aggregation of Data from Different Plant Parts

A core flaw in the DTU evaluations is the failure to differentiate between root, leaf, stem, and berry extracts, despite well-established phytochemical and pharmacological differences. This has led to the erroneous attribution of adverse effects (e.g., cytotoxicity from withaferin A, primarily found in leaves) to root-based products, undermining the validity of the conclusions. The spermicidal activity was determined in vitro tests by mixing *Withania somnifera* stem extract with sperm suspension. The mixture was observed under a microscope for 20 s and examined for motile sperm. The minimum effective spermicidal concentrations of *Withania somnifera* stem extract were found to be 10 mg/million sperm in suspension containing 42.5 sperm count/mL. The authors conclude that 50% ethanol-dried *Withania somnifera* stem extract has an antifertility effect on male rat reproduction, sexual behavior, and epididymal sperm concentration. The oral administration of the extract at 50 mg/kg body weight/day in male albino rats produced antifertility effects. The point is that both the authors and DTU experts do not question the bioavailability of this stem extract and the corresponding oral dose in humans. That is another critical point leading to wrong assumptions and decisions to ban Ashwagandha products. For comparison, the concentration of *Withania somnifera* stem extract in that study was at least 1000-fold higher than that of the blood plasma of *Withania somnifera* root extract, as evident from pharmacokinetic studies and the EFSA assessment report [165]. *Withania somnifera* root extract was investigated after a single oral administration of 500 mg/kg in six non-descript healthy buffalo calves. The mean peak plasma concentration at 0.75 h was 248.16 ± 16.12 μg/mL and was detected up to 3 h, with a mean plasma concentration of 6.55 ± 0.12 μg/mL. That is at least 1000-fold lower than the spermicidal activity. The maximal blood plasma concentrations of withaferin A and withanolide A in mice were found to be 16 and 26 ng/mL, respectively, after oral administration of an aqueous extract of ashwagandha root [165].

3. Selective and Outdated Use of Scientific Literature

Although hundreds of clinical and toxicological studies on Ashwagandha have been published in the past decade, many of which demonstrate a favorable safety profile, the DTU assessments relied heavily on older and animal-based data, some of which lacked relevance to human use. Peer-reviewed safety evaluations, including those by the American Herbal Products Association (AHPA), were omitted.

4. Absence of Peer Review and Transparency

Neither of the DTU reports underwent external peer review. Key methodological details—such as criteria for evidence inclusion, levels of uncertainty, and expert qualifications—were not disclosed, raising concerns about the objectivity and reproducibility of the findings.

5. Regulatory Disparity and Industry Impact

Discrepant evaluations of the same botanical substance by different national authorities—some viewing Ashwagandha as a safe food supplement, others banning it outright—have generated regulatory friction and potential trade barriers. This inconsistency particularly disadvantages producers in countries like India, where the plant has been used safely for centuries.

2.7. Critical Assessment of Common Technical Documentation Submitted by Drug Manufacturers to Drug Authorities

On the other side, the rejections to grant 'well-established use' of some herbal medicines are often based on assessment reports of drug authorities, e.g., EU herbal monograph on *Rhodiola rosea* L., rhizoma et radix [38], which identified serious problems such as:

- The published clinical trials exhibit considerable deficiencies in their quality and show methodological problems.
  - insufficiently characterized herbal preparations,
  - open (label) studies,
  - small sample size,
  - missing ITT analysis, regardless of a detailed description of dropouts and reasons for exclusion in the analysis of an outcome measure,
  - healthy subjects,
  - The efficacy score has not been validated
  - The results from trials on clinical pharmacology are contradictory.
  - There is a lack of independent replications of the single studies.

The sources of inconsistency of the results of various clinical studies of *Rhodiola rosea* L., rhizoma et radix, are due to the authors not adhering to the consolidated standards of reporting trials (CONSORT) recommendations [125] and ICH E6 (R3) Guideline for good clinical practice (GCP)—Step 5 [126]. For example, in a randomized controlled trial, the authors investigated the effect of *Rhodiola rosea* on mental and physical fatigue in nursing students [165,177]. However, the authors did not characterize the product with respect to extraction solvents and dry herb, dry native extract ratio (DER), the content of active markers, and did not provide HPLC fingerprints to ensure consistent quality and reproducible pharmacological activity. The analytical methods were not validated for selectivity, accuracy, and precision [165,177].

The authors declared that placebo capsules containing microcrystalline cellulose and silicon dioxide had the same appearance, odor, and taste as the R. rosea product, which is very unlikely due to their strong specific rose odor, test, and color, particularly when "participants were asked to self-determine their need for one additional capsule (i.e., a half dose), to be taken within four hours of the initial dose [165,177].

The authors have not reported (or assessed) the results of treatment compliance (counting of unused tablets), which is a serious flaw [165,177].

All outcome measures of the study were subjective based on self-assessment questionnaires of QOL in 48 nurses instead of the only doctor having the same unified "standard" [165,177].

The imbalance between the Rhodiola treatment and placebo groups in medication use and physical and emotional health problems has had a significant impact on the results of the study [165,177].

2.8. Other Challenges in Adaptogens Research

It should be noted that some other challenges in adaptogens research are related to the insufficient characterization and standardization of certain active constituents, including the pyrazole alkaloid withasomnine, Supplement S2, found in Withania root preparations [43,178,179], which is known for its sedative properties. New studies are required to demonstrate the reproducibility of well-characterized Ashwagandha-containing products.

Another poorly studied subject is the content of cyanogenic terpenoid lotaustraline identified in *Rhodiola rosea* roots [73,180,181], which should be standardized for its content in *Rhodiola rosea* preparations to ensure reproducible and consistent results in various clinical trials [182], Supplements S3 and S4.

3. Pharmaceuticals vs. Nutraceuticals and Dietary Supplements

3.1. Regulatory Classification, Purpose of Use, Dose and Potency, Labeling and Claims

The requirements for pharmaceuticals [16–19,154,157,183–205] and dietary supplements [158,206–233] of botanical origin differ significantly in terms of regulatory oversight, quality standards, safety and efficacy requirements, manufacturing practices, intended use, health and functional claims, and supported health functions [194–221,223], see Supplement S5 and Tables 4 and 5. Table 6 shows the key differences in the requirements for botanical-origin pharmaceuticals and dietary supplements under FDA (United States) vs. EMA (European Union) regulations. Table 7 includes selected true adaptogens with Pharmacopeial Recognition and some putative adaptogens, such as Eurycoma and Sideritis, which were claimed as adaptogens in publications [107–113].

Table 4. The comparison of differences in requirements for pharmaceuticals and dietary supplements of botanical origin.

Category	**Pharmaceuticals [16–19,154,157,183–205]**	**Dietary Supplements [158,206–233]**
Regulatory Oversight	Very strict	Lenient
Regulated by	Strictly regulated by drug authorities (e.g., FDA *, EMA) **	Governed by food supplement laws (e.g., DSHEA *** in the U.S., EFSA **** in the EU).
Pre-market approval	Required (clinical trials, IND, NDA, etc.)	Not required; must follow labeling and safety guidelines.
Evidence of Safety and Efficacy	Required clinical + preclinical	Not required; General safety only
Efficacy	Must be proven through rigorous clinical trials	No requirement to prove efficacy before marketing
Safety	Extensive safety data required (nonclinical + clinical)	Only required to ensure general safety; no clinical trials mandated
Quality Standards	High	Moderate
Identity and purity	Must meet strict pharmacopoeial standards (e.g., USP †, EP ††)	Less stringent, basic identity and purity testing is often enough, focus on identity, purity, and composition
Standardization	Active ingredients must be quantified and consistent	Often contains a range of components; standardization is not always required
Contaminants (e.g., heavy metals, microbes)	Tightly controlled with established limits	Limits exist, but are less strictly enforced
Batch-to-batch consistency	Mandatory and validated	Expected but not strictly enforced
Manufacturing Requirements	Pharmaceutical grade, GMP	Food GMP
GMP Standards	Must follow pharmaceutical GMP (e.g., ICH Q7 †††, EU GMP, Part 211)	Must follow food-grade GMP (e.g., FDA Part 111), which are less stringent
Process validation	Mandatory for all critical manufacturing steps	Not required for all processes
Change control and documentation.	Detailed documentation and validation are required.	Documentation is required, but it is generally simpler.

Table 4. *Cont.*

Category	Pharmaceuticals [16–19,154,157,183–205]	Dietary Supplements [158,206–233]
Consistency of Botanical Source Specifics	Standardized	Variable
Botanical identity	Must be rigorously confirmed and controlled	Often confirmed, but methods may vary in rigor
Extraction process	Fully validated and standardized	May vary; often not standardized
Complex mixtures	Defined active constituents or fractions used	Often, a whole plant/extract with variable composition
Labeling Claims and Doses	Indications for use in diseases	Health supporting claims
Health claims	Treat/cure diseases; medicine list "Dosage" based on age, weight, or condition. Can make therapeutic claims (e.g., "treats depression")	Support health functions; Supplements list "Suggested use" or "Serving size". Cannot make disease claims; only "structure/function" claims (e.g., "supports mood")
Labeling accuracy	Must match approved documentation	Must be truthful and not misleading, but with less scrutiny
Regulatory Classification	• Regulated as a medicine or therapeutic product. • It can be used for specific health conditions with evidence to support it. • Subject to stricter quality, efficacy, and safety controls. • May contain higher or more standardized doses.	• Regulated as food in most countries (e.g., by the FDA in the U.S.). • Intended for general health support (e.g., to "maintain" or "support" function). • Cannot claim to treat, prevent, or cure diseases. • Doses are often lower to avoid therapeutic claims or side effects.
Purpose of Use	Medicines are designed for therapeutic effect and are often used for shorter-term or targeted purposes.	Supplements aim to provide nutritional support and are typically used on a long-term basis.

FDA *, EMA **, DSHEA *** in the U.S., EFSA ****, USP †, EP ††, ICH Q7 †††.

Table 5. The comparison of differences in requirements for pharmaceuticals and dietary supplements of botanical origin in Sweden.

Product Type	Herbal Medicinal Products	Botanical Dietary Supplements
Regulator	Swedish Medical Products Agency	Swedish Food Agency,
Key Legislation:	under EU Directive 2001/83/EC and national provisions	○ under EU food law Directive 2002/46/EC on food supplements ○ LIVSFS 2023:3—Swedish Food Agency's national regulation
Classification:	○ Herbal Medicinal Products ○ Traditional Herbal Medicinal Products	○ Plant extracts ○ Must have physiological effects
Definitions:	○ *Herbal substances*: Whole or parts of plants, algae, fungi, or lichens. ○ *Herbal preparations*: Extracts, powders, distillates, etc.	
Approval Needed	Yes	No (registration only)
Approval Requirements	○ Must be registered or authorized before sale. ○ Traditional herbal products require bibliographic evidence of safety and plausible efficacy over at least 30 years (15 in the EU). ○ Full marketing authorization demands clinical and preclinical data, similar to conventional drugs.	○ No pre-market approval needed, but food business operators must be registered. ○ Products must be safe, properly labeled, and not misleading. ○ Health claims must comply with Regulation (EC) No. 1924/2006.
Claims Allowed	Treat/cure diseases	Support health functions (not a cure)

Table 6. FDA (United States) vs. EMA (European Union) regulations.

Aspect	FDA (U.S.) [196–198,206–221]	EMA (EU) [157,158,183–195,222–233]
Governing Bodies	- Pharmaceuticals: Center for Drug Evaluation and Research (CDER) - Supplements: Center for Food Safety and Applied Nutrition (CFSAN)	- Pharmaceuticals: European Medicines Agency (EMA) - Supplements: Regulated at member state level (e.g., Germany: BfArM, France: ANSM)
Applicable Legal Frameworks	- Drugs: FD&C Act, 21 CFR - Supplements: Dietary Supplement Health and Education Act (DSHEA, 1994)	- Drugs: Directive 2001/83/EC - Supplements: Food Supplements Directive (2002/46/EC), national laws
Botanical Drugs	Defined as botanical drug products, subject to full NDA or IND path (e.g., Veregen®, Mytesi®)	Herbal medicinal products (HMPs), classified into:—Well-established use (WEU)—Traditional use (THMP)—Full marketing authorization
Supplements (Botanical)	Treated as foods, not drugs. No pre-market approval. No efficacy proof required.	Also treated as foods, but the EU is more restrictive on claims. Heavily influenced by EFSA assessments.
Quality Standards for Botanicals	Encourages use of USP monographs and FDA Botanical Drug Guidance (2004). Must define active constituents or marker compounds.	Uses European Pharmacopeia (Ph. Eur.) monographs. Strict on identity, purity, and standardization. The Herbal Medicinal Products Committee (HMPC) oversees scientific guidelines.
Clinical Evidence (Botanical Drugs)	IND → NDA process: requires full clinical trials unless eligible for accelerated approval.	WEU: requires published literature and some clinical data. THMP: based on 30 years of traditional use (15 in the EU), with nonclinical safety evidence only
Labeling (Supplements)	Structure/function claims allowed: "supports immune health." Must carry a disclaimer: "This product is not intended to diagnose, treat, cure, or prevent any disease."	Health claims reviewed and authorized by EFSA; therapeutic claims prohibited on supplements. Stricter than the FDA.
GMP	- Drugs: 21 CFR Part 210/211- Supplements: 21 CFR Part 111	- Drugs: EU GMP (Annexes)- Supplements: Food GMP (varies by country); less
Unique Points	Allows botanical drug development via standard drug approval paths. Dietary supplements are widely available with relatively light regulation, provided safety is ensured. Botanical Drug Development Guidance has been available since 2004.	Provides a specific regulatory framework for traditional herbal medicinal products (THMPs) via simplified registration. More centralized regulation of herbal drugs via EMA's HMPC. Supplements are subject to tighter control over labeling and claims, often stricter than in the U.S.
Example		
Echinacea supplement	Dietary Supplement, no pre-market approval	Food supplement; cannot claim therapeutic effects
Echinacea extract as a medicine	Must go through the full IND/NDA process	Can qualify as THMP or WEU based on evidence and monograph

Table 7. Countries with Pharmacopeial recognition of selected adaptogens [234–240] and some putative adaptogens, such as Eurycoma and Sideritis [241–243], and their official regulatory status: ✅—Official monographs; ⚠—Dietary supplement use.

Country	Pharmacopeia Monographs	Rhodiola	Ginseng	Withania	Eleuthero-Coccus	Schisandra	Eurycoma	Sideritis
Russia	State Pharmacopeia [189,190]	✅	✅		✅	✅		
China *	Pharmacopeia of PRC -2010 (Eng) [191]		✅		✅	✅		
European Union	EP8 European EMA/HMPC Union herbal monograph	✅	✅	✅	✅	✅		✅
United States	USP, USP Herbal Compendium monograph, AHP	✅	✅	⚠	⚠	⚠		
Germany	Commission E	✅	✅	⚠	✅	✅		

Table 7. *Cont.*

Country	Pharmacopeia Monographs	Rhodiola	Ginseng	Withania	Eleuthero-Coccus	Schisandra	Eurycoma	Sideritis
UK	British Pharmacopoea		✅	⚠	✅			
Mongolia	Mongolian Pharmacopeia	✅			✅	✅		
India *	Indian Herbal Pharmacopeia	✅		✅				
Pakistan	Unani/Ayurvedic Pharmacopeia			✅				
Bangladesh	Unani Pharmacopeia			✅				
Sri Lanka	Ayurvedic Pharmacopeia			✅				
South Korea	Korean Herbal Pharmacopeia		✅		✅	✅		
Japan	Japanese Pharmacopeia	✅	✅		✅ ⚠	✅		
Vietnam	Vietnamese Pharmacopeia		✅				✅	
Lanka								
Australia	Australian Register of Therapeutic Goods (ARTG)			✅				
Malaysia	Malaysian Pharmacopeia						✅	
Indonesia	Indonesia Pharmacopeia						✅	
South Africa	CAM regulatory framework			⚠				
WHO	WHO Monographs		✅	✅	✅			

*—Supplements S6 and S7.

The daily dose of a dietary supplement versus a herbal medicine containing the same active ingredient can differ significantly due to regulatory, intended use, and formulation factors. For example, the daily dose of Eleutherococcus dry root and rhizome is 2–3 g, equivalent to a pharmaceutical preparation of quality [18]. The daily dose of Ginseng dry root is 0.6–2 g, equivalent to a pharmaceutical preparation of quality [19].

Table 5 presents the differences in requirements for pharmaceuticals and dietary supplements of botanical origin in Sweden, which follow EU-wide regulations for botanical products but incorporate national layers through two key agencies: the Swedish Medical Products Agency (MPA) for medicinal products and the Swedish Food Agency for dietary supplements [158,204].

Even if the active ingredient is identical, herbal medicines generally have higher, standardized, and therapeutically justified doses. In contrast, dietary supplements offer lower doses for general wellness and are not intended to treat diseases.

In summary, this section shows the differences between the requirements for the quality of pharmaceuticals and dietary supplements of botanical origin.

Pharmaceutical-grade botanicals typically have standardized doses that are higher, aimed at treating and curing diseases, and are subject to strong regulation and evidence-based research. In contrast, dietary supplements typically have lower, less consistent doses, focusing on wellness and safety to support health and nutrition. They are less regulated, as they are not intended to treat disease.

Dietary supplements typically provide lower, variable doses with less standardization, whereas pharmaceutical-grade ginseng products offer standardized, clinically tested doses for specific therapeutic uses.

Rhodiola rosea exhibits differences in dose depending on whether it is marketed as a dietary supplement or a pharmaceutical/herbal medicinal product (Supplement S4). Rhodiola as a dietary supplement usually comes in lower, less standardized doses. At the same time, as a pharmaceutical herbal medicine, it is administered at higher, clinically validated, and standardized doses for specific conditions, such as stress-related fatigue.

The dosage of ginseng differs significantly depending on whether it is sold as a dietary supplement or as a pharmaceutical-grade herbal medicine. Eleutherococcus products sold as nutritional supplements often have higher variability and may use lower-quality or non-standardized root powder. In contrast, pharmaceutical-quality products are standardized, clinically tested, and typically prescribed at ~300–400 mg/day extract (2–4 g/day root equivalent) for therapeutic purposes. Schisandra supplements typically use lower, non-standardized doses (200–500 mg/day) for wellness purposes, whereas pharmaceutical-quality preparations employ higher, standardized doses (500–1500 mg extract/day or 1.5–6 g dried fruit) to achieve consistent therapeutic effects.

Ashwagandha Dietary supplements usually provide lower, less consistent doses. At the same time, pharmaceutical/medicinal Ashwagandha in India uses higher, standardized, clinically validated doses (often double the typical supplement amount, or even more in traditional powdered form).

In contrast to many herbal medicinal products, such as St. John's Wort, the doses of other well-established adaptogens, including Ginseng, Rhodiola, Eleutherococcus, and Schisandra preparations, are almost within the same range, regardless of their quality grade: pharmaceuticals or dietary supplements (Table 8).

Table 8. The comparison of doses for adaptogenic pharmaceuticals and dietary supplements.

Botanical	Dietary Supplement Dose	Pharmaceutical Dose
Ginseng	100–400 mg/day extract (variable, not always standardized)	200–400 mg/day standardized extract (1–2 g/day root equivalent)
Rhodiola	100–300 mg/day extract (variable)	200–600 mg/day standardized extract (3% rosavins, ~1% salidroside)
Eleutherococcus	300–1200 mg/day crude root or extract (variable)	300–400 mg/day standardized extract (2–4 g/day root equivalent)
Schisandra	200–500 mg/day extract (variable)	500–1500 mg/day standardized extract OR 1.5–6 g/day dried fruit
Ashwagandha	300–600 mg/day extract (often not standardized)	500–1000 mg/day standardized extract (3–6 g/day root powder in Ayurveda)
Rhodiola	100–300 mg/day extract (variable)	200–600 mg/day standardized extract (3% rosavins, ~1% salidroside)
St. John's Wort	100–300 mg/day extract (variable)	900 mg/day standardized extract (hypericin/hyperforin defined)

The reasons for the existing differences came from several issues, including:

- Insufficient product characterization, lack of product standardization, poor and biased reporting that do not meet CONSORT [125] recommendations, poorly conducted clinical studies that do not meet ICH guidelines for GCP requirements [126], and lack of GMP [197,199].
- Complex multi-component botanicals, particularly of fixed combinations of herbal preparations with reproducible and sustainable quantitative and qualitative chemical composition. That is a challenge in analytical chemistry and standardization, ensuring the production of acceptable quality products. Supplement S4. The more components a product has, the more resources and time are spent on quality control, and the higher the product's cost.
- Differences in requirements for manufacturers of medicines and food products in different countries.
- Some tasks and goals of manufacturers and regulatory authorities are different, which can sometimes lead to ambiguous results or conflicts of interest.

In any case, the most effective way to find the best solution to the problem is a scientific and unbiased approach.

3.2. Proposed Solutions

- Establish Internationally Harmonized Guidelines for evaluating botanicals based on their intended use (e.g., pharmaceutical vs. dietary Supplement), incorporating traditional use data alongside modern scientific methods.
- Encourage Peer Review and Transparency in national assessments by mandating public disclosure of methodologies, data sources, and expert affiliations.
- Create a Tiered Evidence Framework that allows differentiated standards of proof for traditional botanical supplements versus pharmaceutical candidates.
- Promote International Scientific Dialogs among regulators, researchers, and industry to develop consensus positions and avoid unilateral bans that may lack scientific rigor.

4. Discussion

Adaptogens are botanicals that trigger the adaptive stress response of the organism by feedback down-regulating mechanisms, resulting in the normalization of physiological functions and supporting homeostasis. As a result, they have nonspecifically targeted multiple effects in the stress system (neuroendocrine immune complex) associated with the cardiovascular and gastrointestinal systems, which play an essential role in stress-induced mental/ brain fatigue, as well as aging-related diseases.

In essence, adaptogens induce adaptability and exhibit adaptogenic effects via adaptive mechanisms where the key role is cortisol targeting corticosteroid receptors. Other intracellular and extracellular mediators of the stress response, such as ATP and GTP, are involved in regulating the activation and inactivation of canonical signaling pathways in physiological processes within the networks of mediators of the stress response.

Network pharmacology studies have uncovered the mechanisms of action of adaptogens, providing insight into how to maintain homeostasis in various stressful conditions and prevent and cure diseases. Therefore, adaptogens are useful both as pharmaceuticals, dietary supplements, and nutraceuticals. In this context, adaptation, like vitamins, is a distinct category of natural products that should be classified as beneficial agents in the borderline between healthy conditions and diseases, both for normalizing physiological functions and curing diseases. In the background of this classification are experienced traditional medicine systems (Ayurveda, TCM, Kampo) [2], Brekman's theory of valeology and pharmacosanation [50,51,244–247], and the elucidation of the mechanism of action of adaptogens through the implementation of network pharmacology analysis/systems biology approaches in adaptogens' research. The interaction between Western and Oriental medical knowledge results in their integration, leading to beneficial symbioses for new drug development. In this context, harmonizing the food and drug regulatory network is essential for human health.

5. Conclusions

Adaptogenic botanicals occupy a complex regulatory space with inconsistent risk assessments. The dual-faced nature of adaptogens necessitates harmonization among Food and Drug regulatory authorities in various countries and the formal recognition of adaptogens as a category of natural products for the prevention of stress-induced brain fatigue, behavioral, and aging-related disorders in individuals with subpar health status. We also conclude that insufficient evidence and differences in the criteria for assessing the quality, efficacy, and safety of botanicals may result in inconsistent results, particularly in clinical studies. The inconsistencies in risk assessments of *Withania somnifera* underscore the broader challenge of regulating botanicals that straddle the food–pharma boundary. Without harmonized standards and transparent methodologies, regulatory decisions risk being unscientific or influenced by conflicts of interest. A more balanced, evidence-informed approach is urgently needed to protect consumer safety without stifling access to beneficial botanicals.

Supplementary Materials: The following supporting information can be downloaded at: https://www.mdpi.com/article/10.3390/ph18091346/s1, Supplements S1–S7 on the website. Supplement S1: *Report NCAG 15/17 H–Hippocampus slice preparation*, **2017**, pp. 1–54; Supplement S2: *ASSAY of sitoindosides VII, VIII and withasomnine in Withania Root*, **2001**, pp. 1–79; Supplement S3: *Progress and the challenges in the phytotherapy research of Rhodiola rosea* L. HMPPA and GA e-Symposium"RHODIOLA ROSEA—PHYTOCHEMICAL, PHARMACOLOGICAL AND CLINICAL EVIDENCE". NOVEMBER 23, **2023**, pp. 1–61; Supplement S4: *Herbal medicine vs Dietary supplement*, **2016**, pp. 1–12; Supplement S5: *Legal and Regulatory Framework for Herbal Medicines;* Association Européenne des Spécialités Pharmaceutiques Grand Public Association of the European Self-Medication Industry Europäischer Verband der Arzneimittel-Hersteller (AESGP): Brussels Belgium, **2010**; pp. 11–21, 51–54, 215–220, 230–240; Supplement S6: National Pharmacopoeia Committee. *Pharmacopoeia of the People's Republic of China*, English ed.; National Pharmacopoeia Committee: Beijing, China, **2010**, pp. 5–6, 209–211, 393–394, Supplement S7: *The Indian Herbal Pharmacopeia;* Revised New Edition 2002; Indian Drug Manufacturers' Association: Mumbai, India, **2002**; pp. 467–489.

Author Contributions: Conceptualization, A.P. and T.L.; writing—preparation of original drafts, A.P.; writing—review and editing, A.P. All authors have read and agreed to the published version of the manuscript.

Funding: This research received no external funding.

Institutional Review Board Statement: Not applicable.

Informed Consent Statement: Not applicable.

Data Availability Statement: Not applicable.

Acknowledgments: The authors received no administrative and technical support or donations.

Conflicts of Interest: Alexander Panossian is self-employed at the research and development company Phytomed AB and has no shares or financial interest in any pharmaceutical company. The author, Alexander Panossian, supported various projects without funding but had received funding in previous years from EuropharmaUSA Inc., Green Bay, Wisconsin, USA, to develop herbal medical products. The author AP declared that they were editorial board members of Pharmaceuticals at the time of submission. This had no impact on the peer review process and the final decision. The author Terrence Lemerond founded Europharma USA Inc., a company that produces herbal dietary supplements. The company had no role in the writing of the manuscript. Both authors, AP, and TL, declare that the research was conducted without any commercial or financial relationships that could potentially create a conflict of interest.

References

1. Panossian, A. Understanding adaptogenic activity: Specificity of the pharmacological action of adaptogens and other phytochemicals. *Ann. N. Y. Acad. Sci.* **2017**, *1401*, 49–64. [CrossRef] [PubMed]
2. Panossian, A.G.; Efferth, T.; Shikov, A.N.; Pozharitskaya, O.N.; Kuchta, K.; Mukherjee, P.K.; Banerjee, S.; Heinrich, M.; Wu, W.; Guo, D.A.; et al. Evolution of the adaptogenic concept from traditional use to medical systems: Pharmacology of stress- and aging-related diseases. *Med. Res. Rev.* **2021**, *41*, 630–703. [CrossRef] [PubMed]
3. Panossian, A.; Lemerond, T.; Efferth, T. Adaptogens in Long-Lasting Brain Fatigue: An Insight from Systems Biology and Network Pharmacology. *Pharmaceuticals* **2025**, *18*, 261. [CrossRef]
4. Lazarev, N.V. General and specific in action of pharmacological agents. *Farmacol. Toxicol.* **1958**, *21*, 81–86.
5. Lazarev, N.V.; Ljublina, E.I.; Ljublina, M.A. State of nonspecific resistance. *Patol. Fiziol. Exp. Terapia* **1959**, *3*, 16–21.

6. Canguilhem, G. Essai sur quelques problèmes concernant le normal et le pathologique. In *The Normal and the Pathological*; Fawcett, C.R.; Cohen, R.S., Translators; Zone Books: New York, NY, USA, 1991; Available online: https://www.undergroundbooks.net/pages/books/11553/georges-canguilhem-michel-foucault-intro/the-normal-and-the-pathological (accessed on 10 February 2025).
7. Anonymous. What is health? The ability to adapt. Editorial. *Lancet* **2009**, *373*, 781. [CrossRef]
8. Cannon, W.B. Stresses and strains of homeostasis. *Am. J. Med. Sci.* **1935**, *189*, 13–14. [CrossRef]
9. Selye, H. Confusion and controversy in the stress field. *J. Hum. Stress* **1975**, *1*, 37–44. [CrossRef]
10. Selye, H. Stress without distress. *Brux. Med.* **1976**, *56*, 205–210.
11. Brekhman, I.I.; Dardymov, I.V. New substances of plant origin which increase nonspecific resistance. *Annu. Rev. Pharmacol.* **1969**, *9*, 419–430. [CrossRef]
12. Wagner, H.; Nörr, H.; Winterhoff, H. Plant adaptogens. *Phytomedicine* **1994**, *1*, 63–76. [CrossRef] [PubMed]
13. Lewis, W.H.; Elwin-Lewis, M.P.F. (Eds.) Panaceas, Adaptogens, and Tonics. In *Medical Botany: Plants Affecting Human Health*, 2nd ed.; JohnWiley & Sons, Inc.: Hoboken, NJ, USA, 2003; Part II, Chapter 18; pp. 608–628.
14. Panossian, A.; Efferth, T. Network Pharmacology of Adaptogens in the Assessment of Their Pleiotropic Therapeutic Activity. *Pharmaceuticals* **2022**, *15*, 1051. [CrossRef] [PubMed]
15. Panossian, A.G. Adaptogens: Tonic herbs for fatigue and stress. *Altern. Compliment. Ther.* **2003**, *9*, 327–332. [CrossRef]
16. Eleutherococcus. In *British Herbal Pharmacopoeia 1996*; British Herbal Medicine Association: Exeter, UK, 1996; pp. 74–75.
17. Ginseng. In *British Herbal Pharmacopoeia 1996*; British Herbal Medicine Association: Exeter, UK, 1996; pp. 89–90.
18. Eleutherococcus. In *British Herbal Compendium*; A Handbook of Scientific Information on Widely Used Plant Drugs; Bredley, P.R., Ed.; British Herbal Medicine Association: Exeter, UK, 1996; Volume 1, pp. 89–91.
19. Ginseng. In *British Herbal Compendium*; A Handbook of Scientific Information on Widely Used Plant Drugs; Bredley, P.R., Ed.; British Herbal Medicine Association: Exeter, UK, 1996; Volume 1, pp. 115–118.
20. Farnsworth, N.R.; Kinghorn, A.D.; Soejarto, D.D.; Waller, D.P. Siberian Ginseng (*Eleutherococcus senticosus*): Current Status as an Adaptogen. In *Economic and Medicinal Plant Research*; Wagner, H., Hikino, H., Farnsworth, N.R., Eds.; Academic Press: London, UK, 1985; Volume 1, pp. 155–215.
21. Farnsworth, N.R.; Waller, D.; Strelkova, L.M. Use of Eleutherococcus senticosus in United States: Problems, prospects and literature update. In *Proceedings of the Second International Symposium on Eleutherococcus*; Far Eastern Scientific Center, USSR Academy of Sciences: Vladivostok, Russia, 1986; pp. 47–51.
22. *EMEA/HMPC/102655/2007*; Reflection Paper on the Adaptogenic Concept. European Medicines Agency: London, UK, 2008; pp. 1–6. Available online: https://www.ema.europa.eu/en/documents/scientific-guideline/reflection-paper-adaptogenic-concept_en.pdf (accessed on 3 September 2025).
23. Panossian, A.; Efferth, T. Entschlüsselung des pleiotropen, therapeutischen Potenzials von Adaptogenen. *Z. Phytother. J. Phytother.* **2025**, *46*, 121–133. [CrossRef]
24. Samuelsson, G.; Bohlin, L. *Drugs of Natural Origin: A Treatise of Pharmacognosy*, 6th ed.; Swedish Academy of Pharmaceutical Sciences: Stockholm, Sweden, 2009; p. 776. Available online: https://www.routledge.com/Drugs-of-Natural-Origin-A-Treatiseof-Pharmacognosy-Seventh-Edition/Samuelsson-Bohlin/p/book/9789198094251 (accessed on 10 February 2025).
25. Winston, D. *Adaptogens: Herbs for Strength, Stamina, and Stress Relief*; Simon and Schuster: New York, NY, USA, 2019; 432p. Available online: https://books.google.se/books/about/Adaptogens.html?id=ZdOPDwAAQBAJ&redir_esc=y (accessed on 10 February 2025).
26. Winston, D.; Maimes, S. *Adaptogens. Herbs for Strength, Stamina, and Stress Relief*; Simon and Schuster: New York, NY, USA, 2007; 336p. Available online: https://www.amazon.com/Adaptogens-Strength-Stamina-Stress-Relief/dp/1594771588 (accessed on 10 February 2025).
27. Yance, D.R. *Adaptogens in Herbal Herbalism, Adaptogens in Medical Herbalism: Elite Herbs and Natural Compounds for Mastering Stress, Aging, and Chronic Disease*; Healing Arts Press: Rochester, NY, USA, 2013; 672p, ISBN 13 978-1-62055-100-4. Available online: https://adaptogensbook.com/ (accessed on 10 February 2025).
28. Brown, R.P.; Gerbarg, P.L.; Graham, B. *The Rhodiola Revolution: Transform Your Health with the Herbal Breakthrough of the 21st Century*; Harmony/Rodale/Convergent: New York, NY, USA, 2004; 260p. Available online: https://www.goodreads.com/book/show/1256256.The_Rhodiola_Revolution (accessed on 10 February 2025).
29. Kuhn, M.A.; Winston, D. *Herbal Therapy and Supplements*; Lippincott Williams & Wilkins: Philadelphia, PA, USA, 2012; Medical—592p; 2000—Medical—430p; Available online: https://books.google.se/books/about/Herbal_Therapy_and_Supplements.html?id=puxU3qzD5_YC&redir_esc=y (accessed on 10 February 2025).
30. Der Marderosian, A.; Beutler, J.A. *The Review of Natural Products*, 6th ed.; Wolters Kluwer Health Kluwer: Waltham, MA, USA; Lippincott Williams & Wilkins: Philadelphia, PA, USA, 2010; 1672p. Available online: https://www.amazon.com/Natural-%20Prod-ucts-DerMarderosian-Lawrence-Paperback/dp/B011DC8AO6/ref=monarch_sidesheet_title (accessed on 10 February 2025).

31. Heinrich, M.; Barnes, J.; Prieto-Garcia, J.; Gibbons, S.; Williamson, E.M. *Fundamentals of Pharmacognosy and Phytotherapy*, 2nd ed.; Elsevier: Amsterdam, The Netherlands, 2012; 4th Edition; Elsevier: Amsterdam, The Netherlands, 2023; p. 340. ISBN 9780323834346.
32. Bone, K.; Mills, S. *Principles and Practice of Phytotherapy*, 2nd ed.; Elsevier: Amsterdam, The Netherlands, 2012; 1056p, ISBN 9780702052972. Available online: https://www.sciencedirect.com/book/9780443069925/principles-and-practice-ofphytotherapy (accessed on 10 February 2025).
33. Panossian, A.; Seo, E.J.; Efferth, T. Novel molecular mechanisms for the adaptogenic effects of herbal extracts on isolated brain cells using systems biology. *Phytomedicine* **2018**, *50*, 257–284. [CrossRef] [PubMed]
34. Panossian, A.; Hamm, R.; Kadioglu, O.; Wikman, G.; Efferth, T. Synergy and Antagonism of Active Constituents of ADAPT-232 on Transcriptional Level of Metabolic Regulation of Isolated Neuroglial. *Cells Front. Neurosci.* **2013**, *7*, 16. [CrossRef]
35. Panossian, A.; Lemerond, T.; Efferth, T. State-of-the-Art Review on Botanical Hybrid Preparations in Phytomedicine and Phytotherapy Research: Background and Perspectives. *Pharmaceuticals* **2024**, *17*, 483. [CrossRef]
36. Panossian, A.; Abdelfatah, S.; Efferth, T. Network Pharmacology of Ginseng (Part II): The Differential Effects of Red Ginseng and Ginsenoside Rg5 in Cancer and Heart Diseases as Determined by Transcriptomics. *Pharmaceuticals* **2021**, *14*, 1010. [CrossRef] [PubMed]
37. EMA/HMPC/232100/2011. Assessment Report on Rhodiola rosea L., Rhizoma et Radix. Based on Article 16d (1), Article 16f and Article 16h of Directive 2001/83/EC as Amended Traditional Use. Final. 27 March 2012. Available online: https://magistralbr.caldic.com/storage/product-files/680546566.pdf (accessed on 10 February 2025).
38. EMA/HMPC/24177/2023. European Union Herbal Monograph on *Rhodiola rosea* L., Rhizoma et Radix. Draft—Revision 1. Committee on Herbal Medicinal Products (HMPC). 19 July 2023. pp. 1–6. Available online: https://www.ema.europa.eu/en/documents/herbal-monograph/final-european-union-herbal-monograph-rhodiola-rosea-l-rhizoma-et-radix-revision-1_en.pdf (accessed on 3 September 2025).
39. EMA/HMPC/321232/2012. Assessment Report on Panax ginseng C.A. Meyer, Radix. Based on Article 16d (1), Article 16f and Article 16h of Directive 2001/83/EC as Amended (Traditional Use). Final. 25 March 2014. Available online: https://www.ema.europa.eu/en/documents/herbal-monograph/final-european-union-herbal-monograph-panaxginseng-camey-radix-revision-1_en.pdf (accessed on 3 September 2025).
40. EMA/HMPC/680615/2013. Assessment Report on Eleutherococcus senticosus (Rupr. et Maxim.) Maxim., Radix. Based on Article 16d (1), Article 16f and Article 16h of Directive 2001/83/EC as Amended (Traditional Use). Final. 25 March 2014. Available online: https://www.ema.europa.eu/en/documents/herbal-report/final-assessment-report-eleutherococcus-senticosus-rupr-et-maxim-maxim-radix_en.pdf (accessed on 3 September 2025).
41. Panossian, A.G. Adaptogens in mental and behavioral disorders. *Psychiatr. Clin. N. Am.* **2013**, *36*, 49–64. [CrossRef]
42. Panossian, A.; Gerbarg, P. Potential Use of Plant Adaptogens in Age-related Disorders. In *Complementary, Alternative, and Integrative Interventions in Mental Health and Aging*; Lavretsky, H., Sajatovic, M., Reynolds, C.F., III, Eds.; Oxford University Press: New York, NY, USA, 2016; pp. 197–211.
43. Panossian, A.; Amsterdam, J. Adaptogens in Psychiatric Practice. In *Complementary and Integrative Treatments*; Gerbarg, P.L., Muskin, P.R., Brown, R.P., Eds.; American Psychiatric Association Publishing: Arlington, TX, USA, 2018; 425p, Chapter 8; pp. 155–181. Available online: https://www.appi.org/Complementary_and_Integrative_Treatments_in_Psychiatric_Practice (accessed on 3 September 2025).
44. Amsterdam, J.D.; Panossian, A.G. *Rhodiola rosea* L. as a putative botanical antidepressant. *Phytomedicine* **2016**, *23*, 770–783. [CrossRef]
45. Sarris, J.; Panossian, A.; Schweitzer, I.; Stough, C.; Scholey, A. Herbal medicine for depression, anxiety and insomnia: A review of psychopharmacology and clinical evidence. *Eur. Neuropsychopharmacol.* **2011**, *21*, 841–860. [CrossRef]
46. Darbinyan, V.; Aslanyan, G.; Amroyan, E.; Gabrielyan, E.; Malmström, C.; Panossian, A. Clinical trial of *Rhodiola rosea* L. extract SHR-5 in the treatment of mild to moderate depression. *Nord. J. Psychiatry* **2007**, *61*, 2343–2348. [CrossRef]
47. Soldati, F. Ginseng, Panax. In *Encyclopedia of Dietary Supplements*; Marcel Dekker: New York, NY, USA, 2005; pp. 265–277.
48. Shikov, A.N.; Tsitsilin, A.N.; Pozharitskaya, O.N.; Makarov, V.G.; Heinrich, M. Traditional and Current Food Use of Wild Plants Listed in the Russian Pharmacopoeia. *Front. Pharmacol.* **2017**, *8*, 841. [CrossRef]
49. Panossian, A.; Brendler, T. The Role of Adaptogens in Prophylaxis and Treatment of Viral Respiratory Infections. *Pharmaceuticals* **2020**, *13*, 236. [CrossRef]
50. Brekhman, I.I. *Valeology—The Science of Health*; Physical Education and Sport: Moscow, Russia, 1990; 208p.
51. Brekhman, I.I. Pharmacosanation Medicaments. In *Man and Biologically Active Substances: The Effect of Drugs, Diet and Pollution on Health*, 1st ed.; Pergamon Press: New York, NY, USA, 1980; Chapter 3; pp. 49–59. Available online: https://openlibrary.org/books/OL4425643M/Man_and_biologically_active_substances (accessed on 3 September 2025).
52. Danish Technical University (DTU). *Food Institute's Risk Assessments of Withania somnifera (Ashwagandha) Root*; DTU DOCX No. 19/1030299; Danish Technical University (DTU): Kongens Lyngby, Denmark, 2020.

53. Danish Technical University (DTU). *Food Institute's Risk Assessments of Withania somnifera (Ashwagandha) Root*; DTU DOCX 25/100205; Danish Technical University (DTU): Kongens Lyngby, Denmark, 2025.
54. Ministry of Ayush, Government of India, New Delhi. *Safety of Ashwagandha. (Withania somnifera)*; Report of the Expert Committee Constituted by Ministry of Ayush Govt. of India; Central Council for Research in Ayuredic Sciences, Ministry of Ayush, Government of India: New Delhi, India, 2020; pp. 1–70. Available online: https://ayush.gov.in/images/domains/quality_standards/safetyReportAshwagandha.pdf (accessed on 3 September 2025).
55. Ramadoss, M.S.K.; Koumaravelou, K. Regulatory Requirement Sufficiency for Registration of Traditional Herbal Medicine-Based Products in Association of Southeast Asian Nations Regions: A Model Study with Ashwagandha Tablets. *Indian J. Pharm. Sci.* **2022**, *84*, 501–512. [CrossRef]
56. Patwardhan, B.; Chaturvedi, S.; Tillu, G.; Deshpande, S.; Hegde, B.M. Danish ban on Ashwagandha: Truth, evidence, ethics, and regulations. *J. Ayurveda Integr. Med.* **2024**, *15*, 101028. [CrossRef]
57. Sukardiman; Mutiah, R.; Handayani, R. Potential and mechanisms of indigenous Indonesian medicinal plants in treating sexual dysfunction: A systematic review and pharmacological network overview. *Heliyon* **2025**, *11*, e42501. [CrossRef] [PubMed]
58. Definition of Health. Available online: https://www.publichealth.com.ng/world-health-organizationwho-definition-of-health/ (accessed on 3 September 2025).
59. Panossian, A.; Lemerond, T. *The Milestones of Adaptogens Research and Use in Medicine*; Vide Leaf: Hyderabad, India, 2022; pp. 1–78. Available online: https://videleaf.com/product/the-milestones-of-adaptogens-research-and-use-in-medicine/ (accessed on 3 September 2025).
60. Panossian, A.; Lemerond, T. *ADAPTOGENS: Proven Plant Medicines Scientifically Researched to Regain and Restore Your Health*; TTN PublishingL: Kingwood, TX, USA, 2022; ISBN 978-1-952507-29-8. Available online: https://www.amazon.com/Adaptogens-Proven-Plant-Medicines-Scientifically/dp/1952507294 (accessed on 3 September 2025).
61. Panossian, A.; Wikman, G.; Wagner, H. Plant adaptogens. III. Earlier and more recent aspects and concepts on their mode of action. *Phytomedicine* **1999**, *6*, 287–300. [CrossRef]
62. Panossian, A.G.; Oganessian, A.S.; Ambartsumian, M.; Gabrielian, E.S.; Wagner, H.; Wikman, G. Effects of heavy physical exercise and adaptogens on nitric oxide content in human saliva. *Phytomedicine* **1999**, *6*, 17–26. [CrossRef] [PubMed]
63. Panossian, A.; Wagner, H. Stimulating effect of adaptogens: An overview with particular reference to their efficacy following single dose administration. *Phytother. Res.* **2005**, *19*, 819–838. [CrossRef] [PubMed]
64. Panossian, A.; Wikman, G. Pharmacology of Schisandra chinensis Bail.: An overview of Russian research and uses in medicine. *J. Ethnopharmacol.* **2008**, *118*, 183–212. [CrossRef]
65. Panossian, A.; Wikman, G. Effects of Adaptogens on the Central Nervous System and the Molecular Mechanisms Associated with Their Stress-Protective Activity. *Pharmaceuticals* **2010**, *3*, 188–224. [CrossRef] [PubMed]
66. Panossian, A.; Wikman, G. Evidence-based efficacy of adaptogens in fatigue, and molecular mechanisms related to their stress-protective activity. *Curr. Clin. Pharmacol.* **2009**, *4*, 198–219. [CrossRef] [PubMed]
67. Panossian, A.; Gabrielian, E.; Wagner, H. Plant adaptogens. II. Bryonia as an adaptogen. *Phytomedicine* **1997**, *4*, 85–99. [CrossRef]
68. Panossian, A.; Gabrielian, E.; Wagner, H. On the mechanism of action of plant adaptogens with particular reference to Cucurbitacin R diglucoside. *Phytomedicine* **1999**, *6*, 147–155. [CrossRef] [PubMed]
69. Orekhov, A.N.; Panossian, A.G. Trihydroxyoctadecadienoic acids exhibit antiatherosclerotic and antiatherogenic activity. *Phytomedicine* **1994**, *1*, 123–126. [CrossRef]
70. Serhan, C.N.; Levy, B.D. Resolvins in inflammation: Emergence of the pro-resolving superfamily of mediators. *J. Clin. Investig.* **2018**, *128*, 2657–2669. [CrossRef]
71. Panossian, A.; Seo, E.J.; Efferth, T. Effects of anti-inflammatory and adaptogenic herbal extracts on gene expression of eicosanoid signaling pathways in isolated brain cells. *Phytomedicine* **2019**, *60*, 152881. [CrossRef]
72. Noreen, E.E.; Buckley, J.G.; Lewis, S.L.; Brandauer, J.; Stuempfle, K.J. The effects of an acute dose of *Rhodiola rosea* on endurance exercise performance. *J. Strength Cond. Res.* **2013**, *27*, 839–847. [CrossRef]
73. Panossian, A.; Wikman, G.; Sarris, J. Rosenroot (*Rhodiola rosea*): Traditional use, chemical composition, pharmacology and clinical efficacy. *Phytomedicine* **2010**, *17*, 481–493. [CrossRef]
74. Panossian, A.; Wikman, G.; Kaur, P.; Asea, A. Adaptogens exert a stress-protective effect by modulation of expression of molecular chaperones. *Phytomedicine* **2009**, *16*, 617–622. [CrossRef]
75. Panossian, A.; Wikman, G.; Kaur, P.; Asea, A. Adaptogens stimulate neuropeptide Y and hsp72 expression and release in neuroglia cells. *Front. Neurosci.* **2012**, *6*, 6. [CrossRef]
76. Panossian, A.G.; Dadayan, M.A.; Gevorkian, G.A. The effect of stress and adaptogen cucurbitacin R diglucoside on arachidonic acid metabolism. *Probl. Endocrinol.* **1989**, *35*, 58–61.

77. Wiegant, F.A.C.; Limandjaja, G.C.; Poot, S.A.H.; Bayda, L.A.; Vorontsova, O.N.; Zenina, T.A.; Langelaar-Makkinje, M.; Post, J.A.; Wikman, G. Plant adaptogens activate cellular adaptive mechanisms by causing mild damage. In *Adaptation Biology and Medicine: Health Potentials*; Lukyanova, L., Takeda, N., Singal, P.K., Eds.; Narosa Publishers: New Delhi, India, 2008; Volume 5, pp. 319–332. Available online: https://www.uu.nl/staff/FACWiegant/Publications (accessed on 3 September 2025).
78. Wiegant, F.A.C.; Surinova, S.; Ytsma, E.; Langelaar-Makkinje, M.; Wikman, G.; Post, J.A. Plant adaptogens increase lifespan and stress resistance in C. elegans. *Biogerontology* **2009**, *10*, 27–42. [CrossRef]
79. Hovhannisyan, A.; Nylander, M.; Wikman, G.; Panossian, A. Efficacy of Adaptogenic Supplements on Adapting to Stress: A Randomized, Controlled Trial. *J. Athl. Enhanc.* **2015**, *4*, 4. [CrossRef]
80. Anderson, E.M.; Gomez, D.; Caccamise, A.; McPhail, D.; Hearing, M. Chronic unpredictable stress promotes cell-specific plasticity in prefrontal cortex D1 and D2 pyramidal neurons. *Neurobiol. Stress* **2019**, *10*, 100152. [CrossRef]
81. Panossian, A. Trends and Pitfalls in the Progress of Network Pharmacology Research on Natural Products. *Pharmaceuticals* **2025**, *18*, 538. [CrossRef] [PubMed]
82. Panossian, A.; Abdelfatah, S.; Efferth, T. Network Pharmacology of Red Ginseng (Part I): Effects of Ginsenoside Rg5 at Physiological and Sub-Physiological Concentrations. *Pharmaceuticals* **2021**, *14*, 999. [CrossRef] [PubMed]
83. Panossian, A.; Abdelfatah, S.; Efferth, T. Network Pharmacology of Ginseng (Part III): Antitumor Potential of a Fixed Combination of Red Ginseng and Red Sage as Determined by Transcriptomics. *Pharmaceuticals* **2022**, *15*, 1345. [CrossRef]
84. Chen, K.X.; Jiang, H.L.; Luo, X.M.; Shen, J.H. Drug discovery in postgenome era: Trend and practice. *Chin. J. Nat. Med.* **2004**, *2*, 257–260.
85. Wu, J.; Huang, H.; Chen, G.; Mao, J.; Tian, X.; Zhan, S.; Peng, Z.; Zhu, Y.; Wang, W. Integration of network pharmacology, bioinformatics and experimental verification strategy to discover the pharmacological mechanisms of mogroside acts against pharyngitis. *J. Ethnopharmacol.* **2025**, *344*, 119499. [CrossRef] [PubMed]
86. Noor, F.; Tahir Ul Qamar, M.; Ashfaq, U.A.; Albutti, A.; Alwashmi, A.S.S.; Aljasir, M.A. Network Pharmacology Approach for Medicinal Plants: Review and Assessment. *Pharmaceuticals* **2022**, *15*, 572. [CrossRef]
87. Efferth, T.; Koch, E. Complex interactions between phytochemicals. The multitarget therapeutic concept of phytotherapy. *Curr. Drug Targets* **2011**, *12*, 122–132. [CrossRef]
88. Panossian, A.; Hamm, R.; Wikman, G.; Efferth, T. Mechanism of action of Rhodiola, salidroside, tyrosol and triandrin in isolated neuroglial cells: An interactive pathway analysis of the downstream effects using RNA microarray data. *Phytomed. Int. J. Phytother. Phytopharm.* **2014**, *21*, 1325–1348. [CrossRef]
89. Gao, X.F.; Zhang, J.J.; Gong, X.J.; Li, K.K.; Zhang, L.X.; Li, W. Ginsenoside Rg5: A Review of Anticancer and Neuroprotection with Network Pharmacology Approach. *Am. J. Chin. Med.* **2022**, *50*, 2033–2056. [CrossRef]
90. He, S.; Shi, J.; Chai, H.; Ma, L.; Pei, H.; Zhang, P.; Shi, D.; Li, H. Mechanisms with network pharmacology approach of Ginsenosides in Alzheimer's disease. *Heliyon* **2024**, *10*, e26642. [CrossRef] [PubMed]
91. Liu, C.; Du, L.; Zhang, S.; Wang, H.; Kong, L.; Du, G. Network pharmacology and experimental study of phenolic acids in salvia miltiorrhiza bung in preventing ischemic stroke. *Front. Pharmacol.* **2023**, *14*, 1108518. [CrossRef] [PubMed]
92. Panossian, A.; Seo, E.J.; Wikman, G.; Efferth, T. Synergy assessment of fixed combinations of Herba Andrographidis and Radix Eleutherococci extracts by transcriptome-wide microarray profiling. *Phytomedicine* **2015**, *22*, 981–992. [CrossRef]
93. Panossian, A.; Seo, E.J.; Efferth, T. Synergy assessments of plant extracts used in the treatment of stress and aging related disorders. *Synerg. Res.* **2018**, *7*, 39–49. [CrossRef]
94. Li, S.; Xiao, W. General expert consensus on the application of network pharmacology in the research and development of new traditional Chinese medicine drugs. *Chin. J. Nat. Med.* **2025**, *23*, 129–142. [CrossRef]
95. Li, S.; Zhang, B. Traditional Chinese medicine network pharmacology: Theory, methodology and application. *Chin. J. Nat. Med.* **2013**, *11*, 110–120. [CrossRef] [PubMed]
96. Han, S.; Lv, A.P.; Li, J.; Jiang, M. Application review of network pharmacology in the study of properties theory of traditional Chinese medicine. *J. Basic Chin. Med.* **2019**, *25*, 127–130.
97. Zhou, Z.; Chen, B.; Chen, S.; Lin, M.; Chen, Y.; Jin, S.; Chen, W.; Zhang, Y. Applications of Network Pharmacology in Traditional Chinese Medicine Research. *Evid. Based Complement. Altern. Med.* **2020**, *2020*, 1646905. [CrossRef]
98. Zhang, P.; Zhang, D.; Zhou, W.; Wang, L.; Wang, B.; Zhang, T.; Li, S. Network pharmacology: Towards the artificial intelligence-based precision traditional Chinese medicine. *Brief. Bioinform.* **2023**, *25*, bbad518. [CrossRef]
99. Zhao, L.; Zhang, H.; Li, N.; Chen, J.; Xu, H.; Wang, Y.; Liang, Q. Network pharmacology, a promising approach to reveal the pharmacology mechanism of Chinese medicine formula. *J. Ethnopharmacol.* **2023**, *309*, 116306. [CrossRef]
100. Spanakis, M.; Tzamali, E.; Tzedakis, G.; Koumpouzi, C.; Pediaditis, M.; Tsatsakis, A.; Sakkalis, V. Artificial Intelligence Models and Tools for the Assessment of Drug–Herb Interactions. *Pharmaceuticals* **2025**, *18*, 282. [CrossRef] [PubMed]
101. Berger, S.I.; Iyengar, R. Role of systems pharmacology in understanding drug adverse events. *Wiley Interdiscip. Rev. Syst. Biol. Med.* **2011**, *3*, 129–135. [CrossRef]

102. Young, M.; Hoheisel, J.D.; Efferth, T. Toxicogenomics for the prediction of toxicity related to herbs from traditional Chinese medicine. *Planta Med.* **2010**, *76*, 2019–2025. [CrossRef]
103. Börner, F.U.; Schütz, H.; Wiedemann, P. The fragility of omics risk and benefit perceptions. *Toxicol. Lett.* **2011**, *201*, 249–257. [CrossRef]
104. Aardema, M.J.; MacGregor, J.T. Toxicology and genetic toxicology in the new era of "toxicogenomics": Impact of "-omics" technologies. *Mutat. Res.* **2002**, *499*, 13–25. [CrossRef]
105. Ouedraogo, M.; Baudoux, T.; Stévigny, C.; Nortier, J.; Colet, J.M.; Efferth, T.; Qu, F.; Zhou, J.; Chan, K.; Shaw, D.; et al. Review of current and "omics" methods for assessing the toxicity (genotoxicity, teratogenicity and nephrotoxicity) of herbal medicines and mushrooms. *J. Ethnopharmacol.* **2012**, *140*, 492–512. [CrossRef]
106. Panossian, A. Challenges in phytotherapy research. *Front. Pharmacol.* **2023**, *14*, 1199516. [CrossRef] [PubMed]
107. Wang, S.; Fang, Y.; Xu, Y.; Zhu, B.; Piao, J.; Zhu, L.; Yao, L.; Liu, K.; Wang, S.; Zhang, Q.; et al. The effects of different extraction methods on physicochemical, functional and physiological properties of soluble and insoluble dietary fiber from Rubus chingiiHu. Fruits. *J. Funct. Foods* **2022**, *93*, 105081. [CrossRef]
108. Tambi, M.I. *Eurycoma longifolia* jack: A potent adaptogen in the form of water-soluble extract with the effects of maintaining men's health. *Asian J. Androl.* **2006**, *8*, 49–50.
109. George, A.; Liske, E.; Chen, C.K.; Ismail, S.B. The *Eurycoma longifolia* Freeze-Dried Water Extract-Physta Does not Change Normal Ratios of Testosterone to Epitestosterone in Healthy Males. *J. Sports Med. Doping Stud.* **2013**, *3*, 2.
110. George, A.; Henkel, R. Phytoandrogenic properties of *Eurycoma longifolia* as natural alternative to testosterone replacement therapy. *Andrologia* **2014**, *46*, 708–721. [CrossRef]
111. Talbott, S.M.; Talbott, J.A.; George, A.; Pugh, M. Effect of Tongkat Ali on stress hormones and psychological mood state in moderately stressed subjects. *J. Int. Soc. Sports Nutr.* **2013**, *10*, 28. [CrossRef]
112. Thu, H.E.; Mohamed, I.N.; Hussain, Z.; Jayusman, P.A.; Shuid, A.N. *Eurycoma longifolia* as a potential adoptogen of male sexual health: A systematic review on clinical studies. *Chin. J. Nat. Med.* **2017**, *15*, 71–80. [CrossRef] [PubMed]
113. Leitão, A.E.; Vieira, M.C.S.; Pelegrini, A.; da Silva, E.L.; Guimarães, A.C.A. A 6-month, double-blind, placebo-controlled, randomized trial to evaluate the effect of *Eurycoma longifolia* (Tongkat Ali) and concurrent training on erectile function and testosterone levels in androgen deficiency of aging males (ADAM). *Maturitas* **2021**, *145*, 78–85. [CrossRef]
114. Chinnappan, S.M.; George, A.; Pandey, P.; Narke, G.; Choudhary, Y.K. Effect of *Eurycoma longifolia* standardised aqueous root extract–Physta® on testosterone levels and quality of life in ageing male subjects: A randomised, double-blind, placebo-controlled multicentre study. *Food Nutr. Res.* **2021**, *65*, 5647. [CrossRef] [PubMed]
115. Bhat, R.; Karim, A.A. Tongkat Ali (*Eurycoma longifolia* Jack): A review on its ethnobotany and pharmacological importance. *Fitoterapia* **2010**, *81*, 669–679. [CrossRef]
116. Rehman, S.U.; Choe, K.; Yoo, H.H. Review on a Traditional Herbal Medicine, *Eurycoma longifolia* Jack (Tongkat Ali): Its Traditional Uses, Chemistry, Evidence-Based Pharmacology and Toxicology. *Molecules* **2016**, *21*, 331. [CrossRef]
117. Low, B.S.; Das, P.K.; Chan, K.L. Standardized quassinoid-rich *Eurycoma longifolia* extract improved spermatogenesis and fertility in male rats via the hypothalamic-pituitary-gonadal axis. *J. Ethnopharmacol.* **2013**, *145*, 706–714. [CrossRef] [PubMed]
118. Leisegang, K.; Finelli, R.; Sikka, S.C.; Panner Selvam, M.K. *Eurycoma longifolia* (Jack) Improves Serum Total Testosterone in Men: A Systematic Review and Meta-Analysis of Clinical Trials. *Medicina* **2022**, *58*, 1047. [CrossRef]
119. Henkel, R.R.; Wang, R.; Bassett, S.H.; Chen, T.; Liu, N.; Zhu, Y.; Tambi, M.I. Tongkat Ali as a potential herbal supplement for physically active male and female seniors—A pilot study. *Phytother. Res.* **2014**, *28*, 544–550. [CrossRef] [PubMed]
120. Khanijo, T.; Jiraungkoorskul, W. Review Ergogenic Effect of Long Jack, *Eurycoma Longifolia*. *Pharmacogn. Rev.* **2016**, *10*, 139–142. [CrossRef]
121. George, A.; Udani, J.; Abidin, N.Z.; Yusof, A. Efficacy and safety of *Eurycoma longifolia* (Physta®) water extract plus 690 multivitamins on quality of life, mood and stress: A randomized placebo-controlled and parallel study. *Food Nutr. Res.* **2018**, *62*, 1374. [CrossRef]
122. Farag, M.A.; Ajayi, A.O.; Taleb, M.; Wang, K.; Ayoub, I.M. A Multifaceted Review of *Eurycoma longifolia* Nutraceutical Bioactives: Production, Extraction, and Analysis in Drugs and Biofluids. *ACS Omega* **2023**, *8*, 1838–1850. [CrossRef] [PubMed]
123. Lee, E.L.; Barnes, J. Tongkat Ali/Long Jack. *J. Prim. Health Care* **2022**, *14*, 380–382. [CrossRef]
124. Muniandy, S.; Yahya, H.M.; Shahar, S.; Kamisan Atan, I.; Mahdy, Z.A.; Rajab, N.F.; George, A.; Chinnappan, S.M. Effects of *Eurycoma longifolia* Jack standardised water extract (Physta) on well-being of perimenopausal and postmenopausal women: Protocol for a randomised, double-blinded, placebo-controlled, parallel group study. *BMJ Open* **2023**, *13*, e073323. [CrossRef]
125. Gagnier, J.J.; Boon, H.; Rochon, P.; Moher, D.; Barnes, J.; Bombardier, C.; CONSORT Group. Recommendations for reporting randomized controlled trials of herbal interventions: Explanation and elaboration. *J. Clin. Epidemiol.* **2006**, *59*, 1134–1149. [CrossRef]

126. ICH E6 (R3) Guideline for Good Clinical Practice (GCP)—Step 5, EMA/CHMP/ICH/135/1995 Legal Effective Date: 23 July 2025. Available online: https://www.ema.europa.eu/en/ich-e6-good-clinical-practice-scientific-guideline (accessed on 3 September 2025).
127. Michail, N. 'Incorrect and Misleading': Industry Defends Ashwagandha Root Extract Safety Amid Danish Assessment. 25 May 2023. Available online: https://www.vitafoodsinsights.com/botanicals-herbs/-incorrect-and-misleading-industry-defends-ashwagandha-root-extract-safety-amid-danish-assessment (accessed on 3 September 2025).
128. Indian Express. Denmark's Ban on Ashwagandha Lacks Scientific Rigor. 2024. Available online: https://indianexpress.com/article/cities/pune/denmarks-ban-on-ashwagandha-ban-based-on-2020-report-that-lacks-scientific-rigor-says-ayush-ministry-9435664/ (accessed on 3 September 2025).
129. Paul, S.; Chakraborty, S.; Anand, U.; Dey, S.; Nandy, S.; Ghorai, M.; Saha, S.C.; Patil, M.T.; Kandimalla, R.; Proćków, J.; et al. *Withania somnifera* (L.) Dunal (Ashwagandha): A comprehensive review on ethnopharmacology, pharmacotherapeutics, biomedicinal and toxicological aspects. *Biomed. Pharmacother. Biomed. Pharmacother.* **2021**, *143*, 112175. [CrossRef]
130. Mukherjee, P.K.; Banerjee, S.; Biswas, S.; Das, B.; Kar, A.; Katiyar, C.K. *Withania somnifera* (L.) Dunal—Modern perspectives of an ancient Rasayana from Ayurveda. *J. Ethnopharmacol.* **2021**, *264*, 113157. [CrossRef] [PubMed]
131. Mikulska, P.; Malinowska, M.; Ignacyk, M.; Szustowski, P.; Nowak, J.; Pesta, K.; Szeląg, M.; Szklanny, D.; Judasz, E.; Kaczmarek, G.; et al. Ashwagandha *(Withania somnifera)*—Current Research on the Health-Promoting Activities: A Narrative Review. *Pharmaceutics* **2023**, *15*, 1057. [CrossRef] [PubMed]
132. Khalid, M.U.; Sultan, M.T.; Baig, I.; Abbas, A.; Noman, A.M.; Zinedine, A.; Bartkiene, E.; Rocha, J.M. A comprehensive review on the bioactivity and pharmacological attributes of *Withania somnifera*. *Nat. Prod. Res.* **2025**, 1–25, *Advance online publication.* [CrossRef]
133. Anupama, N.; Rathi, P.; Sharma, A. Clinical safety profile of Ashwagandha root in human trials. *J. Ayurveda Integr. Med.* **2023**, *14*, 100420.
134. Kalaivani, P.; Siva, R.; Gayathri, V.; Langade, D. Ninety-day repeated dose toxicity of Ashwagandha (*Withania somnifera*) root extract in Wistar rats. *Toxicol. Rep.* **2023**, *11*, 189–198. [CrossRef]
135. Tandon, N.; Yadav, S.S. Safety and clinical effectiveness of *Withania Somnifera* (Linn.) Dunal root in human ailments. *J. Ethnopharmacol.* **2020**, *255*, 112768. [CrossRef]
136. Verma, N.; Gupta, S.K.; Tiwari, S.; Mishra, A.K. Safety of Ashwagandha Root Extract: A Randomized, Placebo-Controlled, Study in Healthy Volunteers. *Complement. Ther. Med.* **2021**, *57*, 102642. [CrossRef] [PubMed]
137. Vaidya, V.G.; Gothwad, A.; Ganu, G.; Girme, A.; Modi, S.J.; Hingorani, L. Clinical safety and tolerability evaluation of *Withania somnifera* (L.) Dunal (Ashwagandha) root extract in healthy human volunteers. *J. Ayurveda Integr. Med.* **2024**, *15*, 100859. [CrossRef]
138. Mandlik Ingawale, D.S.; Namdeo, A.G. Pharmacological evaluation of Ashwagandha highlighting its healthcare claims, safety, and toxicity aspects. *J. Diet. Suppl.* **2021**, *18*, 183–226. [CrossRef] [PubMed]
139. Arumugam, V.; Vijayakumar, V.; Balakrishnan, A.; Bhandari, R.; Boopalan, D.; Ponnurangam, R.; Sankaralingam Thirupathy, V.; Kuppusamy, M. Effects of Ashwagandha (*Withania somnifera*) on stress and anxiety: A systematic review and meta-analysis. *Explore* **2024**, *20*, 103062. [CrossRef]
140. Pratte, M.A.; Nanavati, K.B.; Young, V.; Morley, C.P. An alternative treatment for anxiety: A systematic review of human trial results reported for the Ayurvedic herb ashwagandha (*Withania somnifera*). *J. Altern. Complement. Med.* **2014**, *20*, 901–908. [CrossRef]
141. Durg, S.; Shivaram, S.B.; Bavage, S. *Withania somnifera* (Indian ginseng) in male infertility: An evidence-based systematic review and meta-analysis. *Phytomedicine* **2018**, *50*, 247–256. [CrossRef]
142. Pérez-Gómez, J.; Villafaina, S.; Adsuar, J.C.; Merellano-Navarro, E.; Collado-Mateo, D. Effects of Ashwagandha (*Withania somnifera*) on VO2max: A Systematic Review and Meta-Analysis. *Nutrients* **2020**, *12*, 1119. [CrossRef]
143. Chandrasekhar, K.; Kapoor, J.; Anishetty, S. A prospective, randomized double-blind, placebo-controlled study of safety and efficacy of a high-concentration full-spectrum extract of ashwagandha root in reducing stress and anxiety in adults. *Indian J. Psychol. Med.* **2012**, *34*, 255–262. [CrossRef] [PubMed]
144. Langade, D.; Kanchi, S.; Salve, J.; Debnath, K.; Ambegaokar, D. Efficacy and Safety of Ashwagandha (*Withania somnifera*) Root Extract in Insomnia and Anxiety: A Double-blind, Randomized, Placebo-controlled Study. *Cureus* **2019**, *11*, e5797. [CrossRef]
145. Yerram, C.; Jillella, A.; Reddy, V. Effects of Withania somnifera root extract serum application on hair health in healthy adults: A prospective, double-blind, randomized, parallel, placebo-controlled study. *J. Ayurveda Integr. Med.* **2023**, *14*, 100817. [CrossRef]
146. Choudhary, D.; Bhattacharyya, S.; Joshi, K. Body Weight Management in Adults Under Chronic Stress Through Treatment with Ashwagandha Root Extract: A Double-Blind, Randomized, Placebo-Controlled Trial. *J. Evid.-Based Complement. Altern. Med.* **2016**, *22*, 96–106. [CrossRef]
147. Salve, J.; Pate, S.; Khokan, D.; Langade, D. Adaptogenic and Anxiolytic Effects of Ashwagandha Root Extract in Healthy Adults: A Double-blind, Randomized, Placebo-controlled Clinical Study. *Cureus* **2019**, *11*, e6466.

148. Priyanka, G.; Anil Kumar, B.; Lakshman, M.; Manvitha, V.; Kala Kumar, B. Adaptogenic and Immunomodulatory Activity of Ashwagandha Root Extract: An Experimental Study in an Equine Model. *Front. Vet. Sci.* **2020**, *7*, 541112. [CrossRef] [PubMed]
149. Kaur, J.; Seshadri, S.; Golla, K.H.; Sampara, P. Efficacy and safety of standardized Ashwagandha (*Withania somnifera*) root extract on reducing stress and anxiety in domestic dogs: A randomized controlled trial. *J. Vet. Behav.* **2022**, *51*, 8–15. [CrossRef]
150. Devarasetti, A.K.; Bharani, K.K.; Khurana, A.; Anand, S.; Kollipaka, R.; Saranu, V.D.T.; Hanuman, D.D.V.; Addanki, V.K.; Chetlah, V.S.; Banothu, A.K. Adaptogenic Ashwagandha root extract modulates inflammatory markers in feline stress management: A double-blind placebo-controlled clinical trial. *J. Appl. Anim. Res.* **2024**, *52*, 2335921. [CrossRef]
151. Długołęcka, B.; Jowko, E.; Kotowska, J.; Gierczuk, D. Effects of Ashwagandha (*Withania somnifera*) Supplementation on Body Composition and Blood Health Indices in Professional Wrestlers. *Pol. J. Sport Tour.* **2023**, *30*, 26–32. [CrossRef]
152. Langade, D.; Thakare, V.; Kanchi, S.; Kelgane, S. Clinical evaluation of the pharmacological impact of ashwagandha root extract on sleep in healthy volunteers and insomnia patients: A double-blind, randomized, parallel-group, placebo-controlled stud. *J. Ethnopharmacol.* **2020**, *264*, 113276. [CrossRef]
153. Kelgane, S.B.; Jaysing Salve, J.; Sampara, P.; Debnath, K. Efficacy and Tolerability of Ashwagandha Root Extract in the Elderly for Improvement of General Well-Being and Sleep: A Prospective, Randomized, Double-Blind, Placebo-Controlled Study. *Cureus* **2020**, *12*, e7083. [CrossRef]
154. The Indian Herbal Pharmacopeia; Revised New Edition 2002; Indian Drug Manufacturers' Association: Mumbai, India. 2002; pp. 467–478. Available online: https://www.scribd.com/document/59798407/Indian-Herbal-Pharmacopoeia-Vol-i (accessed on 3 September 2025).
155. Withaniae somniferae Radix—Herbal Medicinal Product | European Medicines Agency (EMA). Available online: https://www.ema.europa.eu/en/medicines/herbal/withaniae-somniferae-radix (accessed on 3 September 2025).
156. Public Statement on Withania somnifera (L.) Dunal, Radix. EMA/HMPC/681519/2012. Committee on Herbal Medicinal Products (HMPC). 9 July 2013. Available online: https://www.ema.europa.eu/en/documents/public-statement/final-public-statement-withania-somnifera-l-dunal-radix-first-version_en.pdf (accessed on 3 September 2025).
157. Herbal Medicinal Products and Natural Medicinal Products. Available online: https://www.lakemedelsverket.se/en/permission-approval-and-control/marketing-authorisation/herbal-medicinal-products-and-natural-medicinal-products (accessed on 3 September 2025).
158. Food Supplements. Available online: https://www.livsmedelsverket.se/en/business-legislation-and-control/legislation-food-business/food-supplements (accessed on 3 September 2025).
159. United States Pharmacopeia. *Ashwagandha Root. Dietary Supplement Monographs, Ashwagandha Root*; USP-NF: Rockville, MD, USA, Pharmacopeia ID: GUID-8F4D7EDA-40ED-44A2-A3AD-E13C8E7638BF_2_en-US. [CrossRef]
160. HPLC Analysis of Ashwagandha Supplements Using Alliance™ iS HPLC System. Available online: https://www.waters.com/nextgen/us/en/library/application-notes/2024/hplc-analysis-of-ashwagandha-supplements-using-alliance-is-hplc-system.html (accessed on 3 September 2025).
161. Is Ashwagandha Legal in the UK: Regulations and Availability. Available online: https://oxford-origins.com/blogs/learn/is-ashwagandha-legal-in-the-uk-regulations-and-availability (accessed on 3 September 2025).
162. Ashwagandha: Food Supplements with Potential Health Risks. 10 September 2024. Available online: https://www.bfr.bund.de/cm/349/ashwagandha-food-supplements-with-potential-health-risks.pdf (accessed on 3 September 2025).
163. Australian Register of Therapeutic Goods (ARTG). Available online: https://www.tga.gov.au/products/australian-register-therapeutic-goods-artg (accessed on 3 September 2025).
164. McKeown, M. Why Did Denmark Ban Ashwagandha? 2 June 2023. Available online: https://www.mcgill.ca/oss/article/critical-thinking-health-and-nutrition/why-did-denmark-ban-ashwagandha (accessed on 3 September 2025).
165. Ashwagandha (Withania somnifera) Root. Summary of Safety Data. Food Supple ments Europe. EFSA. March 2023. pp. 1–26. Available online: https://www.npninfo.nl/wp-content/uploads/2025/03/FSE-Ashwaganda-Mar-2023-F.pdf (accessed on 3 September 2025).
166. de Heer, J.A. Risk Assessment of Herbal Preparations Containing Withania somnifera (Ashwagandha). RIVM Letter Report 2024-0029. Available online: https://www.rivm.nl/bibliotheek/rapporten/2024-0029.pdf (accessed on 3 September 2025).
167. A Safety Report on Ashwagandha Root Extract an Evaluation of the Risk Assessment Made by DTU Food Institute 2020. World Ashwagandha Council and Ixoreal Biomed Inc, USA. March 2023. pp. 1–74. Available online: https://drinktr.getonnet.dev/wp-content/uploads/2023/12/3.-Ashwagandha-Safety-Report.pdf (accessed on 3 September 2025).
168. Studies. All Ashwagandha Are Not The same. Available online: https://en.ksm66.se/studier (accessed on 3 September 2025).
169. Gupta, D.P.; Langade, D. Safety Opinion of Standardized Ashwagandha Root Extract. March 2024. Available online: https://cdn.prod.website-files.com/5e68cf7fabaae796200b13dc/65f2d081c085e3ecd906f836_Appendix%202_Safety%20Opinion%20of%20Standardized%20Ashwagandha%20Root%20Extract.pdf (accessed on 3 September 2025).

170. Opinion: Safety Evaluation on the Root Part vs. The Entire Plant/Aerial Parts. Available online: https://cdn.prod.website-files.com/5e68cf7fabaae796200b13dc/65f2d0817311671eb9fe81e0_Appendix%201_SAFETY%20EVALUATION_ROOT%20PART%20VS.%20AERIAL%20PARTS.pdf (accessed on 3 September 2025).
171. KSM66—A Safety Assessment. Available online: https://en.medicinegarden.se/press/genomgang-av-sakerhet-och-kliniska-studier-avseende-ksm66 (accessed on 3 September 2025).
172. Singh, A.; Singh, K.D.; Shekhawat, P.S. Spermicidal activity and antifertility activity of ethanolic extract of *Withania somnifera* in male albino rats. *Int. J. Pharm. Sci. Rev. Res.* **2013**, *21*, 227–232.
173. Gannon, J.M.; Forrest, P.E.; Roy Chengappa, K.N. Subtle changes in thyroid indices during a placebo-controlled study of an extract of *Withania somnifera* in persons with bipolar disorder. *J. Ayurveda Integr. Med.* **2014**, *5*, 241–245. [CrossRef] [PubMed]
174. Sensoril(Ashwaganhda)for Bipolar Disorder. Available online: https://ichgcp.net/clinical-trials-registry/NCT00761761 (accessed on 3 September 2025).
175. Chengappa, K.N.R.; Bowie, C.R.; Schlicht, P.J.; Fleet, D.; Brar, J.S.; Jindal, R. Randomized placebo-controlled adjunctive study of an extract of *Withania somnifera* for cognitive dysfunction in bipolar disorder. *J. Clin. Psychiatry* **2013**, *74*, 1076–1083. [CrossRef]
176. Speers, A.B.; Cabey, K.A.; Soumyanath, A.; Wright, K.M. Effects of *Withania somnifera* (Ashwagandha) on Stress and the Stress-Related Neuropsychiatric Disorders Anxiety, Depression, and Insomnia. *Curr Neuropharmacol.* **2021**, *19*, 1468–1495. [CrossRef]
177. Punja, S.; Shamseer, L.; Olson, K.; Vohra, S. *Rhodiola rosea* for mental and physical fatigue in nursing students: A randomized controlled trial. *PLoS ONE* **2014**, *9*, e108416. [CrossRef]
178. Schröter, H.-B.; Neumann, D.; Katritzky, A.R.; Swinbourne, F.J. Withasomnine. A pyrazole alkaloid from *Withania somnifera* Dun. *Tetrahedron* **1966**, *22*, 2895–2897. [CrossRef]
179. Rajalakshmy, M.R.; Geetha, G. Isolation and identification of withasomnine, withanolides and butein from industrial herbal marc of *Withania somnifera* (L.) Dunal. *Indian J. Nat. Prod. Resour.* **2016**, *7*, 116–124.
180. Akgul, Y.; Ferreira, D.; Abourashed, E.A.; Khan, I.A. Lotaustralin from *Rhodiola rosea* roots. *Fitoterapia* **2004**, *75*, 612–614. [CrossRef]
181. Langeder, J.; Grienke, U.; Döring, K.; Jafari, M.; Ehrhardt, C.; Schmidtke, M.; Rollinger, J.M. High-performance Countercurrent Chromatography to Access *Rhodiola rosea* Influenza Virus Inhibiting Constituents. *Planta Med.* **2021**, *87*, 818–826. [CrossRef] [PubMed]
182. Dimpfel, W.; Schombert, L.; Panossian, A.G. Assessing the Quality and Potential Efficacy of Commercial Extracts of *Rhodiola rosea* L. by Analyzing the Salidroside and Rosavin Content and the Electrophysiological Activity in Hippocampal Long-Term Potentiation, a Synaptic Model of Memory. *Front. Pharmacol.* **2018**, *9*, 425. [CrossRef]
183. *Legal and Regulatory Framework for Herbal Medicines*; Association Européenne des Spécialités Pharmaceutiques Grand Public Association of the European Self-Medication Industry Europäischer Verband der Arzneimittel-Hersteller (AESGP): Brussels Belgium, 2010; pp. 1–245.
184. European Pharmacopoeia (Ph. Eur.). Available online: https://www.edqm.eu/en/european-pharmacopoeia (accessed on 3 September 2025).
185. European Union Monographs and List Entries. Available online: https://www.ema.europa.eu/en/human-regulatory-overview/herbal-medicinal-products/european-union-monographs-list-entries (accessed on 3 September 2025).
186. Final Guideline on Quality of Herbal Medicinal Products/Traditional Herbal Medicinal Products—Revision 3. EMA/HMPC/CHMP/CVMP/201116/20051 Rev. 318. Quality of Herbal Medicinal Products/Traditional Herbal Medicinal Products. January 2022. Available online: https://www.ema.europa.eu/en/documents/scientific-guideline/guideline-quality-herbal-medicinal-products-traditional-herbal-medicinal-products-revision-2_en.pdf (accessed on 3 September 2025).
187. Guideline on declaration of herbal substances and herbal preparations in herbal medicinal products/traditional herbal medicinal products in the SPC. EMEA/HMPC/CHMP/CVMP/287539/2005. 11 March 2010. Declaration of herbal substances and herbal preparations in herbal medicinal products/traditional herbal medicinal products—Scientific guideline. Available online: https://www.ema.europa.eu/en/documents/scientific-guideline/final-guideline-quality-herbal-medicinal-productstraditional-herbal-medicinal-products-revision-3_en.pdf. (accessed on 3 September 2025).
188. Guideline on Good Agricultural and Collection Practice (GACP) for Starting Materials of Herbal Origin—Revision 1. EMA/HMPC/246816/2005 Rev. 1. Good Agricultural and Collection Practice for Starting Materials of Herbal Origin. 9 July 2025. Available online: https://www.ema.europa.eu/en/good-agricultural-collection-practice-starting-materials-herbal-origin-scientific-guideline. (accessed on 3 September 2025).
189. Guideline on Quality of Combination Herbal Medicinal Products/Traditional Herbal Medicinal Products. EMEA/HMPC/CHMP/CVMP/214869/2006. Quality of Combination Herbal Medicinal Products/Traditional Herbal Medicinal Products. 23 June 2008. Available online: https://www.ema.europa.eu/en/quality-combination-herbal-medicinal-products-traditional-herbal-medicinal-products-scientific-guideline (accessed on 3 September 2025).

190. Guideline on Specifications: Test Procedures and Acceptance Criteria for Herbal Substances, Herbal Preparations and Herbal Medicinal Products/Traditional Herbal Medicinal Products—Revision 3. EMA/HMPC/CHMP/CVMP/162241/2005. Specifications: Test Procedures and Acceptance Criteria for Herbal Substances, Herbal Preparations and Herbal Medicinal Products/Traditional Herbal Medicinal Products—Scientific Guideline. 18 January 2022. Available online: https://www.ema.europa.eu/en/specifications-test-procedures-acceptance-criteria-herbal-substances-herbal-preparations-herbal-medicinal-products-traditional-herbal-medicinal-products-scientific-guideline (accessed on 3 September 2025).
191. Herbal Medicinal Products: Scientific Guidelines. Available online: https://www.ema.europa.eu/en/human-regulatory-overview/research-development/scientific-guidelines/multidisciplinary-guidelines/herbal-medicinal-products-scientific-guidelines (accessed on 3 September 2025).
192. Herbal: European Union Herbal Monographs. Available online: https://efsa.onlinelibrary.wiley.com/authored-by/ContribRaw/EFSA+Scientific+Committee (accessed on 3 September 2025).
193. Kroes, B.H. The legal framework governing the quality of (traditional) herbal medicinal products in the European Union. *J. Ethnopharmacol.* **2014**, *158 Pt B*, 449–453. [CrossRef] [PubMed]
194. Peschel, W. The Traditional Herbal Medicine Directive within the European regulatory framework for Herbal Products. *Bol. Latinoam. Caribe Plant. Med. Aromat.* **2007**, *6*, 102–111.
195. Qu, L.; Zou, W.; Wang, Y.; Wang, M. European regulation model for herbal medicine: The assessment of the EU monograph and the safety and efficacy evaluation in marketing authorization or registration in Member States. *Phytomed. Int. J. Phytother. Phytopharm.* **2018**, *42*, 219–225. [CrossRef]
196. Guidance for Industry. General/Specific Intended Use. 1998. Available online: https://www.fda.gov/media/71966/download (accessed on 3 September 2025).
197. Current Good Manufacturing Practice—Guidance for Human Drug Compounding Outsourcing Facilities Under Section 503B of the FD&C Act Guidance for Industry. U.S. Department of Health and Human Services Food and Drug Administration, Center for Drug Evaluation and Research (CDER). Pharmaceutical Quality/Manufacturing Standards (GMP), Revision 2. January 2020. Available online: https://www.fda.gov/media/88905/download (accessed on 3 September 2025).
198. Federal Registers of 23 September 1997 (62 FR 49826), 5 June 1998 (63 FR 30615), and 15 January 1997 (62 FR 2218). Available online: https://www.federalregister.gov/ (accessed on 3 September 2025).
199. ICH: Q 7: Good Manufacturing Practice for Active Pharmaceutical Ingredients—Step 5, CPMP/ICH/4106/00. 2000. Available online: https://www.ema.europa.eu/en/documents/scientific-guideline/ich-q-7-good-manufacturing-practice-active-pharmaceutical-ingredients-step-5_en.pdf (accessed on 3 September 2025).
200. State Pharmacopoeia of the USSR. *State Pharmacopoeia of the USSR*, 14th ed.; Medicina: Moscow, Russia, 2018; Part 2. Available online: https://pharmacopeia.ru/ (accessed on 3 September 2025).
201. Shikov, A.N.; Pozharitskaya, O.N.; Makarov, V.G.; Wagner, H.; Verpoorte, R.; Heinrich, M. Medicinal plants of the Russian Pharmacopoeia; their history and applications. *J. Ethnopharmacol.* **2014**, *154*, 481–536. [CrossRef]
202. National Pharmacopoeia Committee. *Pharmacopoeia of the People's Republic of China*, English ed.; National Pharmacopoeia Committee: Beijing, China, 2010. Available online: https://books.google.se/books/about/Pharmacopoeia_of_the_People_s_Republic_o.html?id=Z49IXwAACAAJ&redir_esc=y (accessed on 3 September 2025).
203. WHO Good Practices for Pharmaceutical Quality Control Laboratories. Annex 1. World Health Organization WHO Technical Report Series, No. 957. 2010. Available online: https://www.who.int/docs/default-source/medicines/norms-and-standards/guidelines/quality-control/trs957-annex1-goodpractices-harmaceuticalqualitycontrol-laboratories.pdf (accessed on 3 September 2025).
204. Jain, S.D.; Shrivastava, S.K.; Agrawal, A.; Gupta, A.K. WHO guidelines for quality control of herbal medicines: From cultivation to consumption. *Int. J. Pharm. Chem. Anal.* **2024**, *11*, 212–225. [CrossRef]
205. Swedish Medical Products Agency. Herbal Medicines. Available online: https://www.lakemedelsverket.se/en/search?q=herbal%20medicines (accessed on 3 September 2025).
206. Dietary Supplement Health and Education Act of 1994 Public Law 103-417 103rd Congress. Available online: https://ods.od.nih.gov/About/DSHEA_Wording.aspx (accessed on 3 September 2025).
207. Andrews, K.W.; Gusev, P.A.; McNeal, M.; Savarala, S.; Dang, P.T.V.; Oh, L.; Atkinson, R.; Pehrsson, P.R.; Dwyer, J.T.; Saldanha, L.G.; et al. Dietary Supplement Ingredient Database (DSID) and the application of analytically based estimates of ingredient amount to intake calculations. *J. Nutr.* **2018**, *148*, 1413S–1421S. [CrossRef]
208. Botanical Drug Development Guidance for Industry. U.S. Department of Health and Human Services Food and Drug Administration, Center for Drug Evaluation and Research (CDER). Pharmaceutical Quality/CMC Revision 1. December 2016. pp. 1–30. Available online: https://www.fda.gov/files/drugs/published/Botanical-Drug-Development{-}{-}Guidance-for-Industry.pdf (accessed on 3 September 2025).

209. Coates, P.M.; Bailey, R.L.; Blumberg, J.B.; El-Sohemy, A.; Floyd, E.; Goldenberg, J.Z.; Gould Shunney, A.; Holscher, H.D.; Nkrumah-Elie, Y.; Rai, D.; et al. The Evolution of Science and Regulation of Dietary Supplements: Past, Present, and Future. *J. Nutr.* **2024**, *154*, 2335–2345. [CrossRef] [PubMed]
210. Dietary Supplement Health and Education Act of 1994. Public Law 103-417 [Internet], 1994. 1994. Available online: https://www.congress.gov/103/statute/STATUTE-108/STATUTE-108-Pg4325.pdf (accessed on 12 March 2025).
211. Dwyer, J.T.; Coates, P.M.; Smith, M.J. Dietary Supplements: Regulatory Challenges and Research Resources. *Nutrients* **2018**, *10*, 41. [CrossRef]
212. Food Labeling; Nutrient Content Claims: Definition for "High Potency" Claim for Dietary Supplements and Definition of "Antioxidant" for Use in Nutrient Content Claims for Dietary Supplements and Conventional Foods. Department of Health and Human Services Food and Drug Administration. 21 CFR Part 101. [Docket No. 95N–0347]. Federal Register/Vol. 60, No. 249/Thursday, December 28, 1995/Proposed Rules. Available online: https://www.govinfo.gov/content/pkg/FR-1995-12-28/pdf/95-31193.pdf (accessed on 3 September 2025).
213. Food Labeling: Requirements for Nutrient Content Claims, Health Claims, and Statements of Nutritional Support for Dietary Supplements. Department of Health AND Human Services Food and Drug Administration. 21 CFR Part 101. Docket No. 95N–0282. Federal Register/Vol. 60, No. 249/Thursday, December 28, 1995/Proposed Rules. Available online: https://www.govinfo.gov/content/pkg/FR-1995-12-28/pdf/95-31193.pdf (accessed on 3 September 2025).
214. Johnston, D. Natural standard herb and supplement reference: Evidence based clinical reviews. *Ulst. Med. J.* **2006**, *75*, 166.
215. Label Claims for Conventional Foods and Dietary Supplements. Available online: https://www.fda.gov/food/nutrition-food-labeling-and-critical-foods/label-claims-conventional-foods-and-dietary-supplements (accessed on 3 September 2025).
216. Ulbricht, C.E.; Basch, E.M. *Natural Standard Herb and Supplement Reference: Evidence-Based Clinical Reviews*; Mosby: Amsterdam, The Netherlands, 2005; 1040p, ISBN 0-323-02994-9.
217. NIH Office of Dietary Supplements: Mission, Origin, and Mandate. Available online: https://ods.od.nih.gov/About/MissionOriginMandate.aspx (accessed on 12 March 2025).
218. NIST Measurements and Standards for Botanical Dietary Supplements. Available online: https://www.nist.gov/programs-projects/measurements-and-standards-botani (accessed on 12 March 2025).
219. ODS Analytical Methods and Reference Materials Program. Dietary Supplement Analytical Methods and Reference Materials Program (AMRM). Available online: https://ods.od.nih.gov/Research/AMRMProgramWebsite.aspx (accessed on 3 September 2025).
220. Pasiakos, S.M.; Kuszak, A.J. Strengthening Dietary Supplement Research: An Expanded Priority for the NIH Office of Dietary Supplements. *Am. J. Clin. Nutr.* **2025**, *121*, 1217–1219. [CrossRef]
221. Understanding Dietary Supplement Claims. Available online: https://www.chpa.org/news/2021/11/understanding-dietary-supplement-claims (accessed on 3 September 2025).
222. Botanicals. Available online: https://www.efsa.europa.eu/en/topics/topic/botanicals (accessed on 3 September 2025).
223. Compendium of Botanicals. Available online: https://www.efsa.europa.eu/en/data-report/compendium-botanicals (accessed on 3 September 2025).
224. EU Register of Health Claims. Available online: https://food.ec.europa.eu/food-safety/labelling-and-nutrition/nutrition-and-health-claims/eu-register-health-claims_en (accessed on 3 September 2025).
225. EUR-Lex. Available online: https://eur-lex.europa.eu/eli/reg/2006/1925/oj/eng (accessed on 3 September 2025).
226. "General Function" Claims Under Article 13.1 of the EC Regulation on Nutrition and Health Claims Structure/Function Claim. Available online: https://www.fda.gov/food/nutrition-food-labeling-and-critical-foods/structurefunction-claims (accessed on 3 September 2025).
227. Guidance on Safety Assessment of Botanicals and Botanical Preparations Intended for Use as Ingredients in Food Supplements. *EFSA J.* **2009**, *7*, 1249. [CrossRef]
228. Health Claims. Available online: https://ec.europa.eu/food/food-feed-portal/screen/health-claims/eu-register (accessed on 3 September 2025).
229. Health Claims. Available online: https://www.efsa.europa.eu/en/topics/topic/health-claims (accessed on 3 September 2025).
230. Nutrition and Health Claims. Available online: https://food.ec.europa.eu/food-safety/labelling-and-nutrition/nutrition-and-health-claims_en (accessed on 3 September 2025).
231. Nutrition Claims. Available online: https://food.ec.europa.eu/food-safety/labelling-and-nutrition/nutrition-and-health-claims/nutrition-claims_en (accessed on 3 September 2025).
232. Regulation (EC) No 1924/2006 of the European Parliament and of the Council of 20 December 2006 on Nutrition and Health Claims Made on Foods. Available online: http://data.europa.eu/eli/reg/2006/1924/oj (accessed on 3 September 2025).
233. EFSA—The European Food Safety Authority. Available online: https://www.efsa.europa.eu/en/about/about-efsa (accessed on 3 September 2025).

234. Ginseng Radix. In *WHO Monographs on Selected Medicinal Plants*; World Health Organization: Geneva, Switzerland, 1999; Volume 1, pp. 168–182.
235. Radix Eleutherococci. In *WHO Monographs on Selected Medicinal Plants*; World Health Organization: Geneva, Switzerland, 2002; Volume 2, pp. 83–96.
236. Fructus Schisandrae. In *WHO Monographs on Selected Medicinal Plants*; World Health Organization: Geneva, Switzerland, 2007; Volume 3, pp. 296–313.
237. Radix Withaniae. In *WHO Monographs on Selected Medicinal Plants*; World Health Organization: Geneva, Switzerland, 2009; Volume 4, pp. 373–391.
238. Upton, R. (Ed.) *Ashwagandha Root. Withania somnifera. Analytical, Quality Control, and Therapeutic Monograph*; American Herbal Phamacopoia and Therapeutic Compendium: Scotts Valley, CA, USA, 2000; pp. 1–26.
239. Upton, R. (Ed.) *Schisandra Berry. Schisandra chinensis. Analytical, Quality Control, and Therapeutic Monograph*; American Herbal Phamacopoia and Therapeutic Compendium: Scotts Valley, CA, USA, 1999; pp. 1–28.
240. Radix Ginseng. In *WHO Monographs on Medicinal Plants Commonly Used in the Newly Independent States (NIS)*; World Health Organization: Geneva, Switzerland, 2010; Volume 5, pp. 141–160.
241. European Union Herbal Monograph on *Sideritis scardica* Griseb.; *Sideritis clandestina* (Bory & Chaub.) Hayek; *Sideritis raeseri* Boiss. & Heldr.; *Sideritis syriaca* L., herba. EMA/HMPC/39453/2015. Committee on Herbal Medicinal Products (HMPC). 2 February 2016. Available online: https://www.ema.europa.eu/en/documents/herbal-monograph/final-european-union-herbal-monograph-sideritis-scardica-griseb-sideritis-clandestina-bory-chaub-hayek-sideritis-raeseri-boiss-heldr-sideritis-syriaca-l-herba_en.pdf (accessed on 3 September 2025).
242. Panossian, A. Herba Sideritis: A putative adaptogen for reducing the risk of age-related cognitive decline and neurodegenerative disorders. *Phytomed. Plus* **2024**, *4*, 100519. [CrossRef]
243. Panossian, A.; Lemerond, T. *Herba Sideritis: Insights from a Herbal Monograph with Particular Reference to Adaptogenic Potential in Neurodegenerative Disorders and Aging-Related Cognitive Decline*, 1st ed.; BP International: London, UK, 2024; pp. 1–58. ISBN 978-93-48119-26-1/978-93-48119-56-8. [CrossRef]
244. Kligman, E.W. Preventive geriatrics: Basic principles for primary care physicians. *Geriatrics* **1992**, *47*, 39–50.
245. Berezovskiĭ, V.A. Valeology and biophysical medicine. *Fiziol. Zh. (1994)* **2010**, *56*, 3–18. [CrossRef]
246. Ilnitski, A.N.; Prashchayeu, K.I.; Trofimova, S.V.; Birjukova, I.V. Preventive geriatrics vs. anti-aging medicine. *Adv Gerontol.* **2015**, *28*, 589–593. [PubMed]
247. Ruzieva, G.A.; Jabborova, E.J. The science of valeology and its significance in modern medicine. *Mod. Educ. Dev.* **2025**, *26*, 127–129.

MDPI AG
Grosspeteranlage 5
4052 Basel
Switzerland
Tel.: +41 61 683 77 34

Pharmaceuticals Editorial Office
E-mail: pharmaceuticals@mdpi.com
www.mdpi.com/journal/pharmaceuticals

MDPI